DICTIONARY OF
MEDICAL
BIOGRAPHY

EDITORIAL BOARD

DICTIONARY OF MEDICAL BIOGRAPHY

Volume 1, A–B

Edited by

W. F. Bynum *and* Helen Bynum

GREENWOOD PRESS

Westport, Connecticut • London

Library of Congress Cataloging-in-Publication Data

Dictonary of medical biography / edited by W. F. Bynum and Helen Bynum.
    p.   cm.
    Includes bibliographical references and index.
    ISBN 0–313–32877–3 (set : alk. paper) — ISBN 0–313–32878–1 (v. 1 : alk. paper) —
    ISBN 0–313–32879–X (v. 2 : alk. paper) — ISBN 0–313–32880–3 (v. 3 : alk. paper) —
    ISBN 0–313–32881–1 (v. 4 : alk. paper) — ISBN 0–313–32882–X (v. 5 : alk. paper)
    1. Medicine—Biography. 2. Healers—Biography. I. Bynum, W. F. (William F.), 1943– . II. Bynum, Helen.
  R134.D57   2007
  610—dc22   2006022953

British Library Cataloguing in Publication Data is available.

Copyright © 2007 by W. F. Bynum and Helen Bynum

Library of Congress Catalog Card Number: 2006022953
ISBN: 0–313–32877–3 (set)
        0–313–32878–1 (vol. 1)
        0–313–32879–X (vol. 2)
        0–313–32880–3 (vol. 3)
        0–313–32881–1 (vol. 4)
        0–313–32882–X (vol. 5)

First published in 2007

Greenwood Press, 88 Post Road West, Westport, CT 06881
An imprint of Greenwood Publishing Group, Inc.
www.greenwood.com

Printed in the United States of America

The paper used in this book complies with the
Permanent Paper Standard issued by the National
Information Standards Organization (Z39.48–1984).

10 9 8 7 6 5 4 3 2 1

CONTENTS

CONTRIBUTORS

Göran Åkerström
Academic Hospital, Uppsala, Sweden
Sandström

Seema Alavi
Jamia Millia University, New Delhi, India
Aziz

Angelo Albrizio
Institut d'Histoire de la Médecine et de la Santé,
Geneva, Switzerland
De Giovanni

W. R. Albury
University of New South Wales, Sydney,
Australia
Bichat, Broussais, Corvisart des Marets, Magendie

Marta de Almeida
Museu de Astronomia e Ciências Afins,
Rio de Janeiro, Brazil
Ribas

Cristina Álvarez Millán
UNED, Madrid, Spain
*Ibn Buṭlān, Al-Majūsī, Ibn al-Nafīs, Al-Rāzī, Ibn Rushd,
Ibn Zuhr*

Stuart Anderson
LSHTM, London, England
Beecham, Holloway, Squibb

Warwick Anderson
University of Wisconsin–Madison, Madison, WI,
USA
Burnet, Cleland

Jon Arrizabalaga
CSIC, Barcelona, Spain
Laguna, Sanches, Torrella

S. N. Arseculeratne
University of Peradeniya, Peradeniya,
Sri Lanka
M. Paul, Wickramarachchi

Mikel Astrain
Universidad de Granada, Granada, Spain
Lardizábal Dubois

Guy Attewell
Wellcome Trust Centre for the History of Medicine
at UCL, London, England
*Medical Traditions in South Asia, Abd ul-Hamīd,
M. Ajmal Khān, M. A'zam Khān, Saīd*

Nara Azevedo
Casa de Oswaldo Cruz, Fundação Oswaldo Cruz,
Rio de Janeiro, Brazil
Cruz

Søren Bak-Jensen
Medical Museion, Copenhagen, Denmark
*Fibiger, Friderichsen, Gram, Hagedorn,
Pindborg, Salomonsen*

Martha Baldwin
Stonehill College, Easton, MA, USA
Dionis

Marta Aleksandra Balinska
Institut national du cancer, Paris, France
Hirszfeld, Rajchman, Śniadecki

Rosa Ballester
Universidad Miguel Hernández, Alicante-Valencia, Spain
Martínez Vargas

Scott Bamber
UNICEF, Bangkok, Thailand
Jivaka

Richard Barnett
Wellcome Trust Centre for the History of Medicine
at UCL, London, England
Godlee, Knox, Long, W. Morton, Read, Simpson, Wakley

Josep Lluís Barona
Universidad de Valencia Blasco, Valencia, Spain
Ramón y Cajal, Trueta i Raspall

Penelope Barrett
Wellcome Trust Centre for the History of Medicine
at UCL, London, England
Li Shizhen

Alexander R. Bay
Chapman University, Orange Campus, CA, USA
Takaki

Elaine Beale
Cherhill, Wiltshire, England
Ingen Housz

Norman Beale
Cherhill, Wiltshire, England
Ingen Housz

Denise Best
California State University, Fresno, CA, USA
Pokrovskaia

Anne-Emanuelle Birn
University of Toronto, Toronto, ON, Canada
Morquio

Carla Bittel
Loyola Marymount University, Los Angeles, CA, USA
Baker, A. Jacobi, M. P. Jacobi, Van Hoosen

Johanna Bleker
ZHGB, Institut für Geschichte der Medizin,
Berlin, Germany
Henle, Schoenlein

Michael Bliss
University of Toronto, Toronto, ON, Canada
Cushing, Dandy

Hans Blom
Erasmus Universiteit, Rotterdam, the Netherlands
Mandeville

Michel Bonduelle
University of Paris, Paris, France
Duchenne de Boulogne, Guillain

Christopher Booth
Wellcome Trust Centre for the History of Medicine
at UCL, London, England
Haygarth, Hurst, Lettsom, Sherlock

Cornelius Borck
McGill University, Montreal, QC, Canada
Berger

Mineke Bosch
Universiteit Maastricht, Maastricht,
the Netherlands
Jacobs

David Bradley
LSHTM, London, England
Macdonald

Gunnar Broberg
University of Lund, Lund, Sweden
Linnaeus

Alejandra Bronfman
University of British Columbia, Vancouver,
BC, Canada
Finlay y Barres, Guiteras Gener

Linda Bryder
University of Auckland, Auckland, New Zealand
Gordon, King, Liley

Chris Burton
University of Lethbridge, Lethbridge, AB,
Canada
Burdenko, Fedorov, Semashko, Solev'ev

Helen Bynum
Shadingfield, Suffolk, England
Halsted, Harinasuta, Rogers, Snow, Steptoe

Ricardo Campos
CSIC, Madrid, Spain
Rubio Gali

Franco Carnevale
Azienda Sanitaria di Firenze, Florence, Italy
Devoto, Ramazzini

Ana María Carrillo
UNAM, Mexico City, Mexico
Montoya Lafragua

Ian Carter
University of Auckland, Auckland, New Zealand
M. Bell

Ramón Castejón-Bolea
Universidad Miguel Hernández, Alicante, Spain
Azúa y Suárez

Rafael Chabrán
Whittier College, Whittier, CA, USA
Hernández

Iain Chalmers
The James Lind Initiative, Oxford, England
Cochrane

Joël Chandelier
Ecole française de Rome, Rome, Italy
Gentile da Foligno

Rethy Chhem
University of Western Ontario, London, ON,
Canada
Yajnavaraha

Indira Chowdhury
Tata Institute of Fundamental Research,
Mumbai, India
*Chopra, Dharmendra, Mukerji, Pandit,
Ramalingaswami, P. Sen, Vakil*

Charlotte Christensen-Nugues
University of Lund, Lund, Sweden
Harpestreng

Amy Eisen Cislo
Washington University, St Louis, MO, USA
Gilbert the Englishman

Catherine S. Coleborne
Waikato University, Hamilton, New Zealand
Manning

Andrea Contini
University of Paris XII, Paris, France
Basaglia

Roger Cooter
Wellcome Trust Centre for the History of Medicine
at UCL, London, England
Braid, Charnley, Gall, R. Jones, Treves, Wells

Anne Cottebrune
Ruprecht-Karls-Universität Heidelberg,
Heidelberg, Germany
Fischer, Wagner

Christopher Crenner
KUMC, Kansas City, KS, USA
*Bowditch, Codman, Edsall, J. Jackson, Jarvis,
Minot*

Anna Crozier
University of Edinburgh, Edinburgh, Scotland
Atiman, Cook, Kasili, Spoerry, C. Williams

Ivan Crozier
University of Edinburgh, Edinburgh, Scotland
*Dickinson, Ellis, Haire, Hirschfeld, C. Mosher,
E. Mosher, Reich, Sanger, Stopes*

Marcos Cueto
Universidad Peruana Cayetano Heredia,
Lima, Peru
*Balmis, Candau, Horwitz Barak, Houssay,
Monge Medrano, Núñez Butrón, Paz Soldán,
Soper*

Michael Z. David
University of Chicago, Chicago, IL, USA
Pavlovskii, Sklifosovskii

Rosalie David
University of Manchester, Manchester,
England
Imhotep

Annemarie de Knecht-van Eekelen
CITO International, Arnhem, the Netherlands
De Lange

Ana Cecilia Rodríguez de Romo
Universidad Nacional Autónoma de México,
Mexico City, Mexico
Arias de Benavides, Bernard, Bustamante Vasconcelos, Chávez Sánchez, Izquierdo Raudón, Liceaga, Martínez Báez, Montaña Carranco

Michelle DenBeste
California State University, Fresno, CA, USA
Pokrovskaia

Michael Denham
Wellcome Trust Centre for the History of Medicine at UCL, London, England
M. Warren

Sven Dierig
Max-Planck-Institut, Berlin, Germany
Brücke, Ludwig

Derek A. Dow
University of Auckland, Auckland, New Zealand
Buck, Gillies, Hercus, G. Robb, Scott

Alex Dracobly
University of Oregon, Eugene, OR, USA
Fournier, Ricord

Jean-Jacques Dreifuss
Centre Médical Universitaire, Geneva, Switzerland
Coindet, Prevost

Ariane Dröscher
University of Bologna, Bologna, Italy
Bassini, Bizzozero, Cotugno, Lombroso, Perroncito, Rasori, Rizzoli

Jacalyn Duffin
Queen's University, Kingston, ON, Canada
Laennec

Marguerite Dupree
University of Glasgow, Glasgow, Scotland
Anderson, Blackwell, Jex-Blake

Achintya Kumar Dutta
University of Burdwan, West Bengal, India
Brahmachari

William Eamon
New Mexico State University, Las Cruces, NM, USA
Nicholas of Poland

Myron Echenberg
McGill University, Montreal, QC, Canada
Brazil, Girard, A. Gregory, Jamot, Simond, Yersin

Wolfgang U. Eckart
Ruprecht-Karls-Universität Heidelberg, Heidelberg, Germany
Büchner, Dietl, Domagk, Sachs, Sauerbruch, Schwalbe, Sennert, Skoda, Wundt, Zeiss

Flávio Coelho Edler
Casa de Oswaldo Cruz, Fundação Oswaldo Cruz, Rio de Janeiro, Brazil
Wucherer

Martin Edwards
Wellcome Trust Centre for the History of Medicine at UCL, London, England
Balint

Kristen Ann Ehrenberger
University of Illinois, Urbana-Champaign, IL, USA
Drake

Antoinette Emch-Dériaz
University of Florida, Gainsville, FL, USA
Tissot

Eric J. Engstrom
ZHGB, Berlin, Germany
Kraepelin

Gunnar Eriksson
Uppsala Universitet, Uppsala, Sweden
Rudbeck

Bernardino Fantini
Institut d'Histoire de la Médecine et de la Santé, Geneva, Switzerland
Baglivi, Bovet, Celli, Dubini, Fabrizi da Acquapendente, Golgi, Grassi, Lancisi, Pacini, Puccinotti, Redi, Sanarelli

F. N. Fastier
University of Otago, Dunedin, New Zealand
Smirk

Morten Fink-Jensen
University of Copenhagen, Copenhagen, Denmark
Bartholin

Michael A. Flannery
University of Alabama at Birmingham, Maylene, AL, USA
J. Jones, Lloyd, McDowell, Newton, Nott, E. Warren, D. Williams

Yajaira Freites
IVIC, Caracas, Venezuela
Balmis, Beauperthuy, Gabaldón, Razetti

Charlotte Furth
University of Southern California, Los Angeles,
CA, USA
Zhu Zhenheng

Namrata R. Ganneri
Independent scholar, Mumbai, India
Joshi, Rakhmabai, Scudder

Michelle Garceau
Princeton University, Princeton, NJ, USA
Chauliac, William of Saliceto

Amy Gardiner
LSHTM, London, England
Burkitt

Nina Rattner Gelbart
Occidental College, Los Angeles, CA, USA
Du Coudray

Toby Gelfand
University of Ottawa, Ottawa, ON, Canada
*Bayle, Bernheim, Bourneville, Charcot, Desault, Hayem,
Lapeyronie, Lasègeu, Péan, Petit, Sée*

Jacques Gélis
University of Paris, Paris, France
Baudelocque

Dario Generali
Edizione Nazionale delle Opere di Antonio Vallisneri,
Milan, Italy
Vallisneri

Norman Gevitz
Ohio University, Athens, OH, USA
A. Still

James Gillespie
University of Sydney, Sydney, Australia
Argyle, Cilento

Florence Eliza Glaze
Coastal Carolina University, Conway, SC, USA
Constantine the African, Gariopontus

Christopher Goetz
Rush University Medical Center, Chicago, IL,
USA
Déjerine, Marie

Asaf Goldschmidt
Tel Aviv University, Tel Aviv, Israel
*Li Gao, Liu Wansu, Qian Yi, Wang Weiyi,
Xu Shuwei*

Christoph Gradmann
University of Oslo, Oslo, Norway
Klebs, Koch, Pettenkofer, Rabinowitsch-Kempner

John L. Graner
Mayo Clinic, Rochester, MN, USA
C. Mayo, W. Mayo

Joanna Grant
London, England
Wang Ji

Monica H. Green
Arizona State University, Tempe, AZ, USA
Trota

Samuel H. Greenblatt
Brown University, Pawtucket, RI, USA
Broca

David Greenwood
University of Nottingham, Nottingham,
England
Florey

Alberto Alonso Guardo
Universidad de Vallodolid, Vallodolid, Spain
Bernard of Gordon

Patrizia Guarnieri
Università degli Studi de Firenze, Florence, Italy
*Bufalini, Cerletti, Chiarugi, Concetti, De Sanctis,
Morselli, Mya*

Annick Guénel
LASEMA, Villejuif, France
Tùng Tôn Thất

Anita Guerrini
University of California, Santa Barbara, CA,
USA
G. Cheyne

Anne Y. Guillou
L'Université de Haute-Bretagne, Rennes, France
Pen

Bert Hall
University of Toronto, Toronto, ON, Canada
Guido da Vigevano

June Hannam
University of the West of England, Bristol, England
R. Paget

Caroline Hannaway
NIH History, Bethesda, MD, USA
Alibert, Cruveilhier, Dunglison, Dupuytren, Louis, Parran

Signe Lindskov Hansen
Copenhagen, Denmark
Finsen

Marta E. Hanson
Johns Hopkins University, Baltimore, MD, USA
Wu Youxing, Ye Gui, Zhang Jiebin

Susan Hardy
University of New South Wales, Sydney, Australia
Gillbee

Mark Harrison
Wellcome Unit for the History of Medicine, University of Oxford, Oxford, England
Carter, Christophers, Fayrer, Martin, Parkes, Ross

Joy Harvey
Independent scholar, Somerville, MA, USA
Bert, Bertillon, Brès, Edwards-Pilliet, Littré, Rayer, Tardieu, Trousseau, Vulpian

Mike Hawkins
Wellcome Trust Centre for the History of Medicine at UCL/Imperial College, London, England
Willis

E. A. Heaman
McGill University, Montreal, QC, Canada
Fleming, Sanderson, Wright

R. van Hee
Universiteit Antwerpen, Antwerp, Belgium
Depage, Vesalius

Jürgen Helm
Martin Luther Universität, Halle-Wittenberg, Halle, Germany
Brunfels, Erxleben, Frank, Gersdorff, Hoffmann, Stahl

John Henry
University of Edinburgh, Edinburgh, Scotland
Caius, Dubois, Fernel, Harvey, Linacre, Lower, Turquet, Winsløw

Volker Hess
ZHGB, Berlin, Germany
Behring, Frerichs, Kraus, Leyden, Traube, Wunderlich

Martha Hildreth
University of Nevada, Reno, NV, USA
Brouardel, Grancher

Caroline Hillard
Washington University, St Louis, MO, USA
Del Garbo, Mondino de' Liuzzi

Gilberto Hochman
Casa de Oswaldo Cruz, Fundação Oswaldo Cruz, Rio de Janeiro, Brazil
Barros Barreto, Chagas, Cruz, Fraga, Penna, Pinotti, Ribas, Wucherer

Hans-Georg Hofer
University of Manchester, Manchester, England
Krafft-Ebing, Wagner-Jauregg

Eddy Houwaart
Vrije Universiteit Medisch Centrum, Amsterdam, the Netherlands
Ali Cohen

Joel D. Howell
University of Michigan, Ann Arbor, MI, USA
Elliotson, Flick, Gerhard, Heberden, Herrick, Lewis

Elisabeth Hsu
University of Oxford, Oxford, England
Chunyu Yi

Christian Huber
Sigmund Freud-Privatstiftung, Vienna, Austria
Breuer, Jung

Rafael Huertas
CSIC, Madrid, Spain
Orfila i Rotger, Rodríguez Lafora

Teresa Huguet-Termes
Universitat Autònoma de Barcelona, Barcelona, Spain
Cardenal Fernández

Frank Huisman
University Medical Center, Utrecht/Universiteit Maastricht, Maastricht, the Netherlands
Einthoven, Hijmans van den Bergh, Loghem, Sylvius

Marion Hulverscheidt
Ruprecht-Karls-Universität Heidelberg,
Heidelberg, Germany
Basedow, Hegar

J. Willis Hurst
Emory University, Atlanta, GA, USA
White

Erik Ingebrigsten
Norwegian University of Science and Technology,
Trondheim, Norway
Holst

Lorentz M. Irgens
University of Bergen, Bergen, Norway
Hansen

Mark Jackson
University of Exeter, Exeter, England
Blackley, Down, Floyer, Freeman, Seguin, Tredgold

Bengt Jangfeldt
Center for the History of Science, Royal Academy of
Science, Stockholm, Sweden
Munthe

Mark Jenner
University of York, York, England
*Chamberlen, Clowes, Glisson, D. Turner, Wiseman,
Woodall*

William Johnston
Wesleyan University, Middletown, CT, USA
*Gotō Konzan, Hanaoka, Manse, Sugita, Yamawaki,
Yoshimasu*

Peter Jones
King's College Library, Cambridge, England
Arderne, Yperman

Eric Jorink
Constantijn Huygens Instituut, the Hague,
the Netherlands
*J. Heurnius, O. Heurnius, Lemnius, Piso,
Swammerdam*

Robert Jütte
Robert Bosch Stiftung, Stuttgart, Germany
*Auenbrugger, Hahnemann, Hirsch, Hufeland, Kaposi,
Rolfink, Rubner*

Oliver Kahl
University of Manchester, Manchester, England
Ibn at-Tilmīdh

Harmke Kamminga
University of Cambridge, Cambridge, England
Eijkman

Amalie M. Kass
Harvard Medical School, Boston, MA, USA
Cabot, Channing, Churchill, Dameshek, Kelly, Sims

Matthew Howard Kaufman
University of Edinburgh, Edinburgh, Scotland
Ballingall, C. Bell, Brodie, Guthrie, Liston, McGrigor

Amy Kemp
Indiana University, Bloomington, IN, USA
Souza

Helen King
University of Reading, Reading, England
*Agnodice, Archagathus, Hippocrates, Machaon,
Podalirius*

Stephanie Kirby
University of the West of England, Bristol, England
Nightingale

Rina Knoeff
Universiteit Maastricht, Maastricht,
the Netherlands
G. Bidloo, Boerhaave

Carl Henrik Koch
University of Copenhagen, Copenhagen,
Denmark
Stensen

Peter Koehler
Wever Hospital, Heerlen, the Netherlands
Babinski, Brown-Séquard, Winkler

Luuc Kooijmans
Universiteit van Amsterdam, Amsterdam,
the Netherlands
Ruysch

Maria Korasidou
Panteion University of Athens, Athens, Greece
Geroulanos, Goudas, Papanicolaou, Vouros, Zinnis

Jan K. van der Korst
Loosdrecht, the Netherlands
Camper, Swieten

Samuel Kottek
Hebrew University, Jerusalem, Israel
Astruc

Simone Petraglia Kropf
Casa de Oswaldo Cruz, Fundação Oswaldo
Cruz, Rio de Janeiro, Brazil
Chagas

Howard I. Kushner
Emory University, Atlanta, GA, USA
Gilles de la Tourette

Ann F. La Berge
Virginia Tech, Blacksburg, VA, USA
Parent-Duchâtelet, Villermé

Paul A. L. Lancaster
University of Sydney, New South Wales, Australia
Gregg

Øivind Larsen
University of Oslo, Oslo, Norway
Schiøtz

Christopher Lawrence
Wellcome Trust Centre for the History of
Medicine at UCL, London, England
*Cheselden, Culpeper, Lind, Mead, Pott, Pringle,
Salk, Sydenham, Trotter*

Sean Hsiang-lin Lei
National Tsing-hua University, Hsinchu, Taiwan
Yu Yan

Efraim Lev
University of Haifa, Haifa, Israel
Asaph

Milton James Lewis
University of Sydney, Sydney,
Australia
Cumpston

Shang-Jen Li
Institute of History and Philology, Academia
Sinica, Taipei, Taiwan
*Bruce, Hobson, Leishman, Lockhart, Manson,
Parker*

Kai Khiun Liew
Wellcome Trust Centre for the History of Medicine
at UCL, London, England
Chen Su Lan

Vivienne Lo
Wellcome Trust Centre for the History of Medicine
at UCL, London, England
Medicine in China

Stephen Lock
Aldeburgh, Suffolk, England
*The Western Medical Tradition, Beecher, Cooper,
Crile, Dale, Doll, Ferrier, Fishbein, Gull, Hart,
Hastings, G. Holmes, Keynes, Mitchell,
Pappworth, Pickles, Ryle, Saunders, Trudeau*

Winifred Logan
Glasgow, Scotland
Stephenson

Brigitte Lohff
Medizinische Hochschule Hannover,
Hannover, Germany
Autenrieth, Baer, Blumenbach, Müller, Oken, Reil

Jorge Lossio
University of Manchester, Manchester, England
Carrión, Espejo, Unanue

Ilana Löwy
CERMES, Villejuif, France
Aleksandrowicz, Bieganski, Biernacki, Korczak

Kenneth M. Ludmerer
Washington University, St Louis, MO, USA
Flexner

Joan E. Lynaugh
University of Pennsylvania Nursing School,
Philadelphia, PA, USA
L. Dock, L. Richards, I. Robb

Kan-Wen Ma
Wellcome Trust Centre for the History of Medicine
at UCL, London, England
Bian Que

Helen MacDonald
University of Melbourne, Carlton, Victoria,
Australia
W. MacKenzie

Andreas-Holger Maehle
University of Durham, Durham/Wolfson Research
Institute, Stockton, England
Moll

Susanne Malchau
Aarhus Universitet, Aarhus, Denmark
Mannerheim, Reimann

John Manton
University of Oxford, Oxford, England
Johnson, Lambo, Schweitzer

Predrag J. Markovic
Institute for Contemporary History, Belgrade, Serbia
Batut, Djordjević, Lazarević, Kostić, Nešić, Štampar, Subbotić

Shula Marks
SOAS, London, England
Gale, Gear, Gillman, Gluckman, Kark, Waterston

José Martínez-Pérez
Universidad de Castilla-La Mancha, Albacete, Spain
Calandre Ibáñez, Jiménez Díaz, Marañón Posadillo

Àlvar Martínez-Vidal
Universidad Autónoma de Barcelona, Barcelona, Spain
Gimbernat i Arbós, Giovannini

Romana Martorelli Vico
Università di Pisa, Pisa, Italy
Lanfranc, Ugo Benzi

J. Rosser Matthews
Williamsburg, VA, USA
Biggs, Bouchard, Bouchardat, Chapin, Greenwood, Hill

Janet McCalman
University of Melbourne, Melbourne, Australia
Balls-Headley, Bryce, Campbell, Macnamara, Scantlebury Brown

Louella McCarthy
University of Sydney, Sydney, New South Wales, Australia
D'Arcy

Laurence B. McCullough
Baylor College of Medicine, Houston, TX, USA
Hooker, Rush

Susan McGann
RCN Archives, Edinburgh, Scotland
Fenwick

James McGeachie
University of Ulster, Newtownabbey, Northern Ireland
Corrigan, Graves, W. Jenner, M. Mackenzie, Stokes, Wilde

Alessandro Medico
Washington University, St Louis, MO, USA
Peter of Abano

Rosa María Medina-Doménech
Universidad de Granada, Granada, Spain
Goyanes Capdevilla, Guilera Molas

Alfredo Menéndez
Universidad de Granada, Granada, Spain
Casal Julián

Sharon Messenger
Wellcome Trust Centre for the History of Medicine at UCL, London, England
Livingstone

Alexandre Métraux
Dossenheim, Germany
S. Freud, Goldstein

Dmitry Mikhel
Saratov State University, Saratov, Russia
Botkin, Erisman, Manassein, Molleson, Ostroumov, Zakhar'in

Bridie Andrews Minehan
Bentley College, Waltham, MA, USA
Ding Fubao, Yen

Consuelo Miqueo
Universidad de Zaragoza, Zaragoza, Spain
Piquer Arrufat

Néstor Miranda Canal
Universidad El Bosque y de la Universidad de Los Andes, Bogotá, Colombia
Vargas Reyes

Jorge Molero-Mesa
Universidad Autònoma de Barcelona, Barcelona, Spain
Sayé i Sempere

Laurence Monnais
Université de Montréal, Montreal, QC, Canada
Medical Traditions in Southeast Asia: From Syncretism to Pluralism

Maria Teresa Monti
CSPF-CNR, Milan, Italy
Spallanzani

Francisco Moreno de Carvalho
Independent scholar, São Paulo, Brazil
Amatus Lusitanus, Orta

Edward T. Morman
Baltimore, MD, USA
Bartlett, H. Bigelow, J. Bigelow, Billings, Da Costa, Pepper, Thayer, Welch

Barbara Mortimer
Edinburgh, Scotland
Sharp

Anne Marie Moulin
CNRS-CEDEJ, Cairo, Egypt
Bordet, Davaine, Laveran, Netter, Roux, Widal

Wolf-Dieter Müller-Jahncke
Hermann-Schelenz-Institut für Pharmazie und
Kulturgeschichte, Heidelberg, Germany
Paracelsus

Jock Murray
Dalhousie University, Halifax, Nova Scotia, Canada
*Abbott, Banting, Bethune, Gowers, Grenfell, Huggins,
J. H. Jackson, Macphail, Osler, Parkinson, Penfield, Selye*

Takeshi Nagashima
Keio University, Tokyo, Japan
Gotō Shinpei, Kitasato, Miyairi, Nagayo, Noguchi, Shiga

Michael J. Neuss
Columbia University, New York, NY, USA
Al-Anṭākī

Michael Neve
Wellcome Trust Centre for the History of Medicine
at UCL, London, England
Beddoes, Gully, Head, Prichard, Rivers, Winslow

Malcolm Nicolson
University of Glasgow, Glasgow, Scotland
Alison, Baillie, Donald, J. Hunter, W. Hunter, Lister, Smellie

Ingemar Nilsson
University of Gothenburg, Gothenburg, Sweden
Acrel

Sherwin Nuland
Yale University, New Haven, CT, USA
Beaumont, Bloodgood, Kubler-Ross, McBurney, Mott, Murphy

Eva Nyström
University of Uppsala, Uppsala, Sweden
Rosén von Rosenstein

Ynez Violé O'Neill
UCLA, Los Angeles, CA, USA
Paré

Diana Obregón
Universidad Nacional de Colombia Edificio Manuel
Ancizar, Bogotá, Colombia
Carrasquilla, García-Medina

Ambeth R. Ocampo
National Historical Institute, Manila, Philippines
Rizal

Guillermo Olagüe de Ros
Universidad de Granada, Granada, Spain
García Solá, Nóvoa Santos, Urrutia Guerezta

Jan Eric Olsén
University of Lund, Lund, Sweden
Gullstrand, Holmgren

Todd M. Olszewski
Yale University, New Haven, CT, USA
Cannon, D. Dock

Willie T. Ong
Makati Medical Center, Makati, Philippines
Acosta-Sison

Giuseppe Ongaro
Ospedale di Padova, Padova, Italy
*Aranzio, Aselli, Bellini, Benivieni, Berengario da Carpi,
Borelli, Cardano, Cesalpino, Colombo, Cornaro,
Da Monte, Eustachi, Falloppia, Malpighi, Mattioli,
Mercuriale, Morgagni, Santorio, Scarpa, Severino,
Tagliacozzi, Valsalva, Zacchia*

Ooi Keat Gin
Universiti Sains Malaysia, Penang, Malaysia
Danaraj, Lim Boon Keng, Wu Lien-Teh

Teresa Ortiz-Gómez
Universidad de Granada, Granada, Spain
Arroyo Villaverde, Soriano Fischer

Abena Dove Osseo-Asare
University of California, Berkeley, CA, USA
Ampofo, Barnor, De Graft-Johnson, C. Easmon

Nelly Oudshoorn
Universiteit Twente, Enschede,
the Netherlands
Laqueur

Caroline Overy
Wellcome Trust Centre for the History of
Medicine at UCL, London, England
Livingstone

Steven Palmer
University of Windsor, Windsor, Ontario,
Canada
*Calderón Guardia, Durán Cartín,
Fernández y Hernández*

José Pardo-Tomás
CSIC, Barcelona, Spain
Monardes

Lawrence Charles Parish
Jefferson Medical College, Philadelphia, PA, USA
Bateman, Duhring, Gross, Hutchinson, Shippen, Willan

Eldryd Parry
Tropical Health and Education Trust, London, England
Burkitt

Adell Patton Jr.
University of Missouri, St Louis, MO, USA
Boyle, J. Easmon, Odeku, Togba

Harry W. Paul
University of Florida, Gainesville, FL, USA
Pasteur, Rothschild

John Pearn
University of Queensland, Brisbane, Australia
Bancroft, Beaney, Coppleson, Fairley, Halford, MacGregor

Steven J. Peitzman
Drexel University College of Medicine,
Philadelphia, PA, USA
Addis, Bright, A. Richards, Scribner

Kim Pelis
National Institutes of Health, Bethesda, MD, USA
Barker, Councilman, Gorgas, Hammond, Nicolle, Reed, T. Smith

Concetta Pennuto
Université de Genève, Geneva, Switzerland
Ficino, Fracastoro

José Morgado Pereira
Universidade de Coimbra, Coimbra, Portugal
Egas Moniz

Jacques Philippon
Salpêtrière-Pitié Hospital, Paris, France
Mondor

Howard Phillips
University of Cape Town, Rondebosch, South Africa
Abdurahman, Barnard, Barry, Naidoo, Orenstein, Xuma

Jean-François Picard
CNRS, Paris, France
Debré, Delay, Hamburger, Leriche, Roussy, Vincent

Mikhail Poddubnyi
Voenno-meditsinskii Zhurnal, Moscow, Russia
N. Bidloo, Buial'skii, Dobroslavin, Gaaz, Inozemtsev, Pirogov, Pletnev

Hans Pols
University of Sydney, Sydney, Australia
Beard, Beers, Bowlby, Burton-Bradley, Grinker, Klein, Laing, Stillé

María-Isabel Porras-Gallo
University of Castilla-La Mancha, Madrid, Spain
Obrador Alcalde

Patricia E. Prestwich
University of Alberta, Edmonton, AB, Canada
Magnan, Moreau de Tours, Morel

Lawrence M. Principe
Johns Hopkins University, Baltimore, MD, USA
Helmont

Armin Prinz
Medizinische Universität Wien, Vienna, Austria
Wenckebach

Cay-Ruediger Pruell
Albert-Ludwigs-Universität, Freiburg, Germany
Aschoff, Cohnheim, Conti, Ehrlich, Rokitansky, Virchow

Constance Putnam
Independent scholar, Concord, MA, USA
Balassa, Bene, Duka, O. W. Holmes, Korányi, Markusovszky, Meigs, Morgan, Semmelweis, G. Shattuck, N. Smith, J. Warren

Emilio Quevedo
Universidad Nacional de Colombia, Bogotá, Colombia
Franco

Sean Quinlan
University of Idaho, Moscow, ID, USA
A. Louis, Quesnay

Camilo Quintero
University of Wisconsin–Madison, Madison, WI, USA
Mutis y Bosio

Roger Qvarsell
University of Linköping, Linköping, Sweden
Huss

Karina Ramacciotti
Universidad de Buenos Aires, Buenos Aires, Argentina
Carrillo, Mazza, Rawson

Mridula Ramanna
SIES College, University of Mumbai, Mumbai, India
Bentley, Choksy, Jhirad, Khanolkar, Lad, Morehead, J. Turner

Matthew Ramsey
Vanderbilt University, Nashville, TN, USA
Civiale, Desgenettes, Fourcroy, Portal, Richerand, Velpeau,
Vicq d'Azyr

Ismail Rashid
Vassar College, Poughkeepsie, NY, USA
Fanon, Horton

Carole Reeves
Wellcome Trust Centre for the History of Medicine
at UCL, London, England
Abt, Battey, Buchan, Budd, Cole, Darwin, Holt, Keen,
Lane, S. Morton, Prout, Rock, Sabin, Scharlieb, Seacole,
Spock, Tait

C. Joan Richardson
University of Texas Medical Branch, Galveston, TX,
USA
Barton

Philip Rieder
Université de Genève, Geneva, Switzerland
Bonet, De La Rive, Le Clerc, Odier, Reverdin, Tronchin

Ortrun Riha
Universität Leipzig, Leipzig, Germany
Isaac Israeli

Julius Rocca
University of Birmingham, Birmingham, England
Aëtius, Aretaeus, Aristotle, Asclepiades, Caelius Aurelianus,
Celsus, Dioscorides, Empedocles, Erasistratus, Herophilos,
Pliny, Scribonius Largus, Soranus, Whytt

Julia Rodriguez
University of New Hampshire, Durham, NH, USA
Aráoz Alfaro, Coni, Grierson, Ingenieros

Esteban Rodríguez-Ocaña
Universidad de Granada, Granada, Spain
Ferrán y Clúa, Pittaluga Fattorini

Volker Roelcke
Justus-Liebig Universität, Giessen, Germany
Alzheimer, Bleuler, Kretschmer, Mitscherlich, Rüdin

Hugo Röling
Universiteit van Amsterdam, Amsterdam,
the Netherlands
Rutgers

Naomi Rogers
Yale University, New Haven, CT, USA
Kenny

Anastasio Rojo
University of Valladolid, Valladolid, Spain
Bravo de Sobremonte, Mercado, Valles

Nils Rosdahl
Medical Museion, Copenhagen Denmark
Madsen

Barbara Gutmann Rosenkrantz
Harvard University, Cambridge, MA, USA
Hardy, L. Shattuck

Leonard D. Rosenman
UCSF, San Francisco, CA, USA
Frugard

Fred Rosner
Mount Sinai School of Medicine, New York,
NY, USA
Maimonides

Lisa Rosner
Richard Stockton College, Pomona, NJ, USA
Bennett, Brown, Christison, Cullen, Ferriar, J. Gregory,
Laycock, Monro, Percival, Withering

Frederic Roy
Université de Montréal, Montreal, QC,
Canada
Suvannavong

Marion Maria Ruisinger
Friedrich-Alexander-Universität,
Erlangen-Nuremberg, Germany
Heister

Han van Ruler
Erasmus Universiteit, Rotterdam,
the Netherlands
Blankaart, Bontekoe, Graaf

Andrea Rusnock
University of Rhode Island, Kingston,
RI, USA
Arbuthnot, Bond, Boylston, E. Jenner, Jurin, Sutton,
Waterhouse

Fernando Salmón
Universidad de Cantabria, Santander, Spain
Arnald, López Albo

Lutz D. H. Sauerteig
University of Durham, Durham/Wolfson
Research Institute, Stockton, England
Blaschko

Walton O. Schalick III
Washington University, St Louis, MO, USA
*Gilles de Corbeil, Henry of Mondeville, John of
Gaddesden, John of Saint-Amand, Peter of Abano, Peter
of Spain, Richard the Englishman, Taddeo, William of
Brescia*

Volker Scheid
University of Westminster, London, England
Ding Ganren, Fei Boxiong, Yun Tieqiao

Aina Schiøtz
Universitetet i Bergen, Bergen, Norway
Evang

William Schneider
Indiana University, Indianapolis, IN, USA
Hirszfeld, Pinard, Richet, Tzanck

Heinz Schott
Rheinische Friedrich-Wilhelms-Universität,
Bonn, Germany
Mesmer

Andrew Scull
University of California San Diego, San Diego, CA,
USA
*Brigham, Cotton, Dix, Earle, Haslam, Meyer, Ray,
Tuke*

Nikolaj Serikoff
The Wellcome Library, London, England
*The Islamic Medical Tradition, Aḥmad, Ibn al-Bayṭār,
Al-Bīrūnī, Clot Bey, Foley, Ḥaddād, Ibn al-Haytham,
Mahfouz, Ibn al-Māsawayh, Meyerhof, Ibn Sīnā, Sournia,
Van Dyck, Waldmeier, Al-Zahrāwī*

Jole Shackelford
University of Minnesota, Minneapolis, MN, USA
Severinus

Sonu Shamdasani
Wellcome Trust Centre for the History of Medicine
at UCL, London, England
*Adler, Forel, A. Freud, Gesell, Janet, Menninger, Putnam,
Sullivan*

Patrick Henry Shea
Rockefeller Archive Center, Sleepy Hollow, NY, USA
Carrel

Sally Sheard
University of Liverpool, Liverpool, England
*Bevan, Beveridge, Chadwick, Farr, Newman, Newsholme,
Shuttleworth, T. S. Smith*

Dongwon Shin
Korean Advanced Institute of Science and
Technology, Taejon, Korea
Choe Han'gi, Heo, Sejong, Yi Jema

Barry David Silverman
Northside Hospital, Atlanta, GA, USA
Taussig

Mark E. Silverman
Emory University, Atlanta, GA, USA
Flint, Hope, J. Mackenzie

Jelena Jovanovic Simic
Zemun, Serbia
*Batut, Djordjević, Lazarević, Kostić, Nešić, Štampar,
Subbotić*

P. N. Singer
London, England
Galen

Kavita Sivaramakrishnan
Public Health Foundation of India, New Delhi,
India
G. Sen, P. Sharma, T. Sharma, Shukla, Vaid, Varier

Morten A. Skydsgaard
University of Aarhus, Aarhus, Denmark
Panum

Jean Louis De Sloover
Erpent (Namur), Belgium
Dodonaeus

David F. Smith
University of Aberdeen, Aberdeen, Scotland
Orr

F. B. Smith
Australian National University, Canberra, Australia
W. Thomson

Thomas Söderqvist
Medical Museion, Copenhagen, Denmark
Jerne

Marina Sorokina
Russian Academy of Sciences, Moscow, Russia
*Al'tshuller, Briukhonenko, Haffkine, Ilizarov, Iudin,
Negovskii, Semenovskii*

David Sowell
Juniata College, Huntingdon, PA, USA
Perdomo Neira

Eduard A. van Staeyen
Leiden, the Netherlands
Guislain

Frank W. Stahnisch
Johannes Gutenberg-Universität, Mainz, Germany
Graefe, Griesinger, His, C. Vogt, O. Vogt, Warburg,
Wassermann

Ida H. Stamhuis
Vrije Universiteit Amsterdam, Amsterdam,
the Netherlands
Quetelet

Darwin H. Stapleton
Rockefeller Archive Center, Sleepy Hollow, NY, USA
Hackett

Jane Starfield
University of Johannesburg, Bertsham, South Africa
Molema, Moroka

Martin S. Staum
University of Calgary, Calgary, AB, Canada
Cabanis

Hubert Steinke
University of Bern, Bern, Switzerland
Haller

Oddvar Stokke
National Hospital, Oslo, Norway
Følling, Refsum

Michael Stolberg
Universität Würzburg, Würzburg, Germany
Bartisch, Fabricius, Fuchs, Platter, Rösslin, Scultetus

Marvin J. Stone
Baylor University Medical Center, Dallas, TX, USA
Coley, Ewing, Farber, E. Graham, Hodgkin, Wintrobe

Hindrik Strandberg
Helsinki, Finland
Willebrand, Ylppö

Karin Stukenbrock
Martin-Luther-Universität Halle-Wittenberg,
Halle, Germany
Brunfels, Erxleben, Frank, Gersdorff, Hoffmann,
Stahl

Charles Suradji
Jakarta, Indonesia
Soedarmo

Akihito Suzuki
Keio University, Yokohama, Japan
Medicine, State, and Society in Japan, 500–2000,
Asada, Baelz, Conolly, Hata, Mori, Ogata, Pompe van
Meerdervoort, Siebold, Yamagiwa

Mika Suzuki
Shizuoka University, Shizuoka, Japan
Ogino, Yoshioka

Victoria Sweet
UCSF, San Francisco, CA, USA
Hildegard of Bingen

Simon Szreter
University of Cambridge, Cambridge,
England
McKeown

Cecilia Taiana
Carleton University, Ottawa, ON, Canada
Lacan

Ian Tait
Aldeburgh, Suffolk, England
Browne

Jennifer Tappan
Columbia University, New York, NY, USA
Trowell

Robert Tattersall
University of Nottingham, Nottingham,
England
Abel, Addison, Albright, Doniach, Hench, Horsley,
Joslin, Minkowski, Starling

Kim Taylor
Kaimu Productions, Shanghai, China
Hatem, Zhu Lian

Manuela Tecusan
University of Cambridge, Cambridge, England
Alcmaeon, Anaximander, Andreas, Democedes,
Democritus, Diocles, Diogenes, Oribasius, Paul
of Aegina, Philistion, Plato, Praxagoras, Rufus

Bert Theunissen
Universiteit Utrecht, Utrecht, the Netherlands
Donders

Michel Thiery
Stichting Jan Palfyn en Museum voor
Geschiedenis van de Geneeskunde, Ghent, Belgium
Palfyn

C. Michele Thompson
Southern Connecticut State University,
New Haven, CT, USA
Lán Ông, Tuệ Tĩnh

Carsten Timmermann
University of Manchester, Manchester, England
*Bauer, Grotjahn, McMichael, Pickering, D. Richards,
Rosenbach*

Tom Treasure
St George's Hospital Medical School, London,
England
*Beck, Blalock, C. E. Drew, C. R. Drew, Favaloro, Gibbon,
Hufnagel*

Ulrich Tröhler
University of Bern, Bern, Switzerland
*Bergmann, Billroth, Kocher, Langenbeck,
Mikulicz-Radecki, Nissen, Quervain*

Arleen Marcia Tuchman
Vanderbilt University, Nashville, TN, USA
Zakrzewska

Marius Turda
Oxford Brookes University, Oxford, England
Babeş, Cantacuzino, Ciucă, Marinescu

Trevor Turner
Homerton University Hospital, London, England
Maudsley

Peter J. Tyler
Edgecliffe, New South Wales, Australia
*W. Armstrong, Bland, Fiaschi, Mackellar, Skirving,
Stuart, Thompson*

Michael Tyquin
Making History, Darlington, New South Wales,
Australia
Dunlop

Tatiana Ul'iankina
Institute of the History of Science and Technology,
Moscow, Russia
Mechnikov, Sechenov

G. van der Waa
Rotterdam, the Netherlands
Gaubius

Lia van Gemert
Universiteit Utrecht, Utrecht, the Netherlands
Beverwijck

Maria Vassiliou
University of Oxford, Oxford, England
Belios, Livadas

Jan Peter Verhave
UMCN, Nijmegen, the Netherlands
Swellengrebel

Joost Vijselaar
Trimbos-Instituut, Utrecht, the Netherlands
Schroeder van der Kolk

Jurjen Vis
Amsterdam, the Netherlands
Foreest

An Vleugels
National University of Singapore, Singapore
Kerr

Hans de Waardt
Vrije Universiteit Amsterdam, Amsterdam,
the Netherlands
Wier

Keir Waddington
Cardiff University, Cardiff, Wales
*Abernethy, Brunton, Garrod, Gee, Lawrence,
J. Paget*

Lisa K. Walker
University of California, Berkeley, CA, USA
Khlopin, Teziakov

John Walker-Smith
Wellcome Trust Centre for the History of
Medicine at UCL, London, England
G. Armstrong, G. Still, Underwood, West

Paul Weindling
Oxford Brookes University, Oxford, England
Verschuer

Dora B. Weiner
UCLA, Los Angeles, CA, USA
Esquirol, Larrey, Percy, Pinel, Tenon

Kathleen Wellman
Southern Methodist University, Dallas, TX, USA
La Mettrie, Patin, Renaudot

Ann Westmore
The University of Melbourne, Parkville, Victoria,
Australia
Cade

James Whorton
University of Washington, Tacoma, WA, USA
Eddy, S. Graham, Kellogg, Lust, B. Palmer, D. Palmer, S. Thomson, Trall

Ann Wickham
Dublin City University, Dublin, Ireland
A. Jones

Elizabeth A. Williams
Oklahoma State University, Stillwater, OK, USA
Boissier de la Croix de Sauvages, Bordeu

Sabine Wilms
Paradigm Publications, Taos, NM, USA
Ge Hong, Sun Simiao, Tao Hongjing

Warren Winkelstein, Jr.
University of California, Berkeley, CA, USA
Emerson, Frost, Goldberger, Hamilton, Kinyoun, Lane-Claypon, Park, Paul, Wynder

Michael Worboys
University of Manchester, Manchester, England
Allbutt, Bristowe, W. W. Cheyne, Moynihan, Simon, Syme

Jill Wrapson
University of Auckland, Auckland, New Zealand
Barnett

Marcia Wright
Columbia University, New York, NY, USA
Park Ross

Rex Wright-St Clair (deceased)
Huntingdon, Hamilton, New Zealand
A. Thomson

Henrik R. Wulff
Medical Museion, Copenhagen, Denmark
Hirschsprung

Ronit Yoeli-Tlalim
Warburg Institute, London, England
Sangye Gyatso, Yuthog Yontan

William H. York
Portland State University, Portland, OR, USA
Despars, Valesco of Tarenta

Benjamin Zajicek
University of Chicago, Chicago, IL, USA
Bekhterev, Korsakov, Pavlov

Soledad Zárate
Universidad de Chile, Santiago, Chile
Cruz-Coke Lassabe

Alfons Zarzoso
Museu d'Història de la Medicina de Catalunya, Barcelona, Spain
Pedro-Pons, Puigvert Gorro

Franz Zehentmayr
Salzburg, Austria
Zhang Yuansu

Barbara Zipser
Wellcome Trust Centre for the History of Medicine at UCL, London, England
Al-Mawṣilī

Patrick Zylberman
CERMES, Villejuif, France
Sand

ACKNOWLEDGMENTS

Kevin J. Downing of Greenwood Publishing Group has been a constant source of support from the inception of this project to its completion—more or less on time. That we have stayed on schedule has been due to the industry of our editorial board and authors.

The area editors responded with enthusiasm to selecting the list of entries for each region and with resignation to the limits we imposed on the total number of people each could include. We know it was a hard task to choose between notable practitioners while also reflecting the diversity of those involved in health care within national contexts. The individually balanced lists they presented to us may be submerged in the alphabetical format of the *DMB*, but its overall richness is due reward for their endeavor.

Having decided who would be included, the editors were next charged with finding authors who could write about them in English. We are indebted to all of them for their excellent decisions in finding authors; for help with the prose, content, and word length; and especially for translating their authors' articles, where this proved to be the best solution to a commissioning problem. We would also like to express our thanks to those who responded when we realized that a region had been underrepresented in our original division of the world and found additional authors beyond their original remit. Among the individual editors, Marcos Cueto extends his thanks to Jorge Lossio; Toby Gelfand to his secretary, Colette ElAhmar; and Walton Schalick to the Robert Wood Johnson Generalist Faculty Scholars Program.

The authors themselves have made this a truly international project. Our email box is unlikely ever again to send and receive from such a number of people in diverse and distant locations. It has been a joy to have this experience. Tribute is due for the way the authors digested the premise of the *DMB* and provided us with entries that encapsulated their subject's contributions with style and feeling while staying within the word limit. Just as the editors went the extra mile to fill gaps, so too several authors wrote additional entries at short notice and some new authors were recruited at the eleventh hour; to these people we are most grateful.

Among the text are many fine illustrations mainly sourced by Carole Reeves from the wonderful resources of the Wellcome Trust. As illustrations editor, Carole did a magnificent job. Much that is new here is due to her knowledge. We would like to thank Tony Woods at the Wellcome Trust for his initial facilitation of the use of the Trust's collections and acknowledge of course the role of Wellcome Trust's Governors. We echo Carole's thanks to Catherine Draycott, Venita Paul, Laurie Auchterlonie, and Chris Carter in the Wellcome Trust Medical Photographic Library; the Wellcome Library staff in general but particularly those in Rare Books and Archives and Manuscripts; Penny Barrett for locating images of early Chinese healers;

Gilberto Hochman for providing images of important South American doctors and scientists; all the authors who diligently and cheerfully sought for rare or unusual images; and the museums, archives, libraries, art galleries, and universities throughout the world who responded promptly and efficiently to requests for images.

Toward the end of the first editing stage, Lesley Beevor's timely editorial assistance helped us take the strain, for which we are very grateful. So, with the entries in and edited, and the pictures sourced, our final thanks are to Susan Yates and her colleagues at Publication Services, Champaign, IL, and Dave Hallows at C.D. Computers, Beccles, Suffolk. Susie has been ever cheerful and helpful, and noticed that we worked a lot of weekends. Dave has provided hardware and software support, and most importantly reassurance that the electronic transmission of large amounts of data back and forth across the Atlantic wouldn't be a problem—not ours anyway.

INTRODUCTION

The study of medicine's past has changed dramatically during the past generation. The older Great Doctors approach has been replaced by a much broader vision of health, disease, and healers. Historians have challenged the vision of medicine as a simple series of discoveries and improvements, leading to the present. Themes that three decades ago had hardly been explored historically now command center stage. Alternative healers, the interaction of Western medicine with indigenous medical systems, the entry of women into the medical profession, nursing, and a host of other topics are now standard fare for monographs and PhD theses. The History of Medicine has become the Social History of Medicine. This in turn is a central component of the way we think about our past and forms part of the mainstream of historical study at a variety of levels. Undergraduates will find these volumes particularly helpful. So will their teachers.

In all this, the individual has maintained his or her historical status. Medical biographies continue to offer windows into the wider medical world, and the broader view of social history of medicine has uncovered the important activities of healers of all stripes. The biographical approach adopted in these volumes reflects best contemporary historical practice. There are many national biographical dictionaries, in which doctors receive some coverage, and a few that have concentrated on medical biography. Historians of science have long had the *Dictionary of Scientific Biography* as an international guide to the figures within the world of science. For major medical figures such as Hippocrates, Galen, Harvey, Pasteur and Koch, there are entries in the *DSB*, indicated in the bibliographies within the present work. Such influential figures are here freshly interpreted, in entries that incorporate the insights of scholarship that has occurred in the generation since the *DSB* was published. Historians of medicine will be well aware that the editors of the *DSB* routinely excluded clinical medicine from their brief, except for such major scientists and doctors who contributed to biomedical science. We believe that the *Dictionary of Medical Biography* complements the *DSB* in its internationalism and breadth of coverage. Since we have focused on medical practice, the overlap is small. There is simply no modern biographical dictionary of medicine in any language that is comparable to the present work, in size or scope. Time and again, readers can find biographies of health professionals of real national importance, whose contributions deserve to be appreciated by a larger audience. To read these volumes, as we have done in several forms during the commissioning and production stages, is to appreciate the complexity and richness of health, medicine, and medical care throughout the world.

From the beginning, our aim was to be cosmopolitan, and we have been fortunate to recruit a distinguished international Editorial Board of medical historians. Individual entries within each geographical area are the product of careful negotiation with Board members, drawing on their formidable expertise. In turn, they have helped recruit a vibrant group of 384 different contributors, drawn from all over the world. Between them, they have written biographies of 1,140 individuals. In many instances, significant doctors and health professionals are presented here in English for the first time. In addition, the authoritative essays at the beginning of Volume I survey the major themes within the principal medical traditions of the world. Specially commissioned for this work, they will help readers appreciate the nuances of the individual biographies that constitute the main body of the volumes that follow.

In planning this volume, we sought to achieve a balance between including as many individuals as possible, within our 1.25 million word limit, and allowing our authors the possibility of assessing their subjects with subtlety. Entries are of three basic lengths and routinely include a bibliography of both primary and secondary sources. Our subjects are individualized, and we have retained our authors' individual voices. By using the geographical listings of Appendix 1 in the final volume, one can construct national and regional histories of clinical medicine. Thus, the importance of political movements for medical practice and ideas, such as the Franco period in Spain, the Russian Revolution in the former USSR, or the Nazi regime in Germany, can be systematically reconstructed through the health professionals who lived through these modern episodes. The richness of the medical traditions of other geographical regions—Southeast Asia, India, China, Japan, Eastern Europe, Latin America, Spain, Italy or the Scandinavian countries—can also be appreciated. At the same time, the principal figures of Western medicine are also comprehensively covered, with fresh interpretations by acknowledged experts.

The development of the medical and surgical specialties within the Western Medical Tradition is also richly represented here, and can be accessed via Appendix 2 in final volume, which lists the entries by fields of activity. Thus, those interested in the major figures within, for example, dermatology, epidemiology, nursing, pediatrics, psychiatry, public health, surgery, and other areas of medical activity will find the entry points in those lists. These lists also group classical, Islamic, and medieval figures included in the volumes, as well as practitioners of Chinese, ayurvedic, traditional Japanese, Vietnamese, and other medical traditions. Contemporary complementary medical systems, such as homeopathy, osteopathy, chiropractic, hydropathy, botanical medicine, and naturopathy, as well as Christian Science, have their voices in these volumes. Appendix 3 listing the entries by their birth and death dates (Imhotep to Kasili) reveals the constancy and change in medicine, health, and disease over the long durée around the world.

The entries in this set can answer many specific questions about the history of health and medicine, but they can also be browsed for pleasure and stimulation. There are sketches here of good doctors and bad, of heroes and victims, of innovators and defenders of the status quo. Some of the subjects live to ripe old ages, some die young, some commit suicide or die violent deaths, some experiment on themselves, others use their patients. Included are doctors who contribute to politics, literature, music, and welfare. Some die rich, some die poor. Each biographical subject offers a window into a range of cultures, medical systems, attitudes to health and illness, and insights into the causes of disease.

W. F. and Helen Bynum
Shadingfield, Suffolk

EDITORIAL NOTES

Editing this reference work with material from many cultures and traditions has been a wonderful education. It has also required us to make a number of editorial decisions about presentation.

We have decided to use a single dating system. Unless otherwise stated, dates are given in the Common Era (CE). For earlier times, the standard abbreviation BCE has been used. Russian birth and death dates before Russian calendar reform have both dates.

For diacritical marks, we have tried to follow the instructions given by our authors. Some have chosen not to use them, so readers will note some inconsistency, but the meaning should always be clear. The computer has had a hand in our alphabetization. Thus surnames with the prefix Mc come after the ordinary Ma's. The list of entries should make individuals easy to find.

The division of bibliographies into primary and secondary sources has generally been straightforward, but sometimes an autobiography is the fullest account of an individual's life, or collected works contain a biographical introduction by the editor. Bibliographies are organized so that primary works are in date order, whereas secondary sources start with the most recent. Where there is a collected work, this appears at the beginning of the bibliography. Titles of journals are often given in shortened form, and should be easily recognized. If readers are in doubt, they should consult the online catalogue of the National Library of Medicine, or reference works such as *World List of Scientific Periodicals*, fourth edn., ed. Brown, Peter, and George Burder Stratton (London, 1963).

In the appendices to the last volume, we have provided lists of the individuals included in *DMB* in chronological order as well as groupings by country and professional specialty. The peripatetic nature of medical life means that many individuals will have more than one country. We have omitted country of birth for individuals who lived there only a short while and concentrated instead on the places where our subjects made their contributions. The number of individuals whose field of activity included 'medicine' was so large that we have omitted this category from the specialty appendix. We have been guided by the headers provided by our contributors, but we have taken the liberty of including other categories when it seemed appropriate.

Like all works of scholarship, this one builds on work that has gone before. The bibliographies attached to each entry relate to the individual in question. More general guides to the contemporary medical historical literature will be found at the end of each of the essays. Two reference volumes not otherwise included can be noted here:

Jeremy M. Norman, ed., *Morton's Medical Bibliography* ('Garrison and Morton'), 5th edn. (Aldershot, Hants., and Brookfield, VT, 1991). This is the latest edition of the 'checklist' that Fielding H. Garrison first published in 1912. It is a valuable bibliography of both primary and secondary texts 'illustrating the history of medicine', and much beloved by booksellers.

Leslie T. Morton and Robert J. Moore, eds., *A Chronology of Medicine and Related Subjects* (Aldershot, Hants., and Brookfield, VT., 1997). This volume draws heavily on 'Garrison and Morton', but its chronological arrangement and information on classic papers and discoveries, and on biographical details of major figures within the history of medicine, offers a different entrée to the field. Both of these works are international in their approach, although more narrowly focused on North America and Europe than *DMB*.

ABBREVIATIONS

AMA	American Medical Association
ANB	*American National Biography*
BA	Bachelor of Arts
BCE	Before Common Era
BCG	Bacillus Calmette-Guérin (tuberculosis vaccination)
BM	Bachelor of Medicine
BMA	British Medical Association
BMJ	*British Medical Journal*
CBE	Commander, The Most Excellent Order of the British Empire
CE	Common Era
ChB	Bachelor of Surgery
ChD	Doctor of Surgery
ChM	Master of Surgery
CIE	Companion, The Most Eminent Order of the Indian Empire
KCIE	Knight Commander, The Most Eminent Order of the Indian Empire
CM	Master of Surgery
CMB	Combat Medical Badge (U.S. Army)
CMG	Companion, The Most Distinguished Order of St Michael and St George
CMO	Chief Medical Officer
CMS	Church Missionary Society
CSI	Companion, The Most Exalted Order of the Star of India
CSIRO	Commonwealth Scientific and Industrial Research Organization (Australia)
DAMB	*Dictionary of American Medical Biography*
DAuB	*Dictionary of Australian Biography* (available online)
DBE	Dame of the British Empire
DBI	*Dizionario Biografico degli Italiani*
DGMS	Director General Medical Service (military)

DMed	Doctor of Medicine
DNZB	*Dictionary of New Zealand Biography* (available online)
DPM	Diploma of Psychological Medicine
DSB	*Dictionary of Scientific Biography*
DSO	Distinguished Service Order (military British)
ECT	Electo-convulsive Therapy
EEG	Electroencephalogram
FAO	Food and Agriculture Organization (United Nations)
FRCP	Fellow Royal College of Physicians
FRCPEdin/FRCPEd	Fellow Royal College of Physicians Edinburgh
FRCS	Fellow of the Royal College of Surgeons
FRCSEdin/FRCSEd	Fellow Royal College of Surgeons Edinburgh
FRS	Fellow of the Royal Society
FRSEdin/FRSEd	Fellow of the Royal Society of Edinburgh
GBH	General Board of Health (England and Wales)
GMC	General Medical Council (UK)
GP	General Practitioner
ICN	International Council of Nursing
ICS	Indian Civil Service
IHB	International Health Board (Rockefeller Foundation)
IMS	Indian Medical Service
IOC	Institute Oswaldo Cruz
JAMA	*Journal of the American Medical Association*
KCSI	Knight Commander, The Most Exalted Order of the Star of India
LLD	Doctor of Laws
LMS	Licentiate in Medicine and Surgery
LRCP	Licentiate of the Royal College of Physicians
LRCPEdin/LRCPEd	Licentiate of the Royal College of Physicians Edinburgh
LRCSEdin/LRCSEd	Licentiate of the Royal College of Surgeons Edinburgh
LRFPS	Licentiate of the Royal Faculty of Physicians and Surgeons of Glasgow
LSA	Licentiate of the Society of Apothecaries
LSHTM	London School of Hygiene and Tropical Medicine
LSMW	London School of Medicine for Women
MA	Master of Arts
MB	Bachelor of Medicine
MBCM	Bachelor of Medicine Master of Surgery
MC	Military Cross
MD	Doctor of Medicine
mg	milligram
MMed	Master of Medicine
MO	Medical Officer
MoH	Medical Officer of Health
MRC	Medical Research Council
MRCNZ	Medical Research Council of New Zealand
MRCOG	Member of the Royal College of Gynaecologists
MRCP	Member of the Royal College of Physicians
MRCS	Member of the Royal College of Surgeons
MS	Multiple Sclerosis
NHMRC	National Health and Medical Research Council (Australia)
NSDAP	National Socialist Party (Nazi Germany)
NSW	New South Wales (Australia)
OAS	Organization of American States
OBE	Officer, The Most Excellent Order of the British Empire
Oxford DNB	*Oxford Dictionary of National Biography* (UK)
PASB	Pan American Sanitary Bureau

PhD	Doctor of Philosophy
QVJIN	Queen Victoria Jubilee Institute of Nursing
RACP	Royal Australasian College of Physicians
RACS	Royal Australasian College of Surgeons
RAMC	Royal Army Medical Corps (UK)
RBNA	Royal British Nurses Association
RCP	Royal College of Physicians
RCPEdin	Royal College of Physicians of Edinburgh
RCS	Royal College of Surgeons
RCSEdin	Royal College of Surgeons of Edinburgh
RMO	Resident Medical Officer
RSTMH	Royal Society of Tropical Medicine and Hygiene
SA	Sturm Abteilung [Storm Section] (Nazi Germany)
SLSAA	Surf Lifesaving Association of Australia
SS	Schutzstaffel [Protective Squadron] (Nazi Germany)
STD	Sexually Transmitted Diseases
UCH	University College Hospital (London, England)
UCL	University College London (England)
UNICEF	United Nations Children's Fund
UNRRA	United Nations Relief and Rehabilitation Administration
WHO	World Health Organization
YMCA	Young Men's Christian Association

LIST OF ENTRIES

Ge Hong
Gear, James H. S.
Gee, Samuel J.
Gentile da Foligno
Gerhard, William Wood
Geroulanos, Marinos
Gersdorff, Hans von
Gesell, Arnold L.
Gibbon, John H.
Gilbert the Englishman
Gillbee, William
Gilles de Corbeil
Gilles de la Tourette, Georges
Gillies, Harold D.
Gillman, Joseph
Gimbernat i Arbós, Antoni de
Giovannini, Giovanni B.
Girard, Georges D.
Glisson, Francis
Gluckman, Henry
Godlee, Rickman J.
Goldberger, Joseph
Goldstein, Kurt
Golgi, Camillo
Gordon, Doris C.
Gorgas, William C.
Gotō Konzan
Gotō Shinpei
Goudas, Anastasios
Gowers, William R.
Goyanes Capdevilla, José
Graaf, Reinier de
Graefe, Friedrich W. E. A. von
Graham, Evarts A.
Graham, Sylvester
Gram, Hans C. J.
Grancher, Jacques-Joseph
Grassi, Giovanni B.
Graves, Robert J.
Greenwood, Major
Gregg, Norman M.
Gregory, Alfred J.
Gregory, John
Grenfell, Wilfred T.
Grierson, Cecilia
Griesinger, Wilhelm
Grinker, Roy R.
Gross, Samuel D.
Grotjahn, Alfred
Guido da Vigevano
Guilera Molas, Lluís G.
Guillain, Georges
Guislain, Joseph
Guiteras Gener, Juan
Gull, William Withey

Gullstrand, Allvar
Gully, James M.
Guthrie, George J.
Hackett, Lewis W.
Ḥaddād, Sāmī I.
Haffkine, Waldemar M. W.
Hagedorn, Hans C.
Hahnemann, Samuel
Haire, Norman
Halford, George B.
Haller, Albrecht von
Halsted, William S.
Hamburger, Jean
Hamilton, Alice
Hammond, William A.
Hanaoka Seishū
Hansen, G. H. Armauer
Hardy, Harriet L.
Harinasuta, K. Tranakchit
Harpestreng, Henrik
Hart, Ernest A.
Harvey, William
Haslam, John
Hastings, Charles
Hata Sahachirō
Hatem, George
Hayem, Georges
Haygarth, John
Ibn al-Haytham
Head, Henry
Heberden, William
Hegar, E. L. Alfred
Heister, Lorenz
Helmont, Jan B. van
Hench, Philip S.
Henle, F. G. Jacob
Henry of Mondeville
Heo Jun
Hercus, Charles E.
Hernández, Francisco
Herophilus of Chalcedon
Herrick, James B.
Heurnius, Johannes
Heurnius, Otto
Hijmans van den Bergh, Abraham A.
Hildegard of Bingen
Hill, Austin Bradford
Hippocrates of Cos
Hirsch, August
Hirschfeld, Magnus
Hirschsprung, Harald
Hirszfeld, Ludwik
His, Wilhelm (the elder)
Hobson, Benjamin
Hodgkin, Thomas

Hoffmann, Friedrich
Holloway, Thomas
Holmes, Gordon M.
Holmes, Oliver Wendell
Holmgren, Alarik F.
Holst, Axel
Holt, Luther E.
Hooker, Worthington
Hope, James
Horsley, Victor A. H.
Horton, J. Africanus B.
Horwitz Barak, Abraham
Houssay, Bernardo A.
Hufeland, Christoph W.
Hufnagel, Charles A.
Huggins, Charles B.
Hunter, John
Hunter, William
Hurst, Arthur F.
Huss, Magnus
Hutchinson, Jonathan
Ilizarov, Gavriil A.
Imhotep
Ingen Housz, Jan
Ingenieros, José
Inozemtsev, Fedor I.
Isaac Israeli
Iudin, Sergei S.
Izquierdo Raudón, José J.
Jackson, James
Jackson, John Hughlings
Jacobi, Abraham
Jacobi, Mary C. Putnam
Jacobs, Aletta H.
Jamot, Eugène
Janet, Pierre
Jarvis, Edward
Jenner, Edward
Jenner, William
Jerne, Niels K.
Jex-Blake, Sophia L.
Jhirad, Jerusha
Jiménez Díaz, Carlos
Jivaka Komarabhacca
John of Gaddesden
John of Saint-Amand
Johnson, Obadiah
Jones, Agnes E.
Jones, Joseph
Jones, Robert
Joshi, Anandi G.
Joslin, Elliot P.
Jung, Carl G.
Jurin, James
Kaposi, Moritz

THE WESTERN MEDICAL TRADITION

In a volume devoted to biographies it would be more politic to agree with Thomas Carlyle's 'history is the biography of great men' than with Tolstoy's 'great men are no more than labels giving names to events'. Yet we also need to remember Peter Medawar's contention that science, including biomedicine, is different. If Mozart had never been born, for instance, then we should have been deprived of *Cosi fan tutte* and the last symphonies, since nobody else could have written the identical works. If, however, Charles Darwin had never been born, then Alfred Wallace or somebody else would have come up with the doctrine of evolution by natural selection. Thus one major theme in science has been the struggle for personal priority. Every year sees queries about the winners of the Nobel Prize, in favor of a rival or a colleague who has done similar work. And over 200 years ago, the French recognized the unfairness of an accolade with the concept of the forty-first Chair—the figure who just fails to be elected to the Académie Française, with its forty members (past occupants include Molière, Descartes, and Proust).

Similar arguments have occurred in biomedicine. William Osler (1849–1919) was one of those clinician–medical historians who saw history as made by men—whereas Max Neuberger tried to find the *Zeitgeist* for each particular period. Hence as a background to the biographies that occupy much of this book, I shall try to sketch some features of the main epochs in Western medicine before con-

sidering some themes that have been constant throughout much of this period, such as losses versus gains, illness as a punishment for sin, the individual versus the population. And my definition of history is taken from Oswei Temkin, who argued that history studies not only ideas but 'deals with great physicians, hospitals, medical colleges, disease and epidemics, quacks, drugs and surgical operations, and with people's thoughts on health, diseases, and cure' (Temkin, 1977, p. 110).

Over time, the geographical area covered by the Western medical tradition has been large, with the predominant geographical area for its development changing with the rise and fall of nations and empires. Thus, dating probably as far back as 2000 BCE, Babylonian clay tablets provide the earliest records, the code of Hammurabi (1750 BCE), for instance, laying down a legal code for medicine, and later tablets being devoted to the symptoms of scurvy or epilepsy, or listing useful drugs. Similarly, the four known medical papyri show that medicine was active in Egypt during much the same period, recording case histories, injuries, or an elaborate pharmacopoeia. Some centuries later, medical thought was to pass to Greece—undergoing major developments including the composition of the *Hippocratic Corpus*—and in the centuries thereafter to Alexandria and thence to Rome. With the fall of the Roman Empire, medical knowledge was preserved by Islam, from which it was recovered for Europe from the twelfth century.

Other medical traditions also stretch back into antiquity, and in their earliest days the various traditions shared many beliefs. Broadly, all saw disease as having some supernatural causes (whether divine displeasure, sorcery, or witchcraft) and hence needed magic as well as medicine for cures. Greek medicine, however, came to deny such causes, ascribing these instead to an imbalance in the body's makeup, which could be restored by the appropriate measures. The emphasis was thus on the individual and his relationship to the environment. Hence, it was at this stage that Western medicine began to diverge from other systems, a move that was accentuated later with the tentative discoveries in anatomy, and much later with the substantive findings in anatomy and physiology. Disease in this system then abandoned humoral theories and became much less focused on the individual and more on the underlying process to the illness, being successively perceived in terms of damage to the organs, then the tissues, and then the cells and their components.

THE HIPPOCRATIC LEGACY: FROM ANTIQUITY TO THE EARLY MODERN PERIOD

> The art has three factors, the disease, the patient, the physician. (Hippocrates, *Epidemics* book I)

For almost all of history, ordinary people have had to rely on self-help and their families and neighbors for treating their ailments. Even when professional care became available, access was restricted to the wealthy, as it still is in many parts of the world. Initially, illness was seen as having supernatural causes—whether malevolent demons (Egypt or Mesopotamia) or the gods (Greece). Hence when medical treatment began to become the province of specialists, it was religiously based, with practitioners such as priests, astrologers, and shamans, together with bonesetters who could treat injuries from work or battle as well as carry out elementary surgery, such as circumcision.

Elaborate pharmacopoeias were developed. Thus, at twenty meters long, the Egyptian Ebers Papyrus not only covered spells and incantations, but also listed such preparations as pills, pastilles, ointments, bandages, and enemata. And just as the Egyptians had a god of medicine, Imhotep, so in the fifth century BCE the Greeks began to erect temples to his counterpart, Asclepius, with the priesthood using herbs and sacred serpents. In a particular form of treatment called Temple Medicine, the patient, after sacrifice and purification, lay down to sleep near the altar of the god, whereupon the remedy for the disease was revealed, either in a dream or by a priest dressed to represent Asclepius. Over 300 such temples were built, with the principal one being at Epidaurus.

In Greece around 450 BCE this approach changed radically. The medicine described by Hippocrates was independent of the supernatural, and patient-centered rather than disease-centered. Coming from Cos and Cnidus, two medi-

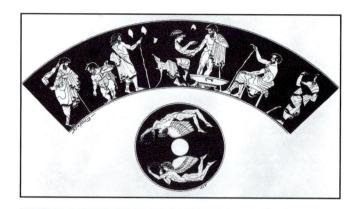

Greek surgery of the fifth century BCE. A doctor bleeds a patient (center) while other patients wait their turn. Watercolor after a painting on an Attic vase (480–460 BCE) in the Louvre, Paris. Iconographic Collection, Wellcome Library, London.

cal schools in Greece that were in active operation by the fifth century, between 420 and 350 BCE the sixty-odd works making up the *Hippocratic Corpus* were written by several authors. A mixture of philosophy, teaching texts, and case notes, the *Corpus* states that man should be regarded as a product of his environment, with diseases having their own individual natures. Building on earlier Greek concepts of the four humors (blood, yellow bile, black bile, and phlegm), it correlated these with the four seasons, the four ages of man (childhood, youth, adulthood, and old age), and the four primary qualities (hot, dry, cold, and wet). By the Roman period, this scheme included further correlation with the four elements (air, fire, earth, and water), the four periods of the day, four colors, and four tastes. Medieval authorities added the four temperaments (sanguine, bilious, melancholic, and phlegmatic) and even the four Evangelists.

Diseases, then, arose from a disturbance of the body's equilibrium—for example, epilepsy was caused by phlegm blocking the passage of air to the brain, whereupon convulsions were caused by the air trying to force its way through. With a conservative outlook, the emphasis of the *Corpus* was on prognosis. Treatment with surgery and drugs should be cautious, with particular concern to do no harm (surgery for bladder stone being forbidden, for example). The main approach was to regulate the diet and to follow regimen—a balance in exercise, sex, bathing, and sleep. The Greeks also took the concept of medical ethics from the Egyptians, with the celebrated Hippocratic Oath laying down codes of conduct for the physician. This concern with the individual patient rather than society at large or the advancement of knowledge is why for so long Hippocrates was as important for medical ethics as for medical practice.

In 367 BCE Aristotle (384–322 BCE), the son of a physician, was sent to Athens to study at Plato's Academy. Plato (427–347/8 BCE) emphasized that there were two types of medical practitioner—one being a 'leech', sometimes an ex-slave, with technical skills, and the other a professional belonging to one of the three (later four) sects that held widely differing views about the nature of illness. He taught that medicine, philosophy, health, and politics were all linked, maintaining that everything must have a purpose. Such so-called teleology was developed by Aristotle, who in between teaching at various academies in Greece also became tutor to the future Alexander the Great. Aristotle was the first to study the observable facts of nature and to try to unify them with an explanation. Thus he established scientific method, a logical approach to problems that was to influence scientific thought for many centuries, even, for example, as late as William Harvey in the seventeenth century.

Possibly because it allowed dissection of the human cadaver, as well as possessing a celebrated library, medicine shifted from Greece to Alexandria in Egypt in the middle of the third century BCE. The medical school established there in 300 BCE enabled great strides to be made in understanding the brain, heart, and nervous and vascular systems. A particular concept developed was pneumatism. Pneuma was an all-pervading vital principle that circulated throughout the body and underwent changes to a form of spirit. Air taken into the lungs passed as pneuma to the heart, where it was converted into vital spirit; this traveled through the arteries to the various organs, enabling them to function. In the brain, vital spirit was converted into animal spirit, which traveled through the hollow nerves and enabled higher functions such as motion and sensation to take place.

With the absorption of Egypt into the Roman Empire and the death of Cleopatra, the Alexandrian school lost its importance and Rome slowly took its place. Nevertheless, at first Greek medicine was wholly dominant, and the first text published in Latin, in 50, was a translation from the Greek. The scene changed dramatically with the arrival of Galen of Pergamum (129–210), an energetic author and self-publicist who had had experience as surgeon to the gladiators. Believing that a good doctor had to be a good philosopher as well as a good practitioner, Galen became physician to the Emperor Commodus in 180 and subsequently to Septimus Severus. Though his teaching was based on the dissection of animals rather than the human cadaver, Galen's influence was enormous, widespread, and long lasting, extending until the seventeenth century. As he himself emphasized, he took over both Aristotle's teleological views and the concepts in the *Hippocratic Corpus*, extending these with his own prolific studies, especially on the skeleton and muscles, nerves, heart, lungs, pulse, and nervous system. For the nervous system he showed how cutting the spinal cord at various levels had different effects, whether instant death at the top of the cord, partial paralysis of the body in the upper part, or paralysis of the legs lower down. In particular, Galen emphasized the therapeutic value of bleeding, which would reduce the excessive humors that had caused illness by accumulating in the body and restore its balances to normal.

Galen also extended pneumatism, teaching that food was absorbed and converted into chyle, which passed to the liver and then to the right ventricle through the vena cava; thereafter some passed to the left ventricle through invisible pores in the septum separating the ventricles. In the liver, the blood was infused with natural spirits, in the left ventricle with vital spirits, and in the brain with a third type, animal spirits. The arteries did not pulsate: instead, blood ebbed and flowed through them, as it did in the veins, nourishing the various tissues.

A totally different aspect of Roman medicine was the development of public health, with the building of aqueducts and sewage systems. The Romans also built hospitals (valetudinaria) where their far-flung troops could be treated. Subsequently, in the fourth century, they introduced hospitals for civilians as well.

After the Arab conquest of Syria, Egypt, and Iraq in the 630s and 640s (in Alexandria 700,000 manuscripts were burned in its library in 641), Western medicine entered a new phase. For several centuries, the classical tradition was preserved in the monasteries, and, though there were a few writers of medical texts, there were no medical professionals or medical training. The body was seen as subordinate to the soul—hence the emphasis shifted to healing by prayer or by miracles wrought at the shrines of numerous saints. For example, St Fillan became the patron saint of the mentally ill, who used to be dipped in his pool at Strathfillan in Scotland and then left wrapped overnight in a corner of the ruined chapel nearby, and several miracles were recorded among patients with throat diseases who traveled to the relics of St Blaise housed at Canterbury Cathedral.

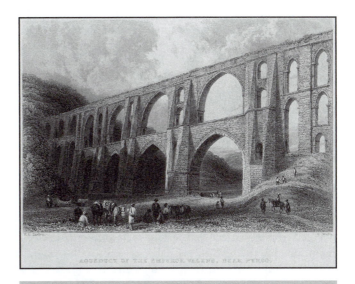

Aqueduct built by the Roman Emperor Valens (364–78), near Pyrgo, Italy. Engraving by Robert Wallis after William Henry Bartlett, 1839. Iconographic Collection, Wellcome Library, London.

The Greek/Alexandrian/Galenic traditions were preserved by Islam. The ideas formulated by the Hellenistic Egyptian sects (later classified as rationalist, dogmatic, and empiricist) were discarded in favor of Galen, whose works were first translated into Syriac, and then into Arabic. These works were then built on by scholars who were all natural philosophers as well as physicians, such as Rhazes (Al-Rāzī), Avicenna (Ibn Sīnā, the Galen of Islam), and Moses Maimonides, many of whom also produced writings of their own. Extensive pharmacopoeias with many new agents were another feature of Islamic medicine, and were subsequently introduced into Europe when the major Arabic texts were translated back into Latin.

Around 1100 the West was becoming increasingly prosperous, while the sharp increase in population was forcing the migration of people from the countryside into the towns, which grew rapidly larger. At this time medical learning started again in Europe, initially at the new center at Salerno. This part of southern Italy had just been conquered by the Normans, and, unusually, the Salerno school was not staffed entirely by monks and included women medical students. Among the several books produced there was the *Regimen Sanitatis Salernitanum*, a lengthy poem stipulating how to live a healthy life as well as listing remedies for illness. A lack of religious dominance tended to be a feature of those newly arising universities that created faculties of medicine—as at Bologna from the late twelfth century.

Another feature was the development of hospitals. In Europe and the Near East (as in Jerusalem) there had long been small set ups, usually hostels without medical staff, that served the needs of pilgrims to the various shrines. Conversely, in Byzantium (St Sampson's in Constantinople, founded around 550) and Islam (Baghdad, founded some time later), larger facilities had featured large staffs offering a variety of treatments. One suggestion is that the returning Crusaders copied the example of Constantinople; thus by 1231 (twenty-seven years after they had sacked the city) the Hôtel-Dieu in Paris had over 200 beds and a large complement of medical and ancillary staff, and in 1288 Santa Maria Novella in Florence had 230 beds. Elsewhere, however, hospitals were much smaller.

In their early years the new medical schools attracted only a few students, given the length of the course (that at Salerno, for instance, lasted five years, preceded by three years' study of logic) and with much of the teaching being devoted to memorizing the ancient texts and writing commentaries on them. But, crucially, several of the schools started to introduce a practice not seen since the Alexandria school: dissection of the human cadaver for teaching anatomy. Dissection raised several difficulties. Not only was there a shortage of cadavers (so that permission had to be sought to anatomize executed criminals), but these tended to decay rapidly (so that dissection was scheduled

for the winter and in a sequence studying first those parts most likely to decay). Moreover, the Church disapproved of dissection, though it did not forbid it: medico-legal autopsies were routine in Italy, and in the 1350s the Pope temporarily relaxed any proscription in the hope of finding the cause of the Black Death.

Of the medical schools, Bologna was the first to teach by dissection in 1315, Montpellier in 1387, Padua in 1429, and Paris in 1484, but it was slow to be adopted elsewhere, such as in England and Germany. Such dissections were public ceremonies, with the professor seated above the cadaver, reading from a treatise in Latin while below an assistant carried out the procedure and another identified particular structures with a wand. In 1537 the Church finally officially accepted the need for dissection as part of medical teaching.

Medieval Europe came to be dominated by its experience of plague, or the Black Death, which between 1347 and 1351 killed more than 25 percent of Europeans. Probably originating

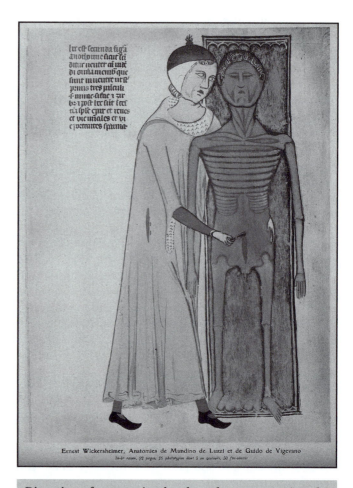

Dissection of an emaciated cadaver by an anatomist who makes an abdominal incision with a scalpel. Facsimile from the *Liber Notabilium* (1345), a manuscript by Guido de Vigevano in the Musée Condé, Chantilly. Collotype, 1926. Iconographic Collection, Wellcome Library, London.

in China, and then spreading along the Silk Road and the Pilgrims' Way to Mecca, it was brought to Europe by Italian soldiers returning from war in the Crimea. The bacterium responsible, *Yersinia pestis*, was spread by rat fleas, and the outbreak combined three types of plague (bubonic, with inflamed lymph nodes; septicemic, with infection of the blood stream; and pneumonic, spread by coughing). The medical response was to institute quarantine (initially at Ragusa (now Dubrovnik) part of the Venetian empire, for thirty days and subsequently elsewhere for a more effective forty days) and at first to house the victims in lazarettos, which had been isolation units for leprosy sufferers. The response of the population was to seek penitence, as by self-flagellation, but also to find scapegoats—particularly the Jews, who were massacred in several cities. Plague was to recur at intervals until the pandemic of 1664–65, The Great Plague (killing over 100,000 people in London, graphically recorded by the diarist Samuel Pepys), after which it virtually disappeared from northern and western Europe. On the eve of the scientific revolution, plague was still explained and understood in a manner that the Hippocratics shared; when this was no longer the case, the new enterprise of modern biomedicine had evolved.

THROUGH SCIENTIFIC REVOLUTION INTO ENLIGHTENMENT

The Renaissance was characterized by a rekindled enthusiasm for everything Greek, with the philosopher Erasmus (1466–1536) making new translations into Latin of several works by Galen, first printed in 1490. With the new thirst for ancient Greek knowledge came a questioning of its authority and then a questioning of nature. One enthusiasm was for anatomy: several new texts were published, though most of these perpetuated the ideas of

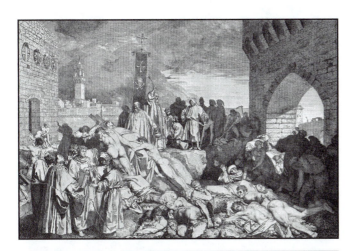

The Black Death of Florence, 1348, as described in Boccaccio's *Decameron*. Etching by Luigi Sabatelli after himself, *c.* 1820. Iconographic Collection, Wellcome Library, London.

Galen. Painters were among the first to realize that they needed a detailed knowledge of anatomy to make their figures real. A good example is Leonardo da Vinci's anatomical drawings in his (unpublished) notebooks, of 1487–93 and 1505–10, though most of these still show medieval ideas.

It was left to Andreas Vesalius (1514–64), a Flemish physician who had moved from Paris to Padua as an anatomy teacher, to emphasize the primacy of firsthand observation. Described as the most important of all medical works, the seven books of his *De humani corporis fabrica* (1543), devoted to the various parts of the body, are a masterpiece of Renaissance printing. The illustrations, most by the German artist Jan Stephan van Calcar and said to have been done in Titian's studio, are beautifully and dramatically posed. Vesalius is said to have supervised the actual production himself, selecting the paper, the block-maker for the woodcuts, and the printer in Basel. Crucially, moreover, he came to realize that, apart from the human skeleton (which Galen had studied), all of Galen's other descriptions of the body were based on animal studies, especially the Barbary ape. In the *Fabrica* not only did Vesalius correct the errors, but in his second edition he disputed Galen's description of blood passing from one ventricle to another, writing: 'Not long ago, I would not have dared to diverge a hair's breadth from Galen's opinion. But the septum is thick, dense, and compact as the rest of the heart. I do not, therefore, see how even the smallest particle can be transferred from the right to the left ventricle through it' (quoted in Weatherall, 1995, p. 32)

At the age of twenty-nine Vesalius became physician to Emperor Charles V and then to his son, King Philip II of Spain, and probably found anatomy research difficult. Yet his earlier appointment at Padua had included teaching surgery, and hence the anatomical discoveries were to improve its standards. Surgery had been, and was to remain for some time, a poor relation of medicine. Its mainly low-status professionals, who sometimes worked also as barbers or innkeepers, were refused admission to the universities and had to train by apprenticeships sponsored by the guilds. Others had no formal training at all, but gained experience through practice, often offering procedures such as bonesetting, tooth drawing, or cataract removal.

Nevertheless, in a few schools, including Salerno, surgery was taught alongside medicine, and there had been influential publications, such as *Chirugia magna* (1363) by the Frenchman Guy de Chauliac (1300–68), surgeon to three popes. Though surgical procedures were largely minor, such as bandaging and bleeding, and occasionally the repair of hernia, for battle injuries operative intervention was vital—especially after the introduction of gunpowder in the fifteenth century—and provided a useful if harsh education. Ambroise Paré (1510–90) was a surgeon from the Hôtel Dieu in Paris who spent thirty years intermittently with the French armies and revolutionized military surgery. He substituted an ointment for the boiling oil previously applied to gunshot wounds, used ligatures rather than the red-hot cautery to stop bleeding (paving the way for safer amputation), and designed prostheses, including artificial arms and hands. His textbook of surgery included passages from the *Fabrica*'s new anatomy section specially translated into French, and its influence persisted for the next 200 years—as did Paré's famous saying: 'I dressed the wound but God healed the patient.'

Vesalius's *Fabrica* appeared in the same year (1543) as another influential (posthumous) work, *De revolutionibus urbium coelestium,* by the Pole Nicholas Copernicus— another component in the emerging Scientific Revolution, with its paradigm-challenging heliocentric astronomy. But for medicine the centuries-long Galenic dogma had already been undermined by the Swiss physician Paracelsus (1493/4–1541). Paracelsus was appointed professor of medicine at the University of Basle in 1527 on the recommendation of Erasmus. He angered his colleagues by publicly burning the works of Galen and Avicenna, and also by admitting barber-surgeons to his lectures—which, unusually, were delivered in the vernacular rather than Latin, a key democratization of medical education. Forced to flee from Switzerland after only a year in his post, he went back to wandering throughout Europe.

Paracelsus (the 'Luther of medicine', in Osler's phrase) divided medicine into the remaining Galenists and the new chemists. He believed that the universe (Aristotle's macrocosm) behaved like a chemical laboratory and that physiological and pathological processes in the body (microcosm) were chemical rather than constitutional, as Hippocrates had maintained. All substances could be classified into hidden powers: sulfur (combustible), mercury (volatile), and salt (unchangeable). Hence diseases were better treated with chemical medicines rather than with the traditional herbal remedies. Another of his doctrines was that of 'signatures', which were treatments using substances resembling the diseased parts, for instance, cyclamen for ear disease because its leaf resembles the human ear, or a yellow-colored remedy for jaundice.

In some ways, Paracelsus was a central figure in the emerging Scientific Revolution. Conversely, though he was a firm believer in the Bible, he also introduced mystical and esoteric concepts into his writings, and personally he was an aggressive bully. Even so, he made some important clinical observations, including distinguishing congenital mental defect from acquired mental illness, associating cretinism with thyroid disease, and introducing iron and antimony for treating disease. He also wrote about the use of mercury for treating syphilis, though Islamic physicians had long been using this for common skin diseases.

Controversy still exists about the origin of syphilis. Was it a variant of yaws, another disease caused by the treponema, widespread in the tropics and then endemic in

Europe? Or had it been brought back from the New World in 1493 by Columbus's troops? For in 1495, starting at the siege of Naples, where some of Columbus's men had fought, a new epidemic spread like wildfire across Europe. At first, sufferers developed skin ulcers and rashes, and later on, tissues such as the nose and long bones were destroyed, and finally, they became seriously ill and died. Early in its history the venereal origin was recognized and the condition was given various names—the Neapolitan disease, the French disease, the Spanish disease, the Great Pox, and so on—and these persisted even after 1530 when the Italian physician Girolamo Fracastoro (1476/8–1553) published a poem, *Syphilus,* describing a shepherd punished with the disease by Apollo for insulting him.

Mercury was used as a pill, inunction, or inhalant to try to rid the body of the syphilitic poison in the saliva (the aim being to spit out as much as four pints in twenty-four hours). It was often combined with several days' treatment in a very hot room to do the same by sweating. But, though mercury continued to be used for treatment, it was soon evident that it did not cure syphilis, and from 1518

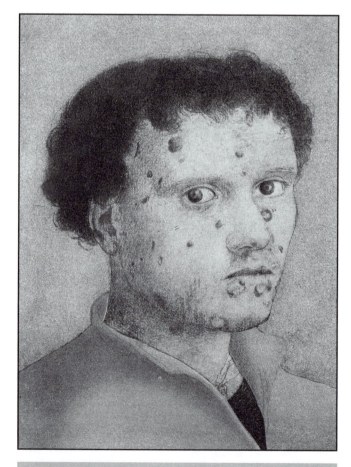

Young man suffering from syphilis. Lithograph after Hans Holbein the Younger, 1523. Iconographic Collection, Wellcome Library, London.

guiacum, a wood from the West Indies, was increasingly used as a less harmful (though equally ineffective) alternative.

Columbus's enterprise may have given Europe syphilis, but in return his men had given the New World the diseases of Europe, among them influenza, smallpox, measles, and typhus. This 'Columbian exchange' reflected how important such illnesses were in agricultural societies. Until around 11,000 years ago, all people had lived as hunter-gatherers and their illnesses, disabilities, and short life expectancy were largely due to food shortages and injuries. With the rise of agriculture in the Near East, people began to settle, at first in villages, some of which grew and became towns, and then, much later, cities. This enabled some infectious diseases to become established and a few existing ones, such as tuberculosis, smallpox, and malaria, to become more important. The result was that life expectancy remained short, with few people surviving beyond the age of forty.

Four features helped the transmission of infectious diseases. Overcrowding, the first, was particularly important for airborne infections, and the second, defective hygiene, which affected water supplies and sewage disposal and produced food contamination, had an important role in intestinal infections, such as typhoid and cholera. The third, malnutrition, lowered resistance to infection. The fourth factor was the new and close contact with farm animals, whose illnesses were sometimes transferred to man, often in a new form. Thus measles is believed to have come from dogs, the common cold from horses, influenza from pigs, and plague from gerbils.

In Western societies, endemic infections produced some population, or 'herd', immunity. But in virgin communities, such as the Amerindians exposed to Columbus's men, illnesses such as influenza and measles turned into explosive and lethal epidemics. Similar dramatic effects were seen in Mexico with Cortés's invasion: between 1518 and 1531 around a third of its population died of smallpox brought by the Spanish troops, none of whom died of this disease. Probably this enabled the conquest to be achieved so easily with so few men. Medicine as well as disease followed the expansion of Europe into the Americas and later the tropics and subtropics of Asia and Africa, and in time Western medicine became part of the apparatus of colonialism.

As early as the fourteenth century the authorities began to set up standards for medical practitioners, who in any case were becoming status-conscious themselves. These moves separated the university-trained practitioners, mainly physicians, from the others—apprenticeship-trained surgeons and midwives and untrained empirics. This movement was particularly active in Germany and Italy, which established colleges of physicians—a move copied in London in 1518. The latter, later given a Royal Charter, was principally concerned with protecting its members' interests, and it was left to a multidisciplinary

academy to spearhead the Scientific Revolution, started by Copernicus and Galileo, in England. Just before Galileo appeared before the Inquisition in 1633, the statesman-philosopher Francis Bacon (1561–1626) (who had delineated the inductive method of scientific reasoning) had described a model for a scientific academy. Bacon was a hero to two outstanding scientists, Robert Boyle (1627–91) and Robert Hooke (1635–1703) (and, curiously enough, also to German philosopher Immanuel Kant, who dedicated his *Critique of Pure Reason* (1781) to him). During the Commonwealth in the 1650s these two Englishmen were founding members of the so-called Invisible College, which became the Royal Society once Charles II had been restored to the throne.

Many of the Royal Society's early studies were in mathematics and astronomy, featuring such authorities as Isaac Newton (1642–1727) and Edmund Halley (c. 1656–1743), but both Boyle and Hooke made contributions of medical importance on the properties of air and the function of the lungs. And it was Boyle who helped overthrow the Aristotelian division of the world into the elements of earth, air, fire, and water. Crucially, moreover, like its French counterpart, the Royal Society started its own journal. Its articles and commentaries became a major method of scientific communication and were widely copied elsewhere.

For medicine the most celebrated discovery of the Scientific Revolution was made by William Harvey (1578–1657), a physician at St Bartholomew's Hospital, London. He became Lumleian Lecturer in Anatomy at the Royal College of Physicians, as well as physician to King Charles I, whom he followed around the country during the Civil War. Harvey had studied in Padua, where he had experimented on living animals, becoming particularly interested in the heart. Two earlier observations made by Realdo Colombo (d. 1558), Vesalius's successor at Padua, were critical for Harvey's research. First, Colombo argued that blood must circulate through the lungs, and, second, he showed that the heart acted with greater force in systole than in diastole.

Harvey was to demonstrate that the heart indeed behaved like a pump, expelling blood received from the veins into the major arteries and thence around the body. Rather than remaining passive receptacles, the arteries pulsated when the heart contracted, and if they were cut blood spurted from them. Moreover, blood did not ooze from the right ventricle to the left ventricle across the cardiac septum. The structure of the valves in the heart and veins could be explained only by blood flowing in one direction. By putting a ligature around the forearm Harvey showed that blood moved toward the heart in the veins and away from it in the arteries. Finally, he calculated that in a short time the left ventricle must eject more blood than was present in the whole body. Hence Harvey had to assume that there was some sort of an anastomosis between the veins and the arteries, promising in *De motu cordis et sanguinis*, the book he published in Frankfurt am Main as late as 1628, that he was busy with such research. Nevertheless, in the interim he was 'obliged to conclude that in animals the blood is driven round a circuit with an increasing circular sort of movement'.

Harvey delayed the publication of his last work, *De generatione animalium*, because he wished to avoid the storm that *De motu cordis* had provoked, though he had made a few ripostes to his critics. But many of his patients deserted him, and his friend John Aubrey, the wit and diarist, was to comment that after *De motu* appeared Harvey 'fell mightily in his Practize and 'twas believed by the vulgar that he was crack-brained'.

The Scientific Revolution ushered in a period of measurement, among the separate inventions being the thermometer, a balance for determining metabolic processes, a method of measuring the blood pressure in animals, and a pulse watch. The Netherlander Antoni van Leeuwenhoek (1632–1723) introduced a primitive microscope, which enabled Hooke to describe cells as the basic structure of plants. This movement chimed in with the views of Frenchman René Descartes (1596–1650), also a philosopher. His philosophy separated the mind from the body, regarding the latter as a machine. Though he argued about some of the detail, Descartes was enthusiastic about Harvey's *De motu*, using its ideas to support his own philosophy. Other developments during the seventeenth century included establishing the identity of the respiratory gases, oxygen and carbon dioxide; studies on digestion in the stomach; and work on 'irritability': how the muscles responded disproportionately to a stimulus, and the connections between the nerves and the brain.

Flanking these discoveries were two explorations of the broader picture of disease. The first came from Thomas Sydenham (1624–89), a Parliamentarian Captain of Horse on the opposite side of the English Civil War to Harvey, who based his practice on clinical observation and his treatment on experience rather than on Galen's teachings. He approached classification of diseases (nosology) rather like a botanist classifying plants, regarding each as an entity rather than a result of the alterations in constitutional factors postulated by Hippocrates. In fact, with Sydenham medieval medicine disappeared, for in his writings he was the first not to pay tribute to Islamic medicine.

The second exploration was in morbid anatomy, by Italian Giovanni Morgagni (1682–1771), a physician at Padua. His book *De sedibus et causis morborum per anatomen indagatis* (1761) recorded the postmortem findings in 700 cases, attempting for the first time to correlate these with the clinical history. He also has priority in describing several lesions, including syphilis of the brain and blood vessels, damage to the heart valves, and tuberculosis of the kidney.

Just as important were the developments in medical teaching. Appointed to the University of Leiden in 1701, Herman Boerhaave (1668–1738) rapidly gained a reputation as an outstanding teacher, with students from all over Europe flocking to the university. His case report of a man who died from a ruptured esophagus inaugurated the now traditional sequence of clinical history, examination, course, and autopsy findings. He also introduced the modern medical curriculum of natural science, anatomy, physiology, and pathology, and was to influence the new Edinburgh and Vienna schools of medicine. In London, William Hunter (1718–83), from Lanarkshire, became first professor of anatomy to the Royal Academy and set up several private anatomy schools in London, the most famous being that in Great Windmill Street. William's brother, John (1728–93), the outstanding surgeon of the era, had his own surgical school in Leicester Square.

Another critical development was the introduction of methods of accurate diagnosis during life. In 1761 Leopold Auenbrugger (1722–1809), a physician in Vienna, described the value of percussion of the chest in diagnosis, though little notice was taken at the time. Fifty years later, his work was translated into French, a little before René Laennec (1781–1826), a physician to the Necker Hospital in Paris, used a roll of paper to listen to a patient's heart. By 1818 he had developed a wooden stethoscope an inch and a half in diameter and a foot long. In a book that also paid tribute to Auenbrugger's work, Laennec described the sounds characteristic of various chest diseases, which could now be recognized as individual conditions.

Such apparently modest discoveries were to mark the beginnings of modern medicine, and took place against a background of change wrought by the French Revolution and the rise of Napoleon. The former closed the medical schools and abolished the role of nuns as hospital nurses, and for a time anybody could pay a small license fee and practice medicine. Nevertheless, with the fall of Robespierre three faculties of medicine were reopened, with professors appointed and paid by the state, and French substituted for Latin in teaching. Most important, starting with the Paris school, the authorities developed a wide-ranging medical curriculum that emphasized practical experience and high standards of competence (Napoleon introduced a strict system of medical licensing in 1803). Given that notable figures—in medicine, surgery, obstetrics, and psychiatry—arose at the time, and that large city hospitals were built, all these developments resulted in Paris becoming the academic powerhouse of European medicine, a status it retained for half a century. Medical students flocked to the French capital from all over the world, while the restored French king put the seal on developments by creating the Academy of Medicine in 1820.

THE BIRTH OF THE MODERN

Nevertheless, important though all these developments were, few directly improved patient care. At the beginning of the nineteenth century, the life expectancy for a male at birth was still what it had been for centuries—well under forty years of age—while a quarter of the population of developed countries was dying from tuberculosis. By 1900, however, life expectancy had risen considerably, through both general measures and the application of specific research findings.

A number of workers appreciated the links between filth and disease. Ignác Semmelweis (1818–65), a Hungarian obstetrician working in Vienna, showed that by merely washing their contaminated hands, medical staff could reduce the death rate in parturient women—but his findings received no publicity. Florence Nightingale (1820–1910) did the same for wounded soldiers in the Crimean War by cleaning up the wards, improving the diet, and introducing trained nursing staff. John Snow (1813–58), a physician-anesthetist, showed how cholera could be spread in contaminated drinking water (thus challenging the centuries-long idea that such diseases were due to miasmas, or contaminated air). Not only did the four major cholera epidemics in the newly industrialized Britain, between 1831 and 1866, provide the impetus for sanitary reform, but there were also the 'Great Stink' of the sewage-laden Thames, which forced the British Parliament to stop sitting, and Frederic Engels's horrifying *The Condition of the Working Class in England* (1845; English trans. 1887). Eventually, then, spurred on by two forceful epidemiologists, William Farr (1807–83) and Edwin Chadwick (1800–90), London and the other large cities introduced piped water and proper sewage disposal. This model was gradually copied throughout the Western world.

Several major discoveries in scientific medicine were interdependent: major surgery was impracticable without anesthesia, and the surgical infection rate was then dramatically reduced by antisepsis, itself arising out of the new germ theory, and much later by asepsis. The claims for priority in the discovery of anesthesia were many. Humphry Davy (1778–1829), the English chemist, had discovered the anesthetic properties of nitrous oxide ('laughing gas') at the Pneumatic Institute in Bristol in the 1790s, and Horace Wells (1815–48), a Connecticut dentist, was to have one of his own teeth extracted using it forty years later. In 1842 the American surgeon, Crawford Long (1815–78), at Jefferson, Georgia, found that ether had similar properties, and five years later James Simpson (1811–70), an obstetrician at Edinburgh, was to substitute chloroform to alleviate the pain of childbirth. The clergy's opposition to such use was undermined when Queen Victoria had it administered by John Snow at the birth of Prince Leopold in 1853.

Many of the great advances in the nineteenth century, however, came from France and the German-speaking countries. British doctors seemed preoccupied with their private patients, and most of their contributions were limited to clinical descriptions, as of the diseases named after Thomas Addison (1795–1860), Richard Bright (1789–1858), and Thomas Hodgkin (1798–1866). London did not even have a university before 1837, and research did not

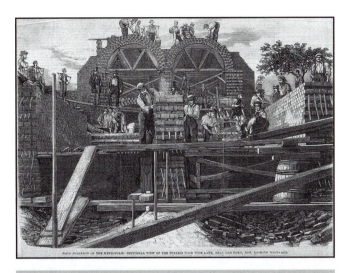

Construction of the great sewage tunnels in London's east end, part of the metropolis's system of sewers, pumping stations, and treatment works built by Sir Joseph Bazalgette during the 1860s. Wood engraving, *c.* 1861. Iconographic Collection, Wellcome Library, London.

figure prominently as an essential part of medicine. Moreover, the strong prejudice against vivisection in animals (present as far back as Samuel Johnson and resurfacing in nineteenth-century public protests) probably inhibited some initiatives. As a result, the mass of itinerant students flocked to the continental centers—at first France and later Germany and Vienna. This applied particularly to those from the United States. Throughout much of the century the quality of medical education there was often abysmal, though at the end of the nineteenth century physicians returned home and transformed standards; thus in 1893 William Welch (1850–1934), who had studied in Berlin, was to energize the medical school at Johns Hopkins University, Baltimore, on German lines.

The French scientist Claude Bernard (1813–78) attracted students from all over the world. Not only was he an outstanding teacher, with a chair at the Sorbonne especially created for him, but he was also the founder of 'experimental medicine'. Without this approach, Bernard maintained, traditional medicine was merely a passive observational science. The scientist should formulate a hypothesis, then devise a study to test it. Using simple experiments, with a superb operative technique, he demonstrated the role of the pancreas in the digestion of fat, the function of the liver, the effect of the nerves on metabolism, and the oxygenation of arterial and venous blood. He also introduced the concept of the *milieu interieur,* whereby the body's internal environment is kept constant by its balancing mechanisms. Bernard's work was complemented by the work on the breakdown of food in the body by German scientists, who were to found the new science of biochemistry.

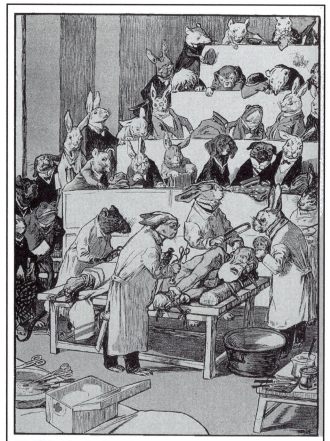

Die Vivisektion des Menschen.
Professor Karnickulus: Nur keine falsche Sentimentalität! Das Prinzip der freien Forschung verlangt es, daß ich diesen Menschen vivisziere zum Heile der gesamten Tierwelt!

Human vivisection. The rabbit says, "Now no phoney sentimentality! The principle of free research requires that I vivisect this human for the health of the entire animal world." Color lithograph, 1910. Iconographic Collection, Wellcome Library, London.

France and the German-speaking countries also made separate though fundamentally important contributions to two important nineteenth-century biomedical concepts: cell theory and germ theory. The first evolved from Morgagni, whose work in morbid anatomy stressed the importance of organs as the seat of disease. Next Marie François Xavier Bichat (1771–1802), a French anatomist, emphasized that diseases affected the tissues (which he was the first to name) rather than the organs. Rudolf Virchow (1821–1902), professor at Berlin and the outstanding pathologist of the nineteenth century—and some claim of all time—put the cell at the heart of pathological processes. Virchow stated that cells rather than the tissues were the site of disease. Earlier German scientists had described various features of the cell, which Virchow brought together in his book *Cellularpathologie* (1858). The body depended on the functioning of its cells, just as the state depended on the work of its citizens; thus a disease such as cancer was akin

to civil war. Such a stance could have been expected from a politician, and that was another of Virchow's roles. Besides taking part in the 1848 revolution, he was a longstanding member of the Berlin City Council and later of the Prussian Parliament, where he frequently opposed the policies of Bismarck.

The French chemist and microbiologist Louis Pasteur (1822–95), a professor at the École Normale, was almost an exact contemporary of Virchow. Initially he disproved the long-held theory of spontaneous generation, showing that fermentation in wine, beer, and milk was due to microorganisms present in the atmosphere. Such souring could be prevented by heating the liquids ('pasteurization'). Pasteur then developed his germ theory by experiments with a disease in silkworms, showing again that this was due to microbial infection and could be prevented. In further studies with infections involving the anthrax and fowl cholera organisms, he could produce immunity by using attenuated preparations (called 'vaccines' in honor of Edward Jenner (1749–1823) of smallpox vaccination fame). Returning to work after a stroke, he attenuated rabid matter from dogs' brains by serially passing it through the spinal cords of rabbits and then using the dried material for a vaccine to treat rabies in people.

The German Robert Koch (1843–1910) built on Pasteur's work, devising methods to identify the bacteria responsible for three important diseases (anthrax, tuberculosis, and cholera) and to grow them on artificial culture media. Thereafter there was an explosion in such discoveries, with bacteriologists all over the world identifying the organisms responsible for serious diseases, including diphtheria, typhoid fever, tetanus, brucellosis, scarlet fever, meningitis, and syphilis.

The final scientist in the great German triumvirate was Paul Ehrlich (1854–1915), a junior colleague of Koch, who was interested not only in immunization but also collaborated with the chemical industry in early work on chemotherapy. By immunizing animals with preparations of killed diphtheria bacilli, he and Emil von Behring produced antitoxin for injection into patients with the disease, which substantially lowered the death rate. Working in a new post in Frankfurt, he then studied agents against trypanosomiasis and syphilis. Though effective, the former proved too toxic, but the latter—his preparation number 606, later named Salvarsan—proved effective against syphilis and was the first cure until the introduction of penicillin in the 1940s.

A nineteenth-century development that involved both French and British contributors was the statistical movement. Statistics originally referred to numerical information about individuals, such as the Egyptian and Roman censuses and the seventeenth century *Bills of Mortality* exploited by John Graunt detailing the weekly burial lists in the London parishes. In France, the Parisian physician

Pierre Louis (1787–1872) tried to introduce a more scientific approach to medicine by analyzing a large series of cases of, in particular, tuberculosis and typhoid. He also conducted one of the first clinical trials, in patients with pneumonia divided into two groups, showing that the time of bleeding had no effect on the outcome of the illness. Eventually he founded a Society of Medical Observation to investigate the efficacy of various treatments; many of these were shown to be useless, with the result that a fashion developed for therapeutic nihilism.

William Farr, a British physician, had studied with Louis and became the pioneer British statistician, helping establish the General Register Office and the classification of diseases and occupations. Nevertheless, the true founder of the modern statistical movement was Karl Pearson (1857–1936), a British mathematician and biologist, who focused on using numerical information to answer specific questions. His pupils were to play an important part in the medicine of the twentieth century.

MORE OF THE SAME? THE TWENTIETH CENTURY

Though much of Ehrlich's work was done in the nineteenth century, he did not introduce Salvarsan until 1910. Similarly, much of the development of diagnostic x-rays, discovered by Wilhelm Roentgen (1845–1923) in 1895, occurred in the early twentieth century, when they were also used in the treatment of cancer. Thereafter, however, Germany—and France—lost much of their pioneering momentum. There were several reasons for this. Like empires, the natural tendency of research conglomerates is to rise and fall. New impetuses were to arise in the English-speaking world. In Britain, in physiology Charles Sherrington (1857–1952), E. D. Adrian (1889–1977), and Henry Dale (1875–1968) showed how nerve impulses were transmitted. In 1902 William Bayliss (1860–1924) and Ernest Starling (1866–1927) discovered the substance secretin, which given its actions they called a hormone—a chemical messenger formed in one place and passing in the blood to influence cell processes elsewhere. In the succeeding decades several new hormones were discovered, notably insulin, which in 1921 was isolated by Canadians Frederick Banting (1891–1941) and Charles Best (1899–1978), thus revolutionizing the outlook in diabetes, transforming it from an acute killer into a chronic disease requiring continuous medical management. In 1912, the British biochemist Frederick Gowland Hopkins (1861–1947) added to the research by the Dutchman Christiaan Eijkman (1858–1930), leading to the discovery of vitamins. A particularly important extension of this work was the discovery in 1926 in the United States of liver extracts, thus enabling the cure of fatal pernicious anemia, a signal of North America's rise to prominence in twentieth-century medicine.

Another factor was the formation of large medical research organizations, mostly in Britain and the United States. With the new emphasis on colonial territories at the end of the nineteenth century (culminating in Ronald Ross's discovery of the life cycle of the malarial parasite, 1898), both France and Britain had set up institutes devoted to tropical medicine. The newer institutes, however, came to have a much broader remit. In 1891 in honor of Pasteur's work on rabies, the British public subscribed the money to build the British Institute for Preventive Medicine (subsequently called the Jenner Institute, 1897, and then the Lister Institute, 1903). Three years later the Rockefeller Institute for Medical Research was founded in New York, also initially concentrating on serum and vaccine research, but crucially as well on raising the standards of medical education and research in the United States. In 1913 the initial charge to the British Medical Research Committee was to study the problems of tuberculosis, but during World War I its activities were diverted to immediate concerns. In 1920, with its name changed to the Medical Research Council, it began to deal with a variety of subjects, including other infectious diseases, serum therapy, and clinical trials. In the United States during World War II, target-directed research had burgeoned, while the vast capabilities in manufacturing had been shown when the British had found it impossible to manufacture penicillin on a commercial scale. Production of the antibiotic, which had been discovered by Alexander Fleming (1881–1955) and developed by Howard Florey (1898–1968) and his team, had had to be transferred to the U.S. pharmaceutical industry. After the war this capacity for research and manufacture continued to increase, with the creation of many research units in the medical schools, and the increased government sponsorship for the expanding National Institutes of Health, as well as the expansion of the pharmaceutical industry.

In Germany, an additional factor in the loss of initiative was political: the postwar depression, the Weimar Republic, and the rise of the Nazi Party. Significantly, the Nobel Prize given to Otto Warburg (1883–1970) for his work on intracellular respiration had been awarded in 1931, before the Nazis assumed power. Later, however, they refused to allow Gerhard Domagk (1895–1964) to accept the Nobel Prize in 1939, awarded for his synthesis of the sulfa drugs (though he collected it in 1947). Again, the exodus from Germany of many medical scientists who were Jewish led to a depletion of its intellectual capital, often to the gain of the host countries.

Medical reform and specialization were two features that started in the nineteenth century, with the pressure to register practitioners and lay down schedules for their training. Specialization was a prominent feature of German medicine, and in France, the United States, and elsewhere, practitioners began to be identified with specific areas of medicine: for instance the superintendents of asylums were among the first

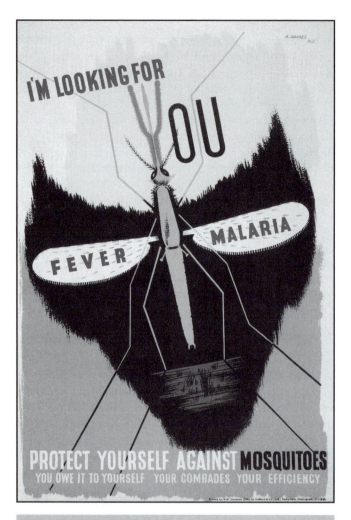

The malaria mosquito forming the eye sockets of a skull represents death from malaria. Poster commissioned by H.M. War Office, 1941, to raise awareness of the cause of malaria among British troops. Color lithograph by Abram Games. Iconographic Collection, Wellcome Library, London. Crown Copyright. Reproduced with permission of the Controller of HMSO and Queen's Printer for Scotland.

to form a specialist group. In 1865 after Joseph Lister (1827–1912) had heard about Pasteur's discovery that antiseptics could kill bacteria, he applied the antiseptic technique during operations using a carbolic spray. This was to greatly increase the number and complexity of surgical operations, and public attention was focused on this specialty when in 1902 the coronation of King Edward VII had to be postponed for him to have the abscess on his appendix drained. Surgical subspecialties developed as techniques and ancillary support improved.

Specialization, however, was to acquire increased emphasis in the twentieth century. During World War I surgery for trauma injuries increased greatly, with the need for more sophisticated anesthesia. The result was a move toward specialization in orthopedics and anesthetics, as

well as in plastic surgery (though this came into its own during World War II), and also to further the new procedure of blood transfusion.

Early in the century, pediatrics had started to devolve from general medicine. Subsequently the main discipline would split further into specialties devoted to chest medicine (tuberculosis particularly), neurology, and cardiology. Other new specialties included diagnostic radiology, radiotherapy, and clinical pathology. Such evolution followed a consistent pattern. Initially there was an informal club, succeeded by an organization with its own secretariat, specialist journal, and regular meetings. And whereas at first most organizations were nationally based, later they tended to come together and form separate regional (European, Nordic, or American) and then international bodies.

Eventually, some bodies acquired academic status and the responsibility for accrediting their members, while the formation of specialties and subspecialties was recognized by those in charge of training and hospital staffing. Moreover, the tendency to split did not stop: initially, for example, professionals might have specialized in general chest surgery, then in cardiac surgery, and later still in pediatric cardiac surgery.

The British perhaps remained committed generalists for the longest; for instance, obstetrics and gynecology was one of the last principal specialties to be delineated by the founding of its typical representative organization—a Royal College—in 1929. Part of the delay was due to intra-professional quarrels, with the surgeons claiming ownership of the specialty, but part was due to its relatively low status. From the beginning of the nineteenth century, many women had been delivered by their general practitioners, but midwives had also had a prominent role in childbirth and there had been very few medically qualified specialist obstetricians. That great British institution—the general practitioner—finally earned Royal College status in 1961.

Two themes from the past continued strongly into the twentieth century. In the first, the ever-reductive emphasis on the organs, tissues, and cells as the seat of disease was extended to the components of the cell. Once the latter had been delineated, in 1953 James Watson (b. 1928) and Francis Crick (1916–2004) demonstrated the double-helix structure of DNA in the nucleus. A subsequent high point was the mapping of the human genome by a combined UK/U.S. commercial/academic team, announced in 2002. Knowledge of the position of various genes has already been used in preventing some genetic diseases, and gene therapy promises to be an important method of treatment in the future.

The second persistent theme was the importance of statistics in prevention and treatment. Karl Pearson lived into the 1930s and his influence extended to Ronald Fisher (1890–1962), Major Greenwood (1890–1949), and Austin Bradford Hill (1897–1991), all of them distinguished statisticians,

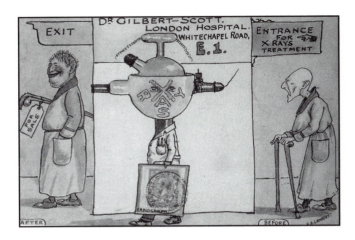

A patient before and after receiving radiotherapy for cancer. Color cartoon by E. A. Lambert, a radiotherapy patient, 1923. Wellcome Photo Library, London.

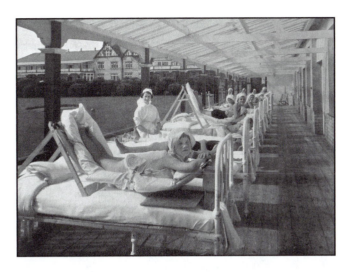

Girls with spinal tuberculosis on a sun verandah after surgery at Stannington Sanatorium, Morpeth, Northumberland. This was Britain's first sanatorium for children with tuberculosis. Photograph, 1930s. Wellcome Library, London.

epidemiologists, or both. Fisher subsequently worked on comparing different strains of wheat at the Agricultural Research Centre at Rothamsted, Hertfordshire in the UK, where he was to introduce the randomized controlled trial. So influenced by this concept was Bradford Hill that he was anxious to introduce it into medicine, particularly given the poor standards of some of the trials in the 1930s. The chance came with three trials: of patulin against the common cold, pertussis immunization, and streptomycin in tuberculosis.

Though not the first to be performed, the last trial was to bring Hill fame and to make the randomized controlled trial the gold standard for such investigations. In 1946 the U.S. government offered Britain, then bankrupt in the aftermath of war, sufficient streptomycin to treat 100 patients with tuberculosis. At that time, 70,000 patients in Britain were dying from the disease every year, and there were four times that number with the disease. Bradford Hill persuaded the tuberculosis committee of the Medical Research Council that the only ethical way of deciding who should be treated was a randomized controlled trial.

Such a decision was to anticipate the new concern with medical ethics, by a few in the profession and many outside it. Previously, ethics had largely been a matter of etiquette between doctors, such as quarrels over the size of their name-plates on the consulting room doors. After World War II the revelations about the Japanese atrocities and the Nazi experiments in the concentration camps had been received with revulsion, and a code of research ethics had been devised to prevent their repetition. Nevertheless, medical researchers thought that such provisions applied to barbarians, and did not consider that their own work might be less than ethical. Two influential publications by Henry Beecher (1904–76) in the United States (1959) and Maurice Pappworth (1910–94) in Britain (1961) showed the extent to which medical research had become a vehicle

for the self-advancement of the scientist rather than being concerned with the patient's cure. Indeed, both writers (an anesthetist and a physician) documented how several of the published procedures had hazarded health, or even life, while informed consent had not been obtained from the patient. The public furor over such disclosure concluded with a new code, the Declaration of Helsinki, defining informed consent and establishing research ethics committees (institutional review boards in the United States) to scrutinize all protocols for research.

In the late 1940s, the increasing number of deaths from lung cancer, previously a rare form of tumor, began to cause concern. Asked to investigate the situation in Britain, Bradford Hill recruited Richard Doll (1912–2005), a gastroenterologist working at the London School of Hygiene and Tropical Medicine. In a series of ever more rigorous reports they showed that unexpectedly this was linked to cigarette smoking, a habit that had become popular during World War I. Their findings were confirmed by similar studies all over the world, and smoking was also found to be linked to other cancers—such as of the lip and mouth, kidneys, and bladder—as well as obstructive lung disease, coronary heart disease, and low-birth-weight babies born to mothers who had smoked during pregnancy.

Governments worldwide were slow to act on these findings, ignoring or even denying the evidence. Nevertheless, they eventually launched campaigns against smoking, and as a result most people in the developed world know of the risks and many have reacted accordingly: in Britain the proportion of adults smoking has fallen from eighty percent in the 1950s to twenty-five percent today. Nevertheless, the debate began, and continues, about how much

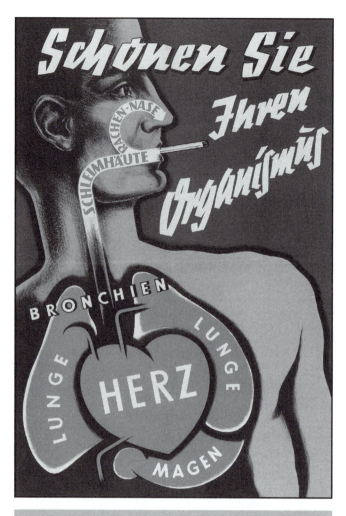

A man smoking a cigarette, showing the route through which the smoke passes to the heart and lungs. German antismoking campaign poster, c. 1900. Color lithograph. Iconographic Collection, Wellcome Library, London.

governments should interfere with individual lifestyles. Given that governments are now concerned as much with the health of populations as of individuals, and largely pay the bills, are they justified in stipulating limits for individuals? For example, should patients with smoking-related arterial disease be refused surgical operations if they refuse to give up the habit? Similar arguments apply to obesity and overindulgence in alcohol, like tobacco a legally obtainable substance.

THE WESTERN MEDICAL TRADITION IN PERSPECTIVE

The Persistence of Ideas

Why have some ideas in Western medicine persisted for so long? Nobody's work persisted longer than Galen's, but this was in a period of copying and transmitting existing knowledge rather than questioning such knowledge and the natural world on which it was supposedly based. The authorities, and particularly the Church, saw any challenge to orthodoxy as heresy—an attitude typified by Galileo, who in public if not in private recanted his heliocentric views. Thus the Salerno school may have taken off because the Church was poorly represented in its staff. Again, perhaps the Reformation principle of studying the Bible firsthand rather than relying on interpretations by priests may have led directly to the questioning attitude that sponsored the Scientific Revolution, with its characteristic penchant for experiment. But Galen's concept of an imbalance that could be treated by restoring balance or wholeness must have remained attractive: even as late as the early twentieth century William Osler, later Regius professor at Oxford, was recommending bleeding in certain cases.

Aristotelianism had also persisted, for, though he disclaimed Galenism, William Harvey went on claiming that everything had a purpose. Thus in his dedication of *De motu* to King Charles I he compared the animal's heart ('the sun of its microcosm') to the king ('the basis of his kingdom, the sun of his microcosm, the heart of the state'). Before we become too Whiggish, however, surely there is a glaring example of dogma, which has persisted into our own times, much as did Galen's ideas for hundreds of years. Sigmund Freud (1856–1939) and the psychoanalysis movement promised much, but delivered virtually nothing for the majority of patients with mental illness. That is not to deny the enormous influence of Freud—described along with Charles Darwin and Karl Marx as one of the three most influential figures born in the nineteenth century—with his ideas for thought, and especially for the arts. But Freud was a philosopher rather than a physician. And, with today's skepticism, it seems doubtful whether his nonvalidated and essentially personal ideas—based on anecdote and speculation in a few carefully selected cases—would ever have passed peer review and been published. In that case, would the bulk of patients with mental illness have been any worse off?

Another persistent theme has been disease as a divine punishment for sin. This was preached for the plague in Ancient Greece, and recurred with later epidemics, especially the Black Death and syphilis. Leprosy, which was prevalent during the Middle Ages but largely disappearing thereafter, was regarded in the same way, with sufferers debarred from contact with healthy people as much for their perceived sinfulness as any infectivity.

In the nineteenth century many clergy preached that cholera was a punishment for the immorality of the working classes, an attitude that was to be revived and modified as 'blaming the victim' to stigmatize homosexuals when HIV infection/AIDS emerged as an epidemic during the 1980s.

We should not be surprised by the persistence of this concept. Thirty years ago a distinguished academic told me about his younger sister, who had developed breast cancer. 'I don't know why she's got it,' he said, 'after all, she's done nothing wrong.'

Successes

To prioritize the advances brought about by Western medicine entails controversial choices, but I would cite four major achievements.

Diagnosis and treatment

Today's system of diagnosis and treatment is both effective and continually evolving. Take the example of how quickly and decisively modern science can be applied to a new problem if the will is there. In 1981 the first reports appeared of a new fatal illness (AIDS), occurring mainly in homosexuals. Within a short time not only had the clinical features been described, but HIV, the causative agent, was identified and also sequenced, with drugs developed to suppress the disease and prolong life.

National health services and international organizations

My second choice is the role of the State in medicine. Can we imagine what medicine would be like without it? (Even in the United States, one Western country where the government has a lesser role, government programs such as Medicare and Medicaid, for the elderly and the indigent, are vital safety nets for millions of people.) In Germany, Bismarck introduced a national insurance scheme as long ago as 1883, as did some of the Nordic countries, New Zealand, and the Soviet Union between the two world wars. Elsewhere, however, access to care was difficult for the non-rich, and in a few countries provision had even regressed, as in Britain, where the relaxed system of parish relief was replaced by the much harsher Poor Laws in 1834. Modern State involvement in prevention and clinical care started gradually, usually with immunization, at first vaccination against smallpox (compulsory in some countries) and later against diphtheria and other infectious diseases when it became available. Often this was linked with tuberculosis dispensaries and maternal and child welfare clinics set up in many countries. And gradually governments also started to pass legislation to address the scandal of many injuries and diseases caused by poor standards in the manufacturing industry and elsewhere.

After World War II, however, most Western countries developed systems of comprehensive health care funded through the State or insurance companies, or both together. A particular priority was improving maternity services and the relief of long-felt minor needs—glasses, dentures, and hernia repair, for example—as well as building new hospitals and health centers. As the sophistication of medicine increased, however, the State became involved in funding ever new developments—whether expensive drugs (starting with streptomycin and continuing with the anti-Parkinsonian agents and the preparations used in oncology) or the buildings needed to house new and complex techniques, such as dialysis, imaging, transplantation, and joint replacement.

As a result, medical science had to continually argue for new resources and to produce figures to convince hard-headed bureaucrats that its requirements were cost-effective. An added feature was the formation of lobbying agencies fighting the cause of a particular disease or working as advocates for a group of patients, such as the mentally handicapped. Given a vigorous public debate, governments could then come to decisions based on hard facts and soft emotions. For example, at one time in Britain selection for dialysis was partly dependent on age. Few patients aged over sixty received such treatment, even though they did in other countries. When the existence of such hidden rationing (a virtual death sentence) emerged, and it was shown that older patients had a good prognosis, the government abolished selection on these grounds.

Inevitably, governments also became concerned with prevention, and again scientific data were needed to introduce radical measures, particularly against the arguments of the skeptics who derided the 'nanny' state. In Britain during World War II, war crash helmets were introduced for motorcyclist dispatch riders; neurosurgeons were concerned about the waste of lives and surgical resources and the protection given by helmets was proven. Later wearing front, then rear, seat belts was made compulsory in cars, with many countries also introducing strict limits on blood alcohol levels. The attack on smoking (campaigns both against the habit and restricting it in public places) came only gradually, years after the seminal work in the 1950s—yet, given that the scientific case was strong, the community gradually came to accept the official moves.

Governments also came together in forming international organizations concerned with health, with the potential at least to work beyond national boundaries. The Red Cross (with its later counterparts the Red Crescent and Red Crystal) was formed in 1864, playing an important part in both peace and war, but—given the scant funding and noncooperation of various countries—the health office of the League of Nations started after World War I achieved relatively little. The World Health Organization, formed by the United Nations in 1948, took care to become independent of its parent body, and has had a substantial role in setting up public health services where these did not exist as well as disease control programs, culminating in the abolition of smallpox in 1979. Other United Nations organizations concerned with health include the Food and Agriculture Organization (FAO) and the United Nations Children's Fund (UNICEF).

Pharmaceutical revolution

The third principal gain has been the revolution in the development of new drugs, such as the cheap, safe, and reliable contraceptive pill. For centuries, women's lives had been dogged by unwanted pregnancies, while contraceptive techniques had been unreliable and unesthetic. The revolutionary development of the pill was another example of how first-class Western medicine works in practice. The basic science was followed by persistent lobbying, then animal studies of a preparation, field trials in populations, and monitoring of community use. Two chemists, E. Russell Marker (1902–95) and Carl Djerassi (b. 1923), synthesized sex hormones (estrogen and progesterone) that could be swallowed. A millionairess pioneer of the American birth-control movement, Margaret Sanger (1879–1966), then lobbied an experimental biologist, Gregory Pincus (1903–67), to study these hormones in animals. Field trials in Puerto Rico showed that both hormones were needed for a contraceptive effect, while community monitoring of the combined pill's use showed that cutting the estrogen content stopped it causing thrombosis. The pill is a superb example of the positive medicalization of life. A healthy woman takes the pill in order to control her life (and health) without the risk of repeated (possibly unwanted) pregnancies, thus maintaining health without there being any illness in the first place.

Among the other agents developed from the 1930s the early sulfa drugs and penicillin meant that for the first time cure of the then two principal sexually transmitted diseases—gonorrhea and syphilis—could be guaranteed. In addition to the antibiotics next introduced against tuberculosis and other infections, a prodigious number of new agents were added: hypotensive drugs, reducing the incidence of disabling stroke and myocardial infarction, with the lipid-reducing statins promising to add to their benefits; antimalarials and antischistosomals (effective against bilharzia); antihistamines; steroids; nonexplosive anesthetics; and agents active against gout, diabetes, and leukemia and other forms of cancer. Ever since the thalidomide tragedy of 1961, in which an apparently safe hypnotic given to pregnant women was to cause deformities in some of their children, the media have tended to be avid to publicize the dangers of drugs. Nevertheless, most people now realize that it is a balance of risk versus benefit and that extensive mechanisms have now been put into place to underpin safety as far as possible.

New surgical procedures

Fourth, there have been the new surgical procedures, themselves made possible by developments in anesthesia (including extracorporeal circulation), blood transfusion, and immunology. As a result, prostheses for hip, knee, shoulder, and finger-joint replacement are available. In addition organs that can now be transplanted include the cornea, kidney, liver, heart, pancreas, and face. And one should not forget the increased sophistication of simpler procedures, such as artificial lens replacement for cataract or restorative dentistry.

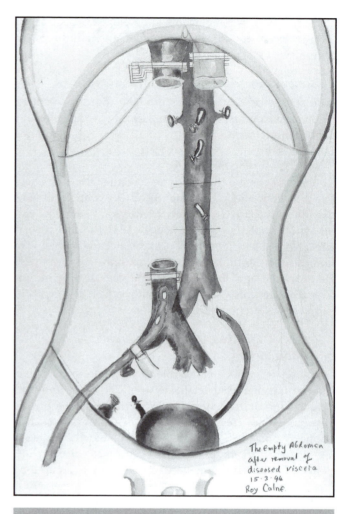

The empty abdomen after removal of diseased viscera during a six-organ transplant (liver, stomach, duodenum, pancreas, ileum, kidneys). Watercolor by the English transplant surgeon, Sir Roy Calne, 1994. Iconographic Collection, Wellcome Library, London.

Failures

Undisputedly, in the development of its science Western medicine has lost some, if not much, of the art. Nowhere is this seen more clearly than in the treatment of mental illness. The older authorities such as Hippocrates saw no difference between mental and physical illness and treated them in the same way. Nevertheless, by Hogarth's time (*The Rake's Progress*, 1735) ordinary lunatics were confined to institutions such as Bedlam, often chained and serving as a spectacle for amused visitors.

Humane treatment of the mentally ill began to return almost simultaneously in France and Britain, with Philippe Pinel (1745–1826) in Paris removing the chains in 1802, and the creation of a few notable institutions such as The Retreat at York (1796). The asylum era has been replaced by the theoretical alternative of community care, which barely exists in practice. Yet mental illness accounts for some 10 percent of all ill health, and, save for the twentieth-century developments of palliative agents for bipolar illness and schizophrenia, little major progress has been made. And the subject does not inspire much sympathy or concern in the general population. Whereas the funding bodies of medical research foundations are bombarded with too many excellent projects to support, they tell of a dearth of applications concerning mental illness. Yet a fundamental breakthrough in the understanding of mental illness, whether prevention or curative treatment, would probably be the most cost-effective discovery that could be made today—certainly since streptomycin and the other drugs emptied the sanatoria of patients with tuberculosis—let alone its revolutionary effects on the sufferers.

The flight from the art of medicine became obvious around the start of the nineteenth century, the French philosopher Michel Foucault (1926–84) argued. Cities such as Paris and Vienna built enormous general hospitals, whose foremost function was to study the features of illness during the patient's life and then its effects on the body after death. The individual behind the patient was forgotten, and what Foucault termed 'the medical gaze' was inaugurated.

Such complaints about the impersonal nature of much of medicine are still heard today, even when the illness itself is cured. Thus alternative medicine, with its perceived 'humanity', has become increasingly popular, with the employment of practitioners such as chiropractors, homeopaths, aroma therapists, and rebirthers. Nevertheless, probably many people assess their own complaints and then choose which type of treatment they will purchase.

Another loser has been the developing world. In the wake of decolonialization, pharmaceutical companies in the developed world have been reluctant to develop new drugs specifically for 'tropical' diseases, unless provided with financial incentives. And there is the high cost of existing agents, highlighted by the emergence of HIV infection/AIDS as a major epidemic in Asia and Africa. Most countries cannot afford the drugs that in the affluent West suppress the process and prolong life. Fortunately, some enlightened philanthropic organizations, such as the Gates Foundation, are attempting to address the problem, and are also encouraging research into other major killers, particularly malaria.

Western medicine has also had a deleterious effect on the developing world, though local practitioners often resent this view. These countries have been tempted to reproduce the complex procedures used in the West (such as heart transplantation), which benefit only the solitary individual who is able to pay. The preferable alternative is to provide general medical care to the community and to lobby for the simple, cheap, and effective methods of improving health in the developing world: piped water supplies, education of women, efficient contraception, and condom use against HIV. Given that many qualified practitioners desert the countryside for the towns, or migrate to the developed world, a large proportion of the population there is denied the help it needs.

A TRIUMPH OF SCIENCE

Ever since Professor Herbert Butterfield warned against 'Whiggish' interpretations of history (1931), writers have been cautious about evaluating the past in the light of the present and claiming that things are better now than they were. Nevertheless, Western medicine has been a conspicuous success, particularly once it based itself squarely on science. Such an evolution has been continual since the Scientific Revolution and is certainly ongoing today, though many details of past work have been forgotten or subsumed in new thinking. In Claude Bernard's words, 'The names of promoters of science disappear little by little, and the further science advances, the more it takes an impersonal form and detaches itself from the past' (Bernard, 1865, English trans. 1957, p. 42).

As in other forms of science, developments in medicine have almost always been based on previous work or ideas. Philosopher of science Thomas Kuhn (1922–96) saw the progression of a topic as occurring in four phases: vagueness, discovery, breakthrough, and consolidation. He also distinguished two types of science: normal and revolutionary. The first type was adding small units of information to what was known already—bricks to the partially built house. Revolutionary science, on the other hand, was much rarer, and involved a 'paradigm shift'—a total change in the community's attitude to a concept. For medicine, this occurred with the discoveries of the circulation of the blood, the structure of DNA, or retroviruses (such as HIV). Nevertheless, even revolutionary science is based on previous thought and work—as witness, for example, the ideas before Harvey, which led to his apparently novel conclusions. There has also been a role for serendipity, as when Edward Jenner in 1796 realized that the milkmaid's harmless cowpox could be harnessed for protective vaccination against smallpox, medicalizing the folk preventive, or William Withering in 1785 recognizing that a crone's self-treatment with foxglove extract could be adopted as digitalis for heart failure. As Louis Pasteur pointed out, 'Chance favors the prepared mind.' The evolution of advances in medicine, then, shares many features with other scientific disciplines.

Nevertheless, weighing all of the above, I would argue that Western medicine emerges as a triumph of science, firmly separating it from the earlier traditions shared with the medicine of other cultures. Think merely of the total abolition of smallpox (1979), with polio and measles potentially next. Western medicine today is very different from what it was yesterday, showing at last all of the characteristics that the sociologist Robert Merton (1910–2003) ascribed to science: universalism, organized skepticism,

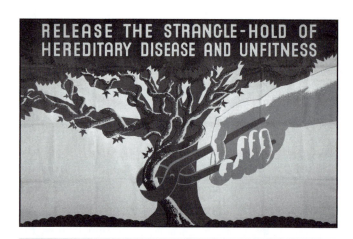

RELEASE THE STRANGLE-HOLD OF
HEREDITARY DISEASE AND UNFITNESS

A parasitic plant, representing hereditary unfitness, is severed near the root to allow the healthy growth of a tree. Eugenics society poster, 1920s. Archives and Manuscripts, Wellcome Library, London. Copyright The Galton Institute, London. Reproduced with permission.

communality, humility, and disinterestedness. In particular, the concern now is as much with the health of populations as of the individual, as the continuing improvement of immunization, the fluoridation of water, and the management of potential serious epidemics (BSE, SARS, avian flu) all show.

Few advances today are made by individuals, and the team contains a variety of disciplines, such as statisticians, sociologists, and methodologists. In medical care, the group has a similarly important role, with the 'greater health profession' achieving parity with the medically qualified. And medicine has become democratized, with patients being told of their diagnosis in simple language and asked to participate in choosing their treatment. Finally, a continuous debate goes on in the media about all aspects of health and disease.

Another important aspect has been that, just as William Harvey discarded Galenism but retained Aristotelianism, so subsequent scientists have shown a canny tendency to cherry-pick. For example, starting with Charles Darwin and Francis Galton (1822–1911), eugenics became a widespread enthusiasm and achieved more than theoretical importance: countries such as the United States, Norway, Sweden, and Denmark all sterilized many people with mental handicap or other conditions. With the horrors of the extreme position taken by the Nazis, however, the concept quietly disappeared from the public domain into the history books. Yet its essence survives in contemporary genetics, whether in counseling or the operative procedures to ensure that embryos are unaffected by an inherited condition.

Modern medicine has continued the tradition of self-experimentation, the sixteenth-century study by Santorio Santorio (1561–1636) on his own metabolism being mir-

rored in the twentieth century by Werner Forssman (1904–79), who passed a catheter into his own heart (1929), or Barry Marshall (b. 1951), who swallowed a culture of *Heliobacter pylori* to prove that these organisms were the cause of gastric ulcer rather than the then-blamed stress or irregular meals (1984). Allied to this is a new concept: the 'courage to fail'. Early attempts at seemingly impossible procedures, such as open-heart surgery, kidney transplantation, or curing childhood leukemia, all produced disastrous results. Yet, encouraged by the results of prolonged animal research as well as the dismaying prognosis of the untreated condition, the pioneers pressed ahead until success made their methods almost routine.

Here the skeptics have to be refuted. Skepticism about medicine has a long history, from Molière through Pierre Louis and George Bernard Shaw to the Jesuit contemporary Ivan Illich (1926–2002). Merton's 'organized skepticism' came to the fore in the debate in the 1970s started by Birmingham professor of social medicine Thomas McKeown (1912–88). He argued that improvements in health or longevity had little to do with developments in modern medicine. For example, the death rate from tuberculosis had started a continual decline 100 years before the discovery of the first curative agent, streptomycin. And, again, the declining death rate from childhood fevers, such as diphtheria, owed more to rising living standards than to immunization or antibiotics.

Nevertheless, whatever the rigor of some of his arguments, few other experts would go very far with McKeown's thesis. Take, for example, the enormous reductions in British death rates for some common infections for which immunization was introduced: diphtheria, measles, and pertussis. In 1900 these were, respectively, 40, 13, and 12; by the 1960s, they had fallen to 0, 2, and 1 (per 100,000). Another good indicator, the British maternal mortality rate (deaths per given number of births)—which crucially depends on professional competence—was 50.9 per 10,000 births in 1882, 24.7 in 1942, and 1.0, in 1981. If ever there was an argument for specialization, this dramatic reduction shows its effects.

McKeown had also ignored the contribution of scientific medicine to care as much as cure. And perhaps the whole case for the success of Western medicine is not just macrocosmic—large populations having healthy lives into their 70s—but its microcosmic role in the individual when things go wrong. As three U.S. medical academics wrote in the 1990s, 'A person who has not experienced a handicap or limitation of activity that hampers someone else may underestimate its importance to the affected person. But the miseries of depression, shortness of breath, angina, creaky and painful joints, severe pain, disabling headaches, major indigestion, urinary difficulties, toothache and sore gums, fuzzy vision, faulty hearing, paralysis and broken bones would add up to a national disaster without the relief we are able to document' (Loudon, 1997, p. 144).

Whatever its defects, then, few of us would choose to be without the benefits of Western medical science. Perhaps the best words on its success were spoken, almost sixty years ago, by the founder of the British National Health Service, the politician Aneurin Bevan (1897–1960): 'I would rather be kept alive in the efficient if cold altruism of a large hospital than expire in a gush of warm sympathy in a small one' (speech in the House of Commons, 30 April 1946).

Bibliography

Bernard, Claude, 1865. *An Introduction to the Study of Experimental Medicine* (English trans. Greene, H. C., 1957, New York); Blakemore, Colin, and Shelia Jennett, eds., 2001. *The Oxford Companion to the Body* (Oxford); Bynum, W. F., 1994. *Science and the Practice of Medicine in the Nineteenth Century* (Cambridge); Bynum, W. F., Anne Hardy, S. J. Jacyna, Christopher Lawrence, and E. M. Tansey, 2006. *The Western Medical Tradition 1800–2000* (Cambridge); Bynum, W. F., and Roy Porter, eds., 1993. *Companion Encyclopedia of the History of Medicine* 2 vols. (London); Conrad, Lawrence I., Michael Neve, Vivian Nutton, Roy Porter, and Andrew Wear, 1995. *The Western Medical Tradition 800 BC to AD 1800* (Cambridge); Cooter, Roger, and John Pickstone, eds., 2002. *Medicine in the Twentieth Century* (Amsterdam); Crosby, Alfred W., 1986. *Ecological Imperialism: The Biological Expansion of Europe, 900–1900* (New York); Diamond, Jared, 1997. *Guns, Germs and Steel: A Short History of Everybody for the Past 13,000 Years* (London); Duffin, Jacalyn, 1999. *History of Medicine: A Scandalously Short Introduction* (Toronto); Kiple, Kenneth F., ed., 1993. *The Cambridge World History of Human Disease* (Cambridge); Lock, Stephen, John M. Last, and George Dunea, eds., 2001. *The Oxford Illustrated Companion to Medicine* (Oxford); Loudon, Irvine, ed., 1997. *Western Medicine: An Illustrated History* (Oxford); McKeown, Thomas, 1988. *The Origins of Human Disease* (Oxford); McNeill, William H., 1977. *Plagues and Peoples* (Oxford); Nutton, Vivian, 2004. *Ancient Medicine* (London); Porter, Roy, 1997. *The Greatest Benefit to Mankind: A Medical History of Humanity from Antiquity to the Present* (London); Risse, Guenter, 1999. *Mending Bodies, Saving Souls: A History of Hospitals* (Oxford, New York); Temkin, Owsei, 1977. *The Double Face of Janus and Other Essays in the History of Medicine* (Baltimore); Wangensteen, Owen H., and Sarah D. Wangensteen, 1978. *The Rise of Surgery: From Empiric Craft to Scientific Discipline* (Minneapolis, Folkestone); Weatherall, David, 1995. *Science and the Quiet Art: Medical Research and Patient Care* (Oxford).

Stephen Lock

THE ISLAMIC MEDICAL TRADITION

Islam is a monotheistic religion that arose in the seventh century CE. It is characterized by acceptance of the doctrine of submission to God and to Muḥammad as the last Prophet of the one and only God. Starting from the seventh century, the so-called Islamic world expanded rapidly. Nowadays it counts approximately 1.5 billion people, who live in both hemispheres: on the Arab peninsula, in Africa, South Asia, Europe, Southeast Asia, and the Americas. The present article deals with the development of the Islamic medical tradition in the Arab Near East and neighboring countries: Iran, Central Asia, and Turkey.

In the medieval period, the Arabs developed a medical tradition that is ranked among the most important in the Eastern and in the contemporary Western world. It significantly influenced modern medicine and the medical sciences in various aspects, ranging from explaining many important medical phenomena, such as the pulmonary blood circulation, to systematizing the medical botanical terminology and introducing some surgical instruments. This tradition originated partly from the pre-Islamic beliefs and healing practices of the indigenous population of the Arab peninsula. It was also enriched, during the Arab conquests of the eighth and ninth centuries, by the medical knowledge of the population of the conquered countries, such as Byzantium and Sasanid Iran, which was often far superior to that of the nomadic Arabs. The Arabic language played a crucial role in the subsequent development of the

Islamic medical tradition. Because the language in which the last Revelation, the Holy Koran, was sent to the Prophet Muḥammad, it was considered as the religious language for all the Muslims. In such capacity it became widely learned and known, the lingua franca for the whole 'Islamic world'. Very quickly Arabic became the language of the sciences and arts, spoken from the Chinese border to the Spanish cities. In many ways, Arabic influenced the vocabulary of the languages of the conquered people, and in a number of instances, the indigenous languages; e.g., Syriac and Coptic were irrevocably abandoned in favor of Arabic, which became in the East what Latin represented in the West. As a specialist 'medical' language, Arabic has been successfully employed over centuries and is widely used today.

THE RISE OF ISLAMIC MEDICINE

To describe medicine and medical practice the Arabs traditionally use the root *ṬBB*. In the pre-Islamic and early Islamic periods, this root and its derivatives referred more to esoteric matters rather than to medical treatment. Therefore, the word *maṬBuB* ('healed') means that someone was afflicted by a spell rather than the recipient of medical care. Equally, the word *ṬaBiB* meant not a medical doctor, but a purveyor of incantations, spells, and other 'religious' services. This is not surprising, since magical medicine among the pre-Islamic Arabs was considered a specialization. Later, with the advent of Islam, the magical approach to medicine was reflected in the role of Islamic scripture, i.e., the Holy Koran. People were quick to conclude that, as God's word, the Koran must possess powers that could be used in magical chants and incantations or in various 'compound medicines'. Such medicines, which might use water with a piece of Koranic text in it for curing various diseases or be applied as an analgesic during labor, were widespread even at the beginning of the twentieth century in the Ottoman Empire (present-day Lebanon). A little-known twentieth-century author, Bishara as-Ṣaiqali, in his work called 'Selections from the Writings of the Ancient Doctors' provided a wide range of such 'remedies'.

The use of the Holy Koran as a component of magical medicine, however, was not universally approved. Many Muslims opposed both the use of the Koran for charms and the trend of presenting the Prophet Muḥammad as a purveyor of such remedies. In the early centuries of Islam, this opposition caused active medical discussions, which partly sought to understand many pre-Islamic Bedouin medical practices from the Islamic point of view. The Islamic critics did not target medicine; moreover, medical practice as such was considered to be reputable. Rather they aimed to curb certain beliefs that were considered repugnant to religious sensibilities. The outcomes of these discussions varied. Although the boundaries of medicine as both science and practice were not identified, some practices contradictory to the Koran disappeared, while others—as well as the beliefs connected to them—remained. Talismans for protection against disease, for example, continued to be widely recommended: books on magic were transcribed even in the mid-twentieth century. Likewise, the *jinn*, a malicious spirit created from a smokeless flame, never ceased to figure as a cause for diseases. Despite the acceptance of humoral medicine, based upon the teachings of Hippocrates and Galen, the pluralistic framework of Islamic medicine continued as one of its most characteristic features.

In describing the Islamic medical tradition, modern scholars stress the fact that during the early centuries of Islam a number of factors contributed to the revival of the humoral medicine. First, an educated elite with broad interests and financial resources, capable of funding scholarship and collecting books, developed and subsequently grew. Second, religious concerns, which could be addressed from the point of view of human health, disease, and healing, represented issues to which the medical works could contribute significantly. Third, the existence of a literary corpus in languages other than Arabic served as a focus for scholarly work.

AN EXERCISE IN TRANSLATION

The first phase of the Islamic medical tradition focused on translations of classical medical and scientific texts from Greek, Syriac, and Pahlavi into Arabic. This major translation movement began in the reign of the caliph Hārūn ar-Rashīd (r. 786–809) and achieved its heyday during the reign of his son and successor, caliph al-Ma'mūn (r. 813–833). Al-Ma'mūn, a learned and educated man, was confronted with the unavoidable task of uniting and consolidating his authority over a vast empire that was suffering from civil wars, autonomist tendencies in various provinces, controversies over influences on nascent Islamic culture, and sociopolitical problems focusing on fiscal policy and the legitimate sphere of imperial authority. It was against this background that caliph al-Ma'mūn took up the cause of *al-Mu'tazila,* an expanding circle of speculative theologians seeking to articulate Islamic doctrine in a systematic fashion on rationalist foundations. In Baghdad at the end of his reign in 832, an institution called *Bayt al-Ḥikma* (usually translated 'House of Wisdom' or, more correctly, the 'House of the Right Decision') was established. Here scholars supervised by the members of Munajjim family worked to collect and to translate into Arabic a broad range of non-Arabic and non-Islamic works, which could contribute to the tasks set by the regime. Christians dominated the translation work, by virtue of their knowledge of Greek and Syriac as languages, which they used for their worship.

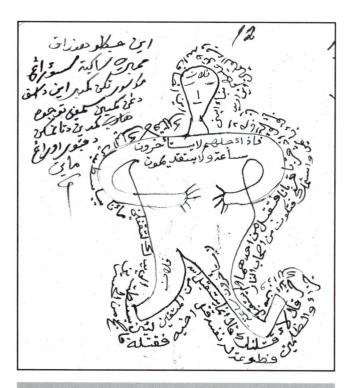

Malayan black magic charm intended to curse its recipient with a fatal illness. Surrounding the human figure are incantations and spells in Arabic, written in the language of Djinns and Syaitan (demonic spirits). Ink on paper, nineteenth century. Wellcome Malayan MS 2, Wellcome Library, London.

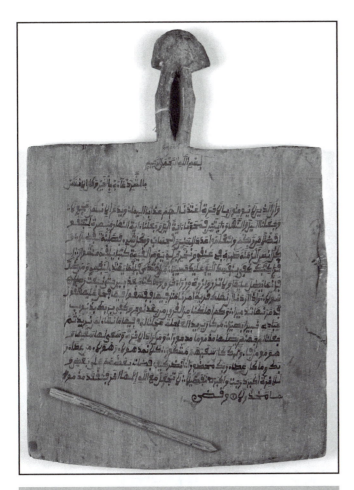

Sudanese wooden talisman and pen. Inscriptions are verses from the Koran. Ink on wood, early twentieth century. Wellcome Library, London.

Page from *Al-A `da' al-alima* [Pain in the Limbs], an Arabic translation of a work by Galen, eighteenth century. Wellcome Arabic MS 402, folio 67B, Wellcome Library, London.

The most important figure in the translation movement was Ḥunayn ibn Ishāq (known in the Latin West as Johannitius, 809–73), a Nestorian Christian, who, according to some accounts, traveled widely, collected Greek and Syriac manuscripts, built up a team of translators, and laid down the linguistic foundation of translations from Greek into Arabic. Ḥunayn's efforts helped to shape a new, precise, professional terminology, which was essential for the further development of the medical sciences. The output of this translation movement was vast. Hundreds of texts on various aspects of science in Greek, Syriac, and Pahlavi were translated into Arabic. A translation from the Greek and Syriac of the *corpus Galenicum* towered over the works rendered into the language of the Prophet Muḥammad.

This movement saved for posterity many Greek texts that otherwise could have been lost, shaped the Arabic medical literature for centuries to come, and provided an impetus for revival of the Greek humoral medicine in an Islamic context. The invention and frequent use of paper (the first paper mill was constructed in Baghdad around the year 800 by Ḥarun ar-Rashīd) contributed enormously to the development of the translation movement and dissemination of knowledge, as did the application of the diacritical dots to the 'cursive' Arabic script. Arabic written without diacritics was like a score in music: it was not possible to read the text without knowing beforehand what this text was about, since many letters were written similarly. After the dots were introduced, it became possible to distinguish between separate letters, i.e., to read the previously unknown text.

RESEARCH AND FURTHER WRITING

From the tenth century onward, the literary medical output of the Islamic authors changed. By the late ninth century, Islamic medical practitioners and researchers faced a completely new situation. They had received access to the bulk of the world's best medical writings translated into Arabic. The availability of texts, with their newly shaped professional medical terminology, had became an instrument that made possible original medical research. This research went on for several hundred years and resulted in thousands of monographs on various topics. Among the early writings contributing to the rise of medical research, modern historians of the Arabic Islamic medical tradition have singled out a treatise: 'On smallpox and measles' by al-Rāzī (known in the Latin West as Rhazes, 865-925/932), who dealt with questions of pathology, diagnosis, therapeutics, and *materia medica*. Rhazes gave an accurate description of these diseases, and for measles he proved that its specificity was appropriate to a certain age.

The quantity of the newly produced medical works rapidly increased and necessitated the need for a more synthetic and systematized writing. This gave rise to one of the most important literary achievements in the field of the Arabic science: the medical compendium. This style of medical work also proved to be important for mastering the special material it contained. Even the Arabic script with diacritics was not convenient for scholarly writing: in rendering of a number of letters, it used additional diacritic dots,

Title page from Avicenna/Ibn Sīnā, Ab 'Ali al-Ḥusayn b. abd Allāh b. Sīnā, *Arabum medicorum principis...* Venice, 1595. Rare Books, Wellcome Library, London.

which if omitted by negligence or ignorance could completely change the meaning of the written text. The famous polymath Abū Rayhān al-Bīrūnī (973–1048/1050) noted and stressed this inconvenience as early as the tenth century. In order to avoid misinterpretation, the students learned the scholarly texts by heart. Usually the medical compendia contained only essential information, which made committing it to memory easier. To further facilitate this process, the compendia's text was shortened and frequently rhymed. Among the most widely known compendia are those by al-Rāzī, al-Mājūsī (known in the Latin West as Haly Abbas, d. *c.* 994), and Ibn Sīnā (known in the Latin West as Avicenna, 980–1037). All these works were swiftly translated into Latin—Rhazes' as *Liber nonus ad Almansorem*, Haly Abbas's as *Liber totius medicine necessaria continens quem sapientissimus . . .*, and Avicenna's as *Arabum medicorum principis / Avicennae* [Canon of Medicine]. These compendia served as medical textbooks until the seventeenth century.

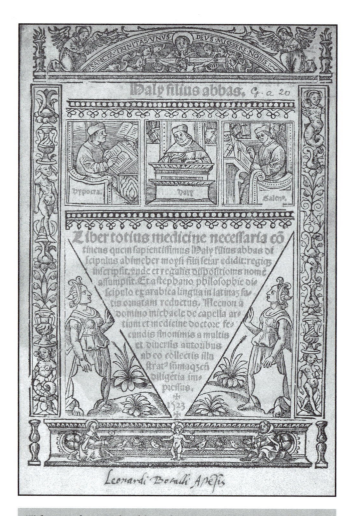

Title page from Haly Abbas/al-Mājāūsī, 'Alī b. al-'Abbās, *Liber totius medicine necessaria . . .* Lyons, 1523. Rare Books, Wellcome Library, London.

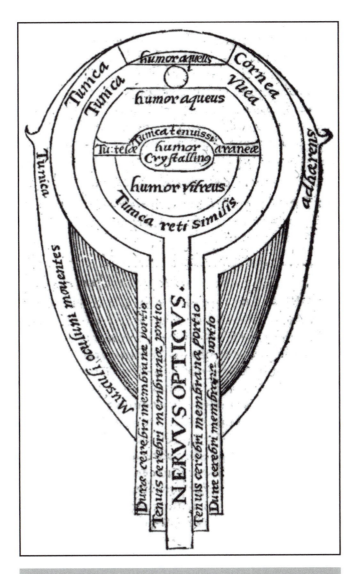

Schematic diagram of the eye showing all the anatomical layers (tunics). Woodcut from Alhazen/Ibn al-Haytham Abū 'Ali al-Ḥasan Ibn al-Ḥasan al-Basrī al-Miārī, *Opticae thesaurus Alhazeni Arabis . . .* Basel, 1572. Rare Books, Wellcome Library, London.

Islamic authors' accumulation and strict systematization of medical knowledge had an important impact on its further development. Because it occasionally helped to show discrepancies found in the writings of the Ancients, Islamic doctors did not consider the Greek authors to be infallible authorities. They were not shy to express doubts about various aspects of their teachings and sometimes collected these doubts in books, such as the 'Doubts about Galen's views', written by al-Rāzī.

PRACTICE INFORMS THE TEXTS

Constant medical practice combined with observations added to the further development of medical knowledge. In

ophthalmology, scholars from Ḥunayn ibn Ishāq to Ibn al-Haytham (known in the Latin West as Alhazen, 965–1039/1041) widened the information on the anatomy of the eye and more generally developed the science of optics. Knowledge of medical botany was enriched by the travels and efforts of the botanists, such as Ibn al-Bayṭār (*c.* 1197–1248). In surgery, new procedures were described in ophthalmology; serious abdominal injuries, previously thought to be fatal, were successfully tackled; and use of animal gut as a suturing material was suggested. Cataract surgery was particularly significant. New or improved designs for medical instruments were introduced, among them scissors, trocars, syringes, lithotrites, and obstetric forceps. A further development occurred in medical illustration, especially with regard to the *Tashrih-i Manṣūrī* (the 'Mansurian Anatomy'), written by Ibn Ilyās in 1396. This work provides full-body illustrations showing the layout of a skeleton, nerves, muscles, veins, and arteries. This was a significant step forward, as medieval surgery possessed rather rudimentary knowledge of the internal systems of the human body.

One area where the achievements of the Islamic medical tradition are still little appreciated is that of contagion. Before the early modern period, the epidemiological distinctions between infection and contagion were not established. The Galenic tradition almost entirely ignored its existence. In early Islamic times, the notion became a focus of religious controversy: Could there be a mode of disease causation that allowed sickness to spread from one person to the next regardless of their level of virtue in a worldview dominated by an all-powerful God? It was argued that, without God, there could be nothing, not even contagion, and this would not be spread indiscriminately. Yet the evidence of leprosy and mange among camels seemed to contradict the absence of contagion. The dispute over a reliance on older, pre-Islamic ideas, which also included such ideas as the interpretation of bird behavior as a means of telling the future, and a specific reading of passages in the Koran may well have driven physicians such as Ibn Qutayba (d. 889) to defense of contagion.

Of equal importance to the achievements of the Greco-Roman medicine was the development of the so-called Prophetic Medicine (*Ṭibb an-nabī*). The collections of *hadīth* (traditions relating to the words and deeds of the Prophet Muḥammad) were used in debates over important issues, including medicine. It was noticed that humoral medicine would sometimes prescribe a drug that would violate Islamic law, for example animal bile or alcohol. The question in such an instance would be 'Does the prohibition apply to someone whom the substance might cure?' Such questions would recall identical or analogous situations with which the Prophet or one of his companions had allegedly dealt. Prophetic Medicine also dealt with important issues concerned with the beginning of life. It would be wrong to consider this type of medicine in opposition to the Greco-Roman humoral teachings. It simply reflects the

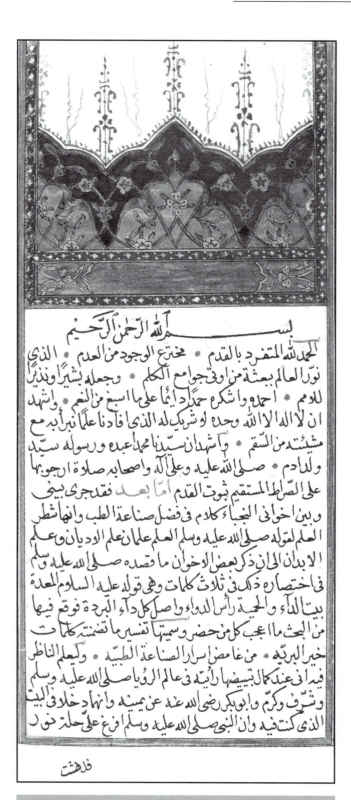

Illuminated page from Abū 'Abd Allah Muḥammad as-Sanūsī, *Tafsīr ma tadammanathu Kalimat Hayr Gal-bariyyat min Ğamid Asrar as-Sina 'at at-Tibbiya* [Commentary on what the Sayings of the Best of Creation contain about the Depth of the Secrets of the Art of Medicine], nineteenth century. Wellcome Arabic MS 446, folio 1B, Wellcome Library, London.

ongoing interest in medical issues among a religiously educated public familiar with the medical chapters and traditions in the early *hadīth* collections who were combining humoral medical axioms, aphorisms, etc. with popular folklore or common-sense traditions. Bishara as-Ṣaiqali, for instance, collected passages from the *hadīth* collections and a series of 'prescriptions' about healing by using the New Testament and the Book of Psalms along with advice based on the teaching of humoral medicine of the Ancients.

MEDICAL EDUCATION

The qualification and level of services of Islamic medical practitioners greatly varied. In the early centuries Jews, Christians, and other non-Muslims dominated the profession, chiefly because of the long tradition of medical learning within the ecclesiastical hierarchy. Many leading clerics in the towns were physicians; medical help was also administered in monasteries. Even in the thirteenth century, the figure of the Christian doctor was widely respected. The senior Syrian Jacobite cleric, the *maphrian* Gregory Bar Hebraeus (known in Arabic as Abū al-Faraj, 1226–86), although a prolific writer and historian, was considered by his contemporaries to be a great astronomer and a skillful doctor. His death was mourned by Muslims and Christians of various denominations.

The example of Gregory Bar Hebraeus—an ecclesiastical authority, a philosopher, and a medical practitioner—shows that in the medieval Islamic period the criteria for being a member of the medical profession were relatively weak. Many doctors were universally educated and along with medicine excelled in philosophy, mathematics, astronomy, and other disciplines. Maimonides (Rabbi Moses ben Maimon, or Rambam, 1135–1204), Ibn Rushd (known in the Latin West as Averroes, 1126–98), and Ibn Sīnā considered themselves to be philosophers rather than physicians. According to Ibn Sīnā, learning medicine was 'not difficult at all', and sufficient knowledge could be acquired merely by a course of self-education. This point of view was advocated by another famous autodidact, the eleventh-century medical practitioner 'Alī ibn Riḍwān from Cairo. In other cases, medical knowledge was acquired by training in a barber shop or with another doctor. Such practices continued: the famous French doctor Antoine Barthélémy (better known as Clot Bey, 1793–1866) received his first medical training under his father's comrade, a retired army surgeon. In many cases, the medical profession was considered as a hereditary skill, and the specialist knowledge was frequently transmitted from father to son.

The venues for medical training varied greatly. The most popular sites were teachers' own homes. Mosques—general sites of textual learning—also provided a place and resources for learning medicine, especially as the *madrasas* developed. Once hospitals were widespread, they were logical

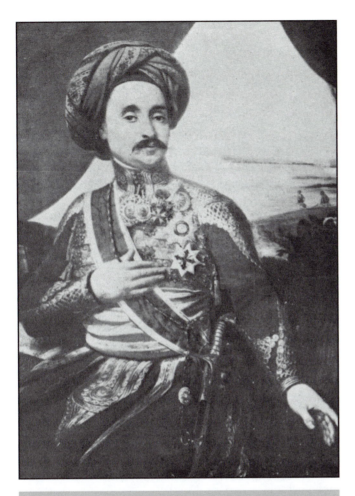

Clot Bey. Halftone reproduction from Naguib Bey Mahfouz, *The History of Medical Education in Egypt*, Cairo, 1935. Wellcome Library, London.

venues for medical education: patients were available and many hospitals had libraries of medical books. Teaching methods varied considerably, but it is clear that medical education concentrated on written texts. Many students must have entered medical practice without even having treated a patient. Mistakes made by ignorant physicians were portrayed by the eleventh-century author Abū 'Alā Sa'id b. al-Ḥasan, who showed that students of medicine were often unaware not only of the medical terminology, but also of the main symptoms of diseases. Ibn Abī Uṣaibi'a, the author of a lengthy manual of medical biographies, mentioned a remarkable incident related by Thābit b. Sinān, the son of the famous physician Sinān ibn Thābit ibn Qurra (d. 942). In 931, when the caliph of Baghdad learned that somebody had died at the hands of an incompetent doctor, he ordered that the authority to practice in Baghdad could be granted only to those whom Sinān had examined. About 860 candidates applied during the first year. Among them was an elderly gentleman, who confessed that he did not possess any training in medicine and could hardly read or write, but pleaded with Sinān not to

deprive his family of their livelihood by denying him permission to practice medicine. Sinān agreed, under the condition that he would only prescribe ordinary medications and treat simple maladies. The next day the man's son appeared before Sinān and was also authorized to practice on similar conditions. Such examinations were, however, rare; more frequently the doctors who wished to practice in the market place were examined ad hoc by the market inspector, the *mukhtasib*, who for these purposes used a special manual with questions about various aspects of medicine, the answers to which the applicant was supposed to know.

Access to physicians varied. Often doctors received their patients in their homes and people had to queue in front of their doors. Wealthy patients could afford a doctor's visit, and some doctors even stayed in their patients' houses until they were properly cured. An examination of a patient included palpation of the body parts, questioning of the patient, and scrutiny of the pulse and urine. It was thought advisable to seek a second or a third opinion. Payment was made upon conclusion of the treatment, and fees varied widely. If the patient died, his family could institute proceedings against the doctor if they felt that he had committed serious mistakes. Popular knowledge of medicine in medieval Islam was rather high: a tenth-century author, the Christian Ibn Buṭlān (d. 1066) from Baghdad, wrote a manual on buying slaves. Obviously based on a common medical knowledge, shared with his readers, he provided a list of typical symptoms that a buyer should look out for in order to prevent an unscrupulous vendor from trying to sell an ill or pregnant slave.

HOSPITALS

The hospital was a crowning achievement of Islamic medical practice. In Arabic it was called *bīmāristān* from the Persian, and in later Arabic works it was occasionally confused with the word *mānāstīr* (monastery). The Arabs traced the origin of this institution to Hippocrates, who is said to have made a *xenodocheion*, i.e., a 'lodging for strangers' for the sick in a garden near his house. Hospitals, however, were not a feature of life in classical antiquity. The foundation of the first Islamic hospital is attributed to the caliph Walīd I (r. 705-715) in Damascus. According to other evidence the first was founded in Baghdad by Jibra'il ibn Bakhtishu' on the orders of Hārūn ar-Rashīd (r. 786–809). By the twelfth century, the hospital had become an essential feature of large Islamic towns.

Establishing a hospital was an act of personal charity, usually connected with setting aside the revenues from specified properties as a religious trust (*waqf*). Hospitals were complex institutions with facilities for women, inpatients, and outpatients. Designated wards served for different procedures and categories of patients, e.g., the mentally ill. The patients were treated in the hospitals free of charge;

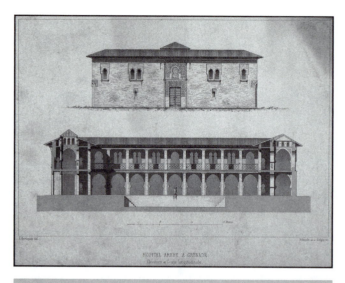

The Arab Hospital, Granada, Spain. Steel engraving by Ribault and J. J. Sulpis after Francisco Enriquez, c. 1750. Iconographic Collection, Wellcome Library, London.

in some cases, provision was made for poor inmates to receive their care, lodging, and board without any payment. The hospitals were sites of learning and often the responsibility of eminent specialists. Thus al-Rāzī is frequently mentioned in connection with the hospital founded by 'Adūd ad-Dawla, which was opened in 982, shortly before the latter's death. It is said that al-Rāzī chose the site by causing a piece of meat to be suspended in every part of the city to discover where there was least putrefaction, and also that 'Adūd ad-Dawla selected him from more than a hundred doctors as first director. However, this is an anachronism, since al-Rāzī had died fifty years earlier, as has been already noted by the medieval historians. The explanation for the anachronism may be the similarity in the script of the *Bimaristan* al-Adudi founded in al-Rāzī's lifetime.

Islamic hospitals, however, should not be regarded as having played the leading role in health care in medieval Islam, because their effective function was the demonstration and promotion of ideas of charity. This becomes clear when one compares traditional Islamic hospitals, the concept of which was exported to medieval Europe, with the first hospital on the Western model founded in Egypt by Clot Bey in the nineteenth century. This hospital, the first aimed to combat severe health problems in the Egyptian army, returned an institution based on a very different concept to its homeland.

MEDICAL BIOGRAPHY IN THE ISLAMIC MEDICAL TRADITION

Individuals played key roles in the Islamic medical tradition, as in everywhere else in the world. However, the history of Islamic medicine to a major extent deals with people and their relationships, i.e., doctors and patients and their reciprocal contacts rather than with the medical inventions. Islamic medical biography was very rarely a subject of separate scholarly study. Partly this was due to linguistic issues: in classical Arabic the word 'biography' as a direct equivalent to the Greek *biographia* does not exist. Usually *biographia* was translated periphrastically as *ta'rīkh hayat* (history of life) or *sīrat hayat* (events of life). The meaning of the Greek word *bios* as 'mode of life', 'sequence of events of a human life' lacks any direct equivalent in Arabic. This fact was obviously well understood by the Arabs themselves: in referring to the *bios* (*vita*) of Christian saints they did not translate the Greek word into Arabic, but simply transliterated it: *bīyūs*.

These linguistic and cultural differences mean that where a 'European mind' referred to a 'biography' as a literary genre, the classical 'Arabic mind' referred to a number of partly overlapping genres, such as *manāqib*, *akhbār*, *faḍā'il*, *mafakhir*, *tarjama*, *ta'rīkh*, and *sira*. Each genre dealt with some different aspect of an individual's life. For biographical descriptions in a broader context, classical Arabic used such terms as *sira* (account of life), *tarjama*, or *ta'rīf*. Other terms were used more specifically. Thus *manāqib* was used predominantly for character traits; *ta'rīkh* meant a listing of death dates; *akhbār* tended to be applied to collections of historical traditions concerning individuals of ethnic or social groups; *faḍā'il* were confined to virtues; *mafakhir* were restricted to the exploits, and *akhlāq* to an innate disposition, or what could also be called 'ethics'. These terms were used in various contexts and could therefore relate to both history and biography.

However, 'biographies' of illustrious people, composed in the various genres mentioned above, occupy a very significant place in classical Arabic literature. The origins of this style of Arabic (Islamic) biography are vague. Some modern researchers suggest that the biographical 'proto-genre' originated from the *hadīth* (a narration about episodes of the Prophet Muḥammad's life). Others attribute its origin to the *akhbār*, where historical information was often conveyed in a narrative.

As early as the eighth century, however, 'biography' developed into an integral part of the classical Arabic literary process and became tightly connected with a so-called group identity. Using the 'division-by-labor' model, or *ṭā'ifa* (a collective, a group entrusted with an exclusive body of knowledge or characteristic activity), biographies were collected and classified by profession, e.g., caliphs, religious practitioners, Koran-readers. The *ṭā'ifa* model became the most productive form for collective biography. The longest catalogue of *ṭā'ifas* is probably given by adh-Dhahabī (d. 1348), who lists forty categories of persons about whom biographies have been written. They range from prophets and kings to lovers, lunatics, and gamblers. His younger contemporary as-Safadī (d. 1362) lists fifteen: Companions of the Prophet, *hadīth*-scholars, caliphs, kings, officials, judges, Koran-readers, scholars, poets, preachers, physicians, astronomers, grammarians, theologians, litterateurs. Modern scholarship shows that *ṭā'ifa* could be an actual occupational group (e.g., judges or inheritance-calculators) as well as an abstract category of 'biographical' subjects (prophets). Like members of a lineage, the members of each *ṭā'ifa* had their single ancestor, the first person to gain the knowledge or to perform the characteristic activity of the group. The *ṭā'ifas*, however, were not stable, and various compilers of biographies listed their representatives differently. For example, Yaqūt al-Ḥamawī (d. 1282) collected under the title al-udaba' (i.e., 'people of culture') biographies of grammarians, lexicologists, genealogists, famous Koran-readers, chroniclers, historians, well-known stationers and scribes, epistolographers, eponymous calligraphers, and others.

Arabic (Islamic) medical biography is scattered among several genres: *tabaqat* (classes), *ta'rīkh* (dates of deaths), and *manāqib* (character traits, virtues). The lives of medical practitioners appear relatively frequently in biographical dictionaries that deal with a very broad range of intellectuals. This is a result of the traditional Arabic attitude to the doctors who were generally considered not as physicians *par excellence*, but as wise men, or *hukamā'* (cf. singular *hakīm*, which denotes a physician and a philosopher), who excelled in other arts besides medicine, e.g. mathematics, philosophy, astronomy, or *adab* (culture—i.e., literature). Therefore, the actual number of classical Arabic works that directly deal with the medical biographies is limited (see Table 1).

The authors Ibn Juljul (*Tabaqāt al-aṭibbā' wa-l-ḥukamā'*) and Ibn Abī 'Uṣaibi'a (*Kitāb 'uyūn al-anbā' fī tabaqāt al-aṭibbā'*) dealt almost exclusively with biographies of medical practitioners. Their titles contain the word *tabaqāt*, i.e., 'classes', which reflects the *ṭā'ifa* principle of arranging material. These classes include the 'ancestors' of the whole profession; i.e., the first class deals with the Hermes Trismegistos (known in the Arabic Tradition as the Three Hermeses), Asclepius, and Apollo and their descendants. In the second class, Ibn Juljul described the lives of Hippocrates, Dioscorides, Plato, Aristotle, Socrates, and Democrates. He restricted the third class to mathematicians and astronomers, including Ptolemy and Euclid. The fifth to the ninth classes consist of doctors who practiced in Alexandria, Syria, North Africa, and Muslim Spain. Similarly in the work by Ibn Abī 'Uṣaibi'a, the biographies of Greek doctors (the ancestors) are followed by other biographies, including those of Syriac, Iraqi, Egyptian, Persian, and Indian physicians.

Although largely dependent on the sources used, an average entry comprised a number of patterns. Thus, both collections of the *tabaqāt* portrayed doctors through their actions rather than giving their physical portraits. Personal information, for instance, details of their origins, education, and families was very limited. In describing illustrious men, the biographers confined themselves largely to their writings, improvements made in medical treatment, and

poems, anecdotes, and sayings by and about them. For example, the 'medical' biography of the first 'Doctor of the Arabs', al-Harith ibn Kalada (who lived in the time of the Prophet Muḥammad) consists of several anecdotes. For instance, when asked by the caliph Mu'awiyah which is the best remedy, al-Harith ibn Kalada is recorded as responding 'the hunger'.

Such anecdotes were thought to be more important than the mere amusement of curious readers: they aimed to portray the members of the professional group of medical practitioners as intelligent and educated people. A sharp mind, a thorough education, and the ability to write in an elegant style were considered necessary prerequisites for successful medical practice. This biographical pattern became very common in the Arabic (Islamic) biographical literature. The fourteenth-century author al-Muwaffaq Faḍl Allāh ibn Abī al-Fakhr Ibn as-Suqa'i al-Kātib an-Naṣrānī (d. 1326) considered it normal that a certain 'Alām ad-Dīn Ibrāhīm ibn Rashīd Abī al-Wahsh ibn al-Hulayqa, the 'doyen of practitioners in Syria and Egypt', was not only an excellent doctor who managed to treat a difficult diphtheria case but also a practitioner of the 'arts of *adab*' (i.e., familiar with literature, a composer of verses, etc.). Sometimes this wide learning was a mere pretence. Thus, the famous medical practitioner and autodidact of the eleventh century 'Alī ibn Riḍwān, in one of his writings, mentioned that the great al-Rāzī demanded each physician should compose a compendium for his own use. This, however, did not have benign consequences: physicians became lazier and were less inclined to study original works by Hippocrates and Galen. Although they possessed these luminaries' books, they did not learn from them, and they earned their livelihood more easily by relying exclusively on their own compendia. The treatment they offered deteriorated; the medical profession lost prestige and was scorned and considered by the public to be only a 'source of income' or a 'profession of the poor'. 'Alī ibn Riḍwān referred to a father who castigated his son thus: 'You are a shame to me because you take up a medical profession'.

The pattern of a universally learned, witty physician dominated the Arabic literature for centuries. In the tenth century, it appeared in an unusual genre in classical Arabic: the autobiography. The great Ibn Sīnā, followed by his pupil Abū 'Ubayd al-Juzjānī, wrote about himself, stressing his scholarly achievements as if he lacked other information about his personal life. According to Abū 'Ubayd al-Juzjānī, Ibn Sīnā personally related his biography (*sira*), which is in fact a series of episodes that highlight Ibn Sīnā's extraordinary memory, his ability to learn endlessly, and his achievements as a medical practitioner and statesman rather than displaying a coherent picture. Abū 'Ubayd al-Juzjānī maintained the usual framework of the biographical genre by this use of anecdotes, and he added a lengthy list of books written by his teacher.

Table 1 Arabic Medical Biographies

Title	Author	Notes
The History	John Grammatikos	Lost
Kitāb adab aṭ-ṭabīb	Isḥāq ibn ʿAlī ar-Ruhawī (ninth century)	Sixteen biographies of Ancient and Islamic doctors
Akhbār al-aṭibbāʾ	Abu al-Ḥasan ibn Ibrahīm ibn ad-Daya	Biographies of ninth-century doctors
Tarīkh al-aṭibbāʾ	Isḥāq ibn Ḥunayn	A short history of the Ancient medicine, with biographies of Ancient doctors in alphabetical order
Kitāb siwān al-ḥikma	Abū Sulaymān Muḥammad ibn Ṭāhir ibn Bahrām al-Sijistānī (d. tenth century)	Lives and sayings of Greek wise men, philosophers, and doctors; the doctors' biographies are collected in the part called *Taʿalīq Ḥikmiya wa-mulah wa-n-nawādīr*
Fihrist	Ibn an-Nadīm (tenth century)	Comprises many biographies of various scholars and intellectuals; a large section deals with doctors and medical practitioners
Tabaqāt al-aṭibbā wa-l-ḥukamāʾ	Sulaymān ibn Ḥassan ibn Juljul (tenth century)	Ibn Juljul was the first to use the *tāʾifa* principle of classification for doctors' biographies
Kitāb manāqib al-aṭibbā	ʿUbayd Allāh ibn Jibraʾil ibn ʿUbayd Allāh ibn Bakhtishuʾ (d. 1032)	Lost
Mukhtar al-ḥikam wa-maḥasin al-kalim	Abu al-Wafaʾ al-Mubashshir ibn Fātik (d. 1049)	Compendium of lives and sayings of Greek doctors
Kitāb an-Nāfiʿ fi kaifiyat taʿlīm ṣinaʿat aṭ-Ṭibb	ʿAlī ibn Riḍwān (d. 1049/50)	Comprises a chapter on the history of medicine; the author mentions biographies of famous doctors, from Hippocrates to al-Rāzī
Kitāb at-taʾrīf bi-ṭabaqāt al-umam	Saʿid ibn Aḥmad ibn ʿAbd ar-Rahmān al-Andalūsī (d. 1070)	Comprises a number of medical practitioners' biographies
Tatimmat siwān al-ḥikma	Zahir ad-Dīn abu al-Ḥasan ʿAlī ibn abi Qāsim al-Baihaqī (d. 1169)	Continues *Kitāb siwān al-ḥikma*, from the caliph al-Maʾmūn and Ḥunayn ibn Isḥāq
Kitāb Ikhbār al-ʿulamāʾ bi-khabar al-ḥukamāʾ	Jamal ad-Din abu-al-Ḥasan ʿAlī ibn Yusuf al-Qiftī (d. 1248)	Better known as the abridged version *al-Muntakhabāt al-muntaqalāt min taʾrīkh al-hukamāʿ* by Muḥammad ibn ʿAlī ibn Muḥammad al-Khātibī al-Zauzanī title; this shorter version comprises 414 biographies of the *hukamāʿ* (wise men), which largely includes medical practitioners.
Kitāb ʿuyūn al-anbāʾ fi tabaqāt al-aṭibbā	Muwaffaq ad-Dīn Aḥmad ibn Qāsim (known as Ibn Abī Uṣaibiʿa, d. 1270)	A source of continuing importance and influence for historians of Arabic medicine and medical biography
Kitāb rauḍat al-afrāḥ wa-nuzhat al-arwāḥ	Muḥammad ibn Mahmud ash-Shahrazuri	

The Arabic biography in its traditional form flourished well into the nineteenth century. Some of the medical historical books, published by Barthélémy Clot Bey in Arabic in the 1830s, were still based upon the traditional patterns: biographies of doctors were mostly considered to be biographies of universally learned and well-educated men, well-known litterateurs, philosophers, calligraphers, and writers—and only then medical practitioners. However, the encounter with Western science and especially Western missionaries started changing the situation.

In the nineteenth century Arabic and Islamic culture was marked by the *al Nahda*, literally an 'awakening' or 'renaissance'. It was partly prompted by an admiration of the modernized West, after encountering European culture with Napoleon's conquest of Egypt. Produced by the interaction of Arab thinkers and Western ideals, *al Nahda* marked the beginning of Arab modernization, or rather the will to modernize. With regard to literature, Arab authors made an effort to adopt the European genres, which included literary biography. The famous litterateur Jurjī Zaydān (1861–1914) made the most important contribution, composing a volume of biographies of eminent people of the nineteenth century. Along with biographies of statesmen, clergymen, and litterateurs, this book included two biographies of medical practitioners active in Lebanon: Cornelius van Dyck and John Wortabet. Such distinguished men, medical practitioners, and missionaries appear in these biographies as more 'human', or rounded, than do their classical counterparts. Jurjī Zaydān was clearly interested in his subjects' medical careers; however, he wrote at length about their childhood and family upbringing, clearly depicting the development of a professional personality. Neither van Dyck nor Wortabet could be placed just among 'educated men' as happened with the biographies of their classical predecessors. The information about their education, which was usually lacking in classical Arabic biographies, was ascribed great importance. Contrary to the traditional classical Arabic static patterns, Jurjī Zaydān introduced a 'diachronical' narrative, giving a balance between personal features and professional development. Jurjī Zaydān's new approach to a doctor or scientist's literary biography was adopted in modern Arabic biographical dictionaries, for example in the biographical dictionary by Aḥmad al-'Alawīna.

THE ISLAMIC LEGACY

The Islamic medical tradition is still very vibrant in the contemporary Middle East and Central Asia, alongside Western medicine, which has become deeply rooted in contemporary Islamic society. Since the mid-nineteenth century, and especially the period after World War I, bearers of Western (initially German or English, now also American or Russian) medical diplomas enjoyed high esteem and a good reputation. The medical institutions in Islamic countries, which arose during the twentieth century, were initially modeled on Western hospitals. Their founders, such as Naguib Mahfouz, tried to make Western medical achievements flourish on Eastern soil. This, however, does not mean that the progress of Western medicine diminished the role played by the region's traditional medicine. In many cases, the Koran and *hadīth* continue to be seen as an effective remedy against disease caused by the *jinn* and evil charms. This is reflected in the flourishing trade of protection amulets (*ṭalasim*) and especially in an influx of literature where traditional methods of healing are widely discussed. A 'pocket advisor', sold by a book-handler (*warrāq*) on the streets of modern Alexandria or in a respectable bookshop in Beirut, indicates the correct Koranic verses to be read in specific cases. It also provides indications of the shrines and other holy places, such as

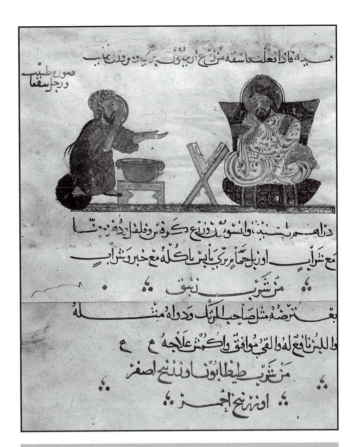

Islamic physician and patient. Arabic manuscript, thirteenth century. Wellcome Library, London.

graves of the holy men, where it would be possible to be cured from disease. This way of healing is especially popular in modern Central Asia, where for example women who want to become pregnant visit a Western (Russian or other) trained doctor and subsequently the grave of a local saint, which is claimed to help.

If one looks at the modern medical practice in Islamic countries and compares it with the situation 1,500 years ago, one still sees a huge market where various forms of healing coexist and compete with each other, now with the new admixture of Western medicine.

Bibliography

Azmi, A. A., 2002. 'Islamic Medicine in India during the Sultanate period (1206–1413).' *Studies in History of Medicine and Science* 18(1): 1–15; Brandenburg, D., 1982. *Islamic Miniature Painting in Medical Manuscripts* (Basel); Conrad, L. I., 2000. 'A Ninth-Century Muslim Scholar's Discussion of Contagion' in Conrad, L. I. and Dominik Wujastyk, eds., *Contagion: Perspectives from Pre-Modern Societies* (Aldershot) pp. 163–178; Conrad, L. I., 1995. 'The Arab-Islamic Medical Tradition' in Conrad, L. I., et al., eds. *The Western Medical Tradition, 800 B.C. to A.D. 1800* (Cambridge) pp. 93–138; Conrad, L. I., 1993. 'Arab-Islamic Medicine' in Bynum, W. F., and Roy Porter, eds., *Companion Encyclopedia of the History of Medicine* 2 vols. (London) pp. 676–727; Cooperson,

M., 2000. *Classical Arabic Biography: The Heirs of the Prophets in the Age of al-Ma'mun.* (Cambridge); Kamal, H., 1975. *Encyclopaedia of Islamic Medicine, with a Greco-Roman Back-ground* (Cairo); Levey, M., 1971. *Substitute Drugs in Early Arabic Medicine: With Special Reference to the Texts of Masarjawaih, al-Razi, and Pythagoras* (Stuttgart); Ibn Qayyim al-Jawziyya, 1998. *Medicine of the Prophet* trans. Johnstone, P. (Cambridge); Müller, A., 1885 'Über Ibn Abi Oçeibi'a und seine geschichte der Ärtzte' in *Actes du 6ème Congrès International des Orientalistes tenu en 1883 à Leide.* 2e partie. Sect. 1: Sémitique (Leiden) pp. 257–280; Rosenthal, F., 1990. *Science and Medicine in Islam: a Collection of Essays* (Variorum series) (Aldershot); Savage-Smith, E., 1996. 'Medicine' in Rashed, R. ed., *Encyclopedia of the History of Arabic Science* (London) vol. iii, pp. 903–962; Savage-Smith, E., F. Klein-Franke, and Zhu Ming. 'Tibb' in *Encyclopaedia of Islam* vol. 10, p. 451b.; Siddiqui, K. A., and M. K. Shafqat Azmi, 1999. 'Islamic Medical Ethics with Special Reference to Moalejat-e-Buqratiya.' *Bulletin of the Indian Institute of History of Medicine* 29(1): 15–27; Syed, I. B., 2002. 'Islamic Medicine: 1000 Years Ahead of Its Times.' *Journal of the International Society for the History of Islamic Medicine (ISHIM)* 1(2): 2–9; Ullman, Manfred, 1978. *Islamic Medicine* trans. Jean Watt (Edinburgh); Yacoub, A. A., 2000. *Responses in Islamic Jurisprudence to Developments in Medical Science* (London).

Nikolaj Serikoff

MEDICINE IN CHINA

INTRODUCTION

Timeline and Early Textual History

Imagining a long empirical tradition dating to a golden age in prehistory is often an integral part of the modern interpretation of traditional medicines. Paleographical inscriptions that date to the Shang dynasty (traditional dates: 1766–1122 BCE) do indeed provide evidence of medical activity on the North China plain, yet pre-modern practice was quite unlike the 'traditional Chinese medicine' (TCM) we see flourishing today in Asia or in Europe and America. From the first medical treatises set down in the late Warring States (fourth to second centuries BCE) to the ten thousand extant pre-Communist (to 1949) medical works listed in the 1991 National Chinese Medicine Union Catalogue, we can trace a rich and diverse medical culture in China.

Many medical practitioners were literate or their work was allied to scholarly traditions and left records through which we can reconstruct their knowledge and practice. Executive power and the competence of the Chinese empire were embodied in a vast ocean of texts produced by the government at every level, and medical practice was not exempt from the bureaucracy of the imperial process. Entry into the higher ranks of the civil service involved passing a series of examinations basically testing knowledge of the Confucian canons. Similarly, there was also a hierarchy in scholarly medicine: in two thousand years of empire social status was increasingly derived from possession, mastery, and ultimately authorship of texts.

The twenty-nine medical titles listed in the bibliographical treatise of *Hanshu* 漢書 (Han History), the official history of the Western Han dynasty (202 BCE to 23), compiled by Ban Gu 班固 (*c.* 97), give us an impression of what kind of medical writing first received imperial sanction in the first century. Among the titles, there are a *Huangdi nei* and *wai jing* 黃帝內/外經 (*Yellow Emperor's Inner/Outer Canon*). These are the first references to the development of a medical canon made up of treatises attributed to the Yellow Emperor. Unfortunately none of the collections listed in the first imperial bibliography is extant in the form or length indicated in Han times, and we know this canon through its editors and from editions based upon a printed version from the twelfth century. Nowadays we have three recensions, circulating as separate books, the title of each beginning with *Yellow Emperor's Inner Canon*: 'The Basic Questions' *Suwen* 素問 , 'The Numinous Pivot' *Ling shu* 靈樞 , and 'The Grand Basis' *Tai su* 太素 . All three texts are varied in content; the first is mainly concerned with medical theory: the body as a microcosm and origins of disease. Some therapy is included, mostly acupuncture (the piercing of the body with stones and needles to move *qi*) and moxibustion, a kind of cautery often using *Artemisia vulgaris* (mugwort), plus a few drug prescriptions. The second text is largely concerned

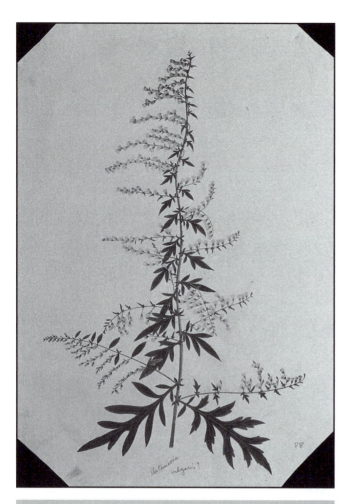

Flowering stem of *Artemisia vulgaris* (mugwort), the dried and ground leaves of which are used in moxibustion. Watercolor, nineteenth century. Iconographic Collection, Wellcome Library, London.

with acupuncture and moxibustion. The third has elements of both. We also know of a 'Bright Hall Canon' *Mingtang jing* 明堂經 dating to circa third century.

Apart from those works whose titles end in the term *jing* 經, not unproblematically translated 'canon' or 'classic', and those texts that are clearly collections of remedies, there are a substantial number of treatises in *Hanshu* concerned with longevity and the pursuit of immortality. These include writing on *daoyin* 導引 (literally 'guiding and pulling', a tradition of therapeutic exercise and breath cultivation designed to condition the inner body and treat pain and other illnesses), on sexual cultivation, on massage, and even on the pursuit of immortality. Many of the healing practices hinted at by these titles were marginalized in later times, or relegated to the religious or alchemical collections.

The medical titles listed in *Hanshu* provide a tantalizing key to medical culture in the early empire. Fortunately in the last few decades archaeologists have also found medical texts on silk and bamboo-strip manuscripts recovered from late

Warring States and early imperial tombs, which restore to us witnesses of some of the otherwise lost genres. The value that wealthy and educated people placed on technical expertise shows in these tomb collections. Manuscript traditions, which survived the advent of printing, tend to tell very different stories to those texts that ultimately made it into print, preserving knowledge of more diverse forms of healing, distinctively local, religious, or associated with the manifold forms of divinatory medical practice. Texts recovered from the Mawangdui 馬王堆 tombs (closed 168 BCE) include treatises on philosophy, astronomy, geography, and politics written on scrolls made of silk and bamboo slips. Seven of these manuscripts describe things medical. Among them are household manuals containing remedies for various illnesses that range from hemorrhoids and convulsions to 'child sprite' and 'ailments of the horse, sheep or snake'. The prescriptions include charms, exorcism, pharmacology, many kinds of heat treatments, and basic surgery. The tombs have also yielded a wide variety of foodstuffs and spices, and the earliest extant specimens of Chinese medical herbs were also found. Recognizable from remains in the tombs are substances still used by physicians today: magnolia, Chinese prickly ash, cassia bark, wild ginger, as well as many fragrant herbs for purifying the air. Other Mawangdui texts describe different forms of self-cultivation, including sexual, breathing, dietary, and callisthenic techniques for prolonging and enhancing life. Sadly, there are no texts in the immortality genre, which remains a mystery.

This essay will begin with a discussion of legendary figures in Chinese medicine and the social processes that had an influence on the formation of the canonical literature and high tradition, before tackling some of the complex issues of the wider culture of healing arts and practitioners in China.

ON MYTH AND MEDICINE

Traditional accounts of the origins of medicine tend to attribute the wisdom of medical classics to the revelations of sages and culture heroes. A survey of the medical aspects of their stories affirms the range of healing traditions in early China. After years of disunity during the Warring States period of the Zhou dynasty (1045–256 BCE), in 221 BCE the brutal war machine of Qinshi Huangdi 秦始皇帝 (259–210 BCE), the first emperor from the state of Qin, brought together the various kingdoms into what we now know as China. His short-lived dynasty was succeeded by the Han ruling house, which while inheriting the Qin realpolitik, distanced itself from the former unpopular regime by claiming to model the new administration after the exemplar of the sage rulers. Imagining a golden age at the beginning of civilization was not new, but Han historians and mythmakers retold the stories for their own time.

Among the ideas attributed to these legendary figures we find theories of statecraft based on the same natural and cosmic principles of Yin 陰, Yang 陽, and the *Wu Xing* 五行 ('Five Agents') that came to infuse classical medical thought. There were five sage emperors, each corresponding to one of the four directions and the center, who together were charged with civilizing a savage world. Without doubt, the most famous as a patron of medicine was the Yellow Emperor. His special responsibility was to model punishments, law, and the calendar after divine patterns thought to be immanent in heaven and earth. He had a role in divination and dividing the seasons and—in what linked him with essential medical arts—a knowledge of the body's relationship with the cycles and phases of nature and the accurate prediction of the progress of disease.

Before the second to third century, medical works were generally not attributed to individual authors. Much of the Yellow Emperor corpus is arranged in the form of a dialogue between the Yellow Emperor himself, represented as a patron of natural philosophy, and his ministers, often Qibo 歧伯, a specialist in acupuncture and other esoteric matters, or Lei Gong 雷公, the Thunder Duke. The tone of these exchanges is one of explanation and authority rather than that of rhetorical persuasion or debate.

The names of the Red Emperor, or *Shennong* 神農 [Divine Farmer], the enigmatic Bian Que, sometimes depicted as a human-headed bird, and the mysterious Bai Shi 白氏, [Mr White] are also common in the titles of medical literature. By calling on the names of these legendary figures from the golden age of pre-history the authors and compilers of early Chinese medical texts conferred a magical authority on their work.

It is in the *Yellow Emperor's Inner Canon* that we find a description of the body's division into twelve distinct 'channels' through which *qi* (the all-pervasive stuff that powers the universe) was thought to move rhythmically around the body. The channels surfaced in the form of the pulse at places where ancient Chinese physicians could examine the condition of the body's *qi* and the organs through which it flowed. A large number of pulse types were distinguished, such as floating, superficial, sunken, and hesitant. This form of diagnosis became the preeminent method of diagnosis for elite physicians throughout imperial China and remains so today for modern practitioners of TCM.

A belief in the empirical spirit of Chinese medicine, that knowledge of the virtues of food and drugs came through trial and error, is enshrined in the legend of the Red Emperor, Shennong 神農. The Divine Farmer's fundamental task was to lead humanity out of a state of hunting and savagery, away from eating raw flesh, drinking blood, and wearing skins, toward an agrarian utopia. Later accounts describe how he thrashed all plants so that they revealed their essential tastes and smells. He then classified those plants, separating those fit for consumption and those used for medicine. Calling upon this tradition of empirical testing his name was evoked in the title of a number of famous

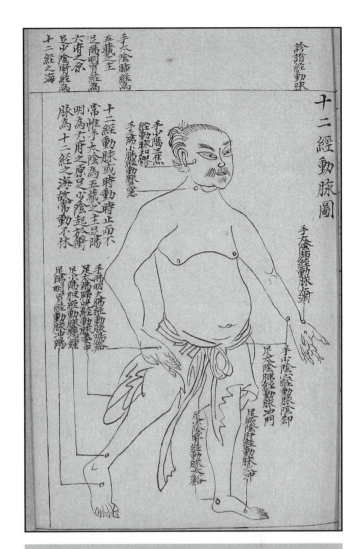

Channel pulses (dongmai) of the twelve channels, each represented by a circle on the body. Ink and brush drawing from Qian Lei, *Renjing jing fulu* (Supplement to the 'Mirror of Humanity' Canon), Ming Dynasty manuscript, 1368–1644. Library of Zhongguo zhongyi yanjiu yuan/Wellcome Library, London.

materia medica beginning with the *Shennong bencao jing* 神農本草經 [Divine Farmer's materia medica; *c.* first century].

It is notable that despite an elaborate view of the functions of the internal organs, early Chinese interest in the study of anatomy is largely conspicuous by its absence. Only during the reign of Wang Mang 王莽 (r. 9–23) do we have records of the careful measuring and weighing of the internal organs of an executed rebel leader. The *Yellow Emperor's Inner Canon* also contains the dimensions and capacities of the organs of the digestive tract and states that (unlike Heaven and Earth) the measurements of humans are easily attained, including those of the internal organs, 'since when they are dead you can cut them open and look'. In twentieth-century China, the lack of almost any surgery since the time of the legendary surgeon Hua Tuo 華佗 (second century) was

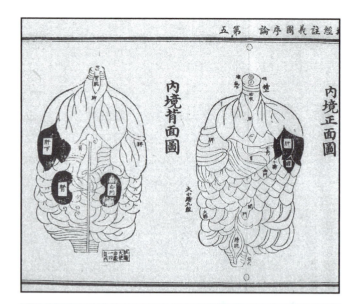

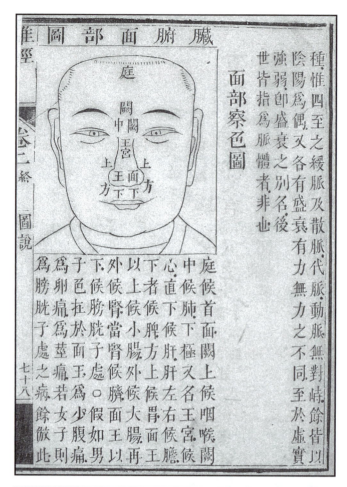

Anatomical illustrations from the Daoist Canon, depicting the internal organs of the chest and abdominal cavities from the back (left) and front (right). Woodcut from Li Jiong, *Huang Di ba shi yi nan jing zuan tu jujie* [Canon of Eighty-one Problems [in the Inner Canon] of the Yellow Lord . . .], vol. 1, Shanghai, 1436–49. Library of Zhongguo zhongyi yanjiu yuan/Wellcome Library, London.

Physiognomy diagnosis chart showing the facial sectors corresponding to the internal organs. Woodcut from Xiong Qinghu, *Bian Que maishu nan jing* [Canon of Problems in Bian Que's Book of the Pulse], vol. 2, Shibi Tang, 1817. Library of Zhongguo zhongyi yanjiu yuan/Wellcome Library, London.

often explained by the fact that medicine had advanced beyond this particular phase of therapy and that such problems should be treated with medicines. But underlying Hua Tuo's legendary use of *mafeisan* 麻沸散 to make his patients as if drunk and unconscious so he could perform abdominal surgery is a suggestion that his skills were founded in the treatment of trauma to the abdomen, and that he did not open up the body on his own volition. After all, he lived through times of great strife and war, and battle victims would have been plentiful (*Sanguozhi* 三國志 [Record of the Three Kingdoms; comp. 285–297]).

Chinese medical theoreticians were clearly not ignorant of the physicality of the body. They simply preferred to visualize a set of physiological functions and relationships subject to regularities perceived in the external world. The body then became amenable to medical intervention, to diagnosis and treatment. It was not a discrete, bounded object in isolation but part of a universe made coherent by the belief in a sympathetic resonance between things deemed to be similar. This kind of medicine, framed in terms of Yin, Yang, and the Five Agents, has been styled the Medicine of Systematic Correspondence (Unschuld, 1985, pp. 51–92).

Representing the rich and vibrant tradition of early Chinese regimen, *Peng Zu* 彭祖 [Ancestor Peng] is reputed to have lived over 900 years through his mastery of sexual cultivation. He was also a patron of those whom the philosopher Zhuangzi 莊子 criticized as 'huffers and puffers', the practitioners of therapeutic exercise and breath cultivation. The physiological (rather than meteorological or topo-graphical) concepts of *qi*, Yin, and Yang developed first in the recording of sexual and breath cultivation and therapeutic exercise before entering mainstream medical literature. Other figures in the world of self-cultivation include the instructresses in the arts of the bedchamber, *Sunü* 素女 [the Plain Girl], and *Xuannü* 玄女 [the Dark Girl]. There are also a group of legendary spirit mediums known as *wu* 巫 who played important roles in healing. Early Chinese society was steeped in worship of divinities and the worlds of departed ancestors and spirits of nature. From well before imperial times the *wu*—male or female diviners, spirit mediums, or ritual specialists—were used at court to avoid and resolve demonic and inauspicious influences and events, and to deal with ancestors, deities, and spirits. Their roles included annual and seasonal exorcisms and sacrifices to nature spirits as a means of dealing with calamities such as drought or floods. At funerals, they brought down the ghosts of the deceased. Often associated with the southern kingdom of Chu

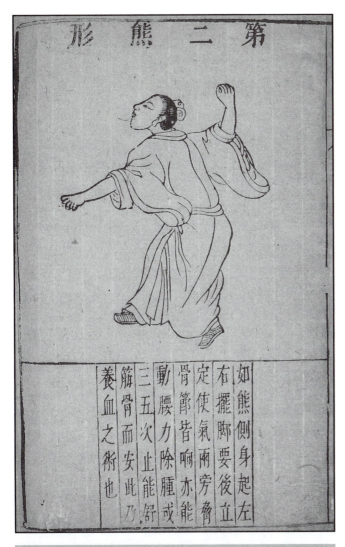

第二熊形

如熊側身起左
右擺腳要後立
定使氣兩旁魯
骨節皆响亦能
動腰力除腫或
三五次而安此乃
養筋骨而安此乃
血之術也

Man performing 'the play of the bear', a form of therapeutic gymnastics based on animal movements, in this case to stretch the sinews and bones and act as a tonic for the blood. Woodcut from Gong Juzhong, *Wanshou danshu* [The Cinnabar Book of Longevity], Ming Dynasty, 1368–1644. Library of Zhongguo zhongyi yanjiu yuan/Wellcome Library, London.

楚, the region exoticized in Han literature, the *wu* gained their reputation from personal skill in the appropriate arts.

Shuowen jiezi 說文解字, a second-century lexical work, stated *wu zhu ye* 巫祝也, 'the *wu* are "invocators"'. In *Zhouli* 周禮, a retrospective work about the bureaucracy of the Zhou dynasty (1045–256 BCE), spirit mediums were listed on the payroll of the Zhou ministry of rites as the last in the pecking order of the ritual specialists. As divination experts, as well as invoking the honorific titles of deities and summoning spirits and ancestors, many aspects of their work could aid in healing. They made proclamations and issued bans to remove sickness and disease, or manipulated effigies to influence the course of an illness. Female *wu* performed ritual dances, prayers, and songs and took their place in healing rituals performed alongside various sorts of priests and physicians.

The *Shanhai jing* 山海經 [Canon of Mountains and Seas; sometime late Warring States—Han] listed fourteen great *wu*. Wu Xian 巫咸 and Wu Peng 巫彭 are the best known. *Shiji* 史記 [Archivist Records] of the historian Sima Qian 司馬遷 (completed *c.* 100 BCE), the most remarkable history ever produced in China, states that Wu Xian and his son were officials at the court of the Shang kings Tai Wu 太戊 (1637–1563 BCE) and Zu Yi 祖乙 (1525–1507 BCE). The third century BCE encyclopedia of ritual and statecraft *Lüshi chunqiu* 呂氏春秋 [Mr Lu's Spring and Autumn, *c.* 239 BCE] associated Wu Peng with medical practice and Wu Xian with divination, although the medicine of the *wu*, as we will later see, often involved divination and communication with the spirits and was therefore not sharply differentiated from other aspects of their work.

THE TRANSMISSION OF MEDICAL KNOWLEDGE AND THE FORMATION OF THE CANON

Sima Qian recorded two biographies of physicians in his archive. Despite having supernatural skills and occasionally a bird's body, Bian Que, like the physician Chunyu Yi, is represented as a *yi* 醫 [scholar physician], in that his status was in part based on the ownership and transmission of medical texts such as those found in the early imperial tombs. Framed in the new medical language of *qi*, Yin, and Yang, some of these texts took on a scriptural quality. They were of a different literary and intellectual quality than the remedy books. But since both physicians prescribed various kinds of decoctions, they no doubt also possessed, used, and passed on collections of *fang* 方 [remedies]. Those deriving status from their collections of remedies were designated *fangshi* 方士 [gentlemen of remedies], probably not a self-referent. The two physicians Bian Que and Chunyu Yi may, for example, have been considered *fangshi* by others. *Fangshi* practice included an eclectic array of medical arts: pharmacological prescriptions, acupuncture and superficial surgical operations, and divination or ritual interdiction all seem to have been a part of their repertoire. Yet, in many respects, we would be unwise to force a hard dividing line between the *yi* and the *fangshi*, for the range of technical texts in the contemporary collections that are extant testifies to a readership with catholic tastes.

Three of the Mawangdui tomb texts are clearly related, in style and content, to treatises contained in the received canons of acupuncture and moxibustion cautery. There are, however, significant differences that are perhaps more interesting than their similarities. First and foremost they spoke mostly of moxibustion and not needle or stone therapy. There were no acupuncture loci for needling, they described different channels from those in the received tradition, and there were no links described connecting the channels to the internal organs. These texts are therefore fascinating for the

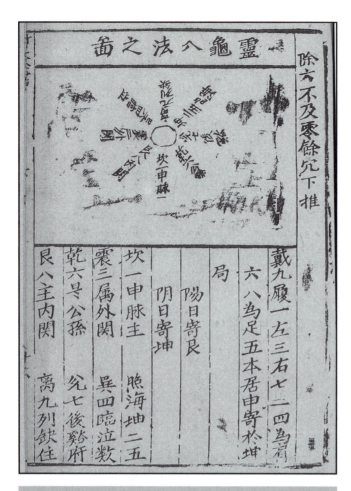

The Eight Techniques of the Spirit Tortoise, a divination procedure to establish the strength or weakness of the patient's blood and Qi, and hence to determine the appropriate course of acupuncture for a particular day and time. Woodcut from Chen Yan, *Xin qie michuan Chang Shan Jing Zhai Yang Xiansheng zhenjiu quanshu* [Complete Secretly Transmitted Texts on Acupuncture and Moxibustion . . .], 1591. Library of Zhongguo zhongyi yanjiu yuan/ Wellcome Library, London.

ence characteristic of particular medical training. Possessing the manuscript itself conveyed a kind of magical status. Perhaps the secrecy with which the texts were passed between generations of physicians or technicians increased their value in the eyes of those educated lay people who collected manuscripts. That may account for the presence of such medical literature in the tombs of elite families and the similarities that exist between one collection and another. The texts contained knowledge, but the material objects themselves transmitted the power that knowledge brought.

Each silk or bamboo scroll might contain one text or a number of units of text transcribed together, the sum of which were often much smaller than the present chapters of the canons. Eventually a lineage of teachers and students

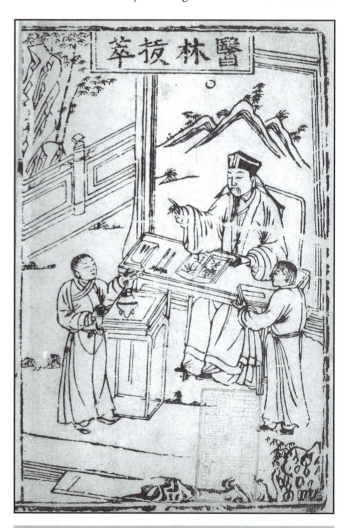

Master physician instructing his students in the arts of acupuncture. One student holds acupuncture needles, the other a medical text, suggesting a balance between theory and practice. Woodcut from Xu Feng, *Tong ren xu shi zhen jiu he ke, Xu shi zhen jiu da quan* [Mr Xu's Great Compendium of Acupuncture], Ming Dynasty, Jinling, 1368–1644. Library of Zhongguo zhongyi yanjiu yuan/Wellcome Library, London.

new light they shed on a critical period in the evolution of classical medical theory; from them it appears likely that the content of the *Yellow Emperor's Inner Canon,* the *locus classicus* for scholarly medicine, may be a product of writings composed during the last years of Warring States to Western Han age—albeit compiled in the following centuries and printed one thousand years later.

The transmission of ancient Chinese medical knowledge was characterized in part by the confidential instruction of these texts, epitomized by the master's ritual conferral of secret medical manuscripts upon his disciple. The text conferral served to confirm the master-disciple relationship and to distinguish physicians that shared the same instructions from others. The ritual of text conferral thus united a distinctive body of texts, the identity of physicians' lineage, and the medical experi-

might possess a large classified collection of scrolls. These would not necessarily be consistent with one another, and some might be designed to explain others in commentarial form. When the lineage ceased to function as previously, the textual collection may also have ceased to change and grow, and thereafter, by accident or design, was treated as canonical.

Toward the end of the Han period individual scholar-physicians began to express their own voice in medical literature. Zhang Zhongjing 張仲景 (c. mid-second to third century), in particular, exerted a remarkable influence on the development of Chinese medical theory. In a preface to the received text attributed to the author, Zhang Zhongjing recounted that after an epidemic decimated his town he wrote two treatises on febrile disease. These were later amalgamated into the much-quoted *Shang Han Lun* 傷寒論 [Treatise on Cold Damage]. His work charts the progress of febrile disease and integrates it with a comprehensive materia medica providing remedies for each stage. Cold damage is a systematic theory of the progress of Yin and Yang in the etiology of febrile illness arising from external attack. During the Song dynasty (960–1279), eight hundred years later, its influence became suddenly widespread. At that time, government officials uncovered the text in the imperial archives when searching for ancient wisdom to apply to increasing outbreaks of epidemic disease. They resurrected and printed an edition that is still published and in use today, and is particularly popular in Japan.

The trend for systematization gained pace during the second century when the question-and-answer format of the Yellow Emperor was further formalized in the *Nanjing* 難經 [Canon of Difficulties], a work that aims to interrogate and explicate many of the assumptions of the Yellow Emperor corpus and 'marks the apex, and also the conclusion, of the developmental phase of the conceptual system known as the medicine of systematic correspondence' (Unschuld, 1986, p. 3). Another notable individual to produce a systematic medical work was Huangfu Mi 皇甫謐 whose third century *Zhenjiu jiayi jing* 針灸甲乙經 [A and B Canon of Acupuncture and Moxibustion] reordered much of the Yellow Emperor's corpus, listing the acupuncture loci in an order that rendered them accessible as a whole.

KNOWLEDGE AND PRACTICE

Ritual, Divination, and the Scholarly Medical Traditions

The importance of divination in Chinese medical history cannot be underestimated. It was an essential skill for finding out the source of an illness, its prognosis, and, most importantly, whether it was wise to treat it (if the patient had a chance of dying). The worlds of language and philosophy, of diviner and physician, were therefore intricately linked. Excavations of the Shang dynasty capital are most famous for the discovery of bronze ritual vessels. But there were also fascinating records of the royal family in the form of a large number of turtle carapace and ox scapulae that had been deliberately cracked with hot rods.

A diviner interpreted the shape of the cracks in response to questions posed by the king. Both question and answer appeared as an inscription beside the cracks. Although most of the questions referred to matters of religious or political significance, some also related to illness in the royal family. Illness might be 'the curse of an ancestor', and the logical remedy, as with any other crisis, was to identify and appease the ancestor with offerings and sacrifice. Apart from these very early divination records, there is not much that tells us about early medical history until the late Zhou period, the Warring States, and the early imperial period (fourth to second centuries BCE).

At this time, diviners were among those *fangshi* and government advisers, such as Confucius and Mencius, who hawked their skills around the courts of the kings. *Fangshi* flocked to the court of the king of Huainan, Liu An 劉安 (?179–122 BCE), which became famous as a center of learning. Medical divination, or iatromancy, often formed a key part of their work. There were a variety of *shushu* 數術 [literally, numbers techniques] numerological calculations that had special significance in medicine. By calculating with divinatory tools one could determine the course and outcome of an illness, the day the illness struck, or the offending or offended ancestor. *Shushu* was a peculiarly Chinese notion of 'numbers' that was mainly used in the computation of 'celestial patterns' at the foundation of the astro-calendrical traditions. It was a pervasive culture that linked knowledge of the movement of the planets, calendar making, choice of auspicious times and places, prediction of the future, setting of ritual times, omenology (watching for eclipses, etc.), and exorcism—all of which also gave it direct application to medical theories, including those implicating demonic causation.

The first emperor had been particularly fond of *fangshi*, who aided him in his pursuit of immortality. Some of them are said to have transmitted the arts of Zou Yan 騶衍. Zou Yan's school, purported to be the institutional origin of the Yin and Yang philosophies, was given a great deal of coverage in the standard histories. And it is in the extant state documents generated by the various advisers, in their military tactics, divination, medical, and religious matters, that we find the earliest records of Yin, Yang, and the Five Agents.

YIN YANG AND THE FIVE AGENTS

Yin and Yang and the Five Agents were two of a number of systems of correlational thinking that came to the fore in the Warring States period and began to dominate in early imperial times. Yin and Yang are not things or substances, but are best thought of as labels or categories. At their most basic Yin and Yang refer to the sunny side and the dark side of a mountain, an analogy that blends crucial spatial and temporal themes. The 'complementary opposition' of Yin/Yang is often expressed in spatial alternation, as in Up/Down or Inner/Outer, or in the expectation that Yin/Yang will be in temporal alternation, as in Day/Night or the Warm/Cold seasons of the year. This in turn led to a more or less limitless set of binary correlations. Something is not spoken of as Yin or Yang either absolutely or in isolation. It derives its status from its relation to other things—thus a man may be Yang in relation to his wife, but Yin in relation to his father.

In the excavated texts from the second century BCE tomb collections, we can see evidence of more sophisticated and sys-

Table 1   The Earliest Extant Yin/Yang Correspondences

Yang	Yin
Heaven	Earth
Spring	Autumn
Summer	Winter
Day	Night
Big states	Small states
Important states	Unimportant states
Action	Inaction
Stretching	Contracting
Ruler	Minister
Above	Below
Man	Woman
Father	Child
Elder brother	Younger brother
Older	Younger
Noble	Base
Getting on in the world	Being stuck where one is
Taking a wife/begetting a child	Mourning
Controlling others	Being controlled by others
Guest	Host
Soldiers	Laborers
Speech	Silence
Giving	Receiving

tematic Yin/Yang correlation. These texts are of broad interest and covered subjects from law and government to treatises on the origins of all things. They show us the degree to which Yin/Yang thinking had begun to penetrate into different areas of specializations. Table 1 shows the earliest extant set of correspondences found in Cheng 稱, the third of four texts that precede the Mawangdui Laozi B, sometimes known as *Huangdi sijing* 黃帝四經 [The Yellow Emperor's Four Canons].

Yin and Yang eventually became fundamental principles in the classification of different physical substances and in the description of human physiological processes, both normal and pathological. There is plenty of evidence of this in the treatises of the *Yellow Emperor's Inner Canon*. In combination with stages in Yin/Yang transformation, which gave definition to annual and diurnal phases of time, Yin/Yang correlations explain changing states of health as well as phases in the etiology of disease, as shown in Table 2. Most significantly, Yin was correlated with dark internal bodily spaces and the organs. Disorders of Yin therefore explained the source and signs of fatal disease, so supporting Yin parts of the body was essential in avoiding or delaying a decline toward death.

By the third century BCE a neat pentic system of correspondences, the *Wu Xing* (Five Agents), began to dominate treatises on ritual and technical thought. For example, *Lüshi chunqiu* suggested changing the emperor's behavior, his diet, ceremonial clothing, and dwelling place according to a calendrical and ritual schedule. The Five Agent correspondences also expanded the correlational basis for interpreting the body with groups of five: five seasons of the year, five flavors, five organs, and so forth, and gave broader definition to the

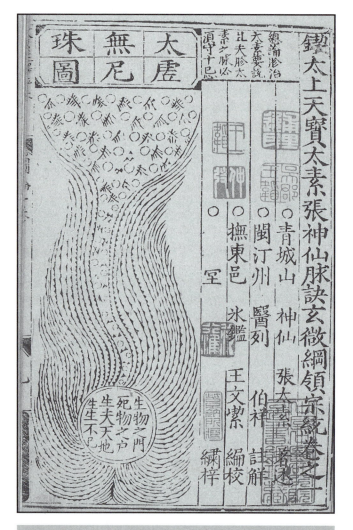

Theory of cosmogony showing the process of generation and transformation through Yin and Yang of the 'Myriad Things' of the universe, from nothingness to being. Woodcut from Zhang Taisu, *Taisu Zhang shenxian maijue xuanwei gangling tongzong* [The Subtle Doctrine of the Secrets of the Pulse of the School of the Immortal Taisu [Great Purity] Zhang], vol. 1, 1599. Library of Zhongguo zhongyi yanjiu yuan/Wellcome Library, London.

Table 2   Yin/Yang in Medicine

Yang	Yin
Outer	Inner
Upper	Lower
Dorsal	Ventral
Qi 氣	*Xue* 血 (Blood)
Vital function	Material substrate
Stimulation	Restraint
Increase, growth	Decrease, decline
Ascent	Descent
Outward orientation	Inward orientation

relationship between the external world and the human body based on a five-fold division of the year. Table 3 gives a selection of those early correspondences.

The correlations set out here embodied the natural (hence proper and beneficial) relations of the body to its environment and gave form and structure to what Joseph Needham termed the 'organismic' universe. We can also appreciate the way the political and social analogies strengthened the representation of the microcosmic body. These were most evident in the Yin and Yang correspondences of the *Yellow Emperor's Four Canons*, that is, Noble/Base or Controlling others/Being controlled by others.

THE IMPERIAL METAPHOR

By the second and first centuries BCE, the empire's physical infrastructure, the geography of the state, and the conduct of its bureaucracy became a key metaphor represented in elite medical writing. Nowhere is this more evident than in the conception of the fourteen channels of the acupuncture body. While the blood vessels and musculature were clearly represented in the contours of the channels, there is much more that we can learn about the origins of the channels from a close reading of the canonical texts. In some treatises in which medical writers

explicitly likened the channels to the great waterways, natural and man-made, of China, they borrowed ideas of physical flow and circulation from the structures of rapid communication and the distribution of materials around the empire. As the agricultural and irrigation systems sustained the great urban centers, so the channel system was the structure conveying nourishment to the body. The internal organs were the body's storehouses and granaries. Obstruction of the channels would lead to blockage, blockage to an excess or insufficiency, which would then render the body vulnerable to illness.

The system of governance in the empire was a mirror to that of heaven, and by logical extension, the organs of the body conformed to the same patterns. The *Basic Questions* stated, 'The heart is the office of the lord and ruler from whence the brilliance of the spirits emerge; the lung is the office of the minister from whence regulation and economies emerge; the liver is the office of the generals of the army, from whence strategies emerge; the gall bladder is the office of the rectifier, from whence judgments and decisions emerge; the chest is the office of minister and envoy, from whence joy and happiness emerge; the spleen and stomach are the bureau of storehouses, from whence the five flavors emerge [author trans.].' Not everyone was convinced of the virtue of following this kind of reasoning to such extremes. By the mid-first century, the over-elaborated correlations attracted mockery and criticism from some corners—most notably from the skeptic Wang Chong 王充 (27–100).

MEDICAL TECHNIQUES

Acupuncture and moxibustion emerged out of a synthesis of older medical practices (such as petty surgery, massage, bloodletting, hot stone treatment, and exorcistic archery) with the new ideas about the nature of the universe that flourished in the late Warring States and early empire. Sharp stone and bone needles and knives survive from Neolithic times, but the tech-

Table 3   *Wu Xing* correspondences

Wood	Fire	Earth	Metal	Water
8	7	5	9	6
Spring	Summer	Late summer	Autumn	Winter
East	South	Center	West	North
Sour	Bitter	Sweet	Acrid	Salty
Goatish	Burning	Fragrant	Rank	Rotten
Jupiter	Mars	Saturn	Venus	Mercury
Wind	Heat	Thunder	Cold	Rain
Wheat	Beans	Pannicled millet	Hemp	Millet
Liver	Heart	Spleen	Lungs	Kidney
Eyes	Tongue	Mouth	Nose	Ears
Anger	Joy	Desire	Sorrow	Fear
Shouting	Laughing	Singing	Wailing	Groaning
Blue-green	Red	Yellow	White	Black
Scaly	Feathered	Naked	Furred	Shelled

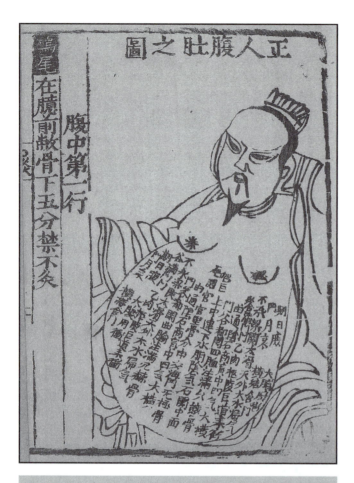

Acu-moxa chart to aid practitioners in recalling the distribution of the abdominal points for acupuncture and moxibustion. Woodcut from Xi Fang Zi, *Xin bian Xi Fang Xi Mingtang jiujing* [Xi Fang Zi's Illuminated Hall Classic of Moxibustion . . .], vol. 1, Shanxi, 1515. Library of Zhongguo zhongyi yanjiu yuan/Wellcome Library, London.

and moving *qi*, although instances of needling to move *qi* were the most common. Needles for moving *qi* were of rare quality, likened to 'fine hair'. Different techniques were also expressed through *bu* 補 and *xie* 瀉 , methods to supplement or drain the body's essences. Thus, from the time of the Yellow Emperor corpus onward we may understand the verb *ci* as referring to the use of different kinds of incisive medical tools.

During the Ming and Qing dynasties acupuncture lost official support, and its importance in elite circles declined rapidly. Physicians such as Zhang Jiebin 張介賓 (1563–1640) and Xu Dachun (1693–1771) noted that there were few well-known acupuncturists to be found in their time. In 1822 the Imperial Academy prohibited the teaching and practice of acupuncture. The reasons for this decline included a dislike of needles among patients, the emergence of gentler therapies such as *tuina* 推拿 (a form of massage), and a preference for herbal medicine. Acupuncture was a manual therapy unsuitable for the scholar-physicians that dominated the field of medicine, and it was practiced instead by external medicine physicians as part of a larger repertoire of petty surgery techniques.

Burned on and over the body, the dried and ground leaves of *ai* 艾 [mugwort; *Artemisia vulgaris*] are first known in apostrophic techniques used to protect the household from attack by demons. *Jiu* 灸 , now translated moxibustion, a form of heat treatment, was one of the earliest and most important methods for treating the channels. By burning mugwort on or over the body, the idea was to stimulate a response theoretically mediated via a system of *jingluo* 經絡 , the primary and secondary networks of the channels in the acupuncture body. The aim was to influence *qi*, to ease pain, and to expel 'wind' or other causes of disease. More accessible and cheaper than needles, it was a popular and widespread treatment. In Han times we know that cautery with mugwort was a part of front-line first aid, used to treat the sick officers and soldiers of the Dunhuang military complex who were unable to consult physicians. Chinese medical practitioners nowadays burn it on the end of metal needles, use cigar-shaped rolls of moxibustion, or roll cones to stimulate particular points or painful parts of the body.

Despite early references to *ai* in a number of therapeutic contexts, we cannot presuppose that it was always *Artemisia vulgaris* used in the practice of pre-modern cautery associated with *jiu*, or that it was widely available. Sui and Tang medical texts included examples of the use of realgar for cautery, and there are cautionary treatises that relate the different types of wood used to prepare or ignite the cautery to various degrees of iatrogenic damage.

ALCHEMY, MEDICINE, AND RELIGION

Religion seemed to play a vital role in preserving elements of continuity between a disintegrating civilization

niques were first linked together with a theory of the channels in Han times, although the accounts described procedures quite unlike the treatments that we know today. Before the Yellow Emperor corpus, records suggest that physicians used stones to pierce the body, to move *qi*, and, equally, to lance abscesses.

One treatise of *Lingshu*, 'Numinous Pivot', known as 'nine needles and nine origins', records the Yellow Emperor expressing dissatisfaction with crude methods associated with stone lancets, implying danger and damage and matching a new set of instruments to various surgical procedures. Yet, despite emphasis on *qi* work, much of the therapy described still involved petty surgery and massage; later discussions of the *yuan zhen* 員針 [round needle] and *pi zhen* 鈹針 [splitting needle]—two of the nine needles described in 'Basic Questions'—continued to refer to treatment for abscesses and bloodletting, respectively. *Ci* 刺 ['piercing'] and *qu* 取 [literally, 'taking'] are common technical designations. Both verbs were used in connection with bloodletting

and its successor, and in medieval China, religious movements became the context within which many medical ideas flourished and were transformed. With the fall of the Han, the political power base shifted from a centralized government, which vested power in a single emperor and an educated elite class that produced scholar-officials, to a broadly linked society of aristocrats with kinship allegiances to ethnic groups from the northern steppes. Despite these social and political transformations, religious structures grew and came to institutional maturity in the cosmopolitan high culture of the Tang period.

In the early part of the first century, millennial cults began to appear in different regions of China, some threatening the authority of the state. Wang Mang's 王莽 (r. 9–23) short-lived Xin dynasty was brought down by a group called the Red Eyebrows. Little is known about their teachings but by the mid-second century groups based around cults of popular healing through confession of sins, spirit possession, and worship of the deified Laozi 老子 [Lord Lao] were active.

In 184, one of these groups, the Yellow Turbans led by Zhang Jue 張角 , rebelled against the Han ruling house. The rebellion was suppressed, but the empire never recovered, finally disintegrating in 220. The Yellow Turbans converted people to their cause through healing practices, including old methods such as incantation and doses of water infused with the ashes of talismans. In 215 the Han general Cao Cao 曹操 obtained submission from a Daoist cult group founded by Zhang Daoling 張道陵, which controlled much of Sichuan, 'The Five Pecks of Rice' movement—so named after the tithe levied for entry. In return for their compliance the group was allowed to continue its teaching, and it became the source of the organized religion of Daoism. To this day, the *Tian Shi Dao* 天師道 [The Celestial Masters] continue to claim direct descent from Zhang Daoling's original church.

The Celestial Masters were healers who taught that illness was caused by sin and could be healed by confession and charity, public works such as road building, and distributing free food. Male or female priests, the highest local officials, would channel celestial powers into a ritual space, the 'chamber of purity'. Important to the Daoist movements of this era was the *Taiping Jing* 太平經 [Canon of Heavenly Peace], an early collection of classic Daoist prescriptions for longevity that included meditation, moral self-cultivation, dietary control, *qi* and breath cultivation, medicinal substances from plants and animals, and talismanic medicine.

The *Shangqing* 上請 [Highest Clarity] Daoist tradition grew out of that of the Celestial Masters. The early history of Daoism is not only one of ritual, meditation, and recluses; it is also very political. Under pressure from the north, the Celestial Masters' northern tradition began to move south, making trouble for local religious people and structures. From the fifth century we find the rise of Shangqing Daoism, which

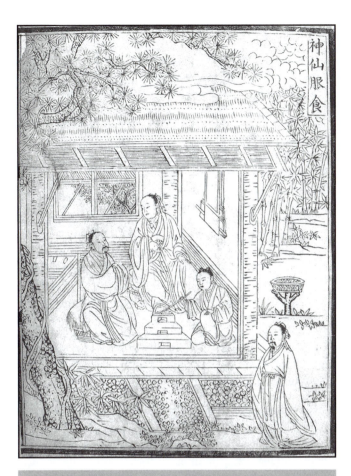

Shenxian fushi (diet of the Immortals). Two men discuss dietetic methods of achieving longevity or immortality while a child stirs an elixir. Woodcut from Hu Shihui, *Yinshan zhengyao* [Principles of Correct Diet], vol. 2, Jing Chang, Ming Dynasty 1368–1644. Library of Zhongguo zhongyi yanjiu yuan/Wellcome Library, London.

can be seen as a reassertion of southern values, guided by Tao Hongjing 陶弘景 (456–536). Tao was a seminal figure in Daoism alchemy and medicine whose mountain retreat became part of the Daoist tradition that enjoyed royal favor with state-sponsored activities—particularly in the alchemical field.

The themes of alchemy, medicine, and high government position recur in the lives of a number of medieval medical writers, the most eminent being Sun Simiao 孫思邈 (581–682), who served fifty years in government service. Sun lived in early Tang times, and was a scholar-physician whose religious and intellectual eclecticism is evident in two monumental medical works that contain demonic medicine, Buddhist incantations, and classical medicine side by side without prejudice. Like Tao he was one of the most important figures in the history of alchemy.

The classic objective of Chinese alchemy was to investigate and understand the universe through examining its material nature. By studying a substance as it moved from its original state and through every stage of transformation, the alchemist and scholar could draw analogies with sequences of time, from the very origin to the end of time, followed by a return to the beginning and the source. Thus, the alchemist would try to speed up time by carefully regulated and repeated heating and cooling in order to turn an imperfect substance into a perfected one—base metal into 'gold'. This was waidan 外丹 [external alchemy].

The alchemist's mastery of the material world included taking drugs as part of the search for physical immortality. Lead, mercury, cinnabar, and arsenic were all minerals used to preserve the physical body in both life and death. Arsenic, when taken over a long period of time, had the effect of nerve poisoning, the symptoms being lapses in consciousness, weakness and heart paralysis, whole body numbness, delusions, and diarrhea. But the gradual nature of the pathology, coupled with bouts of ecstatic hallucination, might have deceived the user as to the nature and outcome of their habit. It has been said that over the course of some three centuries, millions of literati and some of the Tang emperors died of elixir poisoning and that this resulted in the decline of external alchemy.

Whatever the number of fatalities over time, the gentler tradition of *neidan* 內丹 [internal alchemy] ultimately replaced external alchemy. *Neidan* used a language that bore marked similarities to that of external alchemy, but the focus of its practices were the essences of the human person. Trained on perfecting an immortal being within the physical body, adepts of internal alchemy worked on the ingredients of the elixir, that is, their own prime physiological constituents: the *qi*, *jing* 精 [quintessential essence], and *shen* 神 of classical medical theory. Through meditation and visualization, adepts could direct their attention inward and, paradoxically, take ecstatic flights around the cosmos. Charts of the alchemical body used in meditation mirrored the geographical, philosophical, political, and religious realities of China. They show an inner body landscaped with mountain ranges and waterways and sparkling with representations of the sun and moon, the stars, and the constellations. Hierarchies of imperial bureaucracy and administration structured the imagination of the physiological process and the gods and beings that inhabited the body.

In Chinese culture many healing cults existed that came to be labeled Daoist. The work of Daoists in the community was in large part directed toward healing and renewal, protecting people from evil forces and summoning the power of benevolent spirits. They would be called upon to provide protective amulets, talismans, potions, and cures, in addition to performing magic spells and exorcisms. Although the early schools of religious Daoism warned against popular forms of magic many Daoist priests engaged in just such practices and the issue may well have been with sanctioning and restricting a particular pantheon of deities and set rituals. From the Tang dynasty onward and especially under the Song, the organized Daoist churches, and in particular the

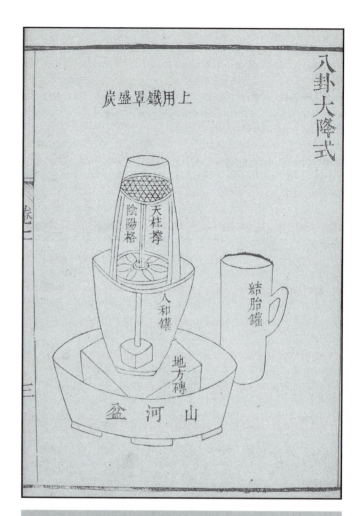

Alchemical refining furnace used to prepare bagua da jiangdan [Eight-Trigram Grand Descending Elixir], a mercuric compound used to treat ulcers, fistulas, and itchy skin conditions. Woodcut from Gao Wenjin, *Waike tushuo* [Pictorial Manual of External Medicine], vol. 2, 1856. Library of Zhongguo zhongyi yanjiu yuan/Wellcome Library, London.

Celestial Masters, were effectively licensed by the emperor to subsume and regulate all these cult groups. Representatives of popular religious healing were not necessarily only Daoists and included a wide range of magico-technicians, for example, *fangshi*, fortunetellers, astrologers, *wu*, and the like. Competition with Buddhism, especially at court, led to both religions appropriating each other's techniques.

From the first century China's growing international trading and cultural contacts had followed land routes through Central Asia, thus spreading Buddhism along the Silk Roads. It is possible that early Buddhism was regarded as a sect of Daoism and that Daoist communities served to spread certain Buddhist symbols and cults. Buddhism articulated a new and pristine vision of the afterlife with the ideal of successive incarnations of the immortal soul, offering prayer and meditation as the primary route to healing and salvation. But the supplication of deities was a common part of popular religion, and as a result Buddha (aka the Medicine King) and the bodhisattvas of healing, as an extension of the local pantheon, were well received and thoroughly sinicized in China.

The reunification of China under the Sui and Tang after hundreds of years of division was a time of great prosperity for both Daoism and Buddhism. Members of the Sui ruling house in particular were great patrons of Buddhism, and Buddhism reached its peak in early Tang as the dominant form of religious expression over the whole of the social spectrum. Court debates between adherents of all the great religious traditions were held under the patronage of the ruling Li family of the Tang dynasty, providing a stimulating and competitive environment that encouraged religious fusion and the general two-way appropriation of healing techniques.

Wealthy monasteries became vibrant cultural and community centers. Some offered low-cost hostels, epidemic relief, and free hospital care, which can be seen in the charitable infirmaries known as the *Beitian fang* 悲田坊 [Fields of Compassion]. Healing was also an effective form of evangelism. But with growing wealth and power came conflict with the state. In the great suppression of Buddhism between 842 and 845, many monastic institutions were shut down, their funds appropriated, and their infirmaries nationalized. Yet, regardless of persecution, religious centers remained an important site for scribal transmission and preservation of medical manuscripts. Much of what we know of medieval Chinese medicine comes from remote monastic communities on the Silk Roads.

Monks and priests of either Buddhist or Daoist affiliation prescribed drugs and dietetic measures, meditative routines, and regulated breathing. Amulets, incantation, and introspection were also a cure for demons and evil gods. Buddhists had a particular focus on healing the sick collectively in order to facilitate their spiritual development, taking the view that illness was an obvious obstruction to enlightenment. Daoists regarded longevity as a vital asset in attainment of the Dao, the true path, and they viewed health as a by-product of inner alchemy with the literal or spiritual goal of becoming immortal. Daoists were also noted for their talismanic cures in which the sick person would drink water or alcohol in which had been dissolved the ashes of documents inscribed with magical characters or formulae. As in India and medieval Europe, the monk and nun healers were often represented as immoral and debauched in Chinese literature. Monks who specialized in treating female illnesses played to the worst of these prejudices.

Important medical figures such as Hua Tuo and Sun Simiao might be honored with posthumous deification within a religious tradition. Medicine gods prevented and cured specific disorders or could be patrons of particular skills. There is a rich tradition of iconography associated with Sun Simiao, who was often depicted with dragon and tiger motifs.

Supplicants would write their requests and place them into the back of the statues.

WOMEN HEALERS

In pre-modern China (usually taken as before *c.* 1840), the status of the practitioner was not necessarily one of power in relation to the patient, and practitioners rarely enjoyed the privilege of their own consultation rooms. Numerous practitioners might be summoned to the bedside, and we frequently find the same practitioners skilled in many kinds of healing arts: scholarly practitioners writing complex prescriptions and reciting incantations, women taking the pulse and performing abortions.

For all that a corpus of literate medical theory had existed from the Han period on, in reality all traditions of practice and practitioners continued to flourish in some form or other throughout imperial times. For reasons of illiteracy and social status, we predictably have very little in the way of writings by medical women themselves. Women healers in early literature were generally subsumed under the category of *wu*, and from the medieval period, Buddhist and Daoist nuns brought spiritual consolation through prayer and incantation and produced charms and potions to be taken at auspicious times.

The existence of women healers and even physicians is documented in local topographies and personal diaries, and their skills are sometimes described by male physicians. Ming dynasty (1368–1644) novels are also a wonderful source for studying medical plurality. One colorful character described in the erotic novel *Jin Ping Mei* 金瓶梅 [The Plum in the Golden Vase] is *Liu pozi* 劉婆子 [Granny Liu]. While the master of the household regarded her as a dangerous empiric, a quack purveyor of old wives' remedies, she was in fact the healer of choice for women and children. She offered services that were similar to the scholar-physicians, felt the pulse, and made equivalent diagnoses without competing with their flamboyant displays of medical erudition and prognosis. Indeed, she had a wider repertoire of techniques—including acupuncture, moxibustion, and exorcism—than the men, who mostly confined their practice to writing complex prescriptions. Certainly, a broad range of skills would have benefited any practitioner in what was often a competitive environment.

Common images of women patients concealed behind screens, gingerly offering their wrist to have their pulse stroked by gentleman doctors illustrated the sense of modesty appropriate to a noble woman. It was the women health-care workers who moved across the boundaries between the private and public world. Beginning in Han times there were, as one might expect, women medical workers in the palace. Officially there are records of female doctors, midwives, and wet-nurses, some known as the *yipo* 醫婆 [physician grannies] or *yifu* 醫婦 [physician matrons].

There were also nuns and spirit mediums as well as those in the business of purveying herbs and substances. At the patients' bedside, the women might compete with male doctors, especially in matters of fertility, reproduction, and presiding over the deathbed, but they were not trained at the Imperial Medical College. There was an apprentice system, and in Ming times they were watched over by the Lodge of Ritual and Ceremony, also known as the Bureau of Nursing Children, which registered, selected, and meted out punishments to women. Being a medical worker in the palace could bring status and title, but the women's work was also subject to intense scrutiny.

MEDICINE AND STATE

Imperial patronage of medicine flourished under a succession of emperors in the Northern Song dynasty (960–1127) as a result of their personal interest and involvement, pressure on the government from successive epidemic outbreaks, together with the emergence of a new class of scholar-physicians, the *ru yi* 儒醫 [scholar-physicians]. Government initiatives included sponsoring the printing of medical works, establishing an Imperial Medical School, and formalizing medical education. There was a widespread initiative to collect local remedies and recipes, which rapidly increased the size of materia medica collections and stimulated a reappraisal of classifications and newly illustrated herbals. Searching for ways to manage the epidemics, physicians and medical theorists reinterpreted and integrated ancient doctrines with contemporary practice. Extending the standardization of medical writing and teaching, Emperor Huizong (r. 1101–26) ordered a distinguished court physician, Wang Weiyi 王惟一 (c. 987–1067), to cast several bronze acupuncture figurines. Conceived as a pedagogical aid, the figurines clearly displayed the circulation networks and labeled each acupuncture location. When the model was covered with a layer of yellow wax and filled with water, medical students had to locate the required acupuncture-loci exactly with a needle, causing water to gush out of the model through the hole.

Beginning at the end of the first millennium, coinciding with the decline of the Tang dynasty and the rise of the Song, the empire underwent rapid and sustained social and economic change. While increased population and wealth brought about a growth in the scholar class in general, the imperial administration—traditionally the most sought after and high-status source of employment—did not expand to provide enough jobs for the increased number of qualified applicants. As a result alternative scholarly careers were sought, and among these medicine was seen as a worthy alternative.

From early (Northern) Song dynasty (960–1125) there was lively political debate about the role and extent of appropriate governance, which came to a head in the later part of the eleventh century when Wang Anshi's 王安石

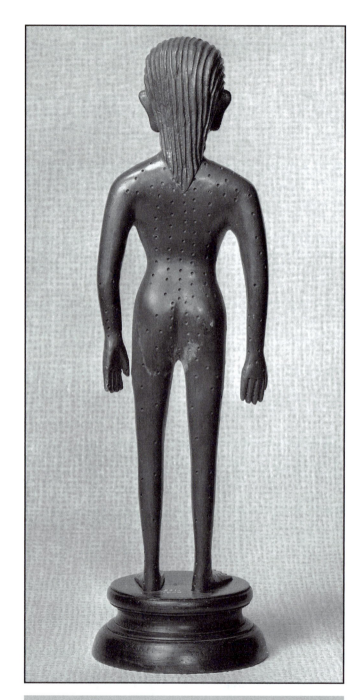

Bronze figurine used in acupuncture and diagnosis, seventeenth century. Wellcome Library, London.

'new policies' were introduced to modernize many areas of agriculture, commerce, finance, and administration. Amid this climate of increased state intervention, in 1057 the Bureau for the Editing of Medical Texts was set up to identify, print, and promulgate a canon of medical writings. This initiative resulted in editions of thirty medical canons and pharmaceutical texts and compendia of remedies, and it was largely responsible for the range to texts available to us today. It was in this period that Zhang

Zhongjing's *Treatise on Cold Damage* was rediscovered and promoted.

Various factors in the Song and Jin (1127–1235) and Yuan (1279–1368) periods had profound implications for the production of medical knowledge. New printing technologies allowed the government to reach a new readership beyond the semi-closed medical lineages that had previously served as the main conduit for the transmission of medical knowledge. The interest in medicine of a succession of Song emperors and their sponsorship of both medical literature and the standardization of medical education were innovations in state intervention that were not surpassed until the public health initatives and professionalization of medicine in the twentieth century. Some officials posted medical texts or medical text inscriptions increasing medical information and the prestige of government. One official forced people in his district to take medicines in order to prove their efficacy.

In an attempt to meet public health needs the government of the Southern Song (1125–75) licensed elite physicians to distribute medicines as relief for epidemics, but no one in their southern districts came to collect the drugs. Officials found that people fled from the sick, forcibly isolating them or abandoning their care to the *wu*, those practitioners specializing in techniques of popular religion. The officials blamed ignorance and 'trust in spirit mediums and demons over officials and medicine'. Some punished local religious healers, destroyed their altars, gave them medical texts, and ordered them to *gaiye* 改業 [change occupations] to farming or medicine.

The growth of a market economy and expanding urban environments supported knowledge networks, and the new elite scholar-physicians had unprecedented opportunities to be involved in the production of texts and new styles of medical praxis. After the Mongol Yuan dynasty (1279–1368) abolished the civil service exams, publishing a medical treatise became one of the ways a gentleman scholar could display his status and 'accumulate virtue'—a public and private, practical, and moral good.

MODERN MEDICAL TECHNOLOGIES FROM EUROPE AND JAPAN AND THE FALL OF THE EMPIRE

The story of the arrival and acceptance of new and foreign medical technologies runs in tandem with the crisis of the late empire in the face of imperialist incursions from Europe, America, and Japan. The Chinese response to a growing awareness of foreign power in all its manifestations was first insularity and protectionism, then desperate but inadequate attempts at reform, followed by collapse in the face of the demonstrable superiority of foreign power. In 1793 Lord George McCartney, a cousin of George III and an experienced diplomat, led a mission to the court of the Qianlong 乾隆 emperor (r. 1736–96). Only with extreme difficulty did he obtain an audience to deliver his gifts, after which the emperor haughtily wrote back to the monarch that, given the riches of the empire, the Chinese had no use for British goods. For his part, McCartney correctly surmised that the Chinese were as hopelessly unprepared as they were oblivious to the impending threat of European intervention.

For a few decades the European nations were distracted by the Napoleonic wars and their aftermath, but by the 1830s Western missionaries and traders were becoming ever more active. Finally, conflict with Britain loomed over the opium trade. After suffering a humiliating naval defeat, the Chinese government acceded to British demands for favorable trade terms. The other European nations and America were eager to follow. Then after a devastating outbreak of revolution during which some fifteen to twenty million people died, the Qing government lost control of central and south China to the rebels during the 1850s. Ironically, the rebellion was led by a Hakka peasant, Hong Xiuquan 洪秀全 (1814–64) who, styling himself as Jesus' brother, preached a novel and egalitarian doctrine derived from a potent mix of Christian and classical Chinese teachings concocted into a grand vision that under his tutelage China would become the *Taiping tianguo* 太平天國 [Heavenly Kingdom of Great Peace], literally heaven on earth.

Against the background of an increasingly frail central power, foreign medical techniques were arriving, in large part, together with Christian missions. After the first Treaty of Tianjin (1858) had granted foreigners freedom to travel and exemption from Chinese law, for the first time missionaries were allowed to own property and reside outside the treaty ports. It was widely acknowledged that free hospitals and clinics drew more converts than preaching; thus by the end of the nineteenth century most large towns would have a mission clinic. Given its appeal to the poor and the association with suspicious foreign doctrines, most wealthy families, who in any case could afford to call for local doctors and had access to a wide range of medical skills and services, looked down on missionary medicine.

From the seventeenth century, there had been Jesuit translations of anatomical texts, but in the absence of demonstrably effective medical techniques, these remained a curiosity until the mid-nineteenth century. The new techniques on offer at that time were mostly surgical and anesthetic, and although spectacular (operations for cataract, stone, removal of cysts and tumors) they allied foreign surgeons to medical artisans rather than to scholar-physicians. China had always had many types of petty surgery: bloodletting, acupuncture, the lancing of boils, suturing of wounds, extraction of projectiles, manipulations for hernia and hemorrhoids, and castration. There were also a handful of new wonder drugs such as quinine and chloroform to add to the vast Chinese materia medica.

Prevention of smallpox provided an important setting for the negotiation of traditional and foreign medical techniques. From the tenth century, symptoms that can retrospectively be identified as smallpox were endemic among

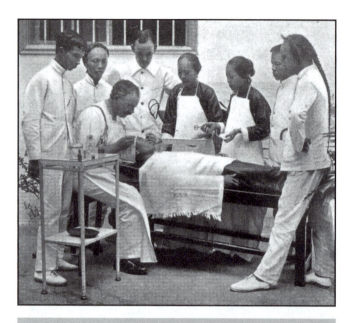

An operation for cataract at Fatshan Hospital performed by an English medical missionary assisted and observed by Chinese staff and students. Half-tone reproduction from A. Tatchell, *Medical Missionaries in China*, 1909. Wellcome Library, London.

children. They were classified as 'cold damage', the syndrome that from Han times had explained febrile disease and other, often contagious, symptoms thought to arise from external attack. But from the sixteenth century, Chinese practitioners in south China had practiced variolation (the deliberate introduction of infected smallpox material from a smallpox sufferer into young children). There were five different forms of variolation, designed to rid the body of 'fetal' poisoning and, accompanied by various rituals, they did prove effective. Fetal poisoning was thought to be an inherited disease attributed in part to disorderly diet, emotions, lifestyle, and sexuality, obliquely indicting the moral condition of the child's mother.

As a result, when Alexander Pearson in 1805 first introduced the Jennerian vaccine into China, there was tension regarding the privately offered variolation, especially in rural areas. Some Chinese charitable institutions offered the vaccine free, but vaccines were hard to come by, distribute, and preserve. The new technique claimed a better theoretical base, easier delivery, and greater safety, allowing mass-institutionalized provision. But both sides believed their techniques caused less suffering and fewer pockmarks, and variolation did not die out until the twentieth century.

Among the increasing numbers of ethnically Chinese bureaucrats in the Manchu administration, there was a core group in favor of the importation and assimilation of Western technology, particularly military. They formed what was known as the Self-Strengthening Movement (1860–95), an essentially conservative program of reform using the slogan 'Chinese learning for our foundation, Western learning for

practical application'. A modest plan for industrialization followed, with the founding of the Jiangnan arsenal in Shanghai and the Fuzhou dockyard. It was in this same spirit that in 1881 the Tianjin Medical School became the first to be established by the government for the teaching of Western medicine.

The defeat by Japan in the war of 1894–95 and the suppression of the Boxer Rising by the concessionary powers in 1900 emphasized the need for reform. Opinions polarized: conservative officials of the failing Qing government continued to reject attempts to modernize their institutions, while for others the modernization of China seemed attainable only by embracing all of Western culture. Many reformers traveled abroad to study science and medicine, notably to Japan, where there had been an effective program of top-down reform since the Meiji Restoration of 1868. In the biographies of great Chinese political reformers and revolutionary authors, there is a remarkable coincidence of medical training.

Beginning at the top, Sun Yatsen 孫中山 (1866–1925), father of the first Chinese revolution, was one of the first graduates of Hong Kong medical school under Sir James Cantlie. As a member of a 'gold rush family' that emigrated to Hawaii, Sun became interested in Christianity. It was in Western educational institutions that Sun developed his progressive and modernizing vision for China. Qiu Jin 秋瑾 (1879–1907) was one of the many revolutionary heroines who broke with tradition and went abroad to study. She left her husband and children behind and went to Japan, where she became very active in the Red Cross. On her return, she encouraged educated women to take up nursing as a profession for the first time. After leading an antigovernment uprising, she was executed. Finally, Lu Xun 鲁迅 (1881–1936) was the most famous of Chinese revolutionary authors. He studied Western philosophy and then medicine in Japan, but finally chose literature over medicine as the most powerful means to improve the underlying condition of his people. Nevertheless, under the influence of Darwin, Huxley, and Spencer he remained dedicated to strengthening their bodies, believing a healthy nation resides in a healthy population. China, in his view, was a 'sick nation' in need of all manner of sustenance.

PUBLIC HEALTH

From before the beginning of the empire there were public health works in China: siting of wells, urban waterways, provision of fresh drinking water, flood control, disaster relief, aesthetic projects, and the distribution of medicines during epidemics under the Tang and Song. Buddhist hospitals had been nationalized for a while during the Tang period. During Song times there was also a rudimentary public health system composed of poorhouses, some public hospitals, and paupers' cemeteries.

Concern with sanitation and public health was a feature of changing China into a modern nation-state, and in part a statement from political reformers about the foreign powers that were oppressing her. Medical missionaries were less concerned with public health than with the demonstration of individual salvation as manifested through their training in curative medicine; no doubt, it aligned somehow with their purpose of gaining conversions to the faith. Thus, public health measures in China were initiated by Chinese who had been educated abroad rather than initiated by foreign doctors themselves. The Cambridge-educated Wu Liande 伍連德 (1879–1960) convinced the imperial government to provide funds for enforcing quarantine during the 1910 pneumonic plague. He went on to play a pivotal role in setting up national health services during the republic.

Testimony to the powerful relationship between political reform and public health in China are the events of 1911. In a year when the very first International Plague Conference was convened in China came the final collapse of the empire. Public health had both a practical and economic imperative. Nineteenth-century campaigners for public health in Europe did so within the background of an economic requirement to keep workers in good health. Foreign approval of a Chinese-run National Quarantine service was a prerequisite for the return of Customs services into Chinese control, and with it the collection of revenue at the ports.

TCM: THE CONSTRUCTION OF TRADITION

From the late nineteenth century onward, physicians of Chinese medicine increasingly advocated the need to modernize their tradition if it was to survive in a rapidly changing society. This included the establishment of Western- and Japanese-style schools, colleges and hospitals, the founding of professional associations, and the publication of learned journals. During this period, traditional medicine also had to defend itself against efforts by more radical modernizers to disband its practice altogether. In 1929, Yu Yan 余巖 proposed a government motion intended to prohibit the practice of traditional medicine. Stimulating a rapid and unexpected reaction, the threat galvanized physicians of traditional medicine to form a united front. At a conference held in Shanghai on 17 March 1929, the decision was made to send a delegation to the capital at Nanjing. They managed to organize the practitioners, defer the motion, protect the integrity of traditional medicine at state level, and thereby usher in a new phase of modern 'traditional' Chinese medicine; 17 March is still commemorated among practitioners in Taiwan and Singapore as 'National Medicine Day'.

At the outset, Chinese Communist Party policy toward traditional medicine was pragmatic. In the absence of any medicine in China's vast rural hinterland they could use all practitioners willing to devote themselves to the service of the 'masses', just so long as they excised all elements of practice deemed superstitious or religious. After 'Liberation' in 1949, new schools for improving traditional medical practitioners began to appear in urban medical training centers. In theory, practitioners had to be licensed in order to practice and pass new training courses and exams. But with a large anatomy and physiology content it was difficult for most to graduate.

By the late 1950s political events were to turn this policy on its head. Chairman Mao Zedong 毛澤東 (1893–1976) was suspicious of the political sympathies of foreign-educated specialists, and with increasing alienation from the Soviet Union he was keen to promote technologies that were local, cheap, and patriotic. He ordered that doctors trained in Western medicine should be taught by the traditional practitioners. From 1954 onward traditional medicine was seen as living evidence of China's cultural genius. Colleges of Chinese medicine were opened in Shanghai, Guangzhou, Chengdu, and Beijing in 1956. In 1958 Chinese medicine was declared a national treasure by the government. But Chinese medicine was not to remain static: it was expected to modernize, scientize, and eventually integrate with Western medicine.

A uniquely Chinese Communist phenomena designed to remedy the lack of health care of any kind—traditional or modern—in the rural hinterland of China was the Barefoot Doctor system, a coordinated public-health program that fitted the prevailing culture of collectivization of property and campaigns to benefit the masses. For three to nine months the Barefoot Doctors, selected according to their political status (workers, peasants, and soldiers with a basic education), trained in the health care centers learning a combination of public health, Western anatomy and physiology, and the collection, preparation, and dispensing of local herbs and medicines. They then combined their daily work in the commune with voluntary medical duties in the field or in factory production teams, and in rotas at the health stations where there were simple consulting rooms and dispensaries. Decentralization of medical care enabled mass immunization projects with a limited people power. Having Mao's characteristic signature, the movement was largely dropped after his death, but a retrospective evaluation of its efficacy has led modern commentators at the WHO to hold it as a model for international development.

In the 1980s Chinese medicine was defined by law as being part of a plural health care system in China and its infrastructure developed further. Since the 1990s, the Chinese government has made stringent efforts to globalize Chinese medicine and to develop its economic potential. Nowadays most medical practitioners have some training in biomedical and traditional medicine. Varying degrees of integration are evident institutionally in the delivery of health care at hospitals, in diagnosis, explanatory models of disease, therapeutic paths, and drug preparations. Some indigenous traditions, such as pharmacotherapy, acupuncture, moxibustion, and massage are on offer in modern hospital and clinical settings, and even in emergency wards. Other traditions are a living part of popular medical knowledge:

elderly people gather in the parks to practice *Tai jiquan* 太機拳 the slow, gentle martial art that moves *qi* and strengthens the spirit. They pass on assumptions about dietary care and tonic medicines. Far from being subsumed under the high tide of a globally powerful biomedicine, according to the WHO estimates in 2002, traditional medicine still accounts for about 40 percent of Chinese health care. Indeed a multimillion dollar trade in prepared Chinese medicines worldwide testifies to a two-way transfer of knowledge and techniques. With mass emigration and the globalization of a plurality of medical traditions, Chinese medicine now survives in many different forms, transforming as it comes into contact with different cultures around the world.

Bibliography

Bray, Francesca, 2000. 'The Chinese Experience' in Pickstone, John V., and Roger Cooter, eds., *Medicine in the Twentieth Century* (Amsterdam) pp. 719–738; Cass, Victoria, 1986. 'Female Healers in the Ming, and the Lodge of Ritual and Ceremony.' *Journal of the American Oriental Society* 106: 233–240; Cullen, Christopher, 1993. 'Patients and Healers in Late Imperial China: Evidence from the *Jingpingmei*.' *History of Science* 31: 126–132; Ebury, Patricia, 1996. *Cambridge Illustrated History of China* (Cambridge); Furth, Charlotte, 1999. *A Flourishing Yin: Gender in China's Medical History, 960–1665* (Berkeley); Goldschmidt, Asaf, 2005. 'The Song Discontinuity.' *Asian Medicine* 1(1): 53–90; Goldschmidt, Asaf, 2001. 'Changing Standards: Tracing Changes in Acu-moxa Therapy during the Transition from the Tang to the Song Dynasties.' *East Asian Science, Technology, and Medicine* 18: 75–111; Grant, Joanna, 2003. *A Chinese Physician: Wang Ji and the 'Stone Mountain Medical Case Histories'* (London); Harper, Donald, 1998. *Early Chinese Medical Literature: The Mawangdui Medical Manuscripts* (London); Hinrichs, T. J., 2003. 'The Medical Transforming of Southern Customs in Song China (960–1279 c.e.)' PhD thesis, Harvard University; Hsu, Elisabeth, ed., 2001. *Innovation in Chinese Medicine* (Cambridge); Hsu, Elisabeth, 1999. *The Transmission of Chinese Medicine* (Cambridge); Yamada, Keiji, 1998. *The Origins of Acupuncture, Moxibustion and Decoction* (Kyoto); Kleinman, Arthur et al., eds., 1975. *Medicine in Chinese Cultures: Comparative Perspectives* (Washington, DC); Kohn, Livia, 2000. *Daoism Handbook* (Leiden); Leung, Angela Ki Che, 1987. 'Organised Medicine in Ming-Qing China: State and Private Medical Institutions in the Lower Yangzi Region.' *Late Imperial China* 8(1): 135–166; Lo, Vivienne, 2002. 'Spirit of Stone: Technical Considerations in the Treatment of the Jade Body.' *Bulletin of SOAS* 65(1): 99–127; Lo, Vivienne, 2001. 'Yellow Emperor's Toad Canon.' *Asia Major* 14(2): 61–99; Lo, Vivienne, and Christopher Cullen, 2005. *Medieval Chinese Medicine* (London); Loewe, M. A. N., 1997. 'The Physician Chunyu Yi and His Historical Background' in Gernet, J., and M. Kalinowski, eds., *En suivant la voie royale. Etudes thématiques* 7. (Paris) pp. 297–313; Lopez, Donald S., ed., 1996. *Religions of China in Practice* (Princeton); Lu, Gwei-djen, and Joseph Needham, 1980. *Celestial Lancets* (Cambridge); Minehan, Bridie Andrews (in press). *The Making of Modern Chinese Medicine* (Cambridge); Needham, Joseph, et al., 1986. *Science and Civilisation in China*, vol. VI, *Biology and Botanical Technology (part 1) Botany* (Cambridge); Scheid, Volker, 2002. *Chinese Medicine in Contemporary China: Plurality and Synthesis* (Durham, NC); Sivin, Nathan, 1994. 'State, Cosmos, and Body in the Last Three Centuries B.C.' *Harvard Journal of Asiatic Studies* 8: 25 (see also http://ccat.sas.upenn.edu/~nsivin/micro.html); Sivin, Nathan, 1987. *Traditional Medicine in Contemporary China* (Ann Arbor); Strickmann, Michel, 2002. *Chinese Magical Medicine* (Stanford); Taylor, Kim, 2005. *Medicine in Early Communist China* (London); Unschuld, Paul, 2003. *Huang di nei jing su wen* (Berkeley); Unschuld, Paul, 1985. *Medicine in China: A History of Ideas* (Berkeley); Wilms, Sabine, 2002. 'The Female Body in Medieval Chinese Medicine: A Translation and Interpretation of the 'Women's Recipes' in Sun Simiao's Beiji qianjin yaofang.' Unpublished PhD thesis, University of Arizona.

Vivienne Lo

MEDICAL TRADITIONS IN SOUTH ASIA

CROSSOVER AND EXCHANGE: INTRODUCING SOUTH ASIA'S MEDICAL TRADITIONS

Ayurveda, unani tibb, siddha of Tamil-speaking areas in the southwest of the Indian peninsula, and gso-ba-rig-pa of Tibet are the four learned medical traditions of South Asia. This chapter will focus mainly on ayurveda and unani tibb, with a review of their foundational texts, theories, and practices. Consideration will also be given to their place in contemporary South Asian societies, although this has been largely transformed in the political economy of health care.

Focusing on the learned traditions is unavoidable because these are accessible through their written sources, but two points need to be made in this regard. First, the division commonly found in writings on medicine in South Asia—the learned as the 'great tradition' versus the popular, or folk, as the 'little tradition', adopted from the study of Indian religions—obscures the reality of the dynamic tension between the learned and the popular domains. The learned is embedded in the popular through the inevitable interactions between the two, which are grounded in common cultures; however, one can also see that by necessity the learned tradition has set itself apart from the local, non-elite practices in order to maintain its privilege as the authoritative domain of medical practice. There are thus significant social dynamics at play in the writing of texts and in the kinds of texts that are being written. Second, it will be clear that the learned tradi-

tions have been historically dynamic—their practices have changed significantly over time. Therefore it is not possible to attempt to understand the contemporary practice of, say, tibb or ayurveda, through the doctrines of the classical texts, even though we are dealing with traditions that have always to some extent looked back, in striving for authenticity, to earlier formulations, whether written or oral, or earlier authoritative figures.

South Asia defines a region that includes Pakistan, India, Tibet, Nepal, Bhutan, Bangladesh, Sri Lanka, and the Maldives. However, this regional geopolitical identification is recent and arbitrary. It embraces a great diversity of peoples whose cultural traditions and social formations may be more appropriately understood according to smaller regional units and which cut across contemporary national/regional boundaries. Ayurveda, tibb, and siddha have all been exported with their diasporas, and in ayurveda's case successfully fed into the 'alternative' health market of Western industrialized countries. Ayurveda, unani tibb, and siddha either took root or evolved within South Asia, but they did not do so in isolation from the cultures and healing traditions of neighboring lands, such as China, Persia, Mesopotamia, and the eastern Mediterranean, all of which influenced the region through overland and maritime trade routes, military campaigns, and migration. This is notably the case with unani tibb, whose name in the Indian subcontinent (*yunani*, 'Ionian' in Arabic) betrays its origin in ancient Greece, introduced to the Indian subcontinent through the written languages of early Islam, Arabic, and Persian. Further influences from beyond the South Asian region are evident in the reworking of Chinese pulse doctrines in tibb (Ming and Klein-Franke, 1998), while Chinese alchemical traditions have been associated with the siddha practices of the Tamils. Moreover, to varying extents the learned traditions of ayurveda, Tibetan medicine, unani tibb, and siddha have been transformed through contact with one another, and all have been equally transformed through contact and engagement over the last three centuries with European capital, culture, and medicine in the colonial era.

At a further level of complexity, these learned traditions have all existed in close dialogue with other local and regional, sometimes less formalized, healing/soteriological practices and traditions, such as herbalist, religious, magical, astrological, tantric, or alchemical. The terms 'crossover', 'exchange', and 'pluralism' may be used to capture the many interactions and overlaps between medical practices and traditions in South Asia within the context of changing political, economic, and social conditions. Nevertheless, ayurveda, unani tibb, and siddha each retain unique characteristics that reflect their diverse origins as therapeutic, intellectual, and social enterprises.

AYURVEDA

Early Ayurveda and Canonical Compendia

Ayurveda is a name that has been applied to a diverse range of practices that are nonetheless linked by common conceptualizations of bodily health and ill-health in relation to environmental contexts. These include the effects of heating, cooling, moistening, and rarefying elements on humans, plants, and minerals. The grounding of ayurveda (Skt. 'knowledge for long living') is understood to lie in a triad of medical compendia, the *Caraka Saṃhitā*, *Suśruta Saṃhitā* and the *Aṣṭāṅgahṛdaya Saṃhitā* of Vāgbhaṭa, which were composed in Sanskrit between the third century BCE and the end of the seventh century. The *Caraka Saṃhitā* has historically been more influential in northern India, while Vāgbhaṭa's work has found greater following in the south of India.

The theoretical core of ayurvedic physiology, as elaborated in *Caraka Saṃhitā* and *Aṣṭāṅgahṛdaya Saṃhitā*, is based on the operation of microcosmic forces (*doṣas*) that govern the state of the body in relation to its environment (in fact there is no division between the body and the world outside it). The three *doṣas*—*vāta* or *vāyu*, *kapha*, and *pitta*—are composed of various combinations of the five elements that pervade all beings: ether, air, fire, water, and earth. *Vāta* is a condensation of ether and air, and is necessary for all kinds of motion and activity in the body. A condition resulting from an imbalance of *vāta*, according to some contemporary interpretations, would be Parkinson's

disease, because of the role that *vāta* plays in motion (Shankar and Unnikrishnan, 2004). *Kapha* is composed of water and earth; it has stabilizing, containing, and lubricating effects on the body. *Pitta*, composed of fire and water, has the potential to transform substances in the body through its heating attributes. The balance of one's particular constellation of *doṣas*, or constitution (*prakṛti*), is the key to health and long life: the excess or deficiency of one or more of the *doṣas* causes illness in the body. Living conditions, seasonal changes, and, in particular, the consumption of food and drink may all disturb the balance of the *doṣas*, depending on the body's ability to 'digest' surrounding influences. The concept of digestion is very important in ayurveda. A strong digestive fire (*āgni*) is produced by well-balanced *doṣas*. According to the *Aṣṭāṅgahṛdaya*, when *vāta* is in excess, the digestive fire becomes erratic. When *pitta* is increased, the fire necessary for digestion becomes intense. When *kapha* is dominant, the fire is dulled. All cases result in the body's inability to assimilate what it is exposed to on a systemic level, leading to illness. The digestion of consumables (food, medicine, drink) through successive 'cookings' and refinement produces, conventionally, the seven *dhātus* (commonly translated as 'tissues' or 'constitutive elements') of the body: nutrient fluid, blood, flesh, fat, bone, marrow, and semen (considered in some texts to be also present in women). Each refinement leads to the production of wastes, such as urine, sweat, and sputum. The imbalance of the *doṣas* may vitiate the bodily tissues or the organs of the body. The function of the vaidya (practitioner) is to restore the body to balance of the *doṣas* or to treat the affected *dhātu*. The difference in approaches may reflect the particular training that the vaidya has received; it may also be understood in terms of the varying geographical influence of the three great compendia previously mentioned. In contemporary ayurveda, the systemic functions of *doṣa* may often be neglected altogether in treatment as the physiological basis of biomedicine and the protocols of biomedical diagnosis supervene.

Historical studies of early ayurveda (e.g., Zysk, 1998; Meulenbeld, 1991–92, 1999) have demystified its origins, running counter to brahmanic-inspired traditions, propounded by some of the classical ayurvedic texts themselves, that trace the revelation of ayurveda through divine and semi-divine sages and intermediaries, originating with the Hindu god Brahmā, and passing ultimately through the divine Dhanvantari to Suśruta (*Suśruta Saṃhitā*), through the sage Ātreya to his pupils Agniveśa and Bhela, to Caraka (the *Caraka Saṃhitā*). Disrupting this interpretation, Zysk has sought to understand the shift from the magico-religious emphasis on healing practices in the *Atharva Veda* (the fourth of the Vedas, the earliest sacred scriptures of Hindu thought) to the broadly 'empirico-rational' paradigm of the ayurvedic texts through the agency of heterodox ascetic traditions in India (Zysk, 1998). Between the eighth and the first centuries BCE, these ascetic traditions detached them-

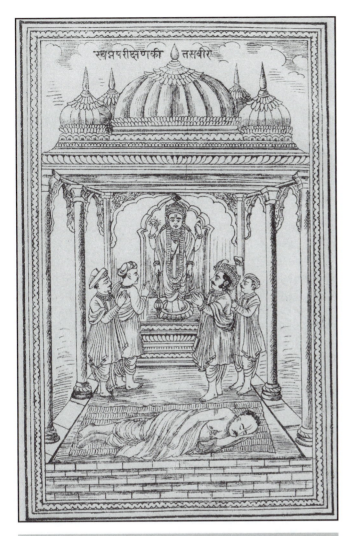

Dhanvantari, God of Ayurvedic Medicine. Ink drawing from Sanskrit MS 172. Asian Manuscripts, Wellcome Library, London.

selves from the socio-religious ideology of social hierarchy and ritual purity characteristic of brahmanic orthodoxy. In this regard, the importance of Buddhism as a favorable milieu for the evolution of ayurveda has been stressed. The development of Buddhist hospices and hospitals in many parts of India and in Sri Lanka is a manifestation of the interest in healing in Buddhist monastic orders. In this early phase, the itinerant ayurvedic practitioner was considered impure and looked upon with suspicion by some brahmin orthodox circles (White, 1996, p. 13). Later, during the Gupta era (320–467), ayurveda became somewhat brahmanized (Zysk, 1998, pp. 47–48).

Notwithstanding this disjuncture posited between vedic and ayurvedic approaches to healing, it is evident that early ayurveda cannot be easily separated from the Vedic matrix (White, 1996, pp. 19–20). The demons and gods of supernatural healing in the Vedas were never expunged entirely from the classical ayurvedic texts, which prescribed ritual

therapies alongside rational forms of intervention (Zimmermann, 1978). As Jean Langford has pointed out, the elimination of fantastic or magical elements in ayurvedic texts in historical writings during the twentieth century has been contingent on the perception of rationality and science as the hallmarks of advanced civilization over the irrationality and superstition of backward cultures. These theories were first developed by early nineteenth-century European scholars during European imperial expansion in South Asia, and were in many cases subsequently taken over by indigenous elites writing about their own culture and traditions, including ayurveda.

The *Caraka Saṃhitā* and the *Suśruta Saṃhitā* were likely the work of many authors and have been successively layered in their historical transmission. The identity of both Caraka and Suśruta has been much disputed, as have their dates. Current scholarship dates Caraka to between 100 BCE and 200 CE, although he was clearly working with an older tradition (Meulenbeld, 1999, IA, p. 114). The *Suśruta Saṃhitā* has been linked with the holy city of Benares, and its revised composition in the form known today likewise spanned several centuries and was probably completed by the fourth or fifth century CE.

Both of these works are vast compendia, covering areas including philosophy, nosology, symptoms, prognosis, pharmacology, food and diet, anatomy, embryology, and therapy, although Suśruta's text puts more emphasis on surgical operations in treatment. Both have been heavily commented upon, abridged, and translated from Sanskrit into vernacular languages in India. The third of the triad of foundational ayurvedic texts was the *Aṣṭāṅgahṛdaya Saṃhitā* of Vāgbhaṭa (seventh century). This work attempted to synthesize the material of Caraka and Suśruta. Vāgbhaṭa was a Buddhist from Sindh whose work was translated into Tibetan, and was also influential in southern India.

In conjunction with the use of the canonical compendia, memory and orality have been at the core of learned ayurvedic traditions. The versified, stylistic nature of the classic texts lends itself to memorizing the multiple correspondences between symptoms, processes, humors, and the intricate taxonomies of foods and remedies of ayurveda to be recalled or reconstituted during clinical practice. It is said that the Aṣṭangavaidayas, a Brahmin subcaste in Kerala for whom the *Aṣṭāṅgahṛdaya* was especially important, used to learn 120 chapters of Vāgbhaṭa's text by heart during their early apprenticeship (Zimmermann, 1978, p. 101).

In the absence of qualifications as such, there were two elements of the ayurvedic profession (and this applies equally to unani and siddha) that were especially important before the new institutional structures of the early twentieth century were implemented: first, adherence to the literary tradition as a carrier of authentic knowledge, and second, and perhaps more important, association with a line of reputed practitioners (as a student/disciple) or a respected occupational caste grouping. Such lineages or groups may or may not have had connections with the learned tradition, depending instead on local knowledge of plants and minerals and other therapeutic techniques, and keeping this knowledge secret within their family or occupational caste.

The Multiplicity of Traditions

Surgery

While the ayurveda of the classical texts reveals approaches to treatment that vary quite significantly—whether it is an emphasis on the effects of drugs, foodstuffs, and lifestyle changes over time, as in Caraka, or an emphasis on surgical procedures, as in Suśruta—major shifts in the practice of ayurveda and highly syncretic trends within the textual tradition itself can be discerned from the tenth century onwards. This conveniently coincides with the onset of the purported centuries-long decline of ayurveda. British Orientalists in the nineteenth century located the authenticity of ayurveda in the classical texts, not in contemporary practice (Langford, 2002), reinforcing their construction of the golden age of classical Hindu civilization and its collapse after the establishment of Muslim rule. T. A. Wise, writing in the 1840s, contrasted 'the ignorance and pusillanimity of the present low-caste surgeons of Bengal' with 'the energy, practical knowledge, and boldness in executing hazardous operations' of the 'ancient Hindu practitioners' (Wise, 1845 1, p. 323). The place of surgery has been taken as a key marker of the perceived decline of elite, learned ayurveda. There is a general consensus among historians of ayurveda that Suśruta's teachings—on studying anatomy through the inspection of decomposing corpses, on midwifery, on detailed surgical techniques—were not expanded in subsequent literature. Possible explanations include the strengthening of brahmanic orthodoxy, ritualization, vegetarianism, and the consolidation of taboos against pollution through contact with bodies, blood, sputum, and excreta, which led elite practitioners to leave the practice of surgery to lower-class practitioners (Jee, 1896, p. 186); the influence of Buddhism (Gupta, 1998); and the political instability caused by Muslim incursions from the northwest from the twelfth century and the subsequent loss of patronage of ayurveda to tibb under Muslim rule (Jee, 1896, p.198; Majumdar, 1971, pp. 262–266). Another reason has also been suggested: that the elusive alchemist and tantric Nāgārjuna (sixth to ninth century), the final redactor of the Suśruta Saṃhitā, removed surgery from the canon (White, 1996, p. 55, citing Arion Roṣu and Priya Vrat Sharma). This may indeed account for why Suśruta's surgery had no literary successors. Moreover, David White interestingly links the demise of surgery with the beginnings of a flourishing field in ayurveda: the therapeutic uses of metals and minerals (rasaśastra), constituting a veritable revolution in ayurveda.

There may also be something in the issue of loss of status in dealing with bodies and their polluting elements. In Ker-

ala, in southwest India, the Aṣṭavaidyas are Nambudiri Brahmins who have been degraded by their professional activities. Francis Zimmermann, however, has argued that the renewed emphasis on the expectant in postclassical times is but a shift in direction (albeit a major one) and should not be construed as the ritualization of ayurveda: violence and nonviolence, meat eating and vegetarianism are, after all, represented in the early texts. The issue of occupational caste is important here. In his study in Kerala, Zimmermann (1978) argues that the polarity between expectant and operative inherent to the texts at some point became expressed in a different kind of polarity, being viewed in terms of the scholarly (e.g., the Brahmin physicians) and the popular (e.g., the Kurup bonesetters attached to the warlike Nayar caste).

A key illustration of the relationship between learned and popular forms of practice is rhinoplasty (the surgical restoration of the nose through skin grafting). In the late eighteenth century a Maratha from Puna working for the British army was captured by Tipu Sultan and had his nose and one of his hands cut off. A member of the brickmaker caste performed the reconstruction and grafting with eminent skill. His dexterity in rhinoplasty caught the attention of British surgeons, and had a profound effect on the course of plastic surgery in Europe. Dominik Wujastyk concluded that due to the sophistication of this procedure 'it would not be possible for the tradition to have persisted purely textually', although similar procedures are mentioned in the Suśruta Saṃhitā (Wujastyk, 1993, p. 764). Moreover, he suggested that it may have been transmitted 'wholly outside the learned practice of traditional Indian physicians', since the surgeon was a member of the brickmaker's caste and probably illiterate. Here we have a fascinating case of the mutuality of textual and oral traditions of practice, but there are other dimensions as well. Rhinoplasty becomes an iconic symbol of ayurveda's sophistication and its ancient surgical knowledge during debates on revivalism among vaids in the twentieth century (see Report of the Committee on the Indigenous Systems of Medicine, Madras, 1925, I, pp. 2, 8). However, the prominence of this procedure arose because of such famous demonstrations, not from Suśruta's descriptions. Was what this brickmaker practiced 'ayurveda'? How does one draw the line between the learned and the popular, the 'great tradition' of the scholarly texts and the 'little tradition' of popular practices?

We learn from this discussion on surgery that there appears to have been a symbiotic relationship between ayurveda as a learned tradition and as a popular practice. This is almost certainly the case in pharmacy as well, as learned physicians had to depend on locally available remedies and the knowledge of people involved in identifying, procuring, distributing, and dispensing medical substances. It is apparent here too that 'ayurveda' has been used strategically, and somewhat elastically, to refer to learned practices of surgery and the scholarly tradition, and to

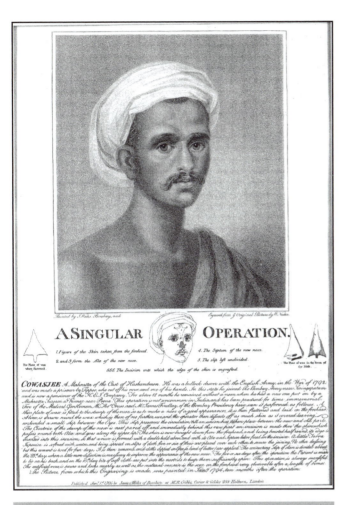

A SINGULAR OPERATION.

Cowasjee, a Mahratta who was captured and mutilated by Tipu Sultan by having his nose and a hand amputated. The nose was replaced from a skin flap brought down from the forehead, an operation thought to have been practiced for centuries in India. Engraving by William Nutter after a painting by James Wales, 1795. Iconographic Collection, Wellcome Library, London.

reflected in an expansive materia medica whose contours have changed markedly over the centuries. The early ayurvedic compendia concentrate on herbal substances but nevertheless contain numerous prescriptions involving the flesh or blood of various animals—the *Caraka Saṃhitā* lists 177 such substances (Wujastyk, 1993, p. 761). These include the cow, held sacred in Hindu scriptures and by orthodox Hindus, but nonetheless part of the materia medica of early ayurvedic medicine. Meats were prescribed for fortifying the body to counteract the loss of blood through injury or bloodletting, or to treat fainting fits (Zimmermann, 1999, p. 159ff.). Meats are mostly culled from the materia medica in later compendia.

From the tenth to the twelfth centuries innovations and experiments in the therapeutic use of minerals and metals begin to find their place in ayurvedic works. This trend is more prominent from the fourteenth century in the discipline of *rasaśastra*, (the medicinal use of metals and minerals), which becomes a fundamental part of ayurvedic practice right down to the present (Subbarayappa, 1971). Mercury began to be widely prescribed internally during the later medieval period (White, 1996, p. 52). White has shown how the growth of tantra and the siddha traditions of heterodox Hindu alchemical cults were entwined with this mineral/heavy metal orientation in ayurveda. Contacts between China and India, via the Silk Road, had a formative influence on Indian alchemy through the encounters between Indian and Tibetan Buddhism and

distinguish them from non-elite realms, and then to reclaim local practices as part of the ayurvedic tradition.

Finally, the decline of surgery within a learned-popular continuum of practice needs to be tempered. Localized surgical practices and their practitioners were certainly valued during postclassical times. Epigraphic evidence points to the royal patronage of the surgeon Aggalayya in eleventh century Andhra (Sastry, 1977). Furthermore, Hindu and Muslim practitioners of surgery received patronage at several Indo-Islamic courts between the sixteenth and early eighteenth centuries (Jaggi, 1997; Sigaléa, 1995).

New directions in pharmacy, diagnosis, and prognosis

The importance in ayurvedic treatment of remedies derived from vegetable, animal, and mineral sources is

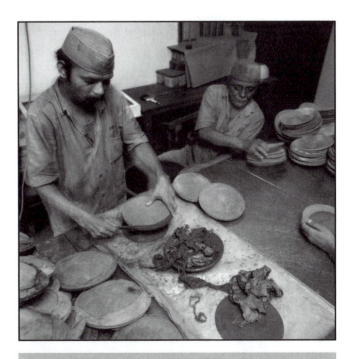

Preparing mercury from cinnabar (mercuric sulfide, HgS), Zandu Pharmaceuticals, Bombay. The mercury will be detoxified by incineration in a clay furnace. Photograph by Mark de Fraeye, Wellcome Photo Library, London.

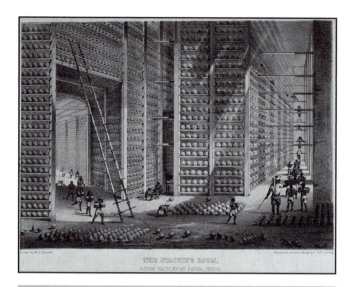

Busy stacking room in the opium factory, Patna, 1850. Lithograph after a drawing by W. S. Sherwill. Iconographic Collection, Wellcome Library, London.

Chinese Taoism. China was the prime source for India's mercury—the substance par excellence, endowed with immortalizing powers. Other important materia medica, such as opium, were introduced to ayurveda through contact with the tradition of unani tibb from the thirteenth century. A further development during this period was the rise of a practice connected with tantra, alchemy and therapeutics—*rasacikitsa*—which thrived especially in south India (where it came to be known as *cittār*, or siddha, in Tamil areas).

New forms of diagnostics and prognostics appear from the tenth century. Urine analysis, not a feature of classical ayurveda, appeared in the work of Vaṅgasena, probably from Bengal, in the eleventh century. During the fourteenth century the diagnostic pulse examination (*nāḍīparīkṣa*) entered ayurvedic traditions. The *Śārṅgadhara Saṃhitā* was the first ayurvedic text to describe how diagnosis can be achieved through the pulse. It has been suggested that this knowledge could have passed from tibb (Rai et al., 1979) or through siddha traditions (Daniel, 1984). Although it has been suggested that pulse was never fully integrated with learned ayurveda (Meulenbeld, 1991–1992, p. 110), pulse reading nevertheless became a fundamental part of practice for a majority of ayurvedic practitioners from Bengal to Kerala. Other innovations after the fourteenth century included an eightfold method of diagnosis and prognosis, which entailed an examination of the patient's pulse, urine, feces, tongue, voice, skin, eyes, and face, as well as their general appearance. The origins of this new and influential method are not currently known, but it is conceivable that they have emerged out of the interrelationships of ayurveda, unani, and siddha therapeutic-alchemical traditions.

Contrary to the assumptions of ayurvedic decline during Indo-Muslim rule in India, ayurvedic literature flourished,

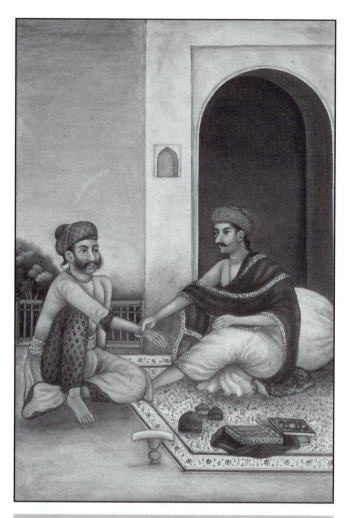

Ayurvedic medical practitioner taking a patient's pulse, c. 1825. Watercolor by a Delhi artist. Iconographic Collection, Wellcome Library, London.

reflecting vibrant social and intellectual Sanskritic currents (Wujastyk, 2003). Influential works include the *Bhāvaprakrāśa* of Bhavamiśra (sixteenth century), which contains the first description of syphilis in an ayurvedic text and the remedy *cobcīnī* (China root). Lolimbarāja's *Vaidya-jīvana*, an extremely popular versified work on therapeutics and materia medica, was the product of Deccani composite culture (Saxena, 2000, p. xxxiv). The author was probably a Maharashtran Brahman, a courtier whose patrons may have included a Muslim ruler. Lolimbarāja married a Muslim woman, Murāsā, apparently the daughter of an official of the sultan of Bijapur, whom he renamed as Ratnakalā and whom he praised in his works for her beauty and learning (Meulenbeld, 2000 2A, pp. 257–262). The encyclopedic *Ṭoḍarānanda*, a section of which was devoted to medicine, was compiled by scholars from Benares under the patronage of Akbar's finance minister, Ṭoḍaramalla (Meulenbeld, 2000 2A, pp. 272–296). Analysis of this literature dating from the sixteenth to the eighteenth centuries is still in its

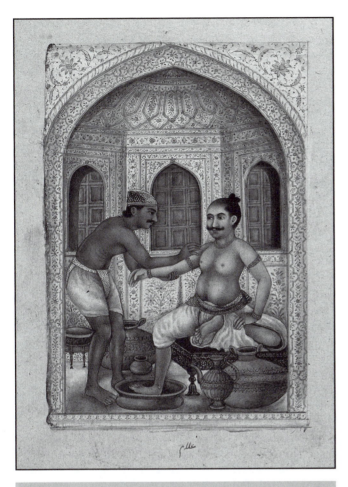

A ghulam, or bath attendant of the Shudra caste, attending to a customer in a Mughal-inspired bath-house. He is applying two Ayurvedic treatments: *snehana* (which includes external oil massage) and *svedana* (which applies hot steam). Gouache painting with pencil by an Indian artist, *c.* 1825. Iconographic Collection, Wellcome Library, London.

early stages, but promises to shed much-needed light on the social historical background of the production of texts and ayurvedic practice, and further contextualize the place of classical learning in postclassical times (Wujastyk, 2003).

It is clear then that there never has been stable, uncontested knowledge within the ayurvedic tradition. Recent work on ayurveda in the twentieth century further exposes the myth of an ayurveda that can be understood historically solely through the logic of its classical expositions. Before we come to this, we turn to another tradition whose postclassical history has also frequently been seen to operate through the theories of its classical texts: unani tibb.

UNANI TIBB

The name 'unani tibb', as this medical tradition has come to be known in South Asia (*yūnānī*, 'Greek' in Arabic, *ṭibb* 'medicine' in Arabic), although it was known as just *ṭibb* or

ḥikmat in medieval Arabic and Persian sources, is at once suggestive of a history of great translocation in time and space. It has been argued that use of the term 'unani' as a means of describing this tradition gained popularity during the nineteenth century among practitioners (*ḥakīms*, *ṭabībs*) who sought to link texts and practices in India that frequently invoke ancient Greek authorities and their Arab and Persian successors as a body of medical knowledge (Speziale, 2005).

From its beginnings in the eighth and ninth centuries, tibb was especially associated with Islam. Under the patronage of early rulers of the ʿAbbasid Caliphate and their expansive imperial ideology—al-Manṣūr (r. 754–775) Hārūn al-Rashīd (r. 786–803), and al-Maʾmūn (r. 813–833)—tibb emerged from a rich heritage of natural philosophy, medicine, and materia medica developed in ancient Greece and Rome, as well as embracing Persian, Indian, and, to a certain extent, Chinese sources. Among the most influential works were those of Galen (second century CE) and the materia medica of the first-century Greek physician Dioscorides. These were among the works translated into Arabic during the eighth and ninth centuries, and which gave tibb its characteristic philosophical and cosmological basis for defining human health and illness. This knowledge, drawn from many sources and traditions, was systematized in a number of works, including *Kāmil al-Ṣināʿa* of al-Mājūsī (d. 994), *al-Ṭibb al-Manṣūrī* of al-Rāzī (d. *c.* 925) and famously in *al-Qānūn fī al-Ṭibb* by the physician and polymath Ibn Sīnā (d. 1037), whose work, through abridgements and commentaries, has been particularly influential in the Indian subcontinent (Abdul Hameed, 1984; Liebeskind, 1997).

Tibb, when seen historically, is a loosely conjoined set of healing practices that have all drawn, to various extents, on the understanding of the body as a site for the interplay of elemental forces—heat, coldness, moisture, and dryness. In pre-modern expositions, the body cannot be separated from its being in the world, akin to ayurveda in some respects. The elements of the macrocosm are intermixed in the microcosm of the body to form humors (*akhlāṭ*), which are four in number: blood—*damm*—(with hot and moist qualities), phlegm—*balgham*—(moist and cold), yellow bile—*ṣafrā*—(dry and hot), and black bile—*saudā*—(dry and cold). Following Galenic theory, each person possesses a specific temperament (*mizāj*), which is characterized by the dominance of one or other of the four humors. Humors are produced through digestion, which is conceived as a process of cooking by the body's innate heat (*ḥarārah ghāridhiyah*). The stomach and the liver are key organs in the transformation of food and drink and the production of humors. The expulsion of wastes and accumulated or vitiated humors is essential for the maintenance of health. Age, gender, the prevailing climate, seasonal change, occupation, habits, food, and drink are all significant factors in the formation of one's temperament, and all are potentially pathogenic. Thus there is a constant dynamic relationship

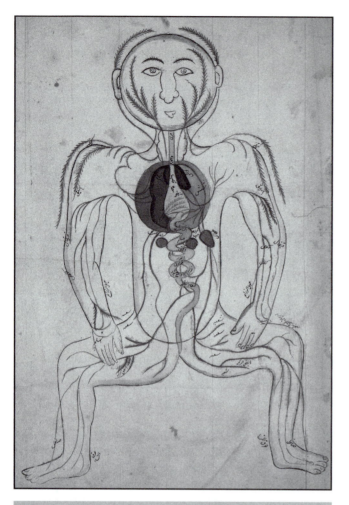

The viscera and venous system with Persian annotations on the image. Diagram comparable to those in Persian MSS of the Zakhira-i Khvarazm Shahi of al-Jurjani and the Tashrih-i Manṣūrī of Manṣūr. Watercolor with pen and ink by a Persian artist, nineteenth century. Iconographic Collection, Wellcome Library, London.

between the body and what it experiences; the physician's role is to bring the body toward a state of equilibrium between humors when one or more factors have caused imbalance and illness has ensued. The restoration of equilibrium may be achieved, as in ayurveda, through the prescription of medicinal substances or dietary and lifestyle changes. Pharmacy in tibb and ayurveda emphasizes the prescription of drugs, singly or more often in combination, of opposite quality to the underlying dominant humor in order to restore balance in the body. Cupping, cauterization, the application of leeches, and especially bloodletting used to be common interventions in tibb, but these procedures have been eclipsed in importance by pharmacy during modern times. It should be emphasized that this description serves to underline some of the key theoretical components of the tibbi tradition. This is, however, a highly diverse tradition, whose theories of natural causa-

tion were often blended with sacral, astrological, and ethical elements, which may be seen as part of an overarching cosmology. The stripping of the sacral was part of the modernization of tibb in India from the late nineteenth century, although many practitioners in this period asserted the cultural significance of religious conviction in the framing of their practice. Ayurveda and tibb have predominantly been male professions (at the formal end of the spectrum of practices), although this trend changed significantly during the twentieth century with the wider educational and professional opportunities that opened up for women in urban India.

Unani Tibb in the Indian Subcontinent

The introduction of tibb to the subcontinent's hinterlands began with the conquest and subsequent establishment of power bases in northwest India by Afghan and Turkic potentates during the twelfth century. Flourishing Indian Ocean trade links between West and South Asia from the eighth century also encouraged the spread of tibb in a localized manner to ports along the coastlines of Malabar and north Travancore on the southwest of the Indian peninsular, as well as to ports in Ceylon (Sri Lanka), such as Beruwela and Galle, and in the Maldives. In Ceylon, tibb transmitted orally and in palm leaf manuscripts written in Tamil and Arabic, remained within families of practitioners. It showed significant acculturation to local traditions following its removal from the Perso-Arab traditions associated with north India. The Perso-Arab scholarly tradition of tibb, associated first in a major way with the courts of the Khaljīs in Delhi (1296–1320), and then their successors, was, however, the principal medium through which tibb came to be known to people in the subcontinent.

Tibb, the Courts, and Islam

The thirteenth-century Mongol invasions of centers of Islamic learning such as Baghdad, Bukhara, Herat, Samarqand, Tabriz, Isfahan, and Rayy and the ensuing political instability of these regions encouraged migration. Physicians and scholars joined the exodus to northern India. The reign of 'Alā al-dīn Khaljī (1296–1316) attracted a number of physicians from these centers, as related by the historian Zīā al-dīn Barnī, who extolled Delhi and his patron's court for the learned men who had come there (Azmi, 2001, p. 327). This trend of migration continued into the Mughal era; for this period, there is evidence of a preponderance of Irani physicians, although there were significant numbers of Hindu physicians and surgeons, particularly during the rule of Akbar (Rezavi, 2001).

Before the nineteenth century, and in pockets into the twentieth century, such as in Hyderabad, tibb was closely linked to the ruling classes and nobility. The relationship of hakīms (practitioners) to the nobility drawn out in historical writings is so inextricably linked that the history of tibb has been widely conceived in terms of the succession of dynasties and rulers—the Delhi Sultanates, the Tughlaqs, Lodīs, Mughals, and Asif Jāhīs. Islam is an additional and fundamental element; all these rulers adopted Islam in various forms. Royal courts and the nobility recruited and patronized tibb, and its practitioners were often employed on a daily or annual basis. The favored practitioners gained rights over land/villages (jāgīrs) from which they assumed the revenue and where they often established their own dispensaries. Tabībs also composed medical treatises under such patronage.

Rulers and nobles from the fourteenth to the early eighteenth century funded the establishment of hospitals (shifā khānah or dār al-shifā, Persian and Arabic for 'place of cure') in regional centers under their control and set up endowments for their maintenance. During the rule of Muḥammad bin Tughlaq (r. 1325–51), the son of the founder of the Tughlaq dynasty of Delhi, there were seventy dispensaries and hospitals near Delhi alone (Jaggi, 1977, p. 108). His successor, Firoz Shāh Tughlaq (r. 1351–88), according to the contemporary chronicler and historian Firishta (1552–1623), is accredited with setting up a further 115 in his dominions, besides other large-scale public works (Azmi, 2001, p. 331). One such hospital described in the Tārīkh-i Firūz Shāhī supplied medicines and free food and drink to the ailing poor of any background (Jaggi, 1977, pp. 111–112). Firoz Shāh Tughlaq himself took a keen interest in medicine and in the running of some of his hospitals, and according to one report, ordered mentally ill patients to be kept in chains in one of his hospitals, where he would personally treat them. In the fourteenth century, hospitals were also set up in Agra, Surat, Malwah, Bhagnagar, and Ahmedabad. During the rule of Aurangzeb, a nobleman founded a hospital in Etawah in the early eighteenth century in which vaids as well as hakīms were employed 'so that they might keep in it valuable and easily available medicines of all kinds together with necessary diet and food for the poor patients' (Jaggi, 1977, p. 195). These hospitals no doubt varied in kind, size, and facilities, but seem to have provided basic accommodation and treatment for the itinerant and the indigent. Some were impressive buildings, such as the dār al-shifā in Hyderabad, founded by Muḥammad Shāh Qūlī in 1595, which could accommodate up to 400 patients in rooms around a central courtyard (Reddy, 1957). India's rulers emulated the precedents set in Baghdad, Damascus, Cairo, Merw, and Rayy. This was no simplistic concern among rulers for 'public health' but a combination of the ideals of Islamic charity with statements of wealth and status.

An important feature of the relationship between tibb and the nobility is the scholarly tradition with its continuous transmission of texts and the numerous permutations of commentaries and abridgements. The tibbi medical tradition remained in close association with, and was in some cases at one with, traditions of the Islamicate world, some scholarly, others mystical—logic (manṭiq), philosophy (falsafa), poetry, ethics (akhlāq), religious studies (dīniyyāt), sufism (taṣawwuf), and astrology ('ilm al-nujūm). Although education in tibb was primarily tutor oriented or hereditary in India, until the late nineteenth century, it was also part of madrasa (Islamic school) education. The famous Nizāmī syllabus included tuition in key texts of tibb's canonical literature: the Sharḥ al-Asbāb of Nafīs ibn 'Iwaḍ, Mūjaz al-Qānūn of Ibn al-Nafīs, and al-Qānūn. The Mughal ruler Akbar is also reported to have ordered that tibb should be included in school curricula (Rezavi, 2001, p. 41).

Tibb in India, however, should not be understood as a profession that was only geared to, or dependent on, courtly culture. S. Nadeem Rezavi shows clearly how unani physicians in the Mughal era established private practices in metropolitan centers, and along with 'bazaar' physicians served a broad spectrum of the community in which they lived (Rezavi, 2001, p. 50f.).

Tibb and Its Engagement with India

We have already mentioned the more or less continuous literary unani tradition with the circulation of key works, written originally in Arabic in West and Central Asia, and commentaries on them. This fact should not obscure an appreciation of the existence of multiple strands of the tibbi tradition in India, as reflected in the works that grew out of local cultures of medical practice. Even in the early periods of tibbi practice in India, hakīms were assimilating local ideas, practices, and materia medica. A courtier of Muḥammad Tughlaq, Zīa Muḥammad Mas'ūd Rashīd 'Umar Ghāznavī, a scholar of Persian, Arabic, and Sanskrit, composed Majmū'ah-i Zīa'ī (Collection of Zia) while in Telengana, a region in present-day Andhra Pradesh. This work was based on well-known writings in the Perso-Arab tibbi tradition, as well as on some ayurvedic works, from which he collected, he wrote, 'those medicines which I thought fit for these countries' (Jaggi, 1977, p. 108). This statement carries particular meaning from the perspectives of tibb and ayurveda, since the temperaments of all things—people, animals, plants, and minerals—were attuned to local environments in terms of their respective attributes of heat, cold, moisture, and dryness. Zīa Ghāznavī also discussed in this work calcination and the preparation of metallic oxides as remedies (Skt. bhasma, Persian kushtajāt) derived from ayurvedic sources, which in the subsequent unani tradition were to become extremely popular. One school of tibb in the early twentieth century, the Takmil ut-tibb in Lucknow, opposed the use of kushtajāt in an attempt to teach tibb without its ayurvedic accretions.

Another Persian work of the fourteenth century, Tibb-i Shihābī, also reflected the syncretic milieu in which new works of unani tibb were being composed (Faruqi, 1985). The family of its author, Shihāb al-dīn b. 'Abd al-Karīm Nāgaurī, had been settled in India for approximately two hundred years at the time of its composition in 1388. Another of his works was commissioned by Muzaffar Shāh I of Gujarat. Apart from being taught by an Afghan physician, Shihāb Nāgaurī also attended yogis (Hindu ascetics) in order to learn ayurveda. In the versified work on pathology and therapeutics, which resulted from his experiences, he adopted local names for drugs and some diseases. He also dealt with processes of calcination. The popularity of this work is evident from the number of copies surviving in various collections, its translation into Urdu in the nineteenth century, and its publication in Kanpur in 1868. Ayurvedic works were also translated into Persian; a translation of the Aṣṭāṅgahṛdaya of Vāgbhaṭa was completed in 1474 under the aegis of Sultān Maḥmūd Shāh of Gujarat. Another work, which was devoted entirely to bringing together knowledge of ayurveda in Persian, was Ma'dan al-Shifā Sikandar Shāhī [The Mine of Cure of Sikandar Shāh], compiled in 1512 with the help of ayurvedic pandits and hakīms by Miyān Bhavah ibn Khavāṣṣ Khān, one of the chief ministers of Sikandar Lodī. In his preface, Miyān Bhavah justified its compilation: 'It is known from experience that the medicine of Greece [ḥikmat-i yūnān] does not suit the constitutions [amzijeh] of the people of India's regions, and that it is not attuned to the climate [āb o havā] of this land. Since the names of the medicinal substances are in Persian and Greek languages their true nature is not known in this country, and they are not commonly found. It therefore became necessary to investigate thoroughly the books of the physicians of India' (Haas, 1876, p. 631).

The interest of ṭabībs in their local environment did not wane. Some of the most accomplished physicians and scholars, such as Rustam Jurjānī (sixteenth century), Muḥammad Akbar Arzānī (eighteenth century), Hakīm 'Alavī Khān (eighteenth century), and Hakīm A'zam Khān (nineteenth century), compiled vast pharmacopoeias and formularies in Persian drawing on their knowledge of simple and compound drugs in local and regional healing traditions. The eighteenth-century texts also mark the incorporation of European drugs into unani pharmacopoeia. Into the late nineteenth and twentieth century, many hakīms in Hyderabad were recognized for their knowledge of Telugu, a Dravidian language of south India, which gave them better access to local knowledge of medicinal substances. Occasionally tibbi works were written in Sanskrit in the eighteenth century, such as the Hikmatparādipa and Hikmatprakāśa of Mahādevadeva (Meulenbeld, 1991–1992), and there is also evidence of tibbi works in Tamil. The social history of tibb in pre-modern, colonial, and postcolonial times is in its infancy and its study in the regional languages and contexts of India still in conception, but these avenues promise to illuminate how tibb has been acculturated into local arenas, removed somewhat from the core domains of practice and learning in the Perso-Arab traditions. Even these, as we have seen, have developed significantly within India, challenging a view, which, linking tibb and Islam, casts them as detached from, or alien to, the subcontinent. The very assumption, and it is a common one, that tibb can be termed Islamic as such, because of its socio-cultural links to the Islamicate world, because the majority of its practitioners are Muslim, and because of a political discourse that originated in the colonial era heavily laden with the assignations of religious community, is one that does not stand up to scrutiny. To see how the exclusive connection of tibb and Islam has been overstated one only has to read of the Hindu tabībs in the Punjab, for example, who in the early twentieth century, at the height of communitarian tensions between Hindus and Muslims in north India, contributed to unani journals. There is no evidence for the assumption that hakīms in private practice have only served their 'community'; in fact the evidence is to the contrary. From the early twentieth century, patient inquiries to the unani journals Rafīq al-Aṭibbā and al-Ḥakīm in Lahore clearly show that people from Hindu and Sikh backgrounds consulted unani tabībs for a range of conditions. With the emergence of the 'nation' in twentieth-century discourse in indigenous medicine, and under the influence of heightened regional and communitarian identity politics, practitioners of tibb, ayurveda, and siddha sought to assert the cultural and symbolic worth of their traditions. Given the rootedness of tibb in India, it is therefore of no surprise that during the twentieth century there have been calls among practitioners to rename 'yūnānī ṭibb' (Greek medicine) as 'Hindustānī ṭibb' (Indian medicine). A well-known ḥakīm of Lucknow, Hakīm Abd ul-Latif, writing in the 1930s made such a claim (Speziale, 2005). Another respected practitioner repeated this as recently as 1998 during his speech at the annual conference of the national organization of unani physicians (All India Unani Tibbi Conference, convened in Delhi, November 1998).

Historically, vaidyas and tabībs in India have coexisted alongside a variety of other healers and modes of practice, and the boundaries between folk and the streams of learned practice have been fluid. Sufi shrines and temples have been places of resort for psychiatric disorders and for fertility complaints (Speziale, 2003; Kakar, 1982). Druggists, itinerant herbalists, adivāsi (tribal) practitioners, Hindu and Muslim ascetics (yogis and faqirs, for instance), traditional birth attendants (dāis), bonesetters, oculists, barber-surgeons, occupational castes of smallpox inoculators (the tikadārs of pre–twentieth-century Bengal, for instance), snake-bite specialists, animal healers, religious guides, and alchemists have all played major roles in forms of localized health care provision throughout India's history. This list should of course include common people, especially women in rural areas, whose knowledge of locally available resources for common ailments and the treatment of children is likely to have been passed down to

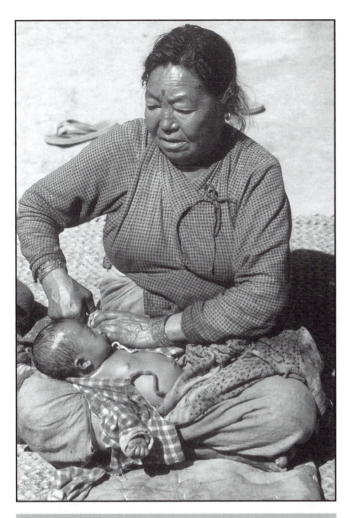

Traditional Nepalese birthing attendant removing a baby's clothing. Photograph by N. Durrell McKenna, Wellcome Photo Library, London.

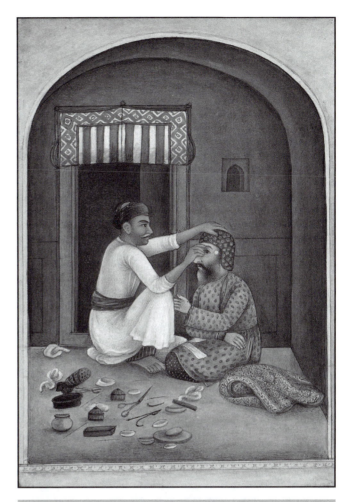

Saīhiya, an eye surgeon, probably performing a cataract operation. Gouache painting with pencil by an Indian artist, *c.* 1825. Iconographic Collection, Wellcome Library, London.

them by their mothers or grandmothers, or through other informal networks.

SIDDHA

In the Tamil country of south India, a form of medical practice known as siddha (Tamil *cittār*) developed out of a web of ascetic, alchemical, and therapeutic traditions. There have been many attempts to show that siddha medical doctrines belonged to high antiquity, but recent scholarship suggests that the majority of siddha medical texts were written no earlier than the sixteenth century (Scharfe, 1999). In these texts the defining characteristics of siddha medical practice are diagnosis by pulse examination and the therapeutic use of minerals and heavy metals, such as lead and mercury, whose poisonous properties are claimed to be eliminated through elaborate processes of 'killing' (*mārana*) the metals (Subbarayappa). Siddha traditions involve eighteen semi-divines and sages, and link Chinese alchemical knowledge to their own through the

semi-historical figure of Bhogar. Trading links between China and the Tamil coast are known to have existed since early in the first millennium. The history of siddha as a medical practice rather than a textual history has not been explored.

Siddha is practiced today in rural and urban areas and has been supported by a state government infrastructure of teaching institutions and dispensaries as a culturally resonant symbol of Tamil ethnic identity. Traditionally siddha was the preserve of certain high castes in hereditary or guru-disciple lines. The knowledge preserved by the lineages of siddha practitioners is guarded by their descendants, reinforcing the power that these practitioners are seen by some to possess. Recent ethnographic studies have pointed to stark divisions between hereditary practitioners, who associate themselves with authentic and effective practice, and the graduates of colleges in Tamil Nadu state teaching siddha in courses heavily weighted with biomedical subjects (Hausman, 1996).

EUROPEAN ENCOUNTERS, MODERNIZING TRENDS

Early Exchanges

Encounters between European physicians in India and their Indian counterparts during the sixteenth century were free of notions of European supremacy, as evident in the work of Garcia da Orta (d. 1563). The tenor of these exchanges changed during the seventeenth and especially the eighteenth and nineteenth centuries, as British colonial rule became consolidated. Increasingly Europeans defined good medical practice in terms of chemical, anatomical, and surgical knowledge, even though the paradigms of health and disease in European and Indian thought were not dissimilar in many respects until the mid-nineteenth century (Pearson, 1995). India's medicinal wealth interested Europeans from the sixteenth century until the nineteenth century. This is reflected in influential works on medicinal drugs written in Portuguese, Dutch, and English during this period. Garcia da Orta compiled his *Colloquios dos Simples e Drogas Mediçinais da India* (1563) in Goa after spending many years learning about the uses of indigenous drugs from numerous physicians and local people. The Dutch botanist Hendrik van Rheede (d. 1691) wrote the *Hortus Malabaricus* with an ayurvedic physician from the Ezhava caste (a lower caste of toddy-tappers in Malabar in littoral southwest India who were nevertheless highly regarded as physicians). This monumental work was published between 1678 and 1703. During the nineteenth century, local knowledge was investigated more systematically. One of the early works of this kind was Whitelaw Ainslie's *Materia Indica* (1826). In the mid-nineteenth century, the British Indian government recognized the economic benefits of substituting the drugs imported from England with drugs grown in India. Through these maneuvers and under the influence of British capital, the drugs of India's medical traditions gradually became divorced from their underlying rationales, which were widely disparaged for their 'stagnation' and lack of scientific pedigree.

Homeopathy and Nature-cure

Strict divisions into colonial and indigenous cannot easily characterize the encounters with European medicine in India. This applies to developments in ayurveda and unani, but homeopathy and nature-cure provide further evidence. Bengal was especially important in the establishment and dissemination of homeopathy in India. Under Rajendra Datta (1818–1889) and his pupil Mahendra Lal Sircar (1833–1904) homeopathy became 'indigenized' in the context of widespread epidemics of cholera and malaria, in the treatment of which 'allopathic' medicines were often seen as ineffective or harmful (Arnold and Sarkar, 2002). Its early practitioners drew on ayurvedic sources and indigenous materia medica. But its appeal lay at the same time in its modernity and rationality, and in its potential to supplant the orthodoxy of allopathic medicine in the colonial context. In independent India homeopathy became associated with the Indian 'Systems of Medicine'. The appeal of nature-cure was somewhat similar. Gandhi, its most famous advocate, espoused nature-cure as a science free from caste hierarchy (in contrast to ayurveda) but which also could be reconciled with his moral-physical ideals of bodily conduct (cleanliness, simplicity, self-control) forming part of his larger scheme of political activism (*satyagraha*) against British rule (Alter, 2000). Nature-cure was untainted by the colonial underpinning of orthodox allopathic medicine. In postcolonial India nature-cure has become a popular option among the urban middle classes for the treatment of chronic ailments. The Ministry of Health in India also supports yoga. This reflects its popular transformation during the twentieth century from a body of meditative and physical practices aimed at spiritual realization and transcendence to one concerned with this-worldly physical and spiritual well being (De Michelis, 2004)

REWORKING MEDICAL TRADITIONS

During the nineteenth century, ayurveda and tibb were reborn as 'systems' of medicine. The practices and epistemologies of tibb and ayurveda were reworked in response to a number of related factors: encounters with European medical practices, culture, and capital in colonial India; the adoption of print technology; widespread social and economic change; the collapse of traditional sources of patronage; and the broader context of the popular mobilization of social, religious, and political movements. Authoritative structures of indigenous medical practice were being challenged. We may take the example of the *tol* system of ayurvedic teaching in Bengal. The tol was a kind of apprenticeship based on a guru–disciple relationship between a *kabirājā* (an occupational caste of ayurvedic physicians in Bengal, literally 'prince of verse', reflecting the ideals of mastery of Sanskrit texts) and his students. This system was gradually eroded during the nineteenth century (Gupta, 1998). The prospect of better employment opportunities and improved financial status after training in newly founded schools of Western medicine is one of the reasons cited for its collapse as young blood was lured (through scholarships and incentives) away from the tols. The new British policy stated in T. B. Macaulay's *Minute on Indian Education* (1835) in part stimulated the reorganization of the ayurvedic profession in Bengal and elsewhere in India (Gupta, 1998; Langford, 2002). Previously the British intention had been to expose the errors of Indian knowledge through their own languages and disciplines; now the British officially abandoned altogether the idea of 'supporting' Indian knowledge, including ayurveda and tibb. In practice, however, there was more ambiguity; concerns about the spread of medical care, plus the need for vaccination and the compilation of vital statistics in rural areas meant that

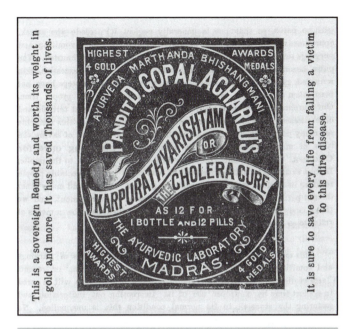

Advertisement for Pandit D. Gopalacharlu's Ayurvedic cholera cure. Halftone illustration from *Ayurvedic Medicines prepared by Ayurveda Marthanda Bhishangmani Pandit D. Gopalacharlu . . .* 1909. Wellcome Library, London.

indigenous medical traditions received some measure of institutional support from provincial governments.

Some indigenous practitioners perceived the change of direction by the British as a watershed, which led to invigorated efforts to organize their profession. Gangadhara Ray Kabiraja opened a tol in Shaidabad (Berhampore), where he educated a number of influential students in the 1830s (Gupta, 1998). Successive generations of his students, such as Gangaprasad Sen, Bijoyratna Sen, and Jaminibhusan Ray, were instrumental in changing the nature of ayurvedic practice in Bengal. These and others, such as Gananath Sen and Chandrakishore Sen, were involved in numerous professional activities: translating key ayurvedic texts into Bengali; publishing journals; opening pharmacies and dispensing ayurvedic drugs along Western lines; introducing disciplines of Western anatomy, surgery and midwifery; and institutionalizing ayurveda in Western-style colleges with integrated curricula. These innovations in Bengali ayurveda were paralleled somewhat in Kerala, where P. S. Varrier established the famous Aryavaidyashala in Kottakal in the early twentieth century in order to commercialize and institutionalize the practice of ayurveda.

During the latter half of the nineteenth century new forms of unani and ayurvedic literature emerged. Journals, self-help pamphlets, and advertising brochures were written in vernacular languages (Hindi, Urdu, Bengali, etc.) by practitioners lacking any formal association with the learned traditions and aimed at those unused to reading about ṭibb or ayurveda. In the case of ṭibb, recent work by Seema Alavi clearly shows how Urdu literature created the bedrock for a

new popularized unani ṭibb and that vernacular newspapers were instrumental in the process of carrying debates about knowledge of ṭibb in the colonial era into the public sphere (Alavi, 2005). Publishing houses, such as Naval Kishor in Lucknow and others in metropolitan centers from Lahore in Punjab to Calcutta in Bengal, were crucial in this dissemination. The flourishing of *ishtihārī atibbā* (advertising physicians) and the success of new classes of physicians using the print medium played an important role motivating elite hereditary unani tabibs to institutionalize their practices in Lucknow, under the leadership of Abd ul-Aziz, who established the Madrasa Takmil ut-Tibb in 1902. The same was largely true in Delhi for another famous family of unani practitioners, the Sharifi, who opened the Madrasa Tibbiya in 1889. Other unani schools were opened in Hyderabad in 1891, in Bhopal in 1902, and later the largest state-run unani hospital and teaching institution in India—the Nizamia Tibbi College in 1939. Unani qualifications, the first of their kind, were issued from Lahore in the 1870s under the aegis of the Punjab government. During a similar period, ayurvedic institutions were also being founded in centers such as Benares, Lahore, Delhi, Jamnagar, Patiala, and Jaipur. This process of institution building was accelerated after legislative reforms in British India in 1919. Some of these colleges taught curricula including Western surgery, anatomy, physiology, pathology, and chemistry, which caused divisions between those who favored integration and those seeking to maintain the integrity of earlier traditions. Practitioners of official ayurveda and ṭibb undertook pharmacological research on their materia medica along the lines of biomedical science, and they had the same institutional structures.

Growing literacy rates during the late nineteenth-century among elites and middle classes also encouraged the emergence of women as professional practitioners of ṭibb and ayurveda. Unani schools, which trained midwives and taught women, were opened in Bhopal, Delhi, and Allahabad during the early twentieth century. Currently there are more women than men training to be unani physicians in Pakistan's most prestigious unani institution, the Faculty of Eastern Medicine at the Hamdard University. This institution was set up by unani's leading advocate in Pakistan, Hakīm Muhammad Said, whose brother Hakīm Abd ul-Hamid had developed the Indian branch of Hamdard (waqf), the largest unani pharmaceutical company and private teaching college in post-Independence India.

There is tension nonetheless in this negotiation of modernity, as revealed in the different domains of authenticity, which exist in parallel and merge. The modern is invoked through the professional qualification, but pulse reading (in ṭibb, ayurveda, and siddha) necessitates experience beyond the technological domain of biomedicine. The distinction between the institutional graduate and the hereditary practitioner becomes stronger in this context, since, in the case of unani, pulse reading is no longer systematically taught in the curricula of unani colleges in India; a similar lack of attention to traditional diagnostic modalities prevails in ayurvedic colleges. Much of unani private practice has also discarded the interventions and diagnostic techniques of earlier periods, such as urine and stool diagnosis, leeching, cupping, enemas, and bloodletting, in favor of pharmacy. For some ayurvedic practitioners the concept of *doṣa* (the three morbid states, the balancing or neutralization of which leads to health) in ayurveda is impervious to the quantification demanded of medical science, but others, such as Gananath Sen, the famous Bengali kabirāj (practitioner) of the late nineteenth and early twentieth century, framed these forces in the language of medical science: *vāyu* ('wind') he equated with the function of cell development; *pitta* ('bile') with metabolism; *kappha* ('phlegm') with cooling and mucal producing functions (Langford, 2002, pp. 150–151).

Contemporary ayurveda and tibb have been shaped by cultural and religious nationalism—ayurveda has come to represent for some a pure, semispiritualized cure for the ills and stresses of modernity (Langford, 2002, pp. 150–151). One common strategy used among tibb's practitioners to find a distinctive place in the medical marketplace has been to project tibb as a natural healing system, whose treatments are devoid of the harmful side effects associated with allopathic pharmaceuticals. Tibb's position, however, is more ambiguous in the sense that it has been projected simultaneously as an Islamic tradition and also a secular 'scientific' discipline. Many of its practitioners complain of marginalization in state-supported health care provision since Independence. Notwithstanding this claim, both tibb and ayurveda have been shaped by the exigencies of state-funded health care provision in colonial and postcolonial India, especially in rural areas. Standardized curricula were introduced following the establishment of the Central Council for Indian Medicine in 1971. These curricula have given little place for instruction in traditional diagnostic skills.

The market has also driven the transformation of ayurvedic and tibbi practices. The commercialization of ayurveda and tibb, begun in the late nineteenth century, has accelerated rapidly during the last thirty years. The brands of ayurvedic and unani pharmaceutical companies Dabur, Zandu and Hamdard (waqf) are household names in the subcontinent, and they are exported throughout the world. Their annual income exceeds the budget granted by the government of India to 'Indian Systems of Medicine' (Bode, 2004). These products are in many ways marginalizing the place of the hakīm and the vaid in their traditional face-to-face encounters with patients, particularly in urban settings. Electuaries, powders, and decoctions may still be made by hakīms, but they are increasingly giving way to over-the-counter products no longer catered to individual temperaments as they once were. The public has also played a significant role in the process of the change from home-produced remedies to mass-produced pharmaceuticals through the purchase of seductive, attractively packaged, standardized products. Nevertheless, hakīms and vaids continue

to occupy an important place in health care provision for South Asia's population in the countryside. In urban areas, they may be seen as 'a last resort' after patients' failures to find a cure through allopathic (Western) medicines, or the first point of call because of a reputation for treating specific conditions. While emergency medicine and the treatment of acute disease has been largely removed from the realm of ayurvedic and unani practice, vaids and hakīms continue to fulfill important and widely sought roles dealing with chronic and degenerative illnesses across all sections of society.

In rural areas, folk medical cultures have been more prevalent than the learned streams of South Asia's medical traditions. It is estimated that in India there are 1.4 million folk healers, and millions of people who possess deep knowledge of home remedies (Shankar and Unnikrishnan, 2004). Such knowledge is embedded in local concepts of lifestyle, diet, and cultural practices. Practitioners of orally transmitted health traditions include traditional birth attendants, bonesetters, a great variety of herbal healers (who may specialize, for example, in the treatment of conditions of the eyes, ears, and skin, nervous disorders, and snake-bites) and those who treat animals. Communities sustain these practices; they have no legal status and exist without the aid of any institution or state support. People resort to them in addition to other medical options that may be available, such as pharmaceutical products. The few microstudies on folk medicinal practices suggest, however, that this knowledge is being eroded. One study found that the average age of practitioners was over forty across many specialisms in a district of Maharashtra (western India), which points to decreasing interest in, or viability of, these practices and will lead to problems in the continued transmission of such orally-based knowledge (cited in Shankar and Unnikrishnan, 2004, p. 10). The erosion of folk knowledge is further indicated by decreasing awareness of the uses of medicinal plants at a popular level, even though once commonly used plants (or rather, derivatives thereof) are now being patented by scientists from outside the region. Darshan Shankar and P. M. Unnikrishnan of the Foundation for the Revitalisation of Local Health Traditions (FRLHT) in Bangalore illustrate this with the case of a plant *kīranzhelli* (Tamil) (*Phyllanthus amarus*) formerly, but not currently, widely used for the treatment of jaundice in southern India and successfully patented in 1987 for the safe treatment of hepatitis B and C. Examples such as this substantiate the authors' claim that the lack of research and support for folk medicinal knowledge reflects on the economic, political, and cultural currents that have informed policymaking decisions on health care in the region, and not on the question of the efficacy of folk uses of medicinal plants. Through documentation, research, and educational activities, the FRLHT is spearheading the effort to awaken interest in folk medical knowledge and put it on the agenda of health policymakers in India, alongside support for the formal medical traditions and biomedical structures.

Bibliography

Abdul Hameed, Hakim, and Hakim Abdul Bari, 1984. 'Impact of Ibn Sina's Medical Work in India.' *Studies in History of Medicine* 8: 1–12; Alavi, Seema, 2005. 'Unani Medicine in the Nineteenth-Century Public Sphere: Urdu Texts and the Oudh Akhbar'. *Indian Economic and Social History Review* 42: 101–129; Alter, Joseph S., 2000. *Gandhi's Body: Sex, Diet, and the Politics of Nationalism* (Philadelphia); Arnold, David, and Sumit Sarkar, 2002. 'In Search of Rational Remedies: Homeopathy in Nineteenth-Century Bengal' in Ernst, Waltraud, ed., *Plural Medicine, Tradition and Modernity, 1800–2000* (London) pp. 40–57; Azmi, Altaf Ahmed, 2001. 'Unani Medicine: Hakims and Their Treatises' in Subbarayappa, Bidare V., ed., *Medicine and Life Sciences in India* (New Delhi) pp. 326–370; Babu, Suresh, 2003. *Over View [sic] of Nāḍīparīkṣā [the pulse study] from Past to Present Times* (Varanasi); Basham, A. L., 1998 (1st publ. 1976). 'The Practice of Medicine in Ancient and Medieval India' in Leslie, Charles, ed., *Asian Medical Systems* (Delhi) pp. 18–43; Bode, Maarten, 2004. 'Ayurvedic and Unani Health and Beauty Products: Reworking India's Medical Traditions.' Unpublished PhD thesis, University of Amsterdam; Daniel, E. Valentine, 1984. 'Pulse as Icon in Siddha Medicine' in Daniel, E. Valentine, and Judy Pugh, eds., *South Asian Systems of Healing* (Leiden) pp. 115–126; De Michelis, Elizabeth, 2004. *A History of Modern Yoga: Patañjali and Western Esoterism* (London); Faruqi, A. H., 1985. 'Tibb-i Shahābī, a Rare Medical Treatise of Tughlaq Period.' *Studies in History of Medicine and Science* 9: 35–42; Gupta, Brahmananda, 1998 (1st publ. 1976). 'Indigenous Medicine in Nineteenth and Twentieth-Century Bengal' in Leslie, Charles, ed., *Asian Medical Systems* (Delhi) pp. 368–378; Haas, E., 1876. 'Ueber die Ursprünge der Indischen Medizin, mit besonderem Bezug auf Suśruta.' *Zeitchrift der Deutschen Morgenländischen Gesellschaft* 30: 617–670; Hausman, Gary, 1996. 'Siddhars, Alchemy and the Abyss of Tradition: "Traditional" Tamil Medical Knowledge in "Modern" Practice.' Unpublished PhD thesis, University of Michigan; Hume, John C., 1977. 'Rival Traditions: Western Medicine and Yunan-i Tibb in the Punjab, 1849–1889.' *Bulletin of the History of Medicine* 51: 214–231; Jaggi, Om Prakash, 1977. *Medicine in Medieval India* (Delhi); Jee, Bhagvat Sinh, 1896. *A Short History of Aryan Medical Science* (London); Kakar, Sudhir, 1982. *Shamans, Mystics and Doctors: A Psychological Enquiry into India and Its Healing Traditions* (New York); Langford, Jean M., 2002. *Fluent Bodies: Ayurvedic Remedies for Postcolonial Imbalance* (Durham); Liebeskind, Claudia, 1997. 'Unani Medicine of the Subcontinent' in van Alphen, Jan, and Anthony Aris, eds., *Oriental Medicine: An Illustrated Guide to the Asian Healing Arts* (Boston) pp. 39–65; Majumdar, R. C., 1971. 'Medicine' in Bose D. M., S. N. Sen, and B. V. Subbarayappa, eds., *A Concise History of Science in India* (New Delhi) pp. 213–267; Meulenbeld, G. Jan, 1991–1992. 'The Many Faces of Ayurveda.' *Ancient Science of Life* 11: 106–113; Meulenbeld, G. Jan, 1999+. *A History of Indian Medical Literature* 5 vols. (Groningen); Ming, Zhu, and Felix Klein-Franke, 1998. 'Avicenna's Links with Chinese Medicine: A Chapter in the History of Sino-Arabic Relations during the Middle Ages.' *Asian Medicine Newsletter* December: 2–5; Pearson, M. N., 1995. 'The Thin End of the Wedge: Medical Relativities as a Paradigm of Early Modern Indian-European Relations.' *Modern Asian Studies* 29: 141–170; Rai, N. P., S. K. Tiwari, S. D. Upadhya, and G. N. Chaturvedi, 1979. 'The Origin and Development of Pulse Examination in Medieval India.' *Studies in History of Medicine* 3: 110–124; Reddy, Subba D. V., 1957. 'Dar us-Sifa Built by Sultan Muhammad Quli: The First Unani Teaching Hospital in the Deccan.' *Indian Journal of History of Medicine* 2: 102–105; Rezavi, S. Nadeem, 2001. 'Physicians as Professionals in Medieval India' in Kumar, Deepak, ed., *Disease and Medicine in Society: A Historical Overview* (New Delhi) pp. 40–65; Roṣu, Arion, 1982. 'Le renouveau contemporain de l'Āyurveda.' *Wiener Zeitschrift für die Kunde Südasiens* 26: 59–82; Sastry, P. V. Parabrahma, 1977. 'Epigraphic Allusion to Surgery in Ayurveda' *Bulletin of the Indian Institute of History of Medicine* 7: 127–130; Saxena, Nirmal, 2000. *Vaidya jīvana of Lolimbarāja: Text, English Translation, Notes, Historical Introduction, Comments, Index and Appendixes* (Varanasi); Scharfe, Hartmut, 1999. 'The Doctrine of the Three Humors in Traditional Indian Medicine and the Alleged Antiquity of Tamil Siddha Medicine.' *Journal of the American Oriental Society* 119: 609–629; Shankar, Darshan, and P. M. Unnikrishnan, eds., 2004. *Challenging the Indian Medical Heritage* (New Delhi); Sharma, Priya Vrat, 1979. 'Contributions of Sharngadhara in the Field of Materia Medica and Pharmacy.' *Studies in History of Medicine* 3: 13–21; Siddiqi, M. Z., 1971. 'The Unani Tibb (Greek medicine) in India' in Bose, D. M., S. N. Sen, and B. V. Subbarayappa, eds., *A Concise History of Science in India* (New Delhi) pp. 268–273; Sigaléa, Robert, 1995. *La Médecine Traditionelle de l'Inde: Doctrines Prévédique, Védique, Āyurvédique, Yogique et Tantrique: les Empereurs Moghols, leurs Maladies et leurs Médecins* (Geneva); Speziale, Fabrizio, 2005. 'Linguistic Strategies of de-Islamization and Colonial Science: Indo-Muslim Physicians and the Yunani Denomination.' *International Institute for Asian Studies Newsletter* 34: 18; Speziale, Fabrizio, 2003. 'Tradition and Modernization of Islamic Psychiatric Care in the Subcontinent.' *International Institute for Asian Studies Newsletter* 34: 30; Subbarayappa, Bidare V., 2001, 'Siddha Medicine' in Subbarayappa, Bidare V., ed., *Medicine and Life Sciences in India* (New Delhi) pp. 427–451; White, David G., 1996. *The Alchemical Body: Siddha Traditions in Medieval India* (Chicago); Wise, T. A., 1845. *Commentary on the Hindu System of Medicine* (Calcutta); Wujastyk, Dominik, 1993. 'Indian Medicine' in Bynum, William F., and Roy Porter, eds., *Companion Encyclopedia of the History of Medicine* (London) pp. 755–778; Wujastyk, Dominik, 2003. 'Indian Medical Thought on the Eve of Colonialism.' *International Institute of Asian Studies Newsletter* 31: 21; Zillur Rahman, Syed, 2001. 'Indian Hakims: Their Role in the Medical Care of India,' in Subbarayappa, Bidare V., ed., *Medicine and Life Sciences in India* (New Delhi) pp. 371–426; Zimmermann, Francis, 1978. 'From Classic Texts to Learned Practices: Methodological Remarks on the Study of Indian Medicine.' *Social Science and Medicine* 12: 97–103; Zimmermann, Francis, 1999 (1st publ. 1982). *The Jungle and the Aroma of Meats: An Ecological Theme in Hindu Medicine* (Delhi); Zysk, Kenneth, 1998 (1st publ. 1991). *Asceticism and Healing in Ancient India: Medicine in the Buddhist Monastery* (Delhi).

Guy Attewell

MEDICAL TRADITIONS IN SOUTHEAST ASIA: FROM SYNCRETISM TO PLURALISM

Everyone has heard of Chinese medicine, Indian Ayurvedic medicine, and Arab-Islamic medicine (*unani*). Most of us are aware that these great systems of medical thought, rooted in Asia, have a rich written corpus of principles and practices perfected over the centuries. They have intersected and enriched one another, and given rise to other medical traditions, which incorporate sociocultural or historical features unique to a given ethnic or national space, e.g., Tibetan, Japanese, or Turkish medicine. What do we know about the Southeast Asian variants of these traditions? To what degree is there a Vietnamese, Thai, Laotian, or Filipino medical tradition?

Many of us will think immediately of the famous Thai massage, or of *jamu*, two of a number of fashionable practices that are part of an increasing Western fascination with so-called natural therapies. This sort of practice, taken out of its therapeutic and cultural context, hardly paints a worthy portrait of a genuine Southeast Asian medical tradition. Such a portrait would be useful because of the revival of traditional medicine under the well-meaning or pragmatic auspices of the World Health Organization (WHO), which since the 1980s has encouraged 'traditional medicine'* in

---

*My choice of terms does not constitute a judgment of any of these medical traditions, or an endorsement of any particular norm. By 'medical tradition' I do not mean to oppose 'tradition' to 'modernity'; I wish to describe in a neutral way the historical medical heritage of a particular sociocultural space. 'Medical system' suggests the cultural and dynamic character of beliefs, knowledge, and practices at the professional and lay levels, interacting in a space open to diverse influences (Kleinman, 1991). The terms 'healer' and 'practitioner' have no pejorative intent but distinguish local practitioners from health professionals created with the rise of nineteenth-century biomedicine.

many national health systems as part of the primary health care initiative. Moreover, we are currently experiencing a widespread rediscovery of traditional medicines, and we are learning what these traditions have to tell us about basic medical principles, disease, and treatment. Finally, a greater knowledge of Southeast Asian medical traditions would be welcome because we are analyzing their contents and proper use as the hegemony of Western biomedicine is contested. Before responding to these questions it is worth noting that the major volumes consulted on 'Asian medical traditions' do not raise these issues and therefore give the impression that Southeast Asia has no medical traditions of its own (Brelet, 2002; Alphen and Aris, 1996; Leslie and Young, 1992; Huard et al., 1978).

SOUTHEAST ASIA: BETWEEN HOMOGENEITY AND HETEROGENEITY

We begin by noting the complex identity of the Southeast Asian region. A product of geopolitical reflections and reflexes, Southeast Asia today contains elements of both homogeneity and heterogeneity, illustrated by a simple listing of the member countries. Viewed historically, Singapore, Vietnam, Myanmar (Burma), Thailand, Malaysia, Indonesia (and East Timor), Brunei, Cambodia, Laos, and the Philippines are countries with artificial and changing borders, constituting a huge ethnic, religious, and cultural mosaic.

The term Southeast Asia came into common use during World War II. Before this, the area was seen as part of the cultural colonies of its large neighbors India and China, particularly India. If we exclude the exceptional case of Singapore, Vietnam is the only country in the region that is part of the *sinic* world, and thus belongs both to Southeast Asia and East Asia. In 1948, Coedès still referred to 'Hinduised states'. These were the products of an Indianization defined by the expansion of a structured culture based on the Indian state and royal leadership, the spread of Buddhist and Hindu faiths, and the use of Sanskrit. This Indianization took on different forms and achieved varied results according to the region in question; this was due partly to the differing impact in time and space of other major cultural factors, particularly religious (Mahayana and Hinayana Buddhism, Islam, Christianity) and philosophical traditions (Confucianism, Daoism).

The extraordinary cultural vehicle of Buddhism, as an agent both of Indianization and of Sinicization, also illustrates the degree to which the region's identity has been shaped by its strategic geographic position, the impact of population movements and human exchanges, and the omnipresence of water providing a multitude of navigable routes. Before the nineteenth century, Southeast Asia was sparsely populated; its inhabitants were concentrated mainly in large cities and areas of wet rice cultivation. With the development of city-states and an increase in commerce and trade, important changes occurred in the region (Reid, 1988). Islam, which made its initial penetration into the Far East in the Malaysian peninsula during the seventh century, became a major political and social force in the region from the fourteenth century onward. These changes, affecting the size and distribution of native populations, and their living and working conditions, were altered again after contact with the West began in the sixteenth century. The immigration of Arab, Chinese, and South Asian people in the wake of the expansion of a European (Iberian, then Dutch, then English) 'capitalistic' economy contributed to the evolution of a 'plural society' (Evers, 2001, pp. 14662–14663).

This plural society incorporates ancient indigenous populations, which have persisted. The native Southeast Asians are divided into five principal ethno-linguistic families, making Southeast Asia one of the richest and most varied regions of the world on this front. There are numerous regional belief systems, including animistic traditions, which continue to influence local social practices. The roller-coaster histories of what are now Vietnam, Cambodia, Thailand, Malaysia, and Indonesia—alternating periods of grandeur and decline continually recasting national boundaries throughout the region—reveal the importance of the internal-external dynamic, even if one agrees with Reid (1988) that up to the pre-modern period, interregional ties were generally more important than ties with people beyond the region. Southeast Asian medicine offers a privileged approach to an understanding of the region's sociocultural diversity and the idea and implications of syncretism. Medical syncretism refers to a medical culture in which the norms associated with several medical systems are added to existing knowledge and practices even as the additions continue to be recognized as such. This gives rise to processes of acculturation but also practices of medical pluralism in which several systems of health care are put into use simultaneously or in succession, according to individual or collective judgments based on representations of illness, health, death, the body, and experience. As Owen (1987, p.17) has indicated, 'a feature of the Southeast Asian's traditional response to disease is syncretism'.

Southeast Asian medicine is characterized by the number of its local traditions, sufficiently varied in time and space to make irrelevant the recent boundaries of the region's nation-states. Such indigenous traditions represent local histories of the diffusion, exchange, and blending of the great traditions with indigenous knowledge, beliefs, and experiences. The object here is not to unravel these complex histories, trying to distinguish imported from local; that is an exercise as meaningless as it is impossible to carry out. It is better to re-examine certain hasty characterizations (such as the frequent identification of Vietnamese with Chinese medicine) and try instead to identify the principal commonalities of these traditions, notwithstanding the distance between medical theories and health practices, and the importance of local conditions for the history and culture of each country.

Our primary resource will be anthropological scholarship on Southeast Asia, a dynamic if scattered research field, resembling the region itself. Such ethnography originated in modern colonial scientific exploration and orientalism, gained momentum in the 1960s, and achieved maturity in the 1990s. It has strengths and weaknesses, providing extremely detailed observations of individual villages or communities (e.g., the superb work of Gimlette, 1939, on the Malay medical world), but at the same time failing to provide even a minimal vision of the whole or place its observations in the kind of chronological order indispensable to historical understanding. The limited historical work on the subject in no way compensates for these lacunae and has been slowed by the limited number of extant written sources about traditions often transmitted orally or in secret. The sources that do exist do little to complete the ethnological work, historical studies having essentially analyzed royal medical traditions and the theories underpinning them.

The available sources set the tone for this essay. It will necessarily be more anthropological than historical and limited to an illustration of the dynamic mix of homogeneity and diversity, as discussed above, for our period extending mostly from the second half of the nineteenth century to today.

NOT ONE BUT MANY MEDICAL TRADITIONS

One common feature in the medical history of Southeast Asia is the absence of a shared theory of medicine despite evidence of all the great Asian medical traditions, especially Ayurvedic medicine, Chinese medicine, and Arab-Islamic medicine. Without attempting to evaluate the specific contributions of each of these traditions (scholarly debates continue over the links between these traditions and the genealogical relationships between Greek, Hippocratic, and other traditions), it is interesting to note that certain scholars also insist on the importance of a fourth tradition, that of Buddhist medicine, in the zone of Southeast Asia comprising Cambodia, Laos, Thailand, and Burma (Chhem, 2001; Souk-Aloun, 2001). This Buddhist medicine, according to these scholars, developed in the shadow of Ayurvedic medicine, following the formalization of Indian Hinayana Buddhism, and was disseminated in the Pali language by monks. Among the important emblems of this medical tradition one finds Jivaka (Komarabhacca), an Indian Buddhist monk of the fifth or sixth century BCE, still considered as the 'father' of Thai traditional medicine.

ROYAL TRADITIONS

These great medical traditions, having come from abroad, were acknowledged in the region as 'royal' urban traditions in the sense that the theories on which they were based, and the ideas that they disseminated, were transmitted and practiced within an elite minority of the population: the royalty and aristocracy, and the higher-ranking administrative and religious authorities. This does not mean that these doctrines had no impact on the population in general, but rather that their strict application was confined to

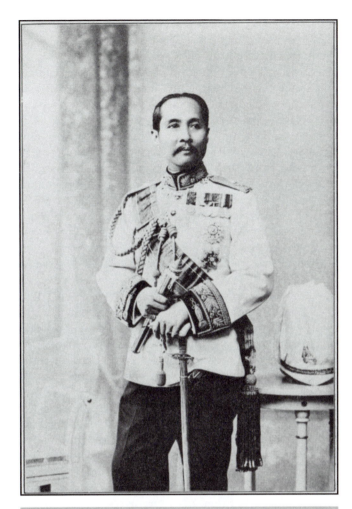

His Majesty King Chulalongkorn of Siam. From *Siam: General and Medical Features*, Bangkok, 1930. Wellcome Library, London.

these elites, and that they remained *relatively* impermeable to the influences of native religions, beliefs, and indigenous practices existing prior to the Indianization, Sinicization, or Islamicization of the region.

Available sources on these royal traditions have suffered the ravages of time, and they possess a sacred character that makes a secular reading difficult, even without the formidable problems of dating the texts (Balinese medical texts, for instance, are inscribed on lontar leaves, the dried fronds of a type of palm). These sources vary in terms of their informative value, depending on the degree of interest in medical science demonstrated by the royal court in question. In Thailand, for instance, it was not until the nineteenth century and the reigns of Rama III (1842–52) and Chulalongkorn (1867–1910) that a body of medical knowledge was made public. During Chulalongkorn's reign, a committee of royal physicians was appointed to collect and edit manuals of traditional medicine. This collection, referred to as *tamra luang* at the time, was kept in the library of the palace, available only to the court physicians. Nonetheless, it became the basic text-book (*Wedchasygsa*) for Thai students in traditional medicine from 1895 onward (Brun and Schumacher, 1987, pp. 6–7).

A large number of Buddhist and Brahmin monks figure among the chief possessors and/or transmitters of medical knowledge. The extant epigraphic sources remain among the most precious sources of information on this elite med-ical world and its workings, despite their almost incestuous nature and consequent bias. In Cambodia, for example, an inscription from Bantay Srei refers to Yajnavaraha, the guru of king Jayavarman V, who was the foremost proponent of the various doctrines, including that of medicine. The Stele of Loley reflects a period from the eighth to the early ninth century and confirms the influence of the king Yasho-varman (the founder of the Angkor site) in creating an atmosphere favorable to the development of Cambodian medicine; the king himself played an important role as a healer on several occasions (Pandey, 1997, pp. 160–163).

The medical treatises that have been preserved, and which contain for the most part formulas (remedies and incanta-tions), information concerning their therapeutic uses, and dis-cussions of certain ailments, reveal the pre-eminence of the Ayurvedic and Buddhist traditions. Among the most famous treatises are two Indonesian manuscripts. The *Serat Kawruh bab Jampi-jampi* [A Treatise on All Manner of Cures] includes 1,734 *Jamu* formulas together with information on their use and 244 entries in the form of prayers. The *Serat Centhini* (known as the 'Centhini's Book'), an encyclopedic poem pro-duced on the orders of a son of Kanjeng Susuhunan Pakubu-wono IV (early nineteenth century), ruler of the central Javanese kingdom of Surakarta, concerns sexual problems but also includes advice on a variety of ailments and their cures. Still, one hesitates to draw firm conclusions about this pre-eminence, given the region's extreme cultural diversity, the interweaving of East Asian medical traditions, and even the accidents of history (e.g., the book burnings carried out by the Chinese Ming dynasty, which occupied Vietnam at the begin-ning of the fifteenth century, in the course of which most Viet-namese medical treatises may well have disappeared).

To probe further into Southeast Asian medical tradi-tions, an undertaking that will also allow us to understand their continuing vitality today, we must turn to popular, rural medicine. Such medicine is not the antithesis of the elite traditions just discussed, but draws upon ancient pre-Buddhist and pre-Hindu cultural strata while adopting a variety of external influences. This process is less compli-cated than it might have been because some of these exter-nal influences already utilized indigenous traditions (Laderman, 1992, pp. 272–274; Golomb, 1985, p. 49).

LAY TRADITIONS

Most scholars agree that the recurring exchanges with India, China, and the Arab world implanted in Southeast Asia certain representations of disease and of healing prac-tices. Itinerant merchants and religious missionaries (often combined in the same person) were eager to make use of their healing arts to convert Southeast Asian populations to their religion (Hart, 1969). Given that their main goal was religious conversion, there was no hesitation about straying from orthodoxy in order to endear themselves to those they sought to convert. Magical, esoteric, and exorcistic prac-tices, myths and the narration of miracles and mysteries, cooption of local polytheistic and animist beliefs: all were grist for the mill (Geertz, 1968). In certain political con-texts, it was the rejection of conversion, and the resulting migrations, that shaped an original medical tradition. For example, in the late tenth century, the influence of Javanese culture began to spread to the neighboring island of Bali, where it found support under the powerful Hindu king-dom of Majapahit. During the mid-fourteenth century, the Javanese kingdom brought Bali under its control. Follow-ing the adoption of Islam and subsequent breakup of the Majapahit Empire in the late fifteenth century, many Jav-anese, including many Brahmin priests, fled to Bali, taking their books and customs with them. Subsequently the pop-ulation of Bali remained isolated until the Dutch coloniza-tion at the turn of the twentieth century. This accident of history apparently explains why Balinese healing—like Balinese culture—frequently mirrors that of Java four hun-dred years earlier (De Beers, 2002, pp.13–14; Connor, 1986, pp. 15–19).

Whether the result of pre-existing native culture, or of the linkage posited by missionaries between the realms of medicine, magic, and religion, foreign proselytizers and native converts apparently shared a holistic approach to man and valorized a constant search for harmony between man (microcosm) and the world (macrocosm), between what the Balinese call the 'small world' (*buana alit*) and the 'great world' (*buana agung*). This worldview resonates with individual and collective health management. A refusal to distinguish between physiology, anatomy, and psychology, and an emphasis on the continuity between body and spirit, championed the idea of the vital breath (Indian *prâna*, Chinese *qi*). This notion is defined differently according to the region or ethnic group in question, but a vital breath possessed by all animate beings bridges the gap between macrocosm and microcosm.

In man, this breath, the motor-force of the bodily fluids, animates the vascular system through the beating of the pulse. Sphygmology (pulse based diagnosis), unknown to Hippocrates but present in Ayurvedic medicine before being adopted by Chinese medicine, came to be the very basis for the diagnosis and prognosis of disease. At the macro level, the vital breath takes the form of the presence of spirits with which man is familiar but which require his careful management. In particular, the omnipresence of the doctrine of souls (Bamber, 1993) sees the material body as inhabited by numerous souls and vital spirits of variable importance: Khmers, for instance, believe that there are

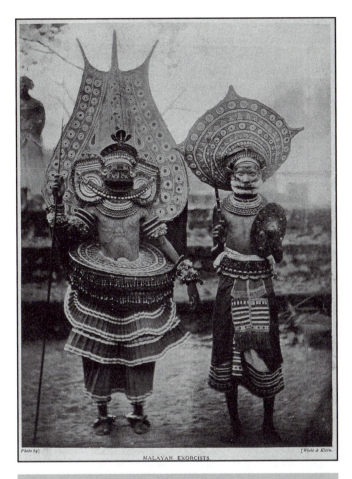

Malaysian exorcists in ritual costume. Process print, late 19th century. Iconographic Collection, Wellcome Library, London.

nineteen souls, the most important of which are found in the head (Chhem, 2001). Even if these souls inhabit the human body, they are not confined to it: they can be captured by witches or by malevolent spirits. This explains certain diseases and justifies certain forms of therapeutic treatment, e.g., the rite of *hauv praloeng*. Westerners would describe these magico-religious concepts (possession rituals, shamanism) as a-medical, but their importance in societies strongly influenced by Hinayana Buddhism (itself influencing certain popular representations of illness and how to treat disease) is not in doubt.

The holistic approach to health in Southeast Asia, and the widely diffused belief in the resonance between the individual and the universe, remind us of the important role in the popular medical traditions of elements related to theories of humors, particularly the theory of elements and the related idea of balance, which determines the existence or absence of disease. The widespread cultural embrace of the opposition of hot and cold and the fundamental role accorded to food in health and medicine came to be added to these original notions, variously shaped by the historical and cultural particularities of the diverse regional societies.

Thus, the Burmese and Lao believe that the thirty-two component parts of the body are grouped under the five Ayurvedic elements (earth, water, fire, air, and ether, or 'wind in empty cavities'), each element linked to a physiological process and internal organs. By contrast, for the Khmer or Thai, there are only four elements (water, fire, earth, and air or wind), as for Hippocrates. Some scholars insist that the fifth element (ether) is secondary rather than absent, particularly in northern Thailand (Brun and Schumacher, 1987) and Laos (Souk-Aloun, 2001, p. 7). Some Khmer communities replace fire and earth by hot and cold, which we also find in traditional Malay medicine. The Indian Tridosa doctrine, found almost everywhere in the region, attributes the origin of diseases to perturbations in the balance of the three bodily humors (bile, wind, and mucus, or phlegm). The wind (volatile and easily influenced in terms of both quantity and quality) constitutes the most vital bodily element throughout the region. It is the origin of the most severe perturbations in the body's balance; it causes serious diseases ('wind illnesses') or those that are diagnostically difficult. The concept of wind illness does not always refer to the same diseases, which range from symptoms of the common cold among Indonesians and Malays to fainting, dizziness, or leprosy among mainland Southeast Asian peoples (Bamber, 1993, p. 430). Among the Redjang of southwestern Sumatra, wind is believed to cause chills, influenza, bronchitis, pneumonia, and other diseases of the broncho-respiratory tract, as well as febrile states, accompanied by headache, muscular discomfort, general lassitude, and loss of strength (Jaspan, 1969, pp. 13–16). In Vietnam and Cambodia, wind illness is the result of the entry of wind into the body according to the Chinese tradition, in which wind is not an element of the human body (Craig, 2002, pp. 44–46). Moreover, we often find in what are called 'pneumatic systems' (Sassady, 1962) a close connection between wind and blood. Blood is recognized as the basic bodily fluid, although the concept of a circulatory system is usually not well understood. The wind may somehow spread anywhere in the body with the blood, producing modifications in its nature, and is potentially pathogenic (Brun and Schumacher, 1987, p. 70).

Turning more specifically to the dominant etiological concepts in the region, we note that disease or imbalance can be either 'personalistic' (i.e., supernatural or specific) or 'naturalistic' (i.e., general or natural). Personalistic etiologies refer to the belief that all misfortune, including disease, is a punishment, resulting from an immoral or antisocial action, or from interpersonal conflicts, via the intervention of ancestors or angry spirits. Consequently, 'bad karma' is often reinterpreted as the result of the hatred of an irritated spirit who causes certain incurable diseases, such as leprosy (Pottier, 1972, pp. 181–182). Naturalistic systems explain illness in impersonal and systemic terms, related to the intervention of natural forces or conditions. Among natural causes of disease we find the influence of the climate and the seasons, the influence of the natural environment, of age, of gender, of life habits (diet, bodily hygiene, excessive consumption of alcohol or of psychotropic drugs), in addition to germs, a theory of disease that came to be accepted with European colonization over the course of the nineteenth century, as we will explore further below.

In addition, certain societies insist on other possible causes of disease: physical abuse of the body or accidents and trauma among the Bisayan Filipinos (Hart, 1969, p. 13), and excessive demands on one's physical or mental energies among the Thai (Golomb, 1985, p. 129). For the Brunei Malays most accidents and some ailments result from *kapunan*. A person in the state of *kapunan*, most commonly resulting from an unfulfilled desire for food, is apt to be harmed, meaning that he or she will encounter whatever harm is lurking nearby (Kimball, 1979, p. 3). The idea of poisoning is also widely shared. In northern Thailand, the word *pid* means poison or venom. Eating the meat of diseased animals introduces *pid* into the body and results in disease: '*Pid* also refers to the less tangible concept of "something with the attribute of poison". . . . Spirits may for example insert *pid* into the body. . . . The presence of *pid* normally results in pain, and the disease is regarded as acute or critical and should be treated with great care' (Brun and Schumacher, 1987, p. 70).

The Thai *pid* prompts us to note again that the boundary between natural and supernatural disease remains imprecise and that one finds the two etiologies in competition in certain explanatory models of disease (Foster, 1976, pp. 773–776). Indeed, multiple etiologies are quite common in the representations of illness: a first cause can bring about a second, explaining the bodily imbalance. This can be worsened by new external or internal perturbing elements (wind, poison, etc.). The introduction of germ theories strengthened the tendency to see multiple explanations, although the idea of contagiousness— by direct contact or through heredity—already existed in the region. This does not mean that no disease is regarded as resulting from a single cause; but at the same time the hierarchy of primary cause (etiology), secondary factors producing disease (pathogeny), and predisposing factors is usually not invoked. Moreover, healers are rarely consistent in their interpretation of this complex causality, an inconsistency reinforced by the belief, widely shared throughout the region by medical practitioners and patients alike, that the experience of illness, as well as the treatment proposed to cure it, is always unique, closely linked to the individual, his activities, his environment, and his personality.

The Thai example of the *pid* also leads to a discussion of the hot/cold dichotomy, which explains illness as resulting from excessive heat or cold in the body. In fact, Southeast Asian people classify most diseases and foods according to this dichotomy, which probably finds its basis in indigenous and quite tenacious representations. The tradition, particular to Southeast Asia, of 'roasting' a woman who has recently given birth (in order for her to regain her strength or 'heat') suggests the ongoing strength of such traditions. In practice this dichotomy is diluted by the existence of intermediary categories used to describe certain foods or remedies with greater precision: 'neutral' (Bisayans, Northern Thais); 'regular' (Malays); 'neutral and bland' (Burmese); and 'neutral and benign' (Vietnamese). In the Malay Peninsula, some foods have the additional qualities of *angin* (air or flatulence) and *bisa* (allergenic or producing an ill effect). The existence of and justification for extra categories are impossible to analyze, as their definitions and uses vary immensely and without apparent logic from community to community, from region to region, and according to the differing availabilities of plants and foods.

What is clear is that the common practice of classifying diseases, foods, and remedies confirms the etiological, therapeutic, and preventive role of diet and particularly of certain foods, and the persistence of the unclear, tenuous distinction between food and medication. For example, for time immemorial, ginger has been used in most Southeast Asian cuisines to prevent certain diseases and to aid digestion, and betel nut chewing (areca nut and lime) is believed to warm the body, freshen the breath, and prevent the penetration of harmful energy through the nose and the mouth.

AN EQUALLY VARIEGATED WORLD OF PRACTITIONERS AND THERAPIES

If variety and variability are the words that best describe Southeast Asian ideas of health and conceptions of disease, the same terms apply equally well to the diversity of healers and their practices. This can be explained again by the history of medical syncretism and pluralism in the region; bearing in mind the intimate connection of the magico-religious with the strictly medical at all levels of the management of illness. It is often difficult to separate these two worlds, as prayers, rituals, amulets, and talismans accompany medical treatments. Shamans often recommend medical treatments, and Thai 'blowers' chant incantations while they put bones back in their proper place. The absence of an accessible written tradition, the importance of secrecy, and private initiation signal the distance from Western ideals, such as delimiting specialties and officially recognizing specialists as professionals who possess certain prerogatives based on specific and exclusive expertise, the result of a uniform education and some form of accreditation. However, the local populations are easily able to recognize the well-defined fields of activity of Southeast Asian medical practitioners.

THE PRACTITIONERS . . .

The world of the Indonesian *balian* (or *belian*) illustrates this reality. Although the term is generally translated

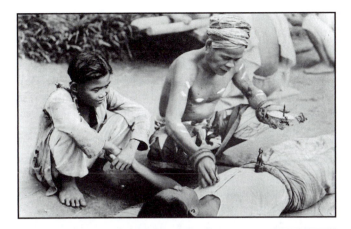

Indonesian *balian* positioning wooden dolls on a sick man's chest and abdomen. The balian's magic will drive the sickness into the dolls. Early 20th century. Wellcome Library, London.

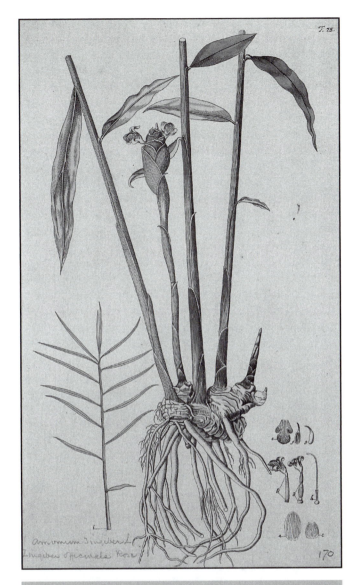

Ginger (*Zingiber officinale Roscoe*); rootstock with flowering stem and separate leaf and flower sections. Line engraving with watercolor after Franz Anton von Scheidl, 1770. Iconographic Collection, Wellcome Library, London.

as 'traditional healer', one should be careful not to adopt a biomedical definition of these healers and their functions. However, the use of this term does tell us that the Balinese perceive a common function among a diverse array of practitioners—a further reminder of the inseparability of the medical and magico-religious worlds. As Connor (1986, pp. 20–23) explains, *balians* are consecrated practitioners who perform many priestly functions, and are often highly esteemed people with some influence in the affairs of the Balinese village. *Balians* operate in a diverse range of healing practices, none of which are mutually exclusive; they include midwives, spirit mediums, masseurs, and bonesetters. They dispense advice, medicines, charms, and instructions for making offerings.

Divining (*matenung*) may be incorporated into their skills. Most *balians* were and still are commoners who are illiterate in classical texts (*usada*); indeed, their social and medical roles declined, at least for the minority close to the ruling elite, after the establishment of the Dutch colonial system.

The education of most Southeast Asian medical practitioners occurred within the private relationship between master and student or father and son, informed by aspects of the healer's individual experience, the transmission of this experience, and the valorization of secrecy. Where manuals and books of remedies do exist, they are still largely the product of private transmission, and have not been rewritten for widespread popular distribution, nor have they undergone critical editing for quality control—hence the extreme difficulty of painting an accurate historical picture of these traditions. Secrecy heals, protects the formulas that work, and establishes the authority and expertise of the healer (Kimball, 1979, p. 3). Other than following a family tradition or responding to community expectations (Golomb, 1985, pp. 75–77), most healers turned to medicine as a result of a personal experience, an illness perhaps (Brun and Schumacher, 1987, p. 45) or evidence of a power to heal or divine (Connor, 1986, p. 23). The degree of secrecy in the process of apprenticeship, practice, and transmission remained variable across the region and probably over time, too, and depended on the healers as well as the knowledge they possessed. Some healers are willing to pass on some of their medical recipes but not their incantations; in certain parts of Indonesia, learned healers (*balian usada*), those conversant with the pertinent classical texts, do not protect their knowledge from the unlearned (Connor, 1986, p. 23).

A tendency to specialization did not give rise to systematization. Many practitioners were sought for their expertise in the management of a particular disease or clientele (e.g., children), or for their mastery of a particular technique (e.g., bone setting, curing snake bites, injections). Other practitioners, usually the most well known, and perhaps the only ones to practice on a full-time basis, often demonstrated multiple fields of expertise. In other cases, it was the practice of his art, and the reception accorded to him by the local clientele, that determined the socio-professional labeling. For example 'in Elah (province of West Nusa Tenggara, Indonesia), there are at least thirty-seven *balian* . . . each of whom has his or her own area of expertise. They cure a wide range of diseases and illnesses, and as well they treat teeth, use massage for an endless list of ailments, deliver babies, produce love magic and sorcery' (Hunter, 2001, pp. 155–156).

Types of specialties tend to repeat themselves from one community or country to another, although there are interesting exceptions resulting from particularities in terms of the explanatory models of disease (nosographic categories unique to a particular community), or of local features, e.g., vegetal, religious, or climatic. In Burma, the *datsayas*, or 'dietists', limit their therapeutic interventions to regulating the patient's diet to restore the humoral balance. Patani Malays recognize a number of therapeutic specialties that they claim can be found only among local Muslims. This claim is linked to the existence of some commonly encountered external disorders, believed to be unique to the community, such as abscesses, boils, cysts, shingles, rashes, and skin discoloration. As a part of their promotion of their own healing tradition over competing Thai and Western ones, Patani Malay practitioners frequently remind patients that only they can treat such local afflictions since only they know how to identify the symptoms properly (Golomb, 1985, pp. 72–73). This last example reminds us of the ethnic and socioeconomic tensions found within this highly diverse world of Southeast Asian healers.

Herbalists are among the most frequently consulted healers in Southeast Asia, although these need to be distinguished from simple remedy vendors. Within the same region or community, there are several types of herbalist. Most often, the herbalist will have learned from his teacher the value of a certain number of substances and formulas (particular to his teacher). Over time, with the development of his practice, an increasing clientele with diverse demands, and success in treating such demands, the herbalist will increase the number of his cures, or develop a specialization. This knowledge will then be handed down to his students. The best known and the most popular herbalists are those capable of identifying medicinal plants and suggesting individualized and effective remedies (often heightened by the use of incantations) adapted to the herbalist's diagnosis made after examining the patient (Golomb, 1985, pp. 127–129; Halpern, 1964, p. 193). Most of the well-known figures in traditional medicine throughout the region were polyvalent healers possessing an impressive literary and religious education in addition to medical knowledge.

This therapeutic elite is exclusively masculine. The very few women working as healers in Southeast Asia concentrate on the management of supernatural illnesses. Connor's work (1986) on Jero Tapakan is an illuminating homage to a female medium in Bali. Alternatively, women function within very narrow specializations, linked to subaltern functions, their practices supplementing the principal interventions of male healers. Often they are midwives or involved in the health of children. In northern Thailand, the 'swinger' is a female practitioner who finds the cause of young children's ailments. Women are also implicated in the harvesting and sale of medicinal herbs. On her daily rounds, the *jamu gendong* usually carries four or five popular *jamu* that maintain or improve health and strength. *Jamu gendong* in Indonesia and especially in Central Java collected and sold herbs, but they never diagnosed disease or treated the sick (De Beers, 2002, pp. 129–130). This does not minimize their usefulness or their social position, which were and continue to be considerable, particularly in providing primary care.

. . . AND THEIR PRACTICES

The diagnostic method used by most practitioners shares some similarities with that of Western biomedicine, even if the theoretical context is quite different. It is based on interrogation and examination of the patient. The interrogation elucidates the patient's history (particularly the medical history), the duration and nature of the symptoms, taboos that might have been broken, and dreams, which might be relevant. The physical examination usually consists of pulse taking on the Ayurvedic model to evaluate the circulation of the vital breath and also to verify the body temperature (usually measured on the forehead or the thorax) or the cooling of the extremities. The eyes, the tongue, the skin, the stools, and the urine can also be part of the examination. While mediums and shamans sometimes obtain such information through divination, some, such as the Bisayan Filipino shamans, also take their patient's pulse. Their taking of the pulse is sometimes metaphorical. Hart recounts in his work 'the shaman most respected by Caticuganers claimed he could diagnose the sickness of a villager by feeling the pulse of the messenger who came to fetch him to the patient' (Hart, 1969, p. 15).

The therapeutic practices employed aimed to restore or protect the patient's normal condition or balance by counteracting the injurious influences impinging upon the body or psyche. Such practices include forms of massage, acupressure/acupuncture, moxibustion, cupping, and coin rubbing, the latter common among Vietnamese populations, certain ethnic minorities such as the Hmongs, and in the Chinese diasporas. Yoga and other 'corporal techniques', along with diet and physical exercises, were all considered valuable tools for preventing disease and maintaining the body's strength. In this respect, it is important to appreciate that certain practices are carried out within

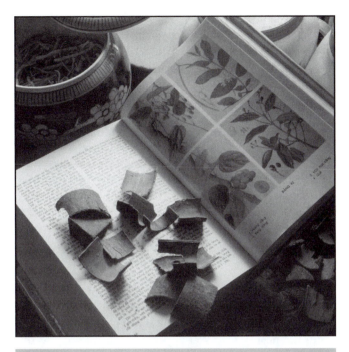

Herbal book and medicinal herbs used in Vietnamese traditional medicine, Hanoi, Vietnam. Photograph by Mark de Fraeye, Wellcome Photo Library.

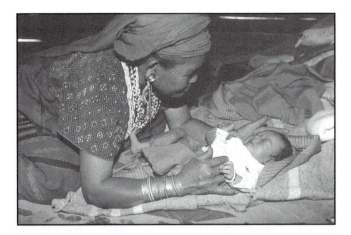

Traditional birthing attendant in rural Thailand wearing the decorative beads and bangles of her profession caresses a baby. Photograph by N. Durrell McKenna. Wellcome Photo Library.

the family and are rarely if ever performed by a qualified practitioner. One might say the same thing of therapeutics, even if the idea that 'a good doctor is one who has effective medicines at his disposal' seems to be widely shared by the peoples of the region. Expertise in the preparation and prescription of remedies is particularly valued, perhaps due to the importance of these arts in the great founding medical traditions, but also to the extraordinary biodiversity of the region.

In certain countries of the region, this biodiversity distinguishes local, even 'national', medical traditions from imported models. The case of Vietnamese medicine is pertinent. Relations and cultural exchanges between China and Vietnam have been governed by a thousand years of colonization from the beginning of the Christian era, and historically the Vietnamese have distinguished Northern medicine, largely influenced by traditional Chinese medicine (*thuốc bắc*), from the more purely Vietnamese and popular Southern medicine. Southern medicine is based on a pharmacopoeia constructed on the basis of local vegetation (*thuốc nam*) by famous pre-modern medical figures such as the monks Tuệ Tĩnh (fourteenth century) and Lán Ông (eighteenth century), authors of compilations of formulas and medical texts that provided the formal bases for Southern medicine. This distinction is to some extent false, and its geographic boundaries open to discussion. Moreover, it has taken on political connotations in the context of the reinvention of tradition after World War II, in Vietnam (Wahlberg, 2006) as well as in other countries of the region, such as Laos (Halpern, 1964, p. 197). Nonetheless, the distinction is worthy of note.

Throughout the region, the dynamic variety of medical formulas and prescriptions is often based on complex combinations of substances (the number of ingredients can vary between regions from two to twenty, with the average being between three and seven), each having a precise role in determining the remedy's function. Prescriptions are unique to each patient and each stage of their illness—taking into account age, general state of health, gender, environment, the moment when the disease manifested itself, etc.—and can be readjusted during the course of treatment. In addition to these highly individual treatments are popular or miracle cures and panaceas supposedly able to cure dozens, indeed hundreds, of ailments. Therapeutic interventions must help to re-establish, slowly but surely, the lost balance rather than launching a frontal attack on the illness or its causes—whence the frequent use, for example, of tonics which make up half of the Sino-Vietnamese pharmacopoeia (Craig, 2002, p. 48). This last quality of the remedy leads us to note the popular distinction made between traditional medications and Western medications and, more broadly, the impact of the introduction and the diffusion of biomedicine in the reconfiguration of the region's medical space, and particularly in use of medications as a part of health care.

THE AMBIGUOUS CONTRIBUTIONS OF MODERN WESTERN MEDICINE

The few historians who have looked at Southeast Asian medical traditions agree that the diffusion of Western scientific medicine, from the second half of the nineteenth century, contributed to their reformulation. Western biomedicine influenced medical practices and the professional and lay ideas underpinning them. The establishment of Western health care systems, albeit rudimentary and adapted to local

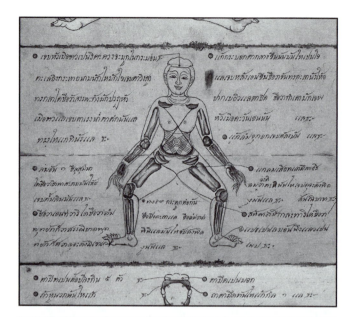

A guide to pressure points on the body for shiatsu massage, from a Siamese pressure massage manual. MS 801, *c.* 1850, Oriental Collection, Wellcome Library, London.

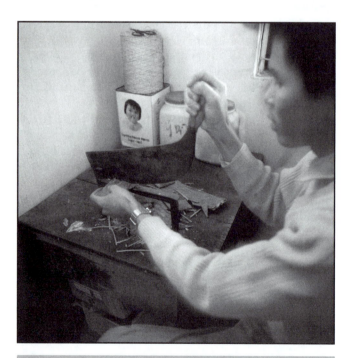

Chopping dried bark in a pharmacy to prepare an individual treatment for a patient, Hanoi, Vietnam. Photograph by Mark de Fraeye, Wellcome Photo Library.

needs, was supported by the colonial experience (Thailand was the only country in Southeast Asia not colonized) and resulted in the dominated peoples, whether they were patients or healers, re-appropriating certain biomedical concepts (Monnais-Rousselot, 1999).

As Owen (1987, pp. 16–22) has noted, although Western medicine may have been beyond the reach of most Southeast Asians, it nevertheless produced changes in the ways in which those even without direct access to biomedicine perceived disease. Germ theories were integrated into indigenous beliefs regarding disease causation, linked in some cases to diseases believed to have come from abroad, to certain supernatural agents, or to prevalent, devastating, and often incurable diseases such as malaria. There appear, too, to have been semantic changes in traditional terms for illness in order to accommodate Western disease categories, e.g., the Thai term *mareng*, which in the past had signified 'deep-seated ulcer' but came to refer to cancer (Bamber, 1993, p. 437). An equal reformulation of the discourse of remedies or of curing occurred. This suggests a certain transformation of the role of treatment and medications, and the introduction of a partial distinction between what is a Western pharmaceutical—chemical, toxic, but also fast-acting, to be used, among other things, for treating infectious diseases (the growing enthusiasm for antibiotics in the post–World War II period would belong to this category)—and a traditional remedy—soft and slow-acting, directed at re-establishing the fundamental balance of the body's elements (Monnais and Tousignant, 2006).

At the same time, these colonial health care systems, which sought to impose biomedicine for both economic and civilizing reasons, also promoted the emergence of new health care professionals. Ad hoc institutions, e.g., the Hanoi Medical School, established in 1902 by the French colonial state in Indochina, educated several hundred Vietnamese in Western medicine (Monnais-Rousselot, 1999, pp. 269–287). Moreover, the requirement for the professionalization of certain types of native healers according to Western standards—particularly the most politically influential elites working in urban areas, and midwives (the primary agents of the diffusion of basic health care in rural areas)—led to the growth of a uniform education in academic institutions and the multiplication of associations and professional orders designed to guarantee the standards of health care practices and self-regulate their members (Connor and Samuel, 2001, pp. 9, 56).

In a less obvious and more ambivalent way, the diffusion of biomedicine also revitalized traditional medicine. In the permeability and openness, syncretism, and voluntary pluralism characterizing the region's societies, we note particularly the arrival of new indigenous treatments linked to the acceptance of Western nosographic categories. Brun and Schumacher (1987, p. 209) explain that they have come across examples of new prescriptions aimed at such new disease concepts as *baw waan* (diabetes) in northern Thailand. Economic and ideological factors, especially the problems of accessibility to Western pharmaceuticals, particularly in countries that have experienced long and painful conflicts over the course of the last few decades (Vietnam or Cambodia), or in regions that continue to suffer ethnic or political marginalization (East Timor), have also led to more systematic research into the value of traditional pharmacopoeias and their ability to treat incurable 'modern' illnesses. The most revealing example is AIDS, the object of 'natural' therapeutic experiments in several countries, including Thailand and Vietnam. Certain new fields of specialization have also emerged for the same reasons within the communities of traditional practitioners. In discussing the Malays and the Thais, Golomb (1985, pp. 74–75) lists 'specialists in blood and circulation problems, cancer specialists, skin specialists, diabetes specialists, specialists in nervous diseases, therapists for sexual problems', in addition to the now familiar herbalists, mediums, and masseurs. This illustrates the increased range of health care available and the partial absorption of apparently useful foreign practices in the syncretic logic.

The introduction of biomedicine has thus followed a similar path as the great religions and the foundational medical theories—Ayurvedic, Chinese, and Islamic. It has evoked the same nuanced and selective process of integration and reformulation, without necessarily changing the magico-religious dimension of the practices (Golomb, 1985, p. 65). Western medicine has also enlarged, often in ambiguous ways, medical pluralism: the possibility of calling on different medical systems simultaneously or in succession.

The current dynamism of Southeast Asian medical traditions is uncontestable. Increasingly, the place of these traditions is being redefined within the framework of 'inclusive' or 'integrative' health care systems, supported by international organizations (WHO, 2002) that determine, together with nation-states, the rules of intervention, thus permitting a certain revalorization of some traditions or those who practice within these traditions (Connor, 1986, pp. 34–36). At the same time, these interventions are carried out according to a logic not always shared by the populations in question. For instance, there is the tendency to develop dual systems, one for rural areas where the diffusion of essential care is entrusted largely to traditional practitioners, working within small, poorly financed structures, while the biomedical doctors and the professionalized elite of traditional practitioners expand the availability of medical care for the affluent urbanites. This multiplies the forms of pluralism, and increases certain risks—e.g., unhappy interactions of various drugs, under-consumption and overconsumption, particularly of antibiotics, and exaggerated self-medication (made worse by the media), all of which are denounced by WHO and by numerous foreign observers. It seems that much remains to be done to promote pluralist medical systems offering an appropriate balance among all of these medical traditions.

Equally, understanding of the medical traditions of Southeast Asia beyond the region is relatively poor and often condemned by the majority of Western health care professionals as nonscientific, useful only for minor afflictions and maladies where orthodox medicine has little to offer. This hostility can be explained above all by ignorance of what is different. Yet there are a growing number of Southeast Asian immigrants in the West, and aspects of these traditions are also welcomed by an increasing number of Westerners, who seek alternatives to a biomedicine perceived as impersonal.

Bibliography

Alphen, J. V., and A. Aris, 1996. *Oriental Medicine. An Illustrated Guide to the Asian Arts of Healing* (Boston); Bamber, Scott, 1993. 'Diseases of Antiquity and the Premodern Period in Southeast Asia' in Kipple, K., ed., *The Cambridge World History of Human Disease* (Cambridge) pp. 425–440; Brelet, C., 2002. *Médecines du monde. Histoire et pratiques des médecines traditionnelles* (Paris); Brun, V., and T. Schumacher, 1987. *Traditional Herbal Medicine in Northern Thailand* (Berkeley); Chhem, R. K., 2001. 'Les doctrines médicales khmères: nosologie et méthodes diagnostiques.' *Siksacakr* 3: 12–15; Coedes, G., 1948. *Les Etats hindouisés d'Indochine et d'Indonésie* (Paris) (2nd ed.); Connor, L. H., 1986. *Jero Tapakan: Balinese Healer* (Cambridge); Connor, L. H., and G. Samuel, eds., 2001. *Healing Powers and Modernity. Traditional Medicine, Shamanism, and Science in Asian Societies* (Westport, CT); Craig, D., 2002. *Familiar Medicine. Everyday Health Knowledge and Practice in Today's Vietnam* (Honolulu); De Beers, S.J., 2002. *Jamu: The Ancient Indonesian Art of Herbal Healing* (Singapore); Evers, H.-D., 2001. 'Southeast Asia: Socio-cultural Aspects' in Smelser, N.J., and P.B. Baltes, eds., *International Encyclopedia of the Social & Behavioral Sciences* (Palo Alto) pp. 14661–14665; Foster, G. M., 1976. 'Disease Etiologies in Non-Western Medical Systems.' *American Anthropologist* 78(4): 773–782; Geertz, C., 1968. *Islam Observed. Religious Development in Morocco and Indonesia* (New Haven and London); Gimlette, J.D., 1939. *A Dictionary of Malay Medicine* (Kuala Lumpur); Golomb, L., 1985. *An Anthropology of Curing in Multiethnic Thailand* (Chicago); Halpern, J.M., 1964. *Government, Politics and Social Structure in Laos: A Study of Tradition and Innovation* (Berkeley); Hart, D. V., 1969. *Bisayan Filipino and Malayan Humoral Pathologies: Folk Medicine and Ethnohistory in Southeast Asia* (Ithaca, NY); Huard, P., J. Bossy, and G. Mazars, 1978. *Les médecines de l'Asie* (Paris); Hunter, C.L., 2001. 'Sorcery and Science as Competing Models of Explanation in a Sasak Village' in Connor L.H., and G. Samuel, eds., *Healing Powers and Modernity. Traditional Medicine, Shamanism, and Science in Asian Societies* (Westport, CT) pp. 152–170; Jaspan, M.A., 1969. *Traditional Medical Theory in Southeast Asia* (Hull); Kimball, L. A., 1979. *Borneo Medicine. The Healing Art of Indigenous Brunei Malay Medicine* (Chicago); Kleinman, A., 1991. 'Concepts and a Model for the Comparison of Medical System as Cultural Systems' in Currer, C., and M. Stacey, eds., *Concepts of Health, Illness and Disease. A Comparative Perspective* (New York) pp. 27–50; Laderman, C., 1992. 'A Welcoming Soil: Islamic Humoralism on the Malay Peninsula' in Leslie, C., and A. Young, eds., *Paths to Asian Medical Knowledge* (Berkeley) pp. 272–288; Leslie, C., and A. Young, eds., 1992. *Paths to Asian Medical Knowledge* (Berkeley); Monnais, L., and N. Tousignant, 2006. 'The Colonial Life of Pharmaceuticals, Accessibility to Health Care, Consumption of Medicines and Medical Pluralism in French Vietnam, 1905–45' *Journal of Vietnamese Studies* 1(1–2): in press; Monnais-Rousselot, L., 1999. *Médecine et colonisation.*

L'aventure indochinoise, 1860–1939 (Paris); Mulholland, J., 1979. 'Thai Traditional Medicine: The Treatment of Diseases Caused by the Tridosa.' *Southeast Asian Review* 3(2): 29–38; Owen, N.G., ed., 1987. *Death and Disease in Southeast Asia. Explorations in Social, Medical, and Demographic History* (Singapore); Pandey, G., 1997. *Traditional Medicine in Southeast Asia and Indian Medical Science* (New Delhi); Pottier, R., 1972. 'Introduction à l'étude des pratiques thérapeutiques lao.' *Asie du Sud-est et du monde insulindien* 4: 173–193; Reid, A., 1988. *Southeast Asia in the Age of Commerce, 1450–1680* (New Haven); Sassady, K. 1962. *Contribution à l'étude de la médecine lao* (Paris); Souk-Aloun, P.N., 2001. *La médecine du bouddhisme Theravada au Laos* (Paris); Wahlberg, A., 2006. 'Bio-politics and the Promotion of Traditional Herbal Medicine in Vietnam.' *Health. An Interdisciplinary Journal for the Social Study of Health, Illness and Medicine* 10(2): 123–147; World Health Organization (WHO), 2002. *WHO Strategy on Traditional Medicine 2002–05* (Geneva).

Laurence Monnais

MEDICINE, STATE, AND SOCIETY IN JAPAN, 500–2000

INTRODUCTION

A common cliché says that Japan is a remarkable society consisting of mediocre individuals. This applies, in an oblique way, to its history of medicine. If one takes the 'great discoveries' approach, the history of Japanese medicine is somewhat lackluster. Nor does a 'great doctors' approach bring Japan to the center stage of the world history of medicine. Looked at, however, from the angle of the social history of medicine, Japan presents truly unique and exciting questions, pertinent to both the agenda in the scholarship of the history of medicine and the present situation of health and medicine in the context of capitalism and globalization. Why did Japan foster one of the earliest vibrant medical marketplaces in the eighteenth century? How did it become the first non-Western nation that adopted Western medicine? Why has it become the nation with the highest life expectancy just fifty years after World War II? The present contribution cannot provide complete answers to these questions. Instead, it puts such questions in historical context by giving a bird's eye view of the history of medicine in Japan over the last 1,500 years.

I have adopted dual frameworks of foreign relations and domestic dynamics to structure my account. One should see Japanese medicine vis-à-vis medicine in other areas of the world, and, at the same time, the place of medicine in Japanese domestic society and culture should be discussed.

A quasi-colonial stance that describes Japanese medicine as subsumed first under Chinese medicine and then under a Western one is avoided. Although influence from abroad was—and remains—a powerful force that molded learned medicine in Japan, Euro- or Sino-centric views of the history of Japanese medicine is of lesser use in its *social* history. A few words are necessary about the use of the word 'Japan', which changed its territorial extent and meanings. I have followed other scholars and adopted the geographical features—the Japanese archipelago—as what is roughly meant by the word.

ANCIENT AND MEDIEVAL PERIODS, 500–1500

Medical historians used to be fond of searching for the earliest precursor of modern medicine. Hippocrates and the *Yellow Emperor's Inner Canon* have enjoyed such a status, respectively, for Western medicine and for Chinese medicine. Recent historiography and scholarship have challenged such views of an epiphany of sophisticated medicine centered around 'foundational' figures or texts, preferring pictures of more gradual and complex change from primitive and supernatural medicine to a sophisticated and naturalistic one. Nevertheless, searching for such a foundational event in the history of Japanese medicine helps, for it reveals two important and perennial features of medicine in Japan. First, a sophisticated medical system was imported to Japan from abroad. Second, the state played a crucial role in the process.

Japan learned its earliest sophisticated medicine from a doctor hailing from a state in the Korean peninsula who visited the court of the Japanese emperor around the fifth century. This event is recorded in both of the two earliest chronicles of Japan, *Kojiki* and *Nihon-shoki*, as happening during the rule of Emperor Jōkyō. We do not know the year of the event. Neither is the name of the invited doctor established. We are fairly certain, however, about the context in which this event took place. The first importation of foreign medical learning was a product of decisions made by the Japanese state. Such a policy was adopted because of the new international order in the Far Eastern peripheries of the mighty Chinese Empires. Japan formed complex relationships with small states in the Korean peninsula. Fierce internal struggles still went on in the unstable Japanese court; the new ideologies of Confucianism and Buddhism created the fluid cultural dynamism. The Japanese court needed foreign connections to acquire advanced knowledge and superior technologies, such as weaving, pottery, and iron-casting. The court also sought cosmologies and philosophies to legitimate and strengthen its still tenuous rule over other powerful clans. The court of the emperor thus eagerly imbibed foreign philosophies, cosmologies, and ideologies from China and Korea. As a part of such strategy, it imported medical theories and practice developed in China via Korea, which were interwoven into the cosmologies of Chinese philosophy and/or Buddhism.

Medical traffic between Japan, China, and Korea was thus established around the early fifth century. During the same century, a physician called Tokoku was invited from a Korean state. He settled in a place that is now Osaka and started a clan specializing in medical practice. In the sixth century, Buddhist cannons were imported, which included substantial medical texts. In 554, a 'doctor' (*hakase*) and two herbalists arrived from Korea, in response to the request of the court. Around the same time, major texts of Chinese classical medicine were brought from China. Prince Shōtoku (574–622), the brilliant and innovative Regent at the court of the Empress Suiko (554–622), adopted vigorous Buddhist policies and established a charitable dispensary annexed to a Buddhist temple in the late sixth century. The Envoy from Japan to China in 608 included two students of medicine, who stayed and studied medicine there. These state policies in the sixth and seventh centuries determined that learned Buddhist and Chinese medical systems would influence medicine in Japan in the subsequent millennium. A substantial number of immigrants from the Korean peninsula and their descendants were organized into medical clans, who must have been major practitioners of learned medicine in Japan.

The state-sponsored implementation of learned medicine imported from abroad culminated in the early eighth century in the medical institutions in the *ritsuryō* system, the governmental structure defined by criminal, adminis-

trative, and civil codes, largely copied from Chinese states. Among the *ritsuryō* codes, the Taihō Code (701) and Yōrō Code (718) were the most important. The Code of Medicine and Diseases (*Ishitsu-rei*) delineated the elaborate structure in which medicine should be taught and administered in the capital and provinces. The central office in the capital was the Bureau of Medicine (*Ten'yaku-ryo*), which hired professors and masters of several branches of medical learning, such as medicine, acupuncture, massage, incantational and exorcistic medicine (*jugon*), materia medica, and gynecology. Each professor taught his subject to between six and forty students, who were admitted to the bureau mainly from the families of medical practitioners. They had to study their subjects for a fixed period of up to nine years, during which time regular examinations monitored their progress. Similar systems of medical education and provision were installed in the provinces. The professors and masters were paid salaries for their service and were honored with court ranks, differing according to the station they occupied. Although they occupied only lowly positions within the hierarchy of state officials, this signaled a clear confirmation of medicine's place as a specialized and learned skill within the bureaucracy of the state. The system also ensured that the complex theories of Chinese and Buddhist medicine were systematically taught to Japanese students by Japanese professors.

By the eighth century, therefore, Japanese medical learning was firmly integrated both in the Japanese state machinery and in the Chinese politico-cultural realm in East Asia. Moreover, reflecting the cosmopolitanism of the vast Chinese Empires, it incorporated elements from numerous parts of the world. The medical cosmopolitanism of Japanese medicine at that time is best exemplified by the collection of medicines that were deposited in the Shōsōin Treasure House in 756. Many of them have survived more than 1,200 years. The collection consisted of about sixty precious and high-quality medicines of Chinese, Indian, Vietnamese, and Central Asian origins. These medicines were actually used to treat the poor, especially in times of epidemics. The medicines that passed through the bodies of the Japanese populace in the eighth century were, at least occasionally, cosmopolitan to a surprising extent.

In the couple of centuries after the creation of the Bureau of Medicine, Japanese state medicine made some major achievements. From the late seventh century on, a series of doctors at the Imperial court or the Bureau of Medicine compiled large-scale compendia of Chinese medical texts. Many of them are now lost. One remarkable exception is *Ishinpō*, an enormous compendium of Chinese medical texts in thirty volumes completed by Tanba Yasuyori (912–95) in 984, which have survived intact. Careful readings of *Ishinpō* have revealed that the editor made many crucial changes to the original Chinese texts in his attempt to adapt the original to local conditions. By the tenth century at the latest, Japanese learned medicine had

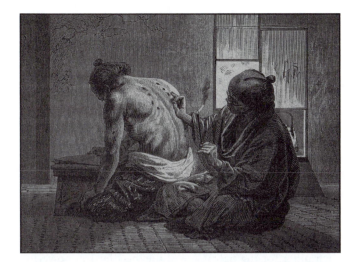

Physician applying moxa to the back of a male patient prior to igniting it with a taper that he holds in his left hand (moxibustion). Moxibustion is often used in conjunction with acupuncture. Wood engraving, nineteenth century. Iconographic Collection, Wellcome Library, London.

matured to become a variation of the Chinese medical system. On the other hand, it is questionable that Japanese patients shared the rational views of diseases expressed in the learned medical system around the time of *Ishinpō*. Contemporary diaries and fictional tales are filled with expressions of more animistic or supernatural views of disease and its cure. The most popular treatment when one became seriously ill was sutra-chanting, and illnesses were routinely attributed to possession by an evil spirit. The medical world of *The Tale of Genji* (1001–1010?) has almost no resemblance with that of *Ishinpō*.

The joining of Japanese medicine with that of the Chinese realm of influence had a darker side: diseases crossed the sea, which had acted as a natural cordon sanitaire. Inhabitants of the Japanese archipelago were drawn into the pool of deadly infectious diseases that had long been established in China and other major centers of civilization on the Eurasian continent. From around the sixth century, chronicles started to record epidemics. The most severe and well-recorded was a smallpox epidemic lasting from 735 to 737. Originating at Dazaifu, then a military base and the diplomatic window to China and Korea, the disease ravaged the country in the following couple of years. Smallpox was imported via the traffic between the continent and the archipelago; its diffusion was certainly helped by the establishment of the nationwide administrative system. This Great Smallpox Epidemic of 735–37 was one of the first of a series of smallpox epidemics that claimed countless lives. Between 750 and 1500, more than thirty outbreaks of smallpox were recorded. These deadly outbreaks, as well as those of measles (about twenty of them being recorded), must have played at least some part in halting the rapid growth of the population since the introduction of agriculture around the third century BCE.

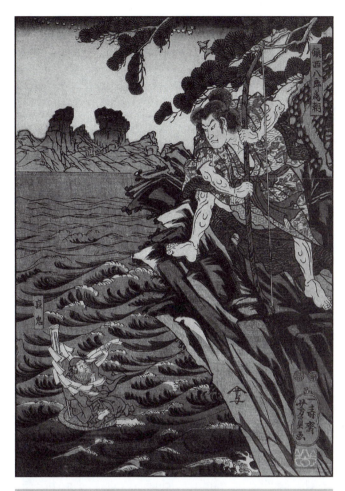

Chinsei Hachiro Tametomo, a legendary hero of the twelfth century, repelling the demon of smallpox from the island of Oshima. Colored woodcut by Utagawa Yoshikazu, *c.* 1850. Iconographic Collection, Wellcome Library, London.

Outbreaks of epidemics persisted throughout the medieval period (*c.* 1100–*c.* 1500), but the grand and elaborate system of state medicine did not. By the tenth century, the *ritsuryō* system exhibited serious signs of disintegration. Central rule was replaced by fragmentary rule under powerful aristocrats, local magnates, and later samurai warrior-rulers. With the disintegration of a nationwide administrative system, the medicine of a centralized government declined. By the eleventh century, appointment to the Bureau of Medicine became a job on paper. Provincial medical offices were discontinued somewhat earlier. The establishment of the Shōgunate in Kamakura (1192), 500 kilometers east of Kyoto (where the Imperial court and the Bureau of Medicine were located), sealed the fate of state medicine. The Kamakura Shōgunate did not develop any coherent and large-scale policy for medical education or provision. When need arose, the warrior-rulers invited court doctors from Kyoto for treatment and later made Kyoto-educated doctors stay in Kamakura. The practitioners of state medicine were thus transformed into personal physicians to the powerful.

The collapse of state medicine, however, did not mean the coming of a medical Dark Age in Japan. By the twelfth century, Japanese society had become complex enough to ensure that maintenance of high medical learning did not depend solely on the state. The largely hereditary nature of medical posts might have had some role in securing the transmission of medical learning for generations. The major new bearers of medical learning were, however, the Buddhist temples, which possessed powerful financial bases, huge political influence, and even military might. After the discontinuation of the official Chinese Envoy in 894, Buddhist temples continued to send their monks to China to study Buddhist learning. In so doing, the temples acted as general centers of learning, including medical knowledge. Major works of medicine in the medieval period were thus written by Buddhist priests and monks: Kajiwara Shōzen (1266?–1337) digested thousands of books and completed Ton'ishō (c. 1302) and Man'anpō (1315–27). These works incorporated new developments in medicine from the Song dynasty in China as well as the author's own practical observations. Eisai (1141–1215), a Zen-Buddhist priest, visited China twice and wrote Kissa Yōjōki [Notes on the regimen and tea drinking] (1211), a seminal work that eventually made tea a national drink. Ninshō (1217–1303), a priest in Singon-Ritsushū, established large-scale and well-organized medical charities for outcasts, lepers, and the poor in the temples in Nara and Kamakura. His institute was reputed to have cured 46,000 sufferers in twenty years.

The decline of state medicine also created a space in which a new social category of medical practitioners emerged. The new medical practitioners were no longer homogeneous public servants employed by the state. Instead, they were a group of heterogeneous people who were paid by their patients. Some were learned monks, as previously mentioned; others were members of established medical families with a long history of appointments as court doctors; others were courtiers who dabbled in medicine; still others were barely literate empirics. The prestige and income of these medical practitioners differed enormously, largely according to the rank and the wealth of the patients they served. Since our evidence is unevenly distributed, our knowledge is largely restricted to those practitioners who served Emperors, aristocrats, courtiers, Shōguns, and other warrior-rulers. Diaries kept by courtiers such as Kujō Kanezane (1149–1207) or Fujiwara Sadaie (1162–1241) reveal that they called in private practitioners for ailments such as beriberi or asthma. Although in principle they should have consulted doctors appointed by the court, they preferred private practitioners who had better reputations. The most detailed records of medical practice around this period were made by Yamashina Kotostugu (1507–76), a courtier who also had an extensive medical practice: he regularly received 'fees' in money and in kind from diverse patients ranging from aristocrats to shopkeep-

ers. Down the social scale, our evidence becomes scanty. There appear, however, signs of the popularization of medicine around the fourteenth century. Ton'isho, a work mentioned above, was written partly in 'kana', or Japanese characters, which are the Japanese equivalent of vernacular languages for the uneducated, while medical texts had been written almost exclusively in 'kanji', or Chinese characters. Likewise, Fukudahō (1460s–70s), a work written by a monk in Kyoto, was also in kana, on the pretext that young doctors needed something other than texts written in kanji.

Medical practice from around the beginning of the medieval period thus started to take place in a medical marketplace, a concept brought to prominence by Roy Porter. Kyoto, the capital full of attractive clients, had a high concentration of medical practitioners competing with each other for the patronage of the wealthy and powerful. Unsuccessful ones might have left the capital for a less competitive environment in the countryside, as depicted in Kaminari [Thunder], a contemporary kyōgen comedy. By mixing intimately with the rich and powerful, medicine now became one of the ways of climbing the social ladder. On the other hand, a medical practitioner's social position meant that he served the rich and powerful individuals, in the same way as craftsmen. Scattered and fragmentary evidence suggests the ambiguity of medical practitioners in terms of their social status; they were regarded as being on a par with other craftsmen, and occupied a lowly status around the court and aristocrats' salons, despite the high court honors they could expect from their patrons.

EARLY MODERN PERIOD, 1500–1850

Japanese medicine in the early modern period (c. 1500–c. 1850) was again profoundly influenced by the state's diplomatic policy as it responded to the new situation in the Far East. The Tokugawa Shōgunate, founded in Edo (now Tokyo) in 1603, completed the so-called seclusion policy

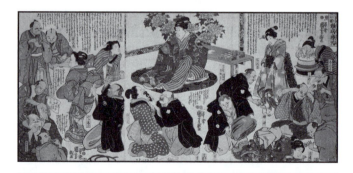

Caricature of patients at a royal court, with conditions such as smallpox, obesity, toothache, venereal disease, and lameness, being treated by quacks—all the figures in black being physicians or surgeons. Colored woodcut by Utagawa Kuniyoshi, c. 1850. Iconographic Collection, Wellcome Library, London.

by the end of the 1630s, mainly to prevent the spread of Christianity among the populace. Trade or traffic with foreign countries was prohibited except at a handful of places and to a handful of authorized people. Any Japanese was forbidden to go abroad without such authorization on the penalty of death. This policy was the Tokugawa Shōgunate's response to the new situation of the world. From the fourteenth century, the Indian Ocean and the South China Sea were the major arenas of international commerce, which the European countries joined in the fifteenth century. By the seventeenth century, Portuguese, Spanish, Dutch, and English merchants as well as those from China were frequent visitors to Japan. A sign of Japanese participation in these arenas of global commerce was the transmission of syphilis, which, whatever its true origin, had almost certainly reached Japan by the 1520s, perhaps through its contact with trading posts in South China (inevitably, it was called 'Chinese pox' by the Japanese). Even under the seclusion policy, cholera first reached Japan early in 1822, during its first pandemic. The point to be emphasized through such examples is that the seclusion policy did not completely isolate Japan, which was constantly touched by the vigorous traffic of the Asian and European merchants. Japan was a secluded society that kept its windows open.

Internally, similar contradictions were rife in the Tokugawa society. The country was divided into about 400 fragments. Semi-autonomous *daimyōs* ruled each domain. The ruling class was samurai warriors, who bore two swords. Normally individuals could not change the status into which they were born. Peasants were bound to the land where they were born and expected to toil upon it until their death. This feudalistic outlook was deceptive, however. It was an extremely mobile society in many aspects. Local *daimyōs* were ordered to maintain their residence in the city of Edo and to live there in alternate years. There was thus constant and massive movement around the country by the elite members of society. Major highways facilitated domestic travel and commerce. Urbanization progressed. Roughly 5 to 6 percent of the Japanese lived in cities with a population greater than 100,000; the comparable figure for Europe was 2 to 3 percent. By 1700, Edo had around one million people, making it the largest city in the world. A dynamic society lay under an apparently feudal institution.

Medicine during the early modern period testified to this dynamism. In terms of medical theory, early modern Japanese medicine was innovative and pluralistic. Doctors preached theories and therapeutics that were sharply and self-consciously different from each other. For the first and arguably the last time in the history of Japanese medicine, we can talk about serious competition between 'schools' of medicine. This medical pluralism was partly due to the weakness of public authority in medical matters and partly due to the so-called seclusion policy. Overwhelmed neither by the state-backed medical teaching nor by foreign

authorities, Japanese doctors competed with each other through their original medical theories.

First to be noted among them is Manase Dōsan (1507–94), who had learned medicine under Tashiro Sanki (1465–1544?) and imbibed from him rationalistic medical theories developed in China by Li Gao (1180–1251) and Zhu Zhenheng (Zhu Danxi) (1282–1358). Manase's teaching became Goseiha (literally meaning 'Later Generation School') medicine, which was the mainstream medical system throughout the early modern period. Goseiha medicine was characterized by its emphasis on mild therapeutics, using complex multidrug treatments. The use of mild but effective remedies impressed the visiting Spanish and was the hallmark of Manase's therapeutics.

More radical, innovative, and controversial was the so-called Kohōha (literally meaning 'Ancient Method School') medicine, started by Nagoya Gen-i (1628–96) and developed by Gotō Konzan (1659–1733). Kohōha doctors rejected systematic and elaborate theories of Goseiha medicine in favor of the simplicity of ancient Chinese medicine. The key text for Kohōha medicine was *Shōkanron*, one of the earliest medical texts in China dating from around the third century. This call for a return to the ancient text was firmly combined with an emphasis on empirical observation. The first anatomy of a human cadaver in Japan was performed in 1754 by Yamawaki Tōyō (1705–62), a leader of Kohōha medicine based in Kyoto, not by a medical practitioner of Western medicine (the similarity between Kohōha medicine and Renaissance medicine has often been pointed out). The theories of Kohōha medicine were simple. Gotō attributed all disease to just one cause, namely the stagnation of *qi* in the body. Yoshimasu Tōdō (1702–73) claimed 'poison' in the body was responsible for all diseases. Their therapeutics was simple and aggressive. Nagata Tokuhon, a sixteenth-century precursor of Kohōha medicine, was reputed to have employed only nineteen recipes, among which powerful purges such as mercury were the most important. Yoshimasu studied the effect of simple drugs, rejecting the routine use of compound medicines. The controversial nature of Kohōha medicine can be gauged by the strong reactions of numerous doctors against Yoshimasu's theory of poison. At the same time, Yoshimasu's book *Ruijuhō* (1765) was a publishing phenomenon, reputed to have sold 10,000 copies in a single month. Kohōha medicine thus epitomized the innovative nature of medicine in the Edo period, which allowed medical theorists to pursue original theory building and therapeutics within the broad framework of Chinese medicine. Fierce controversies and sharp disagreements among Kohōha doctors themselves were a sign that medical theories were now a topic discussed in the public sphere, a phenomenon facilitated by the printing press.

Ranpō (literally meaning 'Dutch style') medicine, or the Western medicine learned from the Dutch, was a late but important addition to this world of dynamic intellectual

ferment. Although its practitioners were in the minority—
the medical census of the 1870s counted that about 15 percent of all medical practitioners identified themselves as
Ranpō practitioners—Ranpō medicine played a disproportionately important role in forging modern Japanese medicine and society in general.

A brave attempt at translating a Dutch anatomy text
with only a modicum of the knowledge of that language
began in 1771, when several doctors attended the dissection of a human cadaver in Edo. Sugita Genpaku (1733–
1817), a physician to a provincial *daimyō*, acted as an able
organizer of the enterprise. Maeno Ryōtaku (1723–1803)
provided knowledge of the Dutch language and scholarly
conscience. *Kaitai Shinsho* [A new book of anatomy] was
published in five volumes in 1774, with high-quality illustrations copied from the original text and other anatomy
books. *Kaitai Shinsho* was an instant success, bringing fame
and a flourishing practice to Sugita. It should be emphasized that the enterprise was purely a private one, with virtually no help from public authorities apart from providing
the original Dutch book. The contrast with the first translation of a Western anatomy text in China around 1720 is
striking: the Chinese translation was done at the request of
the emperor, and the translation was securely held in the
library of the Forbidden City.

Kaitai Shinsho's success was a great enticement to simi-
lar-minded medical practitioners with some access to the
Dutch language, who had long been enchanted by detailed
and realistic illustrations in Dutch medical books but had
been frustrated by their inability to read the text. Further
attempts at translating anatomical and surgical texts with
lavish illustrations quickly followed. One of them, *Ihan
Teiyō* (1805), had fifty-two plates, which were executed by
one of the period's leading engravers. As in Renaissance
anatomy, the flourishing of Ranpō anatomy in Japan intersected with the rise of the visual culture facilitated by printing technology. The atmosphere of this aspect of Ranpō
medicine is best epitomized by the works of Fuseya Soteki
(1747–1811), a doctor-literati who performed a series of
experiments on the kidneys and the urine of animals and
published the results in *Waran Iwa* [Medical discourse
between the Japanese and the Dutch] (1805). This work is
hailed as the first work of experimental physiology in
Japan. At the same time, it was written in an urbane and
non-esoteric spirit, even with a hint of pornographic
appeal. The serious scholarly quest for Western medicine
and science coexisted with a dilettante pursuit of novelty
and intellectual excitement.

The flourishing of various schools in Japanese medicine
was related to the social structure of medical education.
The role of the state in matters related to medicine continued to be small during the early modern period. There was
virtually no attempt to regulate medical practice either at
the Tokugawa Shōgunate or in the provinces. Although
medical schools were established by the Shōgunate and by

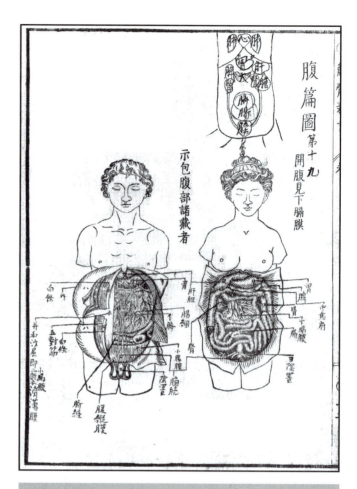

**Anatomical illustrations of male and female torso. Engraving
from *Kaitai Shinsho* (1774), the first translation into Japanese
of Johann Adam Kulmus, *Anatomische Tabellen*. Japanese MS
32, Wellcome Library, London.**

major *daimyōs*, they did not attain eminence. It should be
noted that almost all the famous doctors of the early modern period were individuals who opened their own private
medical schools. Manase Dōsan started Keichin'in in Kyoto
around 1545 and reputedly taught 800 students. After
Dōzan's death, the management of the school was left to his
adopted son, who consolidated the reputation of the flourishing Manase school. Gotō Konzan at Kyoto was reputed
to have taught 200 students, who imitated their teacher's
hairstyle, which eventually became a standard style of medical practitioners. Yamawaki Tōyō attracted so many students in Yōju'in in Kyoto that he drew up regulations for
them. Ōtsuki Gentaku's (1757–1827) Shiba Randō was the
most popular Ranpō private school in Edo. Large concen-
trations of medical students were not restricted to Kyoto
and Edo, the old and new capitals and the centers of learning. Osaka had Ogata Kōan and his famous Teki-juku,
which became, in the 1840s and 1850s, the training ground
of the leaders of Westernization in the Meiji era. Even a
small village in a remote rural corner could attract students
when its medical practitioner became fabulously famous.

That was the case for Hanaoka Seishū (1760–1835), whose celebrated success in a breast cancer operation under a world-first form of general anesthesia attracted hundreds of students to his school in a small village in Kii province. When Dutch medical teaching became a sought-after subject in the nineteenth century, Franz von Siebold (1796–1866) played essentially the same game in Nagasaki. The German doctor opened Narutaki-juku in Nagasaki to teach about fifty Japanese students there.

Part of the reason for the flourishing of various private medical schools was simple: medical practice paid. Much evidence testifies that medical practice was an economically feasible option, which many took. In early nineteenth-century Edo, there were about 2,500 doctors for a population of about one million, the ratio being 400 patients to every one doctor. This is about the same figure found presently in Tokyo. Similarly, Osaka with 300,000 people boasted 300 'eminent doctors' in 1845, listed in the style of a league table of sumō wrestlers. Even the rural and mountainous Yamanashi had a ratio of about 1,000 patients to each doctor in the 1870s. Many of these practitioners must have been part-time. Motoori Norinaga (1730–1801), the greatest Kokugaku scholar, earned roughly half of his income from medical practice and the rest from teaching his Kokugaku students. In the years that saw an epidemic in the area where he lived, his medical earnings doubled that of an ordinary year. Sugita Genpaku received about 130 ryō as a salary of a physician to the *daimyō*, and two to four times as much from his private practice. Several doctors became fabulously rich: Habu Genseki (1762–1848) in Edo and Singū Ryōtei (1787–1858) in Kyoto used their medical income to start commercial banks. For many, if not all, successful practitioners, the key to their success seems to have been the patronage of shōguns and *daimyōs*: appointment as their personal physicians brought not just a stable income, but could lead to fame and huge fortune.

Fame and wealth, however, did not bring high social status to medical practitioners in the Edo period. If compared with Confucian scholars, medics were kept at a much lower social position. In an ideology that put the premium value on serving one's state, medicine was deemed a 'small art', tending only to the body of one's clients. In his early teens, Hashimoto Sanai (1834–59) agonized over his future, as he was destined to a medical career as the son of a medical family. This precocious boy sadly accepted the fate that he should become a man of lowly occupation (i.e., medicine) but found relief in the idea that his true ambition lay elsewhere (in politics).

In rural areas, village officials (wealthy farmers residing in the village) played crucial roles in providing medical care for the people. They needed medical knowledge especially in times of epidemics, and they apprenticed their younger sons to local medical practitioners, doctors at the capital city of the province, or even star teachers of national fame in Edo, Kyoto, and Osaka. At least one of the seventeen

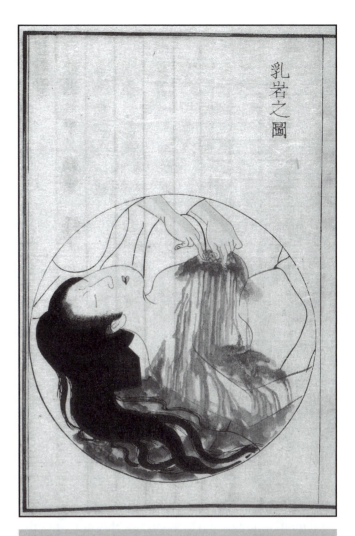

Excision of a cancerous growth from a woman's breast. This treatise made public for the first time the pioneering procedures of Hanaoka Seishū, who performed the operation in 1804 using general anesthetic. Colored block print from Kamata Keishu, *Geka kihai*, 1851. Japanese MS 18 Wellcome Library, London.

original students taught by von Siebold was a peasant hailing from a rural village. When there was no doctor in a village, the village officials invited a medical practitioner to stay and practice.

The ultimate basis for the flourishing of medical practice was demand for medical service by the populace. Much evidence suggests that common people in the Edo period were becoming increasingly health-conscious and sought professional help of one kind or another. A flood of popular manuals for the maintenance of health (*yōjō*) was one of the signs of people's keen interest in self-help regimens. The most famous and enduringly popular was *Yōjō-kun* by Kaibara Ekiken (1630–1714), which told, in a concise and easy style, what to eat and drink, what to wear, and, most famously, how frequently one should copulate. The phenomenal rise in the sales of patent medicine is another tes-

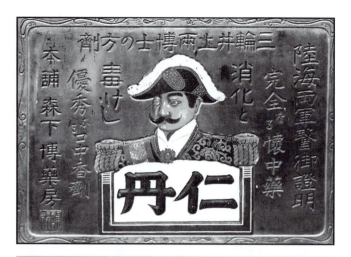

Sign board of an apothecary. Painted and engraved wood, nineteenth century. Wellcome Library, London.

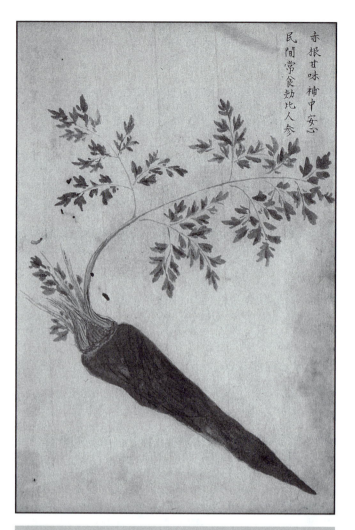

Carrot (*Daucus carota*) root with leaves. Watercolor original of an illustration included in a Japanese book of herbs and vegetables. Iconographic Collection, Wellcome Library, London.

timony to people's demand for professionally produced drugs. These drugs, usually round pills, served for various ailments. Abortion pills were frowned upon, but they were sold under the name of a 'monthly pill' by druggists and peddlers. Fairs and markets were infested by quacks with flamboyant sales dramaturgy; rural villages were served by more trustworthy itinerant merchants. Drugs constituted a huge market, and everyone was keen to take advantage of their potential. Buddhist temples and Shintoist shrines sold their own special brands of medicines, which were popular also as souvenirs for tourist-pilgrims. Cultivation of medicinal plants became a part of major economic policy for the promotion of industry. The Tokugawa Shōgunate ran five physic gardens in Edo, Kyoto, Nagasaki, and Sunpu (now Shizuoka). At least eight provinces had well-tended physic gardens, which acted as regional centers of medical botany and natural history. Local *daimyōs* were keen to develop their own specialty products. Small and poor Toyama province was particularly keen to organize a peddling business, which covered the entire nation as its market. Tsugaru province cultivated poppies for opium. Medicinal plants were also imported from abroad, the most important being Korean carrots. The flourishing drug industry thus involved both public authorities and private producers, urban and rural dwellers, and foreign and domestic trade.

MODERN AND POST-MODERN PERIODS, 1850–2000

Since the emphasis of this essay is on 'traditional' medicine in Japan, I shall give only a sketchy account of its modern and postmodern developments. Yet again, it was a change in the international situation in the Far East and the Japanese response to it that provided a key in ushering Japanese medicine into modernity. The threat of the Western

powers after the Opium War (1840–42) galvanized Japanese intellectuals, many of whom had learned Dutch medicine and had grasped the precarious situation Japan faced. Abandonment of the seclusion policy (1854) under the pressure of the U.S. gunboat diplomacy further inflamed intense disputes and profound turmoil until the overthrow of the Tokugawa Shōgunate in 1867. Through the fierce disputes over the future course of Japan, something very similar to the notion of the imagined community of the nation-state rapidly crystallized. Most active in this remarkable period were the subelites of society, mainly educated samurai of middle to lower ranks. Since this social sector largely overlapped with that to which the upper medical practitioners belonged, many people who had learned medicine, particularly Ranpō medicine, played prominent roles in the overthrow of the Shōgunate. This means that, even before the Meiji Revolution, medicine in the 1850s and 1860s occupied one of the central places in building a strong nation-state able to withstand the onslaught of the Western powers. The chronic frustration of medical practitioners, who had deep inferiority complexes about their 'small art' as previously mentioned, finally found an effective vent: medicine at last looked to make a contribution to dealing with the ills of the body politic.

Several key developments in modernizing Japanese medicine thus happened before the Meiji Revolution. During the period that led to the revolution, local authorities and the national networks of private individuals were more important than the initiatives of the central government. Many provinces built their own hospitals that combined clinical education in Western medicine with medical provision for the poor. The diffusion of vaccination, introduced from Nagasaki in 1849 and spread all over the country in less than ten years, exhibited a similar pattern. Helped by a national network of Ranpō doctors, private medical practitioners often took initiatives in starting vaccination, which was quickly supported by the local authority.

In several medical matters, the powerful central government, which followed the Meiji Revolution of 1868, thus regulated and centralized existing local initiatives in medicine. In other matters, however, the central government was innovative and ambitious. One such matter was the determination to replicate the medical education of German universities in Japan. When the Medical School of the University of Tokyo was founded in 1869, its professors were all German: less than thirty years later, virtually all the departments were headed by Japanese professors, who had studied in German universities. The University of Tokyo then went on to dominate medical education in Japan, by installing its graduates in other prestigious medical schools. The Institute of Infectious Diseases, founded in 1892 with the Koch-trained Kitasato Shibasaburō as its director, became a rival institution to the University of Tokyo. These and other institutions were the home to many discoveries made by Japanese medical scientists. The most famous among them included Shiga Kiyoshi's (1870–1957) discovery of the pathogen of dysentery in 1897 and the experiments on cancer (1915) by Yamagiwa Katsusaburo (1863–1930). By the early twentieth century, Japanese medical scientific communities were capable of fostering world-class research projects.

The Westernization of medical teaching and research was thus achieved first among the agenda of modernizing medicine. In contrast, the modernization of medical practice lagged behind, with compromises and half-measures abounding. After Isei (1874), which was the foundational manifesto for modern medical policy regulated by the state, the government attempted to install a medical licensing system based on the formal education of Western medicine and an examination system to ensure competence. Since the system included only Western medicine in the examination

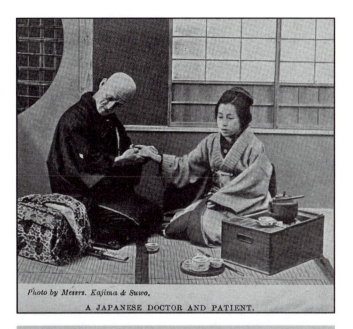

Photo by Messrs. Kajima & Suwo.

A JAPANESE DOCTOR AND PATIENT.

Doctor feeling the pulse of a female patient. Halftone reproduction from a photograph by Messrs Kajima and Suwo, nineteenth century. Iconographic Collection, Wellcome Library, London.

subjects, it met substantial opposition from practitioners of Kanpō (Japanese-Chinese) medicine. Leading Kanpō practitioners, many of whom had connections with former provincial medical schools, put up fierce opposition to the Meiji government's policy of the total Westernization of medical licensing. In the end, their attempt failed when in 1894 parliament rejected the bill for the amendment of the Medical Licensing Act (1884). The victory of the government-led Westernization of medical practice was only partial, however. In 1874, there were about 28,000 medical practitioners, of whom only about 5,200 had learned Western medicine. More than 80 percent of medical practitioners had been trained, if they had been trained at all, in Kanpō medicine. A significant minority were barely literate, due to the almost total lack of regulation of medical practice during the Edo period. The government had to bow to this reality and put the quantity before the quality of medical provision. The resulting system thus had a huge loophole: those who had already practiced medicine were not required to take the examination. This exemption of practitioners from licensing requirements was first adopted in 1875, and retained in subsequent pieces of legislation. In 1882, even the sons of practitioners of Kanpō medicine were granted licenses without examination. This led to a situation in which newly granted medical licenses were based on Western medicine, but the majority of practitioners long remained Kanpō doctors. Even in 1900, more than half of the 40,000 medical practitioners received their license without any examination or attendance at modernized medical schools. The Westernization of medicine did not greatly affect the vested interests of medical practitioners: they continued to be allowed to practice and to make profit at any place of their choice.

Medical provision for those people who could not afford the fees of medical practitioners was also severely limited in the late nineteenth and early twentieth centuries. Public hospitals comparable to European charity hospitals or English voluntary hospitals had not developed in Japan. Koishikawa Yōjō-sho, founded in Edo in 1722 and housing at its height some 170 poor patients, is a famous but isolated exception. When Pompe van Meerdervoort (1829–1908) established a public hospital in Nagasaki, which combined clinical teaching and charitable provision, he was surprised at the rich patients who flocked to the hospital seeking treatment. Similar patterns were repeated later in public hospitals founded by provinces and prefectures in the 1860s and 1870s. By 1877 there were seventy-one public hospitals in Japan, but they were more like today's superior medical centers than charity hospitals in early-modern Europe. The rich patients patronized public hospitals in Japan much earlier than their Western counterparts did. Moreover, the demands of wealthy patients for hospital treatment gave rise to profit-making private hospitals, among which Juntendō Hospital founded in 1875 was the most impressive. Medical entrepreneurs were quick to exploit the situation: between 1877 and 1888, some 300 profit-making hospitals were established. In 1880, there were 241 public hospitals and 122 private ones, while twenty years later in 1899, there were ninety-seven public hospitals and 793 private ones. Hospitals in late-nineteenth and early-twentieth century Japan were typically the symbol of successful private practitioners, rather than the expression of charitable concerns of the elite of society.

With the rapid industrialization and the deepening of accompanying social ills, people started to search for a means to complement the system of medical provision, which consisted almost solely of fee-based service. Such a search was called the 'socialization of medicine', a catchall term that included ideologically diverse policies and schemes. The two early attempts at the socialization of medicine made in 1911 testified to their diversity. The first was Saiseikai, a charitable body established by the government with the help of the Imperial household. Through medical institutions all over the country, it treated 42,000 patients in 1912, 5.4 million in 1926, and 8.8 million in 1935. The second was the nonprofit clinic movement (Jippi-shinryo-jo), a brainchild of two socialist-leaning reformers. It aimed to provide medical treatment to the laboring poor at prices much lower than those fixed by medical practitioners' associations. Despite vehement attacks from medical practitioners, the movement became extremely popular. In 1929, more than 150 clinics and hospitals around the country provided treatment in this way. With diverse concerns and ideological motives as its background, the mixed economy of medical welfare progressed in the 1910s and 1920s. In 1922, the government passed the Health Insurance Act, which covered industrial laborers' medical expenses. By 1935, the Act had about three million individuals insured.

While urban laborers started to benefit from these measures of socialized medicine, peasants and agricultural laborers were left to suffer, often hard hit by violent fluctuations of the price of agricultural products. The shrinking of medical provision in rural areas exacerbated their plight: Japanese medical practitioners were attracted to cities, which left many villages without any practicing doctor. In 1935, cities had 1.3 doctors per 1,000 patients, while the figure for villages was 0.35 doctors per 1,000 patients. About 30 percent of towns and villages had no medical practitioner at all. To facilitate rural workers' access to medical provision, various measures were taken, such as mutual-aid societies in villages. Perhaps the most important breakthrough came in 1938, when the National Health Insurance cast a wider net to include peasants and agricultural laborers. The impetus for National Health Insurance came both from below and from above: while peasants wanted access to medical provision, the government attempted to secure as many healthy soldiers and workers as possible, with the war in China in progress and the increasingly inevitability of war against the United States in their mind.

Although the health status of the Japanese populace started to show signs of improvement from around the 1920s, the present longevity of the Japanese population draws largely on post–World War II developments. During the Edo period, Japanese people seemed to enjoy relatively good health. The infant mortality rate is estimated to have been around 200 per 1,000 live births, which is a low figure for an early modern society. Urban mortality in Edo and other major cities was perhaps not as high as that of comparable European cities in the eighteenth and nineteenth centuries. One historian has attributed this to sophisticated sanitation practices, particularly the disposal of night soil into the agricultural hinterland for fertilizer. From the mid-nineteenth century, the Japanese population started to grow after the stagnation of the previous two centuries: from around 33 million in the 1870s, it grew to 43 million in 1900, and to 60 million in 1925. This increase was, however, perhaps less to do with declining mortality than to rising fertility. In all probability, the health status worsened in the late nineteenth century and the first two decades in the twentieth century. The opening of Japan to foreign trade deprived it of a natural cordon sanitaire, and in the 1880s and 1890s, Japan was hard-hit by a series of epidemics, among which cholera had the most devastating effect. Although cholera subsided after around 1900, in the first half of the twentieth century, life expectancy rose only slightly. S. Ryan Johansson and Carl Mosk have estimated that between 1891 and 1936, the life expectancy of Japanese males rose only slightly, from 42.8 to 46.9 years, while during the same period the comparable figure for England and

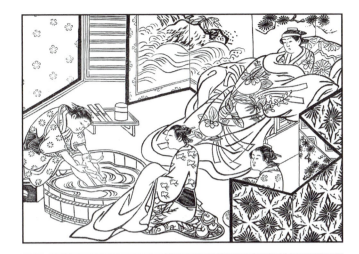

Newborn baby being bathed in a wooden tub while its mother watches from her bed. Halftone reproduction from Heinrich Ploss and Max Bartels, *Das Weib in der Natur—und Völkerkunde* . . . Leipzig, 1913. Wellcome Library, London.

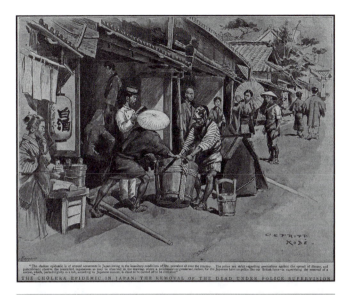

Disposal of the dead under police supervision during a cholera epidemic. The corpse, packed tightly in a wooden tub according to Japanese custom, is carried off to be cremated. Halftone reproduction of a drawing by Meisenbach after Charles Edwin Fripp, *c.* 1890. Iconographic Collection, Wellcome Library, London.

Wales rose by more than ten years.The underdevelopment of the sanitary infrastructure and poor nutrition must have played a large part in keeping Japanese life expectancy low. Mortality from tuberculosis was high, both in urban and rural areas. Johansson and Mosk have pointed a blaming finger at Japan's spending on its huge military budget as a means of achieving its imperial ambitions.

Their speculation sounds more convincing when one observes the phenomenal improvement of health status after Japan's defeat in World War II and the subsequent disarmament. In the fifteen years between 1947 and 1962, the crude death rate almost halved, and infant mortality declined to approximately a third of its former level. It remains a mystery why the rapid improvement of these health indices started in the late 1940s, when millions were facing starvation in the war-ravaged cities. Certainly one of the keys was the introduction of antibiotics, whose domestic production was encouraged by the U.S. army of occupation. The so-called 'Economic Miracle', which was kicked off because of the Korean War in 1950, confirmed the upward trend of the people's health. Various policies of socialized medicine, which had been established before the war in the government's efforts to secure healthy soldiers, were revived and extended. The coverage of insurance plans continued to widen, until in 1961 an insurance plan of one kind or another covered all people in Japan. The rapid improvement of health status continued through the 1970s. Around 1980, the life expectancy of Japanese people became the longest in the world. Since then, Japan has remained the world's healthiest country.

BIBLIOGRAPHY

Fujikawa, Yū, 1980–82. *Fujikawa Yū chosaku-shū* [Collected works of Fujikawa Yū] 10 vols. (Kyoto); Fujikawa, Yū, 1972. *Nihon igakushi* [History of medicine in Japan] (Tokyo); Fujikawa, Yū, 1969. *Nihon shippei-shi* [History of diseases in Japan] (Tokyo); History of Science Publication Society for Japan Academy, ed., 1955–64. *Meiji-zen Nihon igakushi* [History of medicine in Japan before the Meiji period] 5 vols. (Tokyo); Japanese Society for the History of Science, 1965 and 1967. *Nihon kagaku gijutsu-shi taikei* [History of Science and Technology in Japan] 26 vols. [Medicine, vols. 24 and 25] (Tokyo); Kawakami, Takeshi, 1965. *Gendai Nihon iryōshi* [History of medical practice in contemporary Japan] (Tokyo); Sakai, Shizu, 1982. *Nihon no iryōshi* [History of medical practice in Japan] (Tokyo); Shinmura, Hiraku, 1985. *Nihon iryō shakaishi no kenkyū* [A study of Japanese social history of medicine] (Tokyo); Shinmura, Hiraku, 1983. *Kodai iryō kanjin-sei no kenkyū* [A study on ancient medical officials] (Tokyo).

Akihito Suzuki

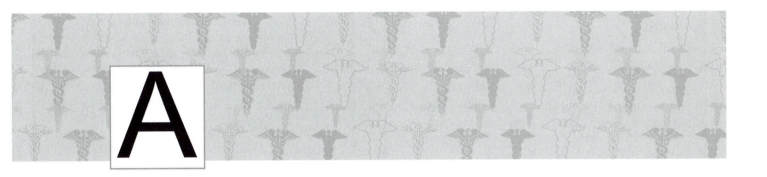

A

ABBOTT, MAUDE ELIZABETH (b. St Andrews East, Quebec, Canada, 18 March 1869; d. Montreal, Canada, 2 September 1940), *pathology, congenital disorders.*

Born Maude Elizabeth Seymour Babin, Abbott lived with her grandmother, Mrs William Abbott, after her parents separated and her mother died of tuberculosis. She later legally adopted the maternal family name. Educated at home and in a small private school, her diary and school record reveal a perceptive, industrious child who was able to win a scholarship to McGill University, which had just begun to admit women to the study of arts. She was elected class president, became editor of the *McGill Fortnightly* and class valedictorian, and at graduation won the Stanley Medal. She said she had fallen in love with McGill, only to be crushed when the medical school did not accept the university policy on women and refused her application. She began an unsuccessful public campaign for admission, and instead was admitted as one of the first three women at Bishop's Medical College in 1890. Although the experience was not a happy one, she graduated MD, CM with highest honors in 1894. It required another public campaign to allow her to complete her clinical studies in the Montreal hospitals.

Abbott spent some years studying pathology in Europe, returning to Montreal in 1897 where she did some private practice, but she yearned for an academic career at McGill. Befriended by McGill professors George Adami and

Charles Martin, she continued her studies in pathology and bacteriology, and was made Assistant Curator of the Medical Museum. She set about reorganizing and cataloguing the museum materials by a method she devised, and although her method became widely used, it was seldom credited to her.

A milestone in her career came in 1898 when she visited Baltimore and attended Sir William Osler's clinical round and his evening conference. He told her she had a fine opportunity at the McGill Museum, and should read Jonathan Hutchinson's article in the 1893 *British Medical Journal* on the nature of a medical museum. A year later she wrote to Osler about a case of cor triloculare that he had identified earlier as one reported by one of the founders of McGill, A. F. Holmes. Osler invited her to write a section on congenital heart disease for his textbook. This began her lifelong interest in congenital heart disease on which she eventually published more than forty-five articles and monographs. Her *Atlas of Congenital Cardiac Disease*, a classification based on more than 1,000 cases, brought her worldwide recognition and became the groundwork for the new field of pediatric cardiac surgery.

In 1907 she founded the International Association of Medical Museums. She was promoted to Curator of the McGill Medical Museum, and appointed Lecturer in Pathology. In 1923 she acquired her highest rank at McGill, Assistant Professor of Medical Research. That same year, after a number of attempts, the Woman's Medical College of Pennsylvania succeeded in recruiting her as Professor of Pathology and Bacteriology; but she accepted the appointment on loan from McGill, and within two years was back in Montreal. She was regarded in her later years as a pioneer in the fight for women's role in medicine. She retired in 1936 and was awarded an honorary LLD from McGill. A scholarship for women was founded in her name.

Aside from her writings on congenital heart disease, she wrote the history of McGill's medical faculty (1902) which did not admit women until 1918; a system of classification of museum specimens (1903); a collection of writings about Osler, a bibliography of his 1,551 writings (1929); and a history of Quebec medicine (1931).

Bibliography

Primary: 1936. *Atlas of Congenital Cardiac Disease* (New York).

Secondary: Waugh, D., 1992. *Maudie of McGill: Dr. Maude Abbott and the foundations of heart surgery* (Toronto); Scriver, J. B., 1966. 'Maude E. Abbott.' in Innis, Mary Quayle ed., *The Clear Spirit: twenty Canadian women and their times* (Toronto); McDermott, H. E., 1959. 'Maude Abbott.' *McGill Medical Journal* 28: 127–152; McDermott, H. E., 1941. *Maude Abbott* (Toronto); *DAMB*.

Jock Murray

ABD UL-HAMĪD   (b. Delhi, India, 14 September 1908, d. Delhi, 23 July 1999); **SAĪD, MUHAMMAD** (b. Delhi, India, 9 January 1920, d. Karachi, Pakistan, 17 October 1998), *hakīms, physicians of unani tibb.*

The brothers Abd ul-Hamīd and Muhammad Saīd expanded their family's pharmacy into the world's largest manufacturers of unani pharmaceuticals—Hamdard Laboratories (*waqf*). They are known in South Asia not only for their commercial success, but also for their commitment to education and for their philanthropic activities.

Abd ul-Hamīd and Muhammad Saīd were the eldest and youngest sons of Abd ul-Majīd and Rābia Begum. The ancestors of one branch of the family had migrated from Kashgar, a vibrant Islamic center on the Silk Road in Chinese Central Asia, at the turn of the seventeenth century. They settled first in Peshawar before moving to Multan and then to Delhi in the nineteenth century. The family had a background in the textile trade. Abd ul-Majīd learned the druggist's trade in the Hindustānī Davākhāna, a relatively large, newly established production base and dispensary for unani medicines set up by Hakīm Ajmal Khān. In 1905 he took a loan of 250 rupees to start up a small pharmacy of his own in the Hauz Qāzī locality of Delhi, an area where there were many druggists' shops. In 1909 regular production of medicines began and two further shops were opened. By 1918, Abd ul-Majīd had expanded his operations under the name Hamdard Davākhāna (*hamdard* means 'sharing pain, empathy' in Urdu, and *davākhāna* is literally 'place of medicine', i.e., dispensary), and in 1920 he

established a manufacturing unit for the production of almond oil. The main building of Hamdard Davākhāna in Lāl Kuān locality was completed in March 1922, shortly before Abd ul-Majīd's untimely death at age forty. Rābia Begum assumed management of the family business and raised the five children. At the time of their father's death Abd ul-Hamīd was thirteen and Muhammad Saīd two. Abd ul-Hamīd's education was interrupted in 1918 by widespread agitation in India over the collapse of the Ottoman Empire and Caliphate (*khilāfat*). After his father's death, Abd ul-Hamīd turned his attention to the study of tibb.

In 1925 he began studies at the Ayurvedic and Unani Tibbiya College in Delhi with the support of his mother and subsequently took over the family's pharmacy business. Abd ul-Hamīd was joined in this enterprise in 1940 by his younger brother Hakīm Muhammad Saīd. Muhammad Saīd graduated from Tibbiya College in 1939, and the two brothers continued to expand Hamdard's operations. They began mass-producing health products that became household names in the subcontinent, such as the cooling summer *sharbat* (medicinal drink) Ruh Afza, the blood-purifier Safi, and the tonic Cinkara. The Partition of India was announced on 3 June 1947. Just over six months later Hakīm Muhammad Saīd left for Karachi in the newly founded Pakistan. Here Muhammad Saīd established the Pakistani branch of Hamdard. Within six years Hamdard had become the leading manufacturer of herbal medicines in Pakistan. Originally a commercial enterprise, in 1948 Hamdard in India was declared a *waqf* (an Islamic religious endowment that emphasizes ideals of public charity). As a result the company became registered as a charity and was therefore exempted from tax. Hamdard converted to *waqf* in Pakistan in 1953 with the formation of the Hamdard Trust. In accordance with the objectives of the *waqf* deeds, Hakīms Abd ul-Hamīd and Muhammad Saīd established several institutions for teaching and research—in unani tibb, biomedicine, nursing, Islamic sciences, and Indo-Islamic culture. The proceeds from the pharmaceutical wing, Hamdard (Waqf) Laboratories, were sown into social and educational projects.

In 1962 Hakīm Abd ul-Hamīd and his associates founded the Institute of History of Medicine and Medical Research, in the following year the Indian Institute of Islamic Studies. In 1972 Hamdard College of Pharmacy was established, and in 1980 Hamdard Tibbi College was incorporated into Jamia Hamdard. Jamia Hamdard acquired the status of a University in 1989. The government of India awarded Hakīm Abd ul-Hamīd the Padma Shri in 1965 and Padma Bhushan in 1991 for his commitment to education, health, and social service. In addition to medical subjects, the current ambit of Jamia Hamdard extends to graduate and postgraduate courses in information technology and business management.

In Pakistan the Hamdard Foundation, under the leadership of Hakīm Muhammad Saīd, became the premier institution for instruction and research in a modernized unani tibb, which incorporated instruction in biomedical pharmacology and other disciplines. Hakīm Saīd founded the Society for Promotion of Eastern Medicine (Anjuman Taraqqi-i-Tibb), which organized a month-long visit to China in 1963. Mao Zedong's promotion of Chinese medicine at this time inspired Hakīm Saīd as a model for the revival of Eastern medical practices (Saīd, 1965). Hakim Muhammad Saīd's ambitions in education were realized in the formation of the large campus Madinat al-Hikmah on the outskirts of Karachi in 1983 and the establishment of Hamdard University Karachi. His engagement with education and health care in Pakistan led to collaborations with national and international bodies, such as UNESCO and WHO. Hakīm Muhammad Saīd was also a prominent political figure. He was the Governor of the Province of Sindh from July 1993 until January 1994.

Hakīms Abd ul-Hamīd and Muhammad Saīd were both prolific writers in Urdu and English. Abd ul-Hamīd was the founder-editor of the journals *Studies in History of Medicine and Science* and *Studies in Islam*. Muhammad Saīd was the founder-editor of *Hamdard Medicus* and *Hamdard Islamicus*, for the promotion of tibb and Islamic culture, respectively. Both hakīms were active in promoting the discipline of medical elementology, in which they attempted to fuse the theories of the four elements in tibb with the elements of modern chemistry. In the work that has resulted from the conferences and publications on this theme, mainstream pharmacological analyses dominate.

In addition to these activities the brothers were practicing hakīms. It was outside his clinic in the early hours of 17 October 1998 that Hakīm Muhammad Saīd was shot dead by unknown assailants. His daughter, Sadia Rashid, subsequently became the chairperson of the Foundation. Hakīm Abd ul-Hamīd died within a year of his brother.

Bibliography

Primary: Saīd, Muhammad, 1965. *Medicine in China* (Karachi); Abd ul-Hamīd, 1967. *Qarabadin-i Hamdard* (Delhi); Saīd, Muhammad, ed., 1970. *Pharmacopeia of Eastern Medicine* (Karachi); Saīd, Muhammad, ed., trans., 1982. *Al-Biruni's book on pharmacy and materia medica* 2 vols. (Karachi); Saīd, Muhammad, ed., 1995. *Essays on science* (Karachi).

Secondary: Bode, Maarten, 2004. 'Ayurvedic and unani health and beauty products: reworking India's medical traditions.' PhD thesis, University of Amsterdam.

Guy Attewell

ABDURAHMAN, ABDULLAH   (b. Cape Town, South Africa, 18 December 1870; d. Cape Town, 20 February 1940), *general practice*.

The grandson of Muslim slaves who had purchased their freedom in the 1820s and son of well-off Cape Town greengrocers, Abdurahman received the best schooling then available in Britain's Cape Colony, despite being neither white nor Christian, thanks to his family's wealth and commitment to Western education. Believing in higher education as an instrument of social mobility, they encouraged him to study further, and in 1889 he entered the University of Glasgow Medical School, where he was influenced by Professor W. T. Gairdner's broadly conceived ideas on public health and the practical implementation of these ideas in Glasgow at the time. Thus, to Abdurahman, susceptibility to disease was due 'largely to the relatively poor environmental and overcrowded conditions under which the majority live, and to the greater degree of under-nourishment to which they are habitually subjected' (*Cape Coloured Population Inquiry*, 1937, ¶523).

Graduating MB ChB from Glasgow University in 1893, he spent the next eighteen months gaining experience in London hospitals before returning to Cape Town, where he opened a general practice in 1895, thereby becoming the first locally born mixed-race 'colored' to do so. His practice blossomed, drawing patients from all race groups in the city's working-class districts where his house calls reimpressed on him the public health lessons he had learned in Glasgow. He took pains to explain to his patients in everyday language the treatment he prescribed, although for their folk remedies he had little tolerance and, as a Muslim, he eschewed the use of medicine containing alcohol. Aware of the poverty of many of his patients, he was careful not to push himself onto them by repeated visits. Consequently, he kept few patient records and rarely did follow-up house calls, declaring that 'a doctor must only call when sent for' (*Cape Times*, 4 April 1912, p. 9).

Formally dressed in suit and fez—a combination that summed up his cross-cultural identity—and traveling in a smart trap (later exchanged for one of Cape Town's first cars), Abdurahman deliberately cut an impressive figure as he made his rounds. His stature in his own 'colored' community and beyond rose rapidly—he quickly became known as 'The Doctor'—and during the bubonic plague epidemic in Cape Town in 1901, he was able to persuade Muslims to accept the tough sanitary controls imposed by the authorities.

His growing reputation also saw him drawn into politics, first as the city's first 'colored' town councilor (1904), then as the president of the African People's Organization (APO), a national political organization fighting for the rights of 'colored' citizens (1905), and finally as a member of the Cape Provincial Council (1914). Not surprisingly, he directed much of his political attention to public health. Yet, despite chairing Cape Town's health, public works and improvements, and streets and drainage committees and devoting less and less time to his own practice (he gave this up in 1929), his greatest achievements in this sphere were quite modest: the introduction of the medical inspection of school pupils, the inclusion of hygiene in the school curriculum, and the creation of a special college to train 'colored' nurses.

For all his powerful championship of the rights of his community, however, he was operating in an environment in which white interests were increasingly prioritized over those of the rest of the population. The crumbs he was able to secure left a new generation unsatisfied, and from the 1930s he and his APO came under growing attacks from this radical quarter. Though his funeral attracted over 30,000 mourners, his APO and gentlemanly means of winning reforms barely survived his death.

Abdurahman was married twice, first (1894–1923) to a Scot, second (1925–40) to a South African. By the former, he had two daughters, by the latter two sons and a daughter.

Bibliography

Primary: 1912. 'Tuberculosis Commission. Dr. Abdurahman's views' *Cape Times*, 4 April, p. 9; Union of South Africa, 1937. *Report of the Cape Coloured Population Inquiry* U.G. 54-1937; 1990. (Van der Ross, R. E., ed.) *Say It Out Loud: The APO Presidential Addresses and Other Major Political Speeches 1906–1940, of Dr Abdullah Abdurahman* (Bellville).

Howard Phillips

ABEL, JOHN JACOB (b. Cleveland, Ohio, USA, 19 May 1857; d. Baltimore, Maryland, USA, 26 May 1938), *experimental medicine, endocrinology.*

Abel was one of the most distinguished biological chemists of his day and the founder of pharmacology in America. Little is known about his early life, but in 1883 he graduated in physiology and chemistry from the University of Michigan. The next year he went to Europe and, in Leipzig from 1884 to 1886, studied physiology under Ludwig and von Frey, histology under His, pharmacology under Boehm, pathology under Strumpell, and inorganic and organic chemistry under Wislicenus. The winter of 1886–87 saw him in Strassburg doing internal medicine with Kussmaul, and he received his MD there in 1888. In 1889–90 he worked with the biochemist v. Necki in Switzerland. Also, he 'walked the wards with von Recklinghausen'. This extremely broad education gave him the background for his wide-ranging chemical research over the next fifty years.

In 1890 he was offered a chair at the University of Michigan to establish a department of pharmacology, but in 1893 was recruited to join the outstanding faculty at Johns Hopkins as the first full time professor of pharmacology where he remained for the next forty-five years. Abel was impressed by the German system of specialist journals, and he introduced it to America. Between 1895 and 1910, he was instrumental in founding the *Journal of Experimental Medicine, Journal of Biological Chemistry*, and the *Journal of Pharmacology and Experimental Therapeutics.*

His interest in the isolation of hormones began around 1895, and he worked on adrenal extracts for the next ten years. He isolated a monobenzoyl form of epinephrine, but

the Japanese chemist, Takamine, isolated the pure compound with a much simpler process and took the credit. In 1909 Abel and Leonard Rowntree studied the phthaleins in the hope of finding an injectable laxative. This never materialized, but the work led to widely used tests of kidney and liver function.

In 1913 Abel became interested in removing substances from the blood of living animals by dialysis, and made an elaborate apparatus with which he could remove salicylic acid and other substances as efficiently as the natural kidney. He also found amino acids in his dialysates, the first proof that they were present in the blood. He also did experiments with 'plasmaphaeresis' in which red cells were separated from the plasma and then reinjected. In his 1914 paper on this topic, he suggested the possibility of blood banks.

Between 1917 and 1924 Abel tried to purify the active principle(s) of the posterior pituitary, but progress was discouraging and he switched to insulin in the aftermath of its discovery in 1921. He became the first person to crystallize insulin in 1925, and established that it was a protein. The idea that a protein could have the unique pharmacological properties of insulin was unthinkable, and led to a long controversy from which Abel emerged victorious. From 1925 to 1932 his laboratory was the center of research into the chemical nature of insulin.

From the many affectionate tributes of his pupils, it is clear that Abel was the archetype of the absent-minded professor. After noting that he was 'a most lovable man', Leonard Rowntree wrote that he 'slept, ate and drank research'; while in the words of Paul Lamson, 'His interest was in the nature of things, the nature of the great chemical laboratory, the living organism'.

Bibliography

Primary: 1957. *John Jacob Abel, M.D.: Investigator, Teacher, Prophet, 1857–1938: A Collection of Papers by and about the Father of American Pharmacology* (Baltimore).

Secondary: Parascandola, John, 1982. 'John J. Abel and the early development of pharmacology at the Johns Hopkins University.' *Bulletin of the History of Medicine* 56: 512–527; Murnaghan, J. H., and P. Talalay, 1967. 'John Jacob Abel and the crystallization of insulin.' *Perspectives in Biology and Medicine* 10: 334–380; Lamson, P. D., 1941. 'John Jacob Abel: a portrait.' *Bulletin Johns Hopkins Hospital* 68:119–157; Voegtlin, Carl, 1939. 'John Jacob Abel.' *Journal of Pharmacology and Experimental Therapeutics* 67: 373–406 (This article includes a full list of his publications); *DAMB; DSB.*

Robert Tattersall

ABERNETHY, JOHN (b. London, England, 3 April 1764; d. Enfield, Middlesex, England, 28 April 1831), *surgery, physiology, anatomy.*

One of the five children of John Abernethy, a merchant, and Elizabeth Weir, Abernethy studied at Wolverhampton grammar school before being apprenticed to Charles Blicke, surgeon to St Bartholomew's Hospital, London. During his apprenticeship he attended lectures at St Bartholomew's, The London Hospital, and William Hunter's anatomy school. Here John Hunter's lectures exerted a considerable influence on him, while William Blizard at The London encouraged his interest in anatomy. At St Bartholomew's he served as assistant surgeon (1787–1815) and senior surgeon (1815–27) and dominated the medical school, lecturing in anatomy (1788–1829) and in surgery (1788–1829).

Although teaching had started at St Bartholomew's before Abernethy was appointed, he had a major impact on the early development of the hospital's medical school and on the nature of medical training in London. He initially gave private lectures in a house near the hospital, but so many students were attracted that the governors built a lecture theater within the hospital in 1791, and an anatomical theater in 1822. Students were drawn to his abruptness, clear and effective manner, and style of teaching that stressed the importance of anatomy, which for him was the foundation of medical knowledge.

Abernethy was not noted for his skill as a surgeon—he disliked operating—but he did enjoy a large, lucrative practice. In his treatment of patients he tended to dismiss contemporary medical practices that emphasized close attention to the peculiarities of the individual case. Heavily influenced by Hunter, Abernethy saw firm distinctions between physic and surgery as misleading, asserting that 'the physician must understand surgery' and 'the surgeon the medical treatment of disease' (Abernethy, 1830, p. 23). He based his ideas on his studies of comparative anatomy, human anatomy and physiology, a combination of experience that distanced him from mere surgical practice. He challenged what he saw as artificial divisions between 'local' and 'constitutional' disease, although he tended to emphasize constitutional over local causes. For Abernethy every aliment was linked to the disorders of digestion. In his work he frequently emphasized the non-surgical aspects of the conditions he described, and argued that close attention to the digestive system was essential for any surgeon.

Frequently brusque and egotistical, Abernethy became embroiled in a number of disputes. Accusations of nepotism in his appointments saw him fall out with the St Bartholomew's governors, damaging the medical school. His dispute with the *Lancet* in 1824 over pirating college lectures not only highlighted the different attitudes toward 'public' and private knowledge, but also resulted in a protracted battle with the journal. Although Abernethy won the dispute, *Lancet* became an enthusiastic critic of St Bartholomew's, frequently condemning the teaching or Abernethy's role.

However, it was his dispute with his former pupil, William Lawrence, which attracted notoriety. In his lectures to the College of Surgeons, Abernethy espoused his Hunterian doctrine that a vital principle animated tissues, vivifying them. He saw life and mind as something 'superadded' to matter, raising mind over neural matter. For Abernethy such a view was essential to keep humanity virtuous. Rather than being a conservative, Abernethy was expressing a speculative Hunterian approach to physiology that many accepted. Lawrence disagreed. In his 1816 lectures to the College he attacked Abernethy's theory. He presented a critique of Hunterian adherence to vital powers, and denied their usefulness as an explanatory model, favoring the experimental physiology of French clinicians. Abernethy saw these views as damaging, responding peevishly in his lectures in the following year. He attacked 'modern sceptics' who espoused French materialism, reasserting his doctrine of vitality and the superiority of British physiologists over continental investigators, whom he castigated as cruel and adding nothing to knowledge. Lawrence was forced to back down to save his position.

Abernethy, despite his influence on the development of English physiology, remained an anatomical surgeon and taught students accordingly. Like his mentor, Hunter, he sought to turn surgery from a craft into a science.

Bibliography

Primary: 1804. *Constitutional Origins of Local Diseases* (London); 1828. *Lectures on Anatomy, Surgery, and Pathology; including Observations on the Nature and Treatment of Local Diseases delivered at St. Bartholomew's Hospital* (London); 1830. *The Surgical and Physiological Works* (London).

Secondary: Lawrence, Susan C., 1996. *Charitable Knowledge: Hospital Pupils and Practitioners in Eighteenth-century London* (Cambridge, UK); Desmond, Adrian, 1989. *The Politics of Evolution: Morphology, Medicine and Reform in Radical London* (Chicago); Thornton, John L., 1953. *John Abernethy: A Biography* (London); *Oxford DNB*.

Keir Waddington

ABT, ISAAC ARTHUR   (b. Wilmington, Illinois, USA, 18 December 1867; d. Chicago, Illinois, USA, 22 November 1955), *medicine, pediatrics.*

Abt was one of twin sons in a family of seven children born to German-Jewish immigrants, Levi Abt and Henrietta Hart. The family, which owned a clothing factory, moved to Chicago (1875), where Abt attended West Division High School, working evenings in a drug store preparing herbal tinctures and popular items. Studying at Johns Hopkins University (1886–69), he was influenced by the clinical research ethos of William Henry Welch, professor of pathology. At Chicago Medical College (1889–91) he extended his pharmaceutical interests by working in the College dispensary. Following graduation and an internship at Chicago's Michael Reese Hospital (1891–92) he toured Europe, studying in London, Vienna, and Berlin.

Returning to Chicago (January 1894), Abt established a practice in internal medicine, but he soon became interested in pediatrics, then a new specialty. He maintained an academic association with Chicago Medical College, becoming an assistant in pediatrics as well as teaching histology and physiology of the nervous system (1894–97). He also served as a district county physician and medical inspector for the Chicago Health Department. In open examination, he earned appointment as the first attending physician in pediatrics, Cook County Hospital (1896). The following year (1897) he became Professor of Diseases of Children at Women's Medical College, Northwestern University, and married Lina Rosenberg, a nurse at Michael Reese Hospital. They had two sons; the elder, Arthur Frederick, also became a pediatrician. Abt moved to Rush Medical College, Chicago (1901), as Associate Professor of Children's Diseases, but returned to Northwestern University Medical School (1909–39) as professor and chairman of the department of pediatrics.

Abt's interests included infant nutrition and the association of artificial feeding with sickness (particularly diarrhea) and death. An advocate of wet nursing over artificial feeding for ailing infants, he was also a founder and first president of the Chicago Milk Commission (1908), which dispensed free fresh milk (from city 'milk stations') to needy mothers. Out of this organization was formed the Infant Welfare Society of Chicago (1911) whose volunteers, including physicians and nurses, offered medical care and parenting advice, as well as making over 40,000 home visits a year. Abt's concern for children's hospital facilities resulted in his election as first president of the Children's Hospital Society of Chicago.

When local philanthropist Edward Morris proposed to endow a children's hospital, Abt and his wife visited pediatric establishments in Europe (1910) to help formulate plans. The resulting Sarah Morris Children's Hospital (1912) was acknowledged as one of the most progressive in the United States. Here was established the country's first premature infant station (1922) under the directorship of Abt's student, Julius Hess. Hess and Abt designed some of the earliest infant incubators, and were among the first pediatricians to establish a role for pediatrics within the obstetric hospital.

Abt was Chairman of the American Medical Association's Section on Pediatrics (1911), serving as its representative in the House of Delegates (1918–35). He prepared a benchmark report on the promotion and sale of infant foods (1925), and published a popular book, *The Baby's Food* (1917). He was a founder of the *American Journal of the Diseases of Children* (1911), and as long-term editor of the *Year Book of Pediatrics* (1902–40), he maintained a comprehensive knowledge of the expanding pediatric literature.

A popular speaker at medical and lay meetings, Abt was noted for an appealing sense of humor. His major edited work, *Abt's Pediatrics* (1923–26), became a classic text. He was President of the American Association for Teachers of the Diseases of Children (1922), the American Pediatric Society (1926), the Chicago Medical Society (1927), and

the Institute of Medicine of Chicago (1933). He was a founder and first president of the American Academy of Pediatrics (1930), and he chaired the Committee on Medical Care for Children at President Hoover's White House Conference (1930). His overseas honors included Chevalier de la Légion d'Honneur (1927) and the one of which he was proudest, honorary membership in the Deutsche Gesellschaft für Kinderheilkunde (1928).

Bibliography

Primary: 1907. (ed.) *Atlas and Epitome of Diseases of Children* (Philadelphia, PA); 1917. *The Baby's Food: Recipes for the Preparation of Food for Infants and Children* (Philadelphia); 1923–26. (ed.) *Pediatrics*, 9 vols. (Philadelphia, PA); 1944. *Baby Doctor* (New York and London).

Secondary: Wiedemann, Hans-Rudolf, 1993. 'The Pioneers of Pediatric Medicine: Isaac Arthur Abt (1867–1955).' *European Journal of Pediatrics* 152(3): 177; Abt, Arthur Frederick, 1965. *History of Pediatrics* (Philadelphia); *DAMB*.

Carole Reeves

ACOSTA-SISON, HONORIA (b. Pangasinan, Philippines, 30 December 1887; d. Manila, Philippines, 19 January 1970), *obstetrics*.

Honoria Acosta-Sison was born in a town in Pangasinan, Philippines. After finishing her high school education, she applied for a government scholarship to continue her education in the United States. Out of 357 applicants, she was chosen as one of the ten who were granted scholarships.

She took her preparatory course at the Drexel Institute and Brown Preparatory School. Afterward, she finished her Doctor of Medicine degree at the Woman's Medical College of Pennsylvania in 1909, making her the first Filipino woman to become a physician. She possessed a strong will and even extended her study to get residency training at the Maternity Hospital in the same institution.

Upon her return to the Philippines, she worked in the Philippine General Hospital, the largest government hospital in the country. Acosta-Sison published research papers on several topics in the *Philippine Journal of Science*, including establishing the normal pelvimetry measures among Filipino women (Acosta-Sison, 1919), and the identification of causes of maternal mortality in the country (Acosta-Sison, 1926). She invented a sagittal pelvimeter and a single-bladed forceps to facilitate the delivery of the fetal head in low cesarean section (Aragon, 1952), a technique she introduced and advocated in the Philippines.

Her accomplishments rivaled those of her male peers. For example, from 1930 to 1938 she wrote forty research papers and a book, *Obstetrics for Nurses* (1936). She became the Head of the Department of Obstetrics at the Philippine General Hospital in 1941. Five years later, she founded and became the first president of the Philippine Obstetrical and Gynecological Society.

Her pioneering efforts earned her more praise. In 1951 she was awarded the Presidential Medal for medical research on the occasion of the fifth anniversary of the Philippine Republic (Acosta-Sison, 1970). In June 1955, President Ramon Magsaysay conferred on her the Presidential Award for being a 'torch bearer in the Feminist Movement,' and in 1959 she was chosen by the Philippine Medical Association as 'The Most Outstanding Practitioner in Manila'.

Clearly, her success has given inspiration to women doctors in the country, but her personality is what endeared her most to her students. Dr. Narciso Cordero, a physiology professor, in his book *To While Away the Hours*, described her as the first Filipino woman physician, first Filipino woman graduate of an American Medical School, first Filipino woman obstetrician, and many other 'firsts'. She reacted with characteristic modesty: 'Why all the fuss? Do you get excited simply because the fellow you have just met happens to be the first born in the family?' (Cordero, 1971).

She was married to Antonio G. Sison, the former Dean of the College of Medicine, University of the Philippines and also Director of the Philippine General Hospital. They had three children: Antonio Jr., Honoria, and Pastora. She quietly passed away on 19 January 1970 at the age of eighty-two, the first Filipina physician and the mother of Philippine obstetrics.

Bibliography

Primary: 1919. (with Fernando Calderon) 'Pelvimetry and Cephalometry among Filipino Women and Newborn Babies: Made on One Thousand Two Hundred Thirty-Seven Cases.' *The Philippine Journal of Science* 14(3): 253–71; 1926. 'Maternal Mortality among Filipinos.' *The Journal of the Philippine Islands Medical Association* 6(10): 321–30; 1970. 'The Story of My Life.' *Journal of the Philippine Medical Association* 46(4): 211–24.

Secondary: Cordero, Narciso, 1971. *To While Away the Hours* (Quezon City, Philippines); Aragon, Gloria T., 1952. 'Honoria Acosta-Sison, M.D.: A Short Biography.' *The Philippine Medical World* 13(3): 63–64.

Willie T. Ong

ACREL, OLOF (b. Österåker, Sweden, 26 November 1717; d. Stockholm, Sweden, 28 May 1806), *surgery*.

Acrel was raised in a clerical family. As a young boy he was sent to the University of Uppsala to study languages and philosophy, but at age sixteen he decided to become a surgeon and moved to Stockholm to study under the barber-surgeon Gerhard Boltenhagen. In 1740 he started a grand European tour of nearly five years. In Paris he studied under Jean-Louis Petit and other eminent surgeons, in Rouen he learned lithotomy with Claude-Nicolas Le Cat, and in London he took advantage of the many hospitals. During the War of the Austrian Succession he enlisted in the French army and soon became an experienced field surgeon. He returned home, still a young man, with the title 'Chirurgien Major'. In Stockholm he passed the examination to qualify as a surgeon and opened a practice.

The Serafimer Hospital, founded in 1752, was the first hospital in Stockholm. It operated under supervision of the Knights of the Order of the Seraphim and served as a training hospital for medical students. Candidates for the post of district medical officer or town or regimental surgeon were required to serve six months to a year at Serafimer. The program for the hospital was taken from two papers to the Royal Academy of Science in 1746 by Olof Acrel and Abraham Bäck—two young men whose experiences in medicine and surgery were acquired in the leading hospitals of Europe. Acrel's paper was titled *The Quickest Way of Establishing and Maintaining a Hospital, so that It May Achieve a Considerable Growth within a Few Years* (in Swedish). Bäck was appointed the hospital's chief medical officer and Acrel was named chief surgeon. Acrel stayed at this unpaid post until 1800, at which time the hospital's beds had increased from eight to 120.

Even before Serafimer Hospital opened, Acrel gave lectures in anatomy and surgery free of charge. In 1755 he achieved the title of professor, although he had earned no university degree; five years later the University of Uppsala awarded him an honorary degree in medicine. This honor was bestowed only after the intense hesitation of Carl Linnaeus, the most influential member of the faculty, who still held deep prejudices against even well-trained modern surgeons.

Acrel established Sweden's modern procedures and techniques in surgery. In 1745 he published his observations on the treatment of wounds in a 300-page monograph that also discussed the medico-forensic aspects of wounds. This monograph has been regarded as the first surgical publication in Sweden. Most of Acrel's many surgical papers were published in the *Proceedings of the Royal Academy of Science*. His two most important collections of cases consisted of notes from the diaries he kept at Serafimer (published 1759; enlarged 1775) in which he described operations to repair hernias, remove stones from the urinary bladder, treat cataracts of the ocular lens, and heal traumatic brain injury.

Acrel belonged to many national and international societies. In 1746 he was elected to the Royal Academy of Science and was its president for three terms. He also held numerous public offices in social and political life; after serving at the court he was elevated to the nobility in 1780. Acrel was appointed the first Director-General of all the hospitals in Sweden (1776).

Acrel was the first doctor in Sweden to combine internal and external medical practice. Although a member of the Society of Surgeons from 1745, he managed to remain above the disputes between surgeons and learned doctors that were common around 1760. He was a most energetic and serious man with a deeply Christian outlook.

Bibliography

Primary: 1745. *Utförlig Förklaring Om Friska Sårs Egenskaper.* [A Detailed Explanation of the Characteristics of Healthy Wounds] Stockholm; 1759. *Chirurgiske Händelser, anmärkte uti Kongl. Lazarettet och annorstädes . . .* [Surgical Cases, Noted in the Royal Hospital . . .] (Stockholm); 1775. *Chirurgiske Händelser, amärkte och smlade uti Kongl. Lazarettet . . .* [Surgical Cases, Noted and Collected in the Royal Hospital] (Stockholm).

Secondary: Kock, Wolfram, 1967. *Olof af Acrel.* (Stockholm); Lindroth, Sten, 1967. *Kungl. Svenska Vetenskapsakademiens historia 1739–1818, I–II.* (Stockholm).

Ingemar Nilsson

ADDIS, THOMAS

ADDIS, THOMAS (b. Edinburgh, Scotland, 27 July 1881; d. Los Angeles, California, USA, 4 June 1949), *internal medicine, kidney disease.*

Addis was the son of Cornelia Beers Campbell and Thomas Chalmers Addis, a Presbyterian clergyman. His early education was at Watson's College in Edinburgh, and his MB ChB (1905) and MD (1908) from the University of Edinburgh. He did hospital training in the UK and postgraduate research work in Berlin and Heidelberg. Following a period as registrar at Leith Hospital in Edinburgh and work at the Laboratory of the Royal College of Physicians of Edinburgh, in 1911 he accepted an invitation from Stanford University School of Medicine, then in San Francisco, to help expand its research work. Addis already had published several papers on blood coagulation and on hemophilia. He became Professor of Medicine in 1920. Following retirement from Stanford in 1948, Addis worked until his death at the Institute for Medical Research at Cedars of Lebanon Hospital in Los Angeles. He served as president of the American Society for Clinical Investigation, and was a member of the National Academy of Sciences.

Tom Addis became a foremost authority on kidney disease, a complete student of the kidney in the clinic and laboratory. Rooted in the nineteenth century, he saw pathology as foundational, so his lifelong program correlated the morbid lesion with both clinical symptoms and functional disturbance. He arrived at a tripartite categorization for chronic renal disease (then known as Bright's disease) with pathologist Jean Oliver; this categorization resembled that of German workers Franz Volhard and Theodor Fahr (*Die Brightsche Nierenkrankheit*, 1914). But Addis believed that his classification was more 'clinical', based on examination of the urine sediment in the living patient. He devised a quantitative method of urine examination (the 'Addis count'), which continued in use into the 1960s. To know the 'extent' of the 'renal lesion' (i.e., the amount of loss of excretory function), he proposed the 'urea ratio', which prefigured the notion of renal 'clearance'. Later in his career, however, he perceived the blood creatinine concentration to serve as a better functional marker,

and some of his last publications deal with simple techniques for measuring this substance.

He recognized that once suffering some insult, kidneys seem to continue to lose mass and physiological capacity even when the inciting disorder, such as glomerulonephritis (an inflammatory process, usually immunogenic, and sometimes induced by streptococcal infection of the throat or skin), has passed. Finally, the patient dies of uremia. The basis for this inexorable progression seemed to Addis the critical question. Following extensive work in the laboratory, he concluded that chronically diseased kidneys simply 'burn out' as compensatory overwork destroys remaining active nephrons. Since the work of the kidneys (in his conception) was expended in excreting the product of protein metabolism (urea), it could be lessened, and renal mass preserved, through a careful limit in dietary protein: this formed the mainstay of his management. This general line of thought was revived by nephrologists of the 1980s, some of whom had discovered Addis's books and articles.

Addis was a far left–leaning progressive—an enthusiast for nondiscrimination, national health insurance in the United States, Republican Spain, and the espoused ideals of Soviet Russia. He conducted his laboratory 'group' as an egalitarian social microcosm in which all contributed ideas. Affluent patients were seen during office hours after the working man. His political views, however, sometimes attracted hostile attention in the years of anticommunist fervor, and probably reduced his influence on future nephrologists. Sharing his politics and serving as his nurse-dietician was Addis's wife, Elesa (Bolton Partridge), whom he married in 1913.

Bibliography

Primary: 1931. (with Oliver, Jean). *The Renal Lesion in Bright's Disease* (New York); 1948. *Glomerular Nephritis: Diagnosis and Treatment* (New York).

Secondary: Lemley, Kevin V. and Linus Pauling, 1994. 'Thomas Addis.' *Biographical Memoirs of the National Academy of Sciences* 63: 3–46; Peitzman, Steven J., 1990. 'Thomas Addis (1881–1949): Mixing Patients, Rats, and Politics.' *Kidney International* 37: 833–840.

Steven J. Peitzman

ADDISON, THOMAS

ADDISON, THOMAS (b. Long Benton, nr Newcastle, England, *c.* April, baptized 11 October 1795; d. Brighton, England, 29 June 1860), *medicine, endocrinology, dermatology.*

Addison's father was a grocer and flour dealer who had higher aspirations for his son. After secondary education at Newcastle grammar school, where he became fluent in Latin, Addison graduated in medicine at Edinburgh in 1815. He moved to London, where he was a pupil of Thomas Bateman (1778–1821), one of the top dermatologists of the day. He became assistant physician at Guy's Hospital in 1824, and full physician in 1837. He was a close colleague of Richard Bright (1789–1858), with whom he published *Elements of Practical Medicine* in 1839. Addison wrote most of it, including the section, 'inflammation of the Caecum and Appendix Vermiformis', an early and remarkably accurate description of appendicitis.

Addison was an expert with the stethoscope, and devoted more attention to diseases of the lungs than to any other area of medicine. Pneumonia had been defined by René Laennec (1781–1826) as 'inflammation of the lung tissue', but in 1843 Addison showed that it was the air spaces that were affected, and described red and gray hepatization.

In 1851, with William Gull (1816–90), he described a twenty-seven-year-old diabetic man with a widespread eruption now known as xanthoma diabeticorum, or xanthomatosis. He founded the department of dermatology at Guy's in 1824, and supervised the making of a series of wax models of skin disorders, which are still extant.

In a paper to the South London Medical Society in 1849, Addison described patients with a peculiar anemia (i.e. weakness), and mentioned that in two of them the only abnormality was disease of the suprarenals. By the time he published his book, *On the Constitutional and Local Effects of Disease of the Supra-renal Capsules* (1855), he had clearly defined two diseases. One was 'a very remarkable form of general anaemia' which 'makes its approach in so slow and insidious a manner that the patient can hardly fix a date to his earliest feeling of that langour which is shortly to become so extreme'. He stressed the absence of weight loss, and that no lesion could be found at autopsy. This disease is now called Addisonian, or pernicious, anemia.

During his investigations, Addison had 'stumbled upon' another disease accompanied by 'anaemia, general languor and debility, remarkable feebleness of the heart's action, irritability of the stomach, and a peculiar change of colour in the skin'. The first five of the eleven patients studied had disease of the adrenal glands, which before then had been thought to be vestigial organs. Confusion between the anemia and the adrenal disease led to a lukewarm reception of Addison's book in England, whereas it was immediately accepted abroad. At a meeting in Paris in 1855, Armand Trousseau (1801–67) proposed the name Addison's disease, which is how it is still known in an age when eponyms are unfashionable.

Addison was noted by his contemporaries for his skill as a diagnostician 'shrewd and sagacious beyond the average of men'. Despite being shy and timid, he was also an outstanding teacher. Unfortunately, he was subject to fits of depression that made him appear haughty and unapproachable. He was not well-known outside of Guy's and never held any office at the Royal College of Physicians. He retired to Brighton in 1860 and three months later committed suicide. When he died, neither the *British Medical Journal* nor the *Lancet* published an obituary.

Bibliography

Primary: 1839. (with Bright, Richard) *Elements of the Practice of Medicine* (London); 1851. (with Gull, W.). 'On a certain affection of the skin. Vitiligoidea, A. Plana, B. Tuberosa.' *Guy's Hospital Reports* 7: 265–276; 1855. *On the Constitutional and Local Effects of Disease of the Supra-renal Capsules* (London); 1868. *A collection of the published writings of the late Thomas Addison, M.D., Physician to Guy's Hospital* (London).

Secondary: Dale, Henry, 1949. 'Thomas Addison, Pioneer of Endocrinology.' *British Medical Journal* ii: 347–352; Hale-White, William, 1935. *Great Doctors of the Nineteenth Century* (London); *DSB*; *Oxford DNB*.

Robert Tattersall

ADLER, ALFRED (b. Penzing, Austria, 7 February 1870; d. Aberdeen, Scotland, 28 May 1937), *individual psychology, psychoanalysis, social medicine.*

From 1888 Adler studied at the Faculty of Medicine in Vienna, where he attended Richard von Krafft-Ebing's course on diseases of the nervous system. He qualified in 1895, after which he set himself up as a general practitioner. In 1897 he married Raissa Epstein, with whom he had four children. He converted from Judaism to Protestantism in 1904 and acquired Austrian citizenship in 1911.

Adler had a deep interest in socialism, and his initial interests lay in the field of social medicine; his first book (1898) was *Gesundheitsbuch für das Schneidergewerbe* [Health book for the tailor trade]. In this work, he presented the thesis that diseases were as much products of society as organically caused, and argued that there was a relationship between diseases and the economic context of any given trade. In 1902 he published some articles on social medicine in Heinrich Grün's journal, *Aerztliche Standeszeitung*, emphasizing the role of prophylaxis.

During this period, Adler began to articulate his concerns in the form of psychology. In 1902 he met Sigmund Freud, and he was one of the initial members of Freud's Wednesday Psychological Society. In 1907 he published a work on organ inferiority, *Studie über Mindwertigkeit von Organen* [Studies on organ inferiority], intended as a contribution to clinical medicine. Therein, he attempted to account for the manner in which diseases were inherited and confined to particular organs, to facilitate the evaluation of disease states. He argued that the inferiority of particular organs gave rise to compensatory phenomena, which expressed themselves psychologically as well as organically. Subsequently, his interests shifted to studying inferiority per se, in terms of individuals' relations to their goals and their environment.

At this time, the formalization of the psychoanalytic movement was taking place. In 1910 Adler became the first president of the Vienna Psychoanalytic Society (VPS), and along with Wilhelm Stekel, co-editor of the new journal *Zentralblatt für Psychoanalyse*. The independence of Adler's theoretical outlook, and his increasing divergence from a number of Freud's theories (which were becoming shibboleths) produced contention. These disputes formed the template for how dissidence came to be managed in the psychoanalytic movement. The fact that some of Adler's criticisms (such as of Freud's overemphasis of the sexual libido) aligned Adler with Freud's detractors, was a serious embarrassment to Freud, given Adler's prominence. Freud's response was to diagnose Adler as paranoid and dismiss his theories as 'heresy'. Following a series of acrimonious debates in Vienna, Adler and his supporters resigned from the VPS in 1911 and formed a 'society for free psychoanalysis', arguing that the unconditional commitment to his theories that Freud demanded was incompatible with science. Dropping Freud's trademark, the society was renamed the 'Society for Individual Psychology'. In his later work Freud would silently reclaim aspects of Adler's theories.

In 1912 Adler published his book *Über den Nervösen Charakter: Grundzüge einer vergleichenden Individual-Psychologie und Psychotherapie* (Eng. edn. 1916), which was marked by his reading of the neo-Kantian Hans Vaihinger's philosophy of fictionalism. Adler stressed the role of social factors, such as birth order, in giving rise to a sense of inferiority, and attempts to compensate for it. Stressing the goal-oriented dimension of life, he claimed that neurotics lived in a fictional world structured by opposites, in particular the masculine and feminine. Thus, the secondary sexual characteristics in neurotic patients led to feelings of inferiority and strivings toward compensation in the form of masculine protest (in both sexes), resulting in a maladaptive lifestyle. Adler stressed the pedagogical role of psychotherapy, and this carried over into a concern with the therapeutic potential of education. In 1914 he founded the *Zeitschrift für Individual-Psychologie*.

With the worsening wartime situation, Adler was mobilized in 1916 and served as an Army physician at military hospitals in Semmering, Cracow, and Grinzig. After the war, he continued to develop his psychological system and attracted followers. He laid increasing emphasis on the therapeutic goal of the development of social feeling as an educational task. Adlerian groups sprang up, and Adler was viewed as part of the triumvirate—Adler, Freud, and Jung—founders of rival and warring schools of depth psychology. A number of Adler's works were directed at a general audience, and he attracted a wide following.

Adler held consultations for teachers and in the 1920s founded a number of educational guidance clinics, kindergartens, and an experimental school in Vienna. In 1926 he became a visiting professor at Columbia University, and came to spend an increasing amount of time in the United States, to which he eventually immigrated. In 1932 he was appointed visiting professor at the Long Island College of Medicine. In 1934 his clinics in Vienna were closed by the government. He died in Aberdeen in 1937, while on a lecture tour.

Bibliography

Primary: 1907. *Studie über Mindwertigkeit von Organen* (Berlin); 1916. *The Neurotic Constitution: Outlines of a Comparative Indi-vidualistic Psychology and Psychotherapy* (New York) [originally published in German, 1912]; 1924. *The Practice and Theory of Individual Psychology* (London); 1938. (ed. Ansbacher, Heinz) *The Individual Psychology of Alfred Adler* (London).

Secondary: Handlbauer, Bernhard, 1998. *The Freud-Adler Controversy* (Oxford); Stepansky, Paul, 1983. *In Freud's Shadow: Alfred Adler in Context* (Hillsdale, NJ).

Sonu Shamdasani

AËTIUS OF AMIDA (b. Amida, Mesopotamia (now Diyarbakir, Turkey); fl. *c.* 530–60), *medicine, ophthalmology, obstetrics, gynecology, pharmacology.*

Aëtius of Amida's birth and death dates are unknown but his period of activity places him at the center of the Byzantine court. He was born in Amida, a city in Mesopotamia, and was educated at Alexandria, one of the best places to receive a medical education. He moved to Constantinople to practice medicine, and his success was such that he was appointed *comes obsequii*, or chief officer in attendance to the person of the Emperor Justinian I (537–67)—an indication that Aëtius was also adept in court politics.

Aëtius is best known for his monumental 'Sixteen Books on Medicine', usually referred to as the *Tetrabiblon*, so called because, in the manuscript tradition, the text is divided into four parts, or *tetrabibli*, most of which have yet to be translated into English. Aëtius's chief interest lay in medical theory, and the lengthy preface to Book I of the *Tetrabiblon* concerns pharmacological theory, derived from Greek physician Galen. However, what elevated Aëtius from being a mere compiler was that he did not simply recapitulate Galenic theoretical pharmacology. Instead, he edited Galen's work into a more readable version, omitting the frequent lengthy digressions that often marred Galen's large body of pharmacological works. The result was a comprehensive and well-ordered synopsis. Galen sought to classify a drug 'by degree' or 'by kind', and Aëtius's chief contribution was to render this system of classification into something relatively straightforward. His success in this can be measured by the fact that his system of classification was used, more or less unchanged, until the nineteenth century. Aëtius's theoretical system was put into practical use in Book II of the *Tetrabiblon*, which listed 418 drugs of plant origin and 195 derived from animal products, earths, and minerals. This list was largely derived from Galen, with contributions from Rufus of Ephesus, Oribasius, and Dioscorides. These medicaments were now sorted on the basis of the classical Greek four elements (the Hot, the Cold, the Wet, and the Dry), and the various medicinal substances were therefore classified on the basis of their heating, cooling, moistening, and drying properties. Book III provided drug recipes; Book IV concerned dietetics; and Books V and VI dealt with humoral theory, prognosis, diagnosis, and treatment, including surgery (featuring an excellent account of an operation for brachial artery aneurysm; Aëtius's own treatise on surgery was lost). Book VII, devoted to sixty-one diseases of the eye, was perhaps the jewel of the *Tetrabiblon*, and provided the best account of ophthalmology until the eighteenth century; it preserved the work of several oculists that would otherwise have been lost (e.g., the treatment of trachoma by Severus, physician to Augustus). Books VIII–XV again returned to the subject of pharmacology, including toxicology, Book XVI concerned obstetrics and gynecology, drawing from Galen, Rufus of Ephesus, Soranus, and Aspasia (an otherwise unknown obstetrician and gynecologist).

Aëtius's scope was truly encyclopedic, and sought to encompass all written medical knowledge through the sixth century. The *Tetrabiblon*'s chief virtue was in its practical codification and systemization of the works of ancient medical authorities. Aëtius and other physicians of the Byzantine epoch, such as Oribasius, are now appreciated for what they were: the embodiment of a Greek medical tradition that they assiduously and judiciously mined and distilled, giving these works enormous longevity and influence.

Bibliography

Primary: Oliveri, Alexander, 1935–50. *Libri medicinales 1–VIII* (Teubner); Ricci, James, 1950. *Aetios of Amida: The Gynaecology and Obstetrics of the VIth Century, A.D.* (Philadelphia and Toronto); Waugh, Richey, 2000. *Ophthalmology of Aëtius of Amida.* Hirschberg History of Ophthalmology Monographs, vol. 8 (Oostende).

Secondary: Scarborough, John, 1984. 'Early Byzantine Pharmacology' in Scarborough, John, ed., 'Symposium on Byzantine Medicine.' *Dumbarton Oaks Papers* No. 38 (Washington, DC) pp. 213–32; Savage-Smith, Emilie, 1984. 'Hellenistic and Byzantine Ophthalmology: Trachoma and Sequelae' in Scarborough, John, ed., 'Symposium on Byzantine Medicine' *Dumbarton Oaks Papers* No. 38 (Washington, DC) pp. 169–86; *DSB*.

Julius Rocca

AGNODICE (fl. third century BCE?), *midwifery.*

Agnodice, 'the first midwife' according to the sole surviving source for her life, was an Athenian virgin at a time when women and slaves were forbidden to learn the art of medicine. No such period can be identified in the historical record, and the preservation of her story in a section of the Latin mythographer Hyginus (probably second century) on 'who invented what' does not add to the modern scholar's confidence in her existence. Hyginus preserved some lost Greek myths, and in a Greek original, her name would have been Hagnodike, meaning 'chaste before justice'. In the context of her story, this name is significant.

Wanting to reduce the death rate in childbirth, which was high because women's modesty prevented them from having male attendants in labor, Agnodice cut off her hair, dressed as a man, and traveled to study medicine under 'a certain Herophilus', a detail that should be understood as an attempt to give the story historicity rather than a clue to the date of the events. She then returned to Athens and built up a successful practice, persuading her embarrassed clients of her true sex by lifting her tunic to expose her lower body (a Greek gesture called *anasyrmos*). When her male rivals lost business as a result of her success, they assumed she was seducing the patients, and brought her to court. Here she again performed *anasyrmos*, showing that as a woman she was not guilty of seduction, but this meant she was subject to a new charge, that of illegal practice of medicine. At this point, her elite patients lobbied the court, and the law was changed so that free-born women could learn medicine.

After the first printed edition of Hyginus was published by Jacobus Micyllus in 1535, the story was popularized and used to provide a precedent for a number of different scenarios in the contested field of early modern midwifery: a female monopoly on midwifery, male midwives (for during the 'ban' on women, they must have existed), or a natural reluctance on the part of women toward practitioners of the opposite sex. The version in the *Child-Birth or, the Happy Deliverie of Women* of Jacques Guillemeau (1550?–1613), a book originally aimed at surgeons, was particularly influential in medicine and, because it appears this was one of the books used by English midwives training under the deputy system, it became familiar to midwives themselves. In Elizabeth Cellier's 1687 proposal for a London college of midwives, extra details—such as witnesses at the trial being paid to give evidence—were transferred to the story from Cellier's own life.

In the modern period, the story of Agnodice has been used by supporters of women's medical education, who emphasized the significance of the story's stress on women learning medicine, rather than merely midwifery. The cross-dressing was recast as showing that women doctors needed a special uniform to demonstrate that they had been properly trained. The version given by Kate Hurd-Mead (1867–1941) suggested that women had previously been midwives, but were banned because they had been performing abortions, and speculated from the inclusion of the name of Herophilus that Agnodice had performed Caesarean sections. This is the version often given in recent histories of women in medicine, and it should be recognized as a fiction. However, Agnodice was invoked as a patron of Caesarean section before Hurd-Mead, in the work of the Parisian anti-Caesarean physician Jean-François Sacombe (1750–1822). In his satirical poem *La Luciniade* he attributed her successful defense before the Athenian court not to her self-display, but to her eloquence.

One further example of the reuse of the story should be mentioned: where Hyginus's story ends with 'free-born women' (Latin *ingenuae*) being permitted to learn medicine, a typesetting error in an eighteenth-century history of medicine led to this becoming 'three women', leading to the idea that there were three 'State midwives' employed in ancient Athens.

Bibliography

Primary: Cellier, Elizabeth, 1687. *To Dr. — an answer to his queries concerning the Colledg of Midwives* in *Writings on Medicine* in Cody, Lisa Forman ed., 2002. *The Early Modern Englishwoman. Printed Writings, 1641–1700*, part 1, vol. 4 (Aldershot); Grant, Mary, 1960. *The Myths of Hyginus* (Lawrence, KS); Hurd-Mead, Kate Campbell, 1938. *A History of Women in Medicine* (Haddam, CT).

Secondary: King, Helen, 1986. 'Agnodike and the profession of medicine' *Proceedings of the Cambridge Philological Society* 32: 53–77.

Helen King

AḤMAD, 'ISSĀ BEY   (b. Rosetta, Egypt, 1876; d. Cairo, Egypt, 1946), *medicine, obstetrics, history of medicine.*

A distinguished medical doctor and historian of medicine, Aḥmad 'Issā attended primary school in his native Rosetta (Rashīd), the Khedival School of Law in Cairo, and then the Medical School in Cairo, where he specialized in obstetrics and gynecology. After graduation, he worked in various hospitals in Egypt and at the beginning of the twentieth century joined the Egyptian Red Crescent. On 21 December 1908 he became one of the founders of the first Egyptian university, the King Fouad University. Aḥmad 'Issā belonged to a diverse group of people with differing socioeconomic status and political affiliations, who were united nevertheless in their belief that the Egyptian university was essential to the social and cultural life of the country.

As well as being a prolific medical writer and a skilled practitioner Aḥmad 'Issā also excelled in the humanities. He studied many languages, including Hebrew, Syriac, Greek, and Latin. His wide knowledge and contacts made him into a leading scholar in the history of science. He was a member of the governing council of The National Library and Archives of Egypt (*Dar al-Kutub*), a founder member of the Arabic Scientific Board in Damascus (*al-Majma' al-'Ilmī al-'Arabī bi-Dimashq*) and various European academies.

The majority of Aḥmad 'Issā's books are written in Arabic. Among them were a university course on gynecology, a treatise on surgical instruments, and a study of uroscopy. European readers are indebted to Aḥmad 'Issā for his fundamental history of *bimaristans* (hospitals) and a multilingual dictionary of the names of plants. Although Eduard Ghaleb's dictionary replaced Aḥmad 'Issā's, it remains one of the primary research tools. A detailed biography of Aḥmad 'Issā Bey has not yet been written. His obituary, published by his colleague Dr Muḥammad Sohby in the *Bulletin de l'Institut d'Egypte* (1947), was translated into Arabic and published in al-Zirkili's bibliographical dictionary.

Bibliography

Primary: 1926. *Dictionnaire des noms des plantes en latin, français, anglais et arabe* (Cairo); 1928. *Histoire des bimaristans (hôpitaux) à l'époque islamique: discours prononcé au Congrés médical tenu au Caire à l'occasion du centenaire de l'École de médecine et de l'Hôpital Kasr-el-Aïni en décembre 1928* (Cairo); 1980. *Tārīkh al-Bīmāristanāt fī al-Islām* [History of Islamic Hospitals] (Beirut); (n.d.) *Ālat al-ṭibb wa-al-jirāḥa wa-al-kaḥḥāla 'inda al-'arab* [Arabic Surgical Instruments and Instruments Used by Apothecaries].

Secondary: Al-'Alawinah, Ahmad, 1998. *Dhayl al-A'lam : qāmūs tarājīm li-ashhar al-rijāl wa-al-nisa' min al-'Arab wa-al-musta'ribīn wa-al-mustashriqīn* [Bibliographical Dictionary of Celebrated Arabs, Men and Women, Orientalists and Specialists in Western Culture] (Jiddah).

Nikolaj Serikoff

ALBRIGHT, FULLER   (b. Buffalo, New York, USA, 12 January 1900; d. Boston, Massachusetts, USA, 8 December 1969), *endocrinology.*

Albright, the father of modern endocrinology, was the son of a wealthy father who made his money from coal, asphalt, and automobiles. After his internship at Massachusetts General Hospital (MGH), Albright spent 1928–29 in Vienna with the skeletal pathologist, Jacob Erdheim. He often talked about Erdheim, whose virtues were that he 'worked hard and was smart as hell', a description that might have been applied to Albright himself. An additional quality of both men was insatiable curiosity. Albright's work was varied and far-reaching, covering the parathyroids, adrenals, and gonads. In an introduction to his bibliography, he wrote: 'In my opinion, my contributions divide into two groups: (a) clinical descriptions and (b) elucidations of pathological physiology.'

Calcium Metabolism

Albright's interest in calcium began as a student; he gave a paper to the Boylston Society of Harvard Medical School on 'the physiology and pathology of calcium'. The minutes taken at that presentation record: 'little known of Ca metabolism. Most advance in the study of metabolism in the next 20 years probably will be in relation to calcium.' Working at Johns Hopkins, Albright and Read Ellsworth described idiopathic hypoparathyroidism for the first time (1929). At this time, hyperparathyroidism was a rare disease. The first curative parathyroidectomy had been done by Mandl in Vienna in 1925, and the first case had been diagnosed in the United States in 1926. This case was Captain Charles Martell, one of the most written-up patients in history, who came into Albright's ambit in 1932 after four unsuccessful operations probing for a tumor. Finally, at the seventh attempt, a retrosternal parathroid adenoma was found. Martell was the subject of Albright's presidential lecture to the Association for the Study of Internal Secretions (1947).

In 1934 Albright and his associates described three patients with hyperparathyoidism due to diffuse hyperplasia of all four glands; that same year, Albright coined the term 'nephrocalcinosis'. In 1937 he described vitamin D-resistant rickets, and later established that the primary action of vitamin D was to increase intestinal calcium absorption. In 1938 he reported five cases of 'a syndrome characterized by Osteitis Fibrosa Disseminata, Areas of Pigmentation and Endocrine Dysfunction with precocious puberty in females', one of the many Albright's syndromes. In 1942 he investigated a young woman with dense skull bones, epilepsy, and hypocalcemia, which could not be corrected with parathyroid hormone. Albright postulated that 'the disturbance was not lack of hormone but a resistance to it'. He speculated that there might be parathyroid antihormones, or 'a deficiency of or interference with some hypothetical substance with which parathyroid hormone reacts'. Seeking an example in nature, he chose the so-called Sebright-Bantam syndrome. Sir John Sebright was an English landowner who, in 1800, had discovered a single bantam rooster with female feathers in his barnyard. He bred this rooster and produced the strain known as Sebright-Bantam. Albright hypothesized, incorrectly as it turned out, that the Sebright bantam had end organ resistance to testosterone. Nevertheless, his paper introduced the concept of end organ resistance to a hormone.

Albright also established the concept of hormone production from nonendocrine tissue. At a clinicopathological conference (1941) on a fifty-year-old Greek bootblack with a hypernephroma, hypercalcemia, and a single metastasis, Albright made the revolutionary suggestion that the tumor might be producing a parathyroid hormone-like substance, a concept that became established twenty-five years later.

Gonadal Diseases

In 1930 Albright and Dr Joe Meigs set up the Ovarian Dysfunction Clinic, and developed a method of assaying follicle-stimulating hormone (FSH) with which it was possible to distinguish various forms of gonadal dysgenesis. In 1935 Albright wrote a comprehensive description of 'A Syndrome Characterized by Primary Ovarian Insufficiency and Decreased Stature', which is now called Turner's syndrome.

Over the years, Albright had collected a group of men with gynecomastia, small testes, and elevated FSH. Generously, he gave these subjects to Harry Kleinfelter to write up, so that their condition is now known as Kleinfelter's syndrome. In 1941, with Patricia Smith and Ann Richardson, he investigated forty-two cases of osteoporosis, of which forty were in postmenopausal women. Balance studies showed that the women excreted more calcium and phosphate than they took in and that giving estrogens could reverse this. Albright postulated that estrogens lay down reserves of calcium and phosphate in the bones that were mobilized in pregnancy and lactation, and that those women whose bones outlive their ovaries often have 'too

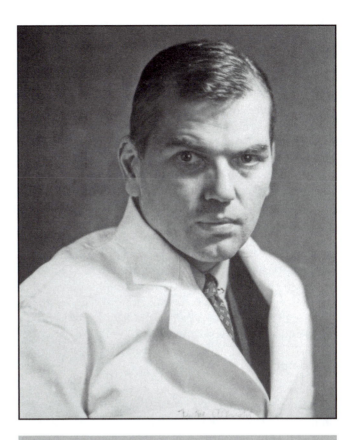

Fuller Albright. Photoprint, courtesy of the National Library of Medicine.

little bone'. He called this 'postmenopausal osteoporosis', and suggested estrogen treatment.

He showed that dysmenorrhea and ovulation could be prevented by giving estrogen, and predicted that this could be used for contraception. This statement, made in 1945, became known as Albright's Prophecy and, being too politically sensitive for the time, remained buried in a book chapter on menstrual disorders.

Adrenal Glands

Albright's sorting out of adrenal diseases is less well remembered than his work on calcium, but was equally influential for contemporaries. One of his maxims was that one had to measure something—or at least someone else had to, because he never did any laboratory work. In 1941 his fellow, Russell Fraser, showed that the cause of impaired glucose tolerance in Cushing's syndrome was insulin resistance. A test for 17-ketosteroids was developed, and Albright deduced that they were the end products of secretions from both the testes and adrenals. Since normal 17-ketosteroid excretion was fourteen mg in men and only nine in women, he hypothesized that nine mg came from the adrenals and five mg from the testes.

In his 1942 Harvey lecture on Cushing's syndrome, he outlined its 'Pathological Physiology, Its Relationship to the

Adrenogenital Syndrome and Its Connection with the Reaction of the Body to Injurious Reagents ("Alarm Reaction" of Selye)'. He clearly stated that all forms of Cushing's syndrome were caused by hyperfunction of the adrenal cortex, something we now take for granted but which was then in doubt, because Cushing had suggested that it was due to 'pituitary basophilism'. Albright deduced that the adrenal cortex produced two hormones: the catabolic 'S', or sugar, hormone, and another, which stimulated growth, the nitrogen, or 'N', hormone. The N hormone was responsible for virilism in the adreno-genital syndrome, and for the growth of axillary and pubic hair in both sexes. Part of the evidence for the latter was that when he rubbed testosterone ointment into one axilla of a patient with hypopituitarism, it stimulated the growth of hair in that axilla but not the other.

Prophetically, he suggested that if a steroid could be found which was not an androgen, it would suppress adrenal androgens and thus be a treatment for the adrenogenital syndrome. Five years later compound S, or hydrocortisone, was found to have just such an effect.

Personality

In his witty presidential address to the American Society for Clinical Investigation (1944), Albright described his philosophy of clinical investigation. The 'do's' included 'do look at the problem from all points of view'; 'do measure something'; and 'do develop a theory'. According to his associates, he had an amazing capacity for collecting facts from other disciplines and developing hypotheses which could be tested. Nevertheless, he was never a slave to his theories and used to say, 'these concepts are subject to change without notice'.

The 'do not's' included: 'do not be a lone wolf investigator'; 'do not be a slave to your theory'; and 'do not wake up some fine morning in an executive job. Do not show too much administrative ability. Whatever you do, do not become a Professor of Medicine or head of a department.' Albright never held any administrative position and was lucky to have been given free rein and supplied with funds by Dr James Howard Means, who believed in backing the man, not the project. Albright was also lucky to have use of the metabolic research ward at MGH, one of the first facilities of its kind, which had opened in 1925.

Albright's career was cruelly affected by Parkinsonism, which began in 1936. By 1956 he was so incapacitated that he decided to undergo experimental chemopallidectomy. Unfortunately, this led to hemorrhage and akinetic mutism, which lasted until his death thirteen years later.

Bibliography

Primary: 1936. (with Aub, J. C., and W. H. Bauer) 'Hyperparathyroidism—a common polymorphic condition, as illustrated by 17 proved cases from one clinic.' *Journal of the American Medical Association* 102: 1276; 1937. (with Butler, A. M., A. O. Hampton, and P. H. Smith). 'Syndrome characterized by osteitis fibrosa disseminata, areas of pigmentation and endocrine dysfunction, with precocious puberty in females.' *New England Journal of Medicine* 216: 727–746; 1942. (with Burnett, C. H., P. H. Smith, and W. Parson) 'Pseudo-hypoparathyroidism—an example of the 'Seabright-Bantam syndrome': report of three cases.' *Endocrinology* 30: 922–932; 1942–43. 'Cushing's syndrome: its pathological physiology, its relationship to the adreno-genital syndrome and its connection with the problem of the reaction of the body to injurious agents ("Alarm reaction" of Selye).' *Harvey Lecture Series* 38: 123–186; 1948. (with Reifenstein, Edward C., Jr.) *The Parathyroid Glands and Metabolic Bone Disease: Selected Studies* (Baltimore).

Secondary: Howard, J. A., 1980–1. 'Fuller Albright: the endocrinologists' clinical endocrinologist.' *Perspectives in Biology and Medicine* 24: 374–381; Leaf, A., 1976. 'Fuller Albright.' *Biographical Memoirs National Academy of Sciences* 48: 3–22; Axelrod, L., 1970. 'Bones, stones and hormones: the contributions of Fuller Albright.' *New England Journal of Medicine* 283: 964–970; *DAMB*.

Robert Tattersall

ALCMAEON OF CROTON (fl. Crotona [now Crotone, Italy], 490–430 BCE), *anatomy, physiology.*

A Pre-Socratic physician-physicist, Alcmaeon of Croton illustrated the overlapping of boundaries among philosophy, natural science, and medicine in antiquity. He was known for his influential view that health and disease result from the balance and imbalance of the elementary forces of moisture, dryness, coldness, wetness, bitterness, and the like (Aëtius); for the view, which would become a major focus of controversy, that the site of consciousness was the brain (Plato and Aëtius); for his distinctive theory of sense perception, involving the role of *pneuma* (Theophrastus); for supposed experiments in dissection, especially of the optic nerve (Chalcidius); and for ideas in embryology and in the physiology of sleep.

Alcmaeon's chronology is controversial. Aristotle's discussion in *Metaphysics* 1 (Chapter 5) would suggest that he was an approximate contemporary of Empedocles, Anaxagoras, Leucippus, and Democritus. This placement corresponds to the range of problems encountered in Alcmaeon's work, so the dates tentatively proposed (between 490 and 430 BCE) are equally plausible. An earlier dating, in the late sixth century BCE, seems by comparison anachronistic. That dating was based on late reports of an association between Alcmaeon and the Pythagoreans, including Pythagoras himself, who is said to have taught him (Diogenes Laertius, Iamblichus); but such reports are not reliable without confirmation from a source like Aristotle.

Alcmaeon held that sense perception was monitored by the brain through channels that connected it to the organs of vision, hearing, smell, and taste. He claimed that the transportation of air or breath (*pneuma*) to the brain along these channels was essential, at least for hearing and smell: 'we smell by drawing in the breath to the brain through the nostrils at the same time as we breathe'. But it is not known if and how *pneuma* was supposed to act in producing sensation. A fragment from Theophrastus's *On Sense-Perception* showed how the production of vision was explained. The textual details are disputed, but Alcmaeon resorted to a notion of reflection and to the elemental constituents of the eye—the watery (transparent) and the fiery (luminous). Whether *pneuma* and its channels featured in this account or not, Alcmaeon, like the other Pre-Socratics, clearly focused on elements, and not on anatomical structures.

A less reliable report (by Chalcidius) described Alcmaeon as the first anatomist who dared to perform something between a 'dissection', an 'operation', and an 'excision' (cutting out?) of the eye—which would place him in the illustrious company of the Hellenistic anatomist Herophilus. Hence Alcmaeon has been appraised as a pioneering experimentalist in anatomy and the true Father of Medicine. But such views are overly optimistic. There is no evidence that he ever traced the courses of the optic nerves in the skull, conducted any empirical investigations to discover links between the brain and the organs of sense, or was even involved in any dissection at all.

Alcmaeon discussed the order of formation of the embryo's and the egg's parts and nourishment. (The white of an egg, he thought, was its milk.) He believed that sleep and wakefulness were due to a reflux of blood, followed by its return to the surface—views shared later by some Hippocratics and by Aristotle, which did not entail (as had been supposed) any awareness of a distinction between arteries and veins.

Bibliography

Primary: 1951–52. Diels, H. and W. Kranz. *Die Fragmente der Vorsokratiker*, 6th ed. (Berlin).

Secondary: Lloyd, G. E. R., 1991. 'Alcmaeon and the Early History of Dissection' in Lloyd, *Methods and Problems in Greek Science* (Cambridge) pp. 164–93; Harris, C. R. S., 1973. *The Heart and the Vascular System in Ancient Greek Medicine. From Alcmaeon to Galen* (Oxford); Stella, L. A., 1938–39. 'L'importanza di Alcmeone nella storia del pensiero greco'. *Atti della reale Accademia Nazionale dei Lincei* (Memorie ser. 6) 8: 237–87; Wellmann, M., 1929. 'Die Schrift *peri hieres nosou* des Corpus Hippocraticum' *Sudhoffs Archiv für Geschichte der Medizin* 22: 290–312; *DSB*.

Manuela Tecusan

ALEKSANDROWICZ, JULIAN   (b. Krakow, Poland, 20 August 1908; d. Krakow, 18 October 1988), *hematology.*

In 1998 the Polish journal *Gazeta Wyborcza* conducted a poll to identify the most famous citizens of the city of Krakow. The winners were Pope John Paul II (1920–2005), Art Nouveau painter and playwright Stanislaw Wyspianski (1869–1907), and physician Julian Aleksandrowicz. Aleksandrowicz's popularity, unusual for a clinician and medical researcher, can be related to admiration for his professional skills (he was regarded as one of the great Polish doctors of the post–World War II era), combined with appreciation for his pioneering studies on the environmental determinants of illness in Poland.

Aleksandrowicz spent all his life in Krakow. Born into an assimilated Jewish family, he studied medicine at the Jagellonski University. After graduating from medical school in 1933, he worked at St. Lazarus hospital in Krakow, where he specialized in hematology. During the war he was a physician in the Krakow ghetto. In his memoirs from this period, he provided unique testimony of Jewish life under Nazi occupation. Thanks to his contact with the Polish underground, he was able to escape during the liquidation of the ghetto in 1943. He then joined the Armia Krajowa (Interior Army) resistance, where, under the pseudonym of 'Dr. Twardy', he made important contributions to the resistance's activity. Today a street in Krakow carries the name of Dr. Twardy.

After the war, Aleksandrowicz joined the academic staff of the Jagellonian University's medical school, where he spent his entire academic career. Professor of internal medicine and head of the hematology department, he was a prolific researcher, interested mainly in hematological and immunological disorders. His department specialized in studies of leukemia, and introduced to Poland new therapies for treating this disease. Aleksandrowicz also studied the role of the thymus in immune disorders, and the effects of nutrition on hemopoiesis, the immune system, and the brain. His work on nutrition led to pioneering studies on the physiological role of magnesium.

Aleksandrowicz's popularity outside academia stemmed mainly from his involvement in ecological issues. Krakow is situated in the center of a heavily industrialized region. In the post-World War II era, the city suffered from very high levels of pollution. Aleksandrowicz was initially interested in the links between industrial pollution and the rising incidence of childhood leukemia. He enlarged the scope of his studies and investigated the environmental determinants of health and disease. These studies demonstrated clear-cut correlations between levels of air pollution and the incidence of numerous pathologies. Aleksandrowicz did not oppose progress per se, but strongly denounced its excesses. Human beings, he explained, seem to increasingly suffer from a specific form of mental disease—what he called 'dementia rationalis', a push to the uncontrolled and ever-expanding production and consumption that threaten the fragile equilibrium between humans and the natural world.

Aleksandrowicz started to promote this point of view in the 1950s and 1960s, a period during which the Polish communist state glorified intensive industrialization. Official posters of that time proudly depicted landscapes adorned with smoking chimneys, a visible symbol of progress and the promise of a brighter future. Aleksandrowicz is remembered as one of the first Poles to show that just the opposite was true: chimney smoke promised a much darker future for those forced to breathe it.

Bibliography

Primary: 1951. *Hematology of Infectious Diseases* (in Polish) (Warsaw); 1963. *Leukemia* (in Polish) (Warsaw); 1963. *Pages from the Diary of Dr. Twardy* (in Polish) (Krakow); 1979. *Ecological Consciousness* (in Polish) (Krakow); 1985. *Medical Studies and Medical Ethics* (Krakow).

                                                               Ilana Löwy

ALI COHEN, LEVY   (b. Meppel, the Netherlands, 6 October 1817; d. Groningen, the Netherlands, 22 November 1889), *public health, history of (Jewish) medicine.*

Ali Cohen was born in the small Dutch town of Meppel. The oldest son of Ali Salomon Cohen and Golda Noach ten Brink, he was raised in poverty in a religious Jewish family. Levy Cohen's remarkable intelligence and the financial assistance of a school inspector enabled him to attend the 'Latin School'. In 1836 he enrolled at Groningen University as a medical student, graduating MD in 1840. The same year, he started his medical practice in Groningen as a doctor serving the Jewish poor. Shortly afterward, he changed his family name to Ali Cohen.

In the 1840s, Ali Cohen became part of the Jewish intellectual elite of Groningen as well as the scientific and political elite of the city, which was still quite uncommon in those years. While a moderate romanticism in literature, science, and medicine was still *en vogue*, he became involved in geological, botanical, and historical research of the Dutch northern provinces. In 1845, Ali Cohen started research activities in the clinic of J. Baart de la Faille. Three years later, he became the editor of the *Nieuw practisch tijdschrift voor de geneeskunde,* a well-known medical journal for nongraduated practitioners (the *heelmeesters*) dating to the 1820s. From 1848 onward, Ali Cohen was fully committed to local and national causes of public health.

Ali Cohen was cofounder of the Dutch Society of Medicine in 1849. In the 1850s and 1860s, he was an active member of an influential committee on medical statistics. With Amsterdam physicians J. Zeeman and L. J. Egeling, he laid the foundations of modern Dutch epidemiology, developing nationwide statistical and topographical research on mortality (in general) and cholera (in particular). Ali Cohen was soon regarded as among the most prominent of sanitary reformers. In 1857, he joined the initiative to establish a new Dutch medical journal, the *Nederlandsch Tijdschrift voor Geneeskunde* (still in publication). Until the 1870s, he oversaw topics related to *medicina politica* and *hygiena publica.*

In 1853 Minister of the Interior J. R. Thorbecke requested Ali Cohen and Amsterdam medical doctor J. Penn to prepare a comprehensive reform of Dutch medical legislation, although their advisory role ended when conservative agitation caused the government to fall. When Thorbecke returned to office in 1862, Ali Cohen and Penn were more successful. With their help, Thorbecke succeeded in enacting four new medical laws which established the first Dutch national Inspectorate of Health, regulated medical practice, concentrated medical education at the university level, and grounded medical education on the solid basis of the natural sciences.

Ali Cohen became provincial inspector of public health, first in Overijssel and Drente (1866), later in Groningen and Friesland (from 1869 until his death in 1889). Ali Cohen wrote numerous books, articles, and reports addressing issues of public health, and also discussing Jewish culture and the emancipation of the Jews. He was the editor of the first handbook on public health in the Netherlands, to which he contributed substantial chapters.

Bibliography

Primary: 1852. 'Over openbare gezondheidsregeling, de gevolgen van hare verwaarlozing en de noodzakelijkheid van hare invoering hier te lande.' *Nieuw practisch tijdschrift voor de geneeskunde in al haren omvang.* Nieuwe reeks 4: 252–300; 1872. *Handboek der openbare gezondheidsregeling en der geneeskundige politie, met het oog op de behoeften en de wetgeving van Nederland* 2 vols. (Groningen).

Secondary: Nicolai, Henk, 2004. 'Ter gedurige herinnering' in *Leven en werken van Levy Ali Cohen 1817–1889* (Zutphen); Houwaart, E. S., 1997. 'Gronings romanticus en nationaal hervormer: de hygiënist Levy Ali Cohen (1817–1889)' in Huisman, Frank and Catrien Santing, eds., *Medische geschiedenis in regionaal perspectief. Groningen 1500–1900* (Rotterdam) pp. 101–130; Houwaart, E. S., 1994. 'Medical Statistics and Sanitary Provisions: a New World of Social Relations and Threats to Health.' *Tractrix. Yearbook for the History of Science, Medicine Technology and Mathematics* 5: 1–33; Houwaart, E. S., 1991. *De hygiënisten. Artsen, staat en volksgezondheid in Nederland 1840–1890* (Groningen).

                                                            Eddy Houwaart

ALIBERT, JEAN-LOUIS   (b. Villefranche-de-Rouergue, France, 2 May 1768; d. Paris, France, 4 November 1837), *clinical medicine, dermatology.*

Jean-Louis Alibert was the son of Pierre Alibert, a local magistrate, and Claudine Alric. He studied in the schools of the Pères de la Doctrine Chrétienne, but his early aspirations to become a priest were thwarted when religious congregations were disbanded in 1792 by the French Revolution. In pursuit of a teaching career, Alibert came to Paris in 1795 to attend the École Normale, which also dissolved. Alibert frequented the salon of Madame Helvétius, where he met Pierre J. G. Cabanis and Pierre Roussel. These men inspired him to study medicine and introduced him to Condillac's sensationalist epistemology. Alibert became a member of the younger generation of Idéologues.

In 1796 he enrolled at the new École de Santé and became secretary general of the newly created Société médicale d'émulation; he published many articles in its *Mémoires*. His MD thesis on pernicious intermittent fevers (1800) was published in several editions. In 1804 and 1814, Alibert published books on therapeutics and materia medica, topics of continuing interest for him.

In 1801 the Hôpital Saint-Louis, formerly an institution for the internment of the poor, became a hospital for patients with chronic and contagious diseases, particularly those of the skin. These ranged from scabies, ringworm, and smallpox to scurvy, syphilis, scrofula, and cancer. Alibert became adjunct hospital physician in 1801 and physician-in-chief on 9 July 1802. At Saint-Louis he had the opportunity to make the extensive investigations of skin disorders that form his enduring contribution. Acclaimed since as the 'father of French dermatology', Alibert's teaching clinic became one of the most popular in Paris with well-attended lectures that featured theatrical elements. His *Description des maladies de la peau observées à l'Hôpital Saint-Louis*, with its splendid and expensive folio color plates, was published in installments beginning in 1806. In 1810 he published a cheaper précis of his findings for students.

In 1815, after the return of the French monarchy, Alibert became a court physician. In 1818 he became Louis XVIII's first physician-in-ordinary. The king's precarious health required Alibert's constant attention and he left his closest student, Laurent Biett, in charge at Saint-Louis. Now an influential figure in medical politics, Alibert was one of the founding members of the Académie Royale de Médecine in 1820. In 1821 he was appointed professor of botany at the Faculty of Medicine and in 1823 he was named titular professor of the first chair of therapeutics and materia medica. That same year, he became an officer of the Légion d'Honneur. Alibert was appointed physician-in-ordinary to Charles X in 1824 and was made a baron in 1827.

In the 1830s Alibert published further important works on dermatology: *Monographie des Dermatoses* (1832), and the summation of his work, *Clinique de l'Hôpital Saint-Louis, ou Traité Complet des Maladies de la Peau* (1833). The latter work includes his often depicted Tree of Dermatoses, a graphic representation of how skin diseases can be organized and classified in a manner derived from botany. Alibert's views on this matter were eclipsed by those of Robert Willan, whose classification of skin diseases proceeded from the first location of the lesion. A prolific author, Alibert also wrote on the nosology of human diseases (1817), and the physiology of the passions (1825).

Bibliography

Primary: 1806. *Description des maladies de la peau observées à l'Hôpital Saint-Louis. Et exposition des meilleures méthodes suivies pour leur traitement* (Paris); 1832. *Monographie des dermatoses, ou, précis théorique et pratique des maladies de la peau* (Paris); 1833. *Clinique de l'Hôpital Saint-Louis, ou traité complet des maladies de la peau* (Paris).

Secondary: Jacyna, L. S., 1998. "Pious Pathology: J.-L. Alibert's Iconography of Disease" in Hannaway, Caroline, and Ann La Berge, eds., *Constructing Paris Medicine* (Amsterdam), pp. 185–219; Brodier, Léon, 1923. *J.-L. Alibert, médecin de l'Hôpital Saint-Louis (1768–1837)* (Paris).

Caroline Hannaway

ALISON, WILLIAM PULTENEY (b. Boroughmuirhead, Scotland, 12 November 1790; d. Colinton, Edinburgh, Scotland, 22 September 1859), *medicine, public health*.

Alison was the son of Archibald Alison, an author and Episcopal clergyman, and Dorothea Gregory, a member of one of Edinburgh's most prominent medical and literary families. Alison graduated MD from Edinburgh University in 1811 and, in 1815, was appointed physician to the New Town Dispensary. Alison's experiences in this post led him to develop a concern for the health and sanitary conditions of the urban poor, and to take a scientific interest in the causes of epidemic disease.

In 1820, Alison was appointed Professor of Medical Jurisprudence to Edinburgh University and began lecturing on 'medical police', which encompassed what is now known as public health. He was elevated to the chair of the Institutes of Medicine in 1822 and, twenty years later, to that of the Practice of Medicine, the most senior position within the Edinburgh medical faculty. His textbook, *Outlines of Physiology*, appeared in 1831 (Edinburgh). Much of Alison's teaching may be seen as distinctively Scottish in character. Drawing upon his knowledge of the metaphysical philosophy of Dugald Stewart (1753–1828), he opposed what he saw as the pernicious materialism of phrenology. As a physiologist he was concerned with the elucidation of broad principles, rather than the incremental accumulation of experimental data. In Alison's view, the purpose of physiology was to assist the practitioner by providing a rational foundation for the practice of medicine, especially therapeutics.

The teaching of 'medical police' had been introduced to Scotland by Alison's older contemporaries, Andrew Duncan father (1744–1828) and son (1773–1832). Alison followed their example by emphasizing that medical investigation should focus not only on individuals but also on populations. Acknowledging that many diseases were difficult to cure, he argued that some of the most serious could be prevented relatively easily. Prevention, moreover, was often most effectively directed at the level of the community. Such concerns led Alison to engage in social and political controversy, particular in connection with the operation of the Poor Law. In England, Edwin Chadwick (1800–90) had advocated reforms of the system for maintaining paupers that were predicated on the assumption that, among the laboring population, ill health occasioned poverty. Alison's analysis of the problem of the urban poor was diametrically opposite. Drawing on the teachings of William Cullen (1710–90), he argued that inadequacies of diet, clothing, and accommodation produced 'debility', leading to increased susceptibility to fever and other diseases. In Alison's view, poverty was the root cause of much of the ill health of the laboring population. The effects of poverty were also moral. Far from spurring the poor to efforts of self help, unremitting destitution eroded their self-respect and rendered them apathetic and feckless.

In Scotland, provision for the poor of each parish had long been the responsibility of the Church. The system was voluntary, and levels of support were uneven and, by European standards, meager. Alison argued both for the reform of the Scottish Poor Law and against the adoption of the Utilitarian English Poor Law in Scotland. He urged that a new Poor Law should provide support for the able-bodied poor to prevent the unemployed worker and his family from being reduced to destitution and disease. Likewise, the sick poor should have access to medical treatment, including food, to enable them to return to work.

Although Alison greatly influenced the framing of the 1845 Poor Law Act, not all of his recommendations were accepted. Provision for the able-bodied poor was not included, but medical assistance was offered to the sick poor. Moreover, benefits could be received under the Act without the recipient having to enter a poorhouse.

Alison was a clinician who saw beyond the ills of the individual patient and began to inquire into the causes and medical effects of, as he put it, 'the grand evil of Poverty itself'. He can, thus, be reasonably regarded as a pioneer of social medicine.

Bibliography

Secondary: Martin, S. M. K., 1995. 'William Pulteney Alison: activist, philanthropist and pioneer of social medicine.' PhD thesis, University of St. Andrews; Pitman, J., 1989. 'William Pulteney Alison.' *Proceedings of the Royal College of Physicians of Edinburgh* 19: 219–224; *Oxford DNB*.

Malcolm Nicolson

ALLBUTT, THOMAS CLIFFORD (b. Dewsbury, England, 20 July 1836; d. Cambridge, England, 22 February 1925), *medicine*.

Allbutt was the son of the Reverend Thomas Allbutt and Marianne Wooler. He was born in Dewsbury and educated at St Peter's School, York, before going up to Gonville and Caius College, Cambridge University, in 1857, where he graduated with a first in the Natural Sciences Tripos. He then studied medicine at St George's Hospital, London, and took his MB at Cambridge in 1861, completing his education with a stay in Paris, where he attended the clinics of Armand Trousseau (1801–67), Guillaume Duchenne (1800–75), and Alfred Hardy (1811–93). While at St George's he became a friend of George Henry Lewes (1817–

78) and his wife Marian Evans (1819–80)—the novelist George Eliot. Allbutt was widely regarded at the model for Dr Tertius Lydgate in Eliot's novel *Middlemarch*. Allbutt's mother was the sister of Miss Margaret Wooler, whose school at Mirfield was attended by the Brontë sisters, who visited the Dewsbury parsonage when Allbutt was a young man. In 1869 Allbutt married Susan England of Headingley, Leeds; they had no children.

Allbutt began his career in Leeds, rapidly developing a successful consulting practice and serving as consultant physician at the Leeds General Infirmary, the Leeds Hospital for Women, and the Leeds Fever Hospital, where he introduced the open-air treatment of typhus fever. Indeed, throughout his career he remained a first-rate clinician, respected by his peers and popular with his patients. However, he gained particular attention in Leeds for his scientific work, primarily for his innovations in clinical thermometry. Although the German physician Carl Wunderlich (1815–77) demonstrated the value of quantitative measurement of bodily temperature over qualitative judgment, it was Allbutt's development of the small thermometer that allowed thermometry to become a mainstay of diagnosis. The standard instruments of the day were nearly twelve inches long; Allbutt's thermometer was six inches long, which was both more portable and also gave more rapid readings. This instrument was developed and made for him by Messrs Harvey and Reynolds of Leeds, and it seems that his work on thermometry was quite independent of the now more famous studies of Wunderlich. Allbutt summarized his work in this field in a much-quoted article in 1870 on 'Medical Thermometry'. He went on to use the new instrument in studies of body heat, taking measurements of foundry workers and of himself when exercising. Allbutt also promoted the use of the ophthalmoscope, and in 1871 published one of the earliest general volumes on the use of this instrument in nervous and other diseases. In recognition of his work on the physical sciences in clinical medicine, he was elected FRS in 1880. He was elected FRCP in 1883, and in 1884 gave the Goulstonian Lectures.

In 1889 Allbutt's life changed when he became a Commissioner in Lunacy, a post he held for three years. He seems to have accepted this position to escape the pressures of his Leeds consultancy, and to be more active in London's professional and scientific circles. He had some relevant background, having undertaken some of his ophthalmic investigations in the laboratory that James Crichton Browne (1840–1938) had established at the West Riding Asylum in Wakefield.

In 1892 Allbutt was offered the Regius Chair of Physic at the University of Cambridge, succeeding Sir George Paget (1809–92). The appointment was seen by some as surprising in that Allbutt had no academic experience; in fact, it took him eight years to gain full access to patients at Addenbrooke's Hospital in Cambridge. From 1896, through the lobbying of Sir Michael Foster (1836–1907), he was able to lecture at the hospital, but his exclusion from the wards remained an issue. Nonetheless, he took an increasing interest in medical education, securing the development of new buildings for the School and promoting innovation in postgraduate studies. At this time he was keen to promote hygiene, preventive medicine, and bacteriology, and in 1898 endeavored to set up a clinical laboratory with Alfredo Antunes Kanthack (1863–98). However, his most prominent work, his lasting legacy, was already in hand—his compilation and editing of *A System of Medicine by Many Writers*. This comprehensive account of the state of modern understanding of all aspects of medicine appeared in eight volumes between 1896 and 1899. The standing of the contributors and the quality of their chapters were testimony to Allbutt's reputation in the profession. He wrote many chapters himself, including those on chlorosis, neurasthenia, and cardiac and aortic diseases. He also penned the chapter on mountain sickness, drawing on his own Alpine experiences. Allbutt was a literary stylist, and his own writings were famously well-crafted, a feature that he brought to the whole *System* through his editorial input. *System* also reflected Allbutt's continuing interest in new developments in medicine; he was an avid reader, and could write authoritatively on a wide range of historical, scientific, medical, and literary topics. In 1904 he published a pamphlet titled *Notes on the Composition of Scientific Papers*, in which he gave advice on the do's and don't's of scientific writing, especially the misuse of words, which he illustrated with examples drawn from his extensive reading. The publication went through three editions, and one historian has described Allbutt as 'the Fowler of Medical Literature'. A second, expanded edition of *System* was published between 1905 and 1911, co-edited with Sir Humphry Rolleston (1862–1944), reflecting a decade of rapid developments in many areas of medicine. This edition included a long section on the history of medicine, which reflected Allbutt's growing research and writing in the field, especially on Greek medicine, which he had studied from the mid-1890s. In 1900 he gave the Harveian Oration on 'Science and Medieval Thought', and in 1904 he lectured at the Congress of Arts and Sciences in St Louis on 'The Historical Relations of Medicine and Surgery'. The culmination of this aspect of Allbutt's oeuvre was his *Greek Medicine in Rome,* published in 1921.

In the 1890s, Allbutt had begun to specialize in cardiac and aortic disease, holding unfashionable views on the origins of angina pectoris, which he set out in 1915 in a book entitled *Diseases of the Arteries Including Angina Pectoris*. He was supportive of the open-air treatment of tuberculosis, and in 1906 was one of the twelve founding physicians of the King Edward VII Sanatorium at Midhurst, Sussex. During World War I, in his late seventies and early eighties, he served as a Lieutenant Colonel in the RAMC and, after the war, was active with German Sims Woodhead (1855–1921) and Pendrill Charles Varrier-Jones (1883–1941) in the establishment of the Papworth Tuberculosis Colony. He published a number of books on tuberculosis with Varrier-Jones.

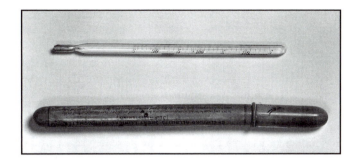

Allbutt's short self-registering clinical thermometer. Wellcome Library, London.

Allbutt was a keen climber and member of the Alpine Club; he also enjoyed walking in the Lake District, often on one of Leslie Stephen's Sunday Trips. He remained active into his eighties, with William Osler (1849–1919) noting that, at eighty-two, he was 'in fine form . . . and cycling 10–15 miles a day'. Allbutt was described by his obituarists as a 'leader of the profession' and, at the time of his death, 'the most prominent and courtly figure in British medicine'. He received many honors: he was knighted in 1907, and in 1920 was the first medical man to join the Privy Council because of his professional work. He received honorary degrees and fellowships, held positions in the RCP, served on the National Insurance Committee, and was President of the BMA in 1920. However, his standing in the profession came from his reputation as a clinician and from the breadth of his contributions to the profession scientifically, socially and politically over many decades.

Bibliography

Primary: 1871. *The Use of the Ophthalmoscope in Diseases of the Nervous System and of the Kidneys* (London); 1870. 'Medical Thermometry.' *British and Foreign Medico-Chirurgical Review* 45: 429–441; 1896–99. *A System of Medicine by Many Writers* 8 vols. (London); 1904. *Notes on the Composition of Scientific Papers* (London); 1915. *Diseases of the Arteries Including Angina Pectoris* (London); 1921. *Greek Medicine in Rome: The Fitzpatrick Lectures on the History of Medicine* (London).

Secondary: Underwood, E. Ashworth, 1963. 'Clifford Allbutt, Scholar-Physician and Historian.' *Proceedings of the Royal Society of Medicine* 56 (Supplement): 11–19; Rolleston, H. D., 1929. *The Right Honourable Sir Thomas Clifford Allbutt KCB: A Memoir* (London); *Oxford DNB*.

Michael Worboys

AL'TSHULLER, ISAAK NAUMOVICH   (b. Livny, Russia, 10 May (22 May), 1870; d. New York, New York, USA, 27 June 1943), *social hygiene, therapeutics.*

Born into a traditional Jewish family in the Russian province of Orel, Isaak Al'tshuller entered the Aleksandr II classical gymnasium in Riga, Latvia. He graduated with a gold medal in 1889, despite the educational restrictions imposed on Jews in the Russian Empire. Because of his brilliant abilities and thanks to a special decree by the Minister of Education, Al'tshuller was admitted to the Department of Natural Sciences at Moscow University, despite the quota that limited the number of Jews who could be enrolled. He advanced into the medical faculty the following year. Although his family had left for New York, Al'tshuller refused to follow them because he was committed to improving the social and political atmosphere in Russia. As an undergraduate, he was active in the liberal movement and worked tirelessly with the medical teams that mobilized to respond to epidemics of cholera.

After graduating from the university in 1894, Al'tshuller declined the opportunity of a scientific career and began a medical practice in the provinces. He became a physician in the *zemstvo* (elective district council) of the small town of Torzok in Tver province. Almost the entire staff of Torzok's hospital was recruited from university-educated physicians with liberal political views who had decided to devote their lives to the enlightenment of the Russian rural population. They established a council for social hygiene and developed a program to teach the basics of community sanitation—one of the earliest Russian initiatives for the reform of the public health system. As often happens in Russia, the project was not implemented because of police persecution of its participants—and Al'tshuller was among the persecuted.

When he contracted tuberculosis, Al'tshuller moved in 1898 to Yalta, on the coast of Crimea, where he settled for many years. The dry mountain air and location on the shore of the Black Sea made Yalta one of the best places for tuberculosis treatment in Russia, and Al'tshuller's medical practice there focused on the problems of tuberculosis patients. He was one of the founders of the Russian section of the International Anti-Tuberculosis League and one of the Russian members of its Central Committee.

A physician with a well-respected reputation, Al'tshuller had a very wide private practice. He treated everyone: autocrats and members of the emperor's family, the Russian artistic and scientific intelligentsia, poor students, and Tatars. Elite patronage helped Al'tshuller to establish a special hospital for physicians, named for Russian Emperor Aleksandr III, and to support the tuberculosis sanatorium, named Yauzlar. He became a personal physician of the famous Russian writers Anton Chekhov, Leo Tolstoy, and Maxim Gorky. He was especially close to Chekhov, who was himself a doctor who wrote extensively about medicine.

Al'tshuller's authority was so high that during World War I he was appointed the head of all Crimean civil and military hospitals, and he administered and coordinated both state and private relief efforts on the peninsula. However, this important public service did not save him from arrest by the Bolsheviks in 1918. A former patient helped Al'tshuller to escape, and in the summer of 1920 he emigrated with his family to Turkey. Later they moved to Berlin and Prague, where Al'tshuller worked for the Russian Red Cross. His son Grigorii, also a well-known physician, became a professor at Charles University in Prague. Al'tshuller spent his last years in the United States, continuing his professional practice and working to bring together Russian and other European refugees. His substantial contributions to the development of local medicine and to the support of medicine in general are representative of the multilateral social and professional activity common among Russian physicians.

Bibliography

Primary: 1930. 'About Chekhov.' *Sovremennye zapiski* XLI: 470–85; 1942. 'Reminiscences about L. N. Tolstoy.' *Novyi zhurnal* 2: 339–59.

Secondary: Solomon, S. Gross, and J. F. Hutchinson, eds., 1990. *Health and Society in Revolutionary Russia* (Bloomington, Indiana, USA); Panina, S. V., 1943. 'Isaak Naumovich Al'tshuller.' *Novyi mir*: 6; 2nd edition, 1996. *Evrei v kulture russkogo zarubezh'ia.* (Jerusalem), 5: 506–14.

Marina Sorokina

ALZHEIMER, ALOIS (b. Marktbreit am Main, Germany, 14 June 1864; d. Breslau, Germany, 19 December 1915), *psychiatry, neuropathology.*

Alzheimer was the son of the lawyer Eduard Alzheimer and his wife, Therese Busch. He attended medical school at the universities of Berlin, Würzburg, and Tübingen and graduated as MD at Würzburg University in 1888. After a short training at the Würzburg anatomical institute with Albert von Kölliker, he commenced work as resident at the Communal Psychiatric Hospital in Frankfurt am Main in December 1888. In 1895, he was promoted to a consultant position and held the responsibility for the neuropathological laboratory. His psychiatric teacher was Emil Sioli, and he also profited from systematic exchanges with his psychiatric colleague Franz Nissl, as well as with the pathologists Ludwig Edinger and Carl Weigert. In March 1903 Alzheimer followed the offer of Emil Kraepelin to join the Department of Psychiatry at Heidelberg University, where he again became a direct colleague of Nissl and started to edit a high-profile publication series on neuropathology. After only a few months, in December 1903, Alzheimer followed Kraepelin to the Psychiatric Department at Munich University to take over the responsibility for the neuroanatomy laboratory. In the same year, he also completed his Habilitation with a study on histopathological criteria for the diagnosis of progressive paralysis. In 1906 Alzheimer was promoted to chief-of-staff and deputy director of the Psychiatric Clinic at Munich University, and in 1909 he received the title of professor extraordinarius. To be able to devote all his work to further research, Alzheimer requested and received the exceptional status of a research associate without salary for the period from 1909 until 1912. In this year, he moved to the University of Breslau, where he was appointed full professor of psychiatry, and director of the Psychiatric Clinic. Suffering from a chronic infection, he died in 1915 at the age of fifty-one.

Alzheimer was one of the leading neuropathologists of his time who, before the emergence of a distinct discipline of neuropathology, worked in the institutional context of psychiatry. He succeeded in establishing the morphological and histological changes in the brain with some psychiatric disorders, notably the form of senile dementia that is today known as Alzheimer's disease—an eponym coined by Emil Kraepelin. Alzheimer also published important contributions to the knowledge of extrapyramidal movement disorders, Huntington's chorea, and specific types of glial cells. Methodologically, he employed a variety of staining techniques to investigate the chemistry of the central nervous system and may thus be understood as one of the initiators of neurochemistry.

Together with his Heidelberg colleague Nissl, Alzheimer edited the influential series *Histologische und histopathologische Arbeiten über die Grosshirnrinde* (from 1904 onward). He was also cofounder (in 1911) and coeditor (1911–15) of the *Zeitschrift für die gesamte Neurologie und Psychiatrie*. He was also a very early proponent of the idea to establish a central German research institute for psychiatry to serve the needs of the public and the nation; this idea was then put into practice by the foundation of the Deutsche Forschungsanstalt für Psychiatrie in 1917, an institution that served as a model for similar psychiatric research institutes worldwide. Among Alzheimer's pupils were Francesco Bonfiglio, Louis Casamajor, Ugo Cerletti, Hans-Gerhard Creutzfeldt, F. Fulci, Alfons Jakob, F. H. Lewy, L. Omorokow, and Gaetano Perusini.

Bibliography

Primary: 1904. *Histologische Studien zur Differentialdiagnose der progressiven Paralyse* (Jena); 1904–1918. (with Nissl, Franz) *Histologische und histopathologische Arbeiten über die Großhirnrinde mit besonderer Berücksichtigung der pathologischen Anatomie der Geisteskrankheiten* 6 vols. (Jena); 1906. 'Ueber einen eigenartigen schweren Erkrankungsprozess der Hirnrinde.' *Neurologisches Centralblatt* 25: 1134–1141; 1911. 'Ist die Einrichtung einer psychiatrischen Einrichtung im Reichsgesundheitsamt wünschenswert?' *Zeitschrift für die gesamte Neurologie* 6: 242–246.

Secondary: Maurer, Konrad, and Ulrike Maurer, 2003. *Alzheimer: The Life of a Physician and the Career of a Disease* (New York); Meyer, J. E., 1961. 'Alois Alzheimer' in Scholz, W., ed., *50 Jahre Neuropathologie in Deutschland* (Stuttgart) pp. 67–78.

Volker Roelcke

AMATUS LUSITANUS, JOÃO RODRIGUES DE CASTELO BRANCO (b. Castelo Branco, Portugal, 1511; d. Salonika, Ottoman Empire (now Greece), 1568?), *medicine, surgery.*

Amatus Lusitanus was a New Christian (i.e., a descendant of the Jewish people forced to convert to Christianity by Manoel I in 1497) in Portugal. He attended the University of Salamanca in Spain, where he received his MD in 1532. In Lisbon he worked as a physician until 1534. The persecution of New Christians during the Inquisition forced Amatus Lusitanus to leave Portugal and begin a life of wandering across Europe. He roamed until his last years in Salonika, in northern Greece, where he was safe from persecution.

The first place he lived outside Portugal was in the Flemish city of Antwerp, between 1534 and 1541. There he published his first medical work, commentaries on the Materia Medica of Dioscorides, published under the name Ioanne Roderico Castelialbi Lusitanus. The work was incomplete because of difficulties in publication.

The next place Amatus lived was Ferrara, in northern Italy. He was invited by the Duke d'Este to occupy the chair of medicine at the university. There Amatus enjoyed the friendship of such scholars as botanists Antonio Musa Brassavola (1500–55) and Johan Falconer and anatomist Giambattista Canano (1515–79). Together, they gave lectures and performed dissections.

The shadows of intolerance continued to influence his life. Persecutions against crypto-Jews in Ferrara, and the invitation to settle in Ragusa (now Dubrovnik, Croatia) led Amatus to leave the town. He was waiting for the definitive call of the Senate of Ragusa. The invitation did not come, and in 1547 he settled at Ancona, a city belonging to the Papal province under Pope Paul III, who showed great tolerance toward Jews and New Christians. He remained in Ancona until 1555, a time very rich in Amatus's intellectual life and medical practice.

He was called to treat very important persons: noblemen, ambassadors, and members of the Pope's family, in many places in Italy. Probably during this period he took the name Amatus (beloved) Lusitanus—perhaps a reference to the former surname of his Jewish family, Haviv.

During his sojourn in Florence 1551 he published his first *Centuria*. This was the most important work of Amatus—a compilation of one hundred medical cases, with commentaries and discussions. Many cases of surgery were recorded, and Amatus, in many places of his work, stressed the duty of the physician to work in concert with the surgeon. In this field, Amatus gave the world the first accounts of an obturator being used to close a perforation in the palate, and of a method of treating empyema by means of an incision in the lower intercostal space, not higher in the chest as was then customary. He also quoted a treatment for strictures of the urethra by introducing bougies at regular intervals. In the next year, 1552, Amatus published in Venice his *Centuria II* and three additional books of the series by 1555. Amatus also brought out a new and enlarged edition of the commentaries on Materia Medica of Dioscorides in 1553.

The ascension of Pope Paul IV in 1555 renewed the anti-Jewish persecutions, and Amatus went to Ragusa that same year. There he published *Centuria VI,* in 1558. From there he went to Salonika, where he joined the local Jewish community and published in 1561 his last *Centuria VII,* which contains an Oath for the Physician. This shows Amatus's great concern for the ethical foundations of medical practice.

The *Centurias* were studied at medical schools in Europe until the eighteenth century.

Amatus died from plague around 1568.

Bibliography

Primary: 1553. *In Dioscoridis Anazarbei de medica materia libros quinque* (Venice); 1566. *Centuriae I–VII* (Venice).

Secondary: Front, Dov. 1998. 'The Expurgation of the Books of Amatus Lusitanus: Censorship and the Bibliography of the Individual Book.' *Book Collector* 47(4): 520–36; Kottek, Samuel S. 1994. 'Amatus Lusitanus in Salonica: The Last Paragraph in Eventful Biography' in Carrillo, Juan L., and Guillermo Olagüe, eds., *Actas del XXXIII Congreso Internacional de Historia de la Medicina: Granada-Sevilla, 1–6 September, 1992* (Seville), pp. 409–16; Friedenwald, Harry, 1944. *The Jews and Medicine* (Baltimore), pp. 332–417.

Francisco Moreno de Carvalho

AMPOFO, OKU   (b. Powmu, Eastern Province, British Gold Coast (now Ghana), 4 November 1908; d. Ghana, 18 February 1998), *general practice, plant medicine.*

Oku Ampofo bridged Western and African culture in both his medical practice and artistic endeavors. Ampofo was the first Ghanaian to receive the Gold Coast Medical Scholarship to study abroad at Edinburgh University. Importantly, he integrated regional plants into his medical practice and collaborated with the World Health Organization (1976–98) and U.S. National Institutes for Health through his Centre for Scientific Research into Plant Medicine (CSRPM). Ampofo's clinical trials with fellow Ghanaian, physician Gilbert Boye, scientifically proved the efficacy of 'Ghana quinine', or *Cryptolepis sanguinolenta,* in combatting falciparum malaria.

Ampofo was born on his father's cocoa estate near Powmu in the Akuapem Mountains. His mother, Akua Adwo, and his father, Chief Kwesi Ampofo, both descended from royal family lines. He learned to value traditional African culture as a child, often spending his mornings at his father's feet during village court proceedings. Chief Ampofo encouraged his son to pursue a mission education, and sent him to Amanase Primary School and Mampong Lower Primary School. Ampofo attended Anum Senior School (1922–25) and Mfantsipim School (1926–29). On a principal's scholarship, he continued his scientific studies at the Prince of Wales College (now Achimota) (1930–32).

Ampofo received the Gold Coast Medical Scholarship to attend the University of Edinburgh in 1932, and completed his training at the Royal Colleges of Edinburgh and Glasgow through private sponsorship (LCRP Edin., LRCS Edin., LRFP&S Glas). After qualifying as a doctor in 1939, he continued studying at the Liverpool School of Tropical Medicine, and interned at the Karolinska Hospital in Stockholm.

Upon returning to Ghana (1940), Ampofo established a private practice in the Akuapem Mountains, and worked tirelessly to provide health care to the rural population. Ampofo headed the committee that established Tetteh Quarshie Memorial Hospital in Mampong-Akuapem, where he served as its first Senior Medical Officer (1961–72). During the 1980s, when many physicians fled Ghana's economic instability, Ampofo remained. In Akuapem he established the Ghana Rural Reconstruction Movement with his brothers, gynecologist D. A. Ampofo and Kwadwo Ohene-Ampofo.

Ampofo was also a member of the 'Alkaloid Group', charged by the National Research Council under Ghana's first president, Kwame Nkrumah, to identify medicinal plant alkaloids. Ampofo's leadership in this area dated to the 1940s when drug scarcity during World War II led him to cooperate with indigenous healers to incorporate plant-based therapies into his practice. As a member of a delegation to the People's Republic of China during Nkrumah's tenure, Ampofo was inspired by Chinese traditional medicine. Members of the Alkaloid Group, including Albert Nii Tackie, joined him in establishing his center for research into plant medicine. In recognition of his contributions to medical research, Ampofo was awarded the Grand Medal by the Government of Ghana (1969), an honorary doctorate (DLitt) by the University of Ghana, Legon (1974), and the Scroll of Honor by the Ghana Academy of Arts and Sciences (1984).

Ampofo chaired the Arts Council of Ghana (1969–72) and the Ghana Museums and Monuments Board (1973–77). His interest in the arts originated during his time in Europe: while studying medicine in Scotland, he had trained simultaneously at the Edinburgh School of Art (1935–39). One of his special interests was in reclaiming African iconography, such as that appropriated by Pablo Picasso and others. After returning to the Gold Coast, Ampofo organized the first Neo-African Art Exhibition in 1945, formed the 'Akuapem Six' Artists Society, and later starred with his wife Rosina in the film *The Boy Kumasenu* (1952). His sculptures stand in front of the Ghana National Theater and Ghana National Museum. His work *Asase Due* [Earth, Condolence] (1965), created to commemorate the assassination of U.S. President John F. Kennedy, is displayed at the Kennedy Center in Washington, D.C.

In his later years, particularly after a spinal injury in 1978, Ampofo's health deteriorated. Nonetheless, he finished writing a memoir and several other publications while continuing to see patients and consult at CSRPM.

Bibliography

Primary: 1983. *First Aid in Plant Medicine* (Accra); 1998. *My Kind of Sculpture* (Accra).

Secondary: Osseo-Asare, Abena, 2005. 'Bitter Roots: African Science and the Search for Healing Plants in Ghana 1885–2005.' PhD thesis, Harvard University; Vieta, Kojo, 1999. *The Flagbearers of Ghana* (Accra, Ghana); July, Robert W., 1987. *An African Voice: The Role of the Humanities in African Independence* (Durham, NC).

Abena Dove Osseo-Asare

ANAXIMANDER (b. Miletus, Asia Minor (now Turkey), *c.* 610 BCE; d. *c.* 545 BCE), *natural philosophy, cosmology, astronomy.*

A Pre-Socratic from Miletus, like Thales, Anaximander was one of the earliest philosophers to be preoccupied with the explanation of natural phenomena through an all-inclusive system. Explanations of the Milesian type were bottom-up, progressing from simple to complex and building speculative cosmologies on one or more elementary principles. Anaximander's cosmology postulated an undifferentiated state—the *apeiron* ('that which is infinite' or 'unbound')—as the ultimate source and constituent of things (*arche*). It was probably born in response to Thales's cosmology, which postulated water. Anaximander raised objections concerning the forces holding earth and water (Aristotle, *Physics* 204b). He dealt with questions of natural philosophy and developed the notions of zoogony, the origin and development of species (including that of man), and meteorology.

According to Plutarch, Anaximander conceived of the universe as developing from the *apeiron*. In his account, matter separated itself from the undifferentiated state by a rotary motion in the vortex; it disposed itself in layers according to weight, the heavy matter going to the center. At any given time, there were an infinite number of worlds undergoing this process, and they succeeded each other (Simplicius). The heavenly bodies were masses of fire surrounded by air and pierced by narrow pipes, which emitted light from the fire within. The earth was a flat-topped cylinder whose diameter was three times its height. Anaximander described the distances between the earth and heavenly bodies in earth-diameters: the stars were nine diameters away, the moon was eighteen diameters away, the sun was twenty-seven diameters away. In explaining meteorological occurrences, Anaximander ascribed a central role to *pneuma* (Aetius and Seneca, fragments A 23–24).

The causal agent responsible for the origin of all things, including the earth and the species inhabiting it, was the interaction of the hot and the moist. Life on earth originated from inanimate matter, namely, from water acted upon by the sun; humans developed from fish; and primitive humans were nursed in the bellies of fish until adolescence. The fetus was frail and protected by a thorny crust.

Anaximander is credited with conceiving a form of the principle of survival of the fittest (Hippolytus, Plutarch, Aetius).

Another notion of vital importance in Anaximander's system was that of balance. He thought that the earth 'remains where it is because of its equal distance from everything' (Aristotle, *On the Sky*, 294a). And in a famous, if obscure, political metaphor, he described the entire cosmos as a balance of forces, equal and opposed, which 'pay the penalty and recompense to one another for their injustice, according to the assessment of time' (Simplicius, *On Aristotle's Physics* 24.19). This is the only direct quotation surviving from Anaximander's work. The difficulty in interpreting it is a warning that all interpretations of Anaximander are controversial, based as they are on fragmentary and decontextualized material.

Bibliography

Primary: Diels, H., and W. Kranz, eds., 1952. *Die Fragmente der Vorsokratiker* (Berlin) I: 81 ff; Kirk, G. S., J. E. Raven, and M. Schofield, eds., 1983. *The Presocratic Philosophers* (Cambridge).

Secondary: Barnes, J., 1979. *The Presocratic Philosophers* (London, Henley, Boston) I: 19 ff; Stokes, M. C., 1971. *One and Many in Presocratic Philosophy* (Washington, DC); Dicks, D. R., 1970. *Early Greek Astronomy to Aristotle* (London); Guthrie, W. K. C., 1962. *A History of Greek Philosophy* (Cambridge) I: 72 ff; Kahn, K. H., 1960. *Anaximander and the Origins of Greek Cosmology* (New York); DSB.

Manuela Tecusan

ANDERSON, ELIZABETH GARRETT (b. London, England, 9 June 1836; d. Aldeburgh, Suffolk, England, 17 December 1917), *medical education, medicine.*

The second of the nine surviving children of Newson Garrett, a self-made businessman of Aldeburgh, Suffolk, and his wife, Louisa Dunnell, Elizabeth Garrett was educated at home and at a boarding school for ladies at Blackheath, Kent (1849–1854). With her friend Emily Davies, who later founded Girton College (for Women), Cambridge, Garrett became a member of the Langham Place circle of middle-class women at the core of the emerging mid-Victorian women's movement. Her younger sister, Millicent Fawcett (1847–1929), became leader of the constitutional women's suffrage movement.

In 1859, through the Langham Place circle, she met Elizabeth Blackwell, the only woman on the General Medical Council's new medical register. Inspired by Blackwell and supported by her father, she obtained a medical education and a registrable medical qualification. Barred from admission as a medical student to a university or London teaching hospital, she completed the required courses as a private student of teachers from recognized medical schools, and passed the examination for the Licence of the Society of Apothecaries. In 1865 her name was entered on the medical register, the second woman and first British-trained woman;

no more women were added until 1876. In 1870 she became the first woman to obtain an MD from the University of Paris. Admitted to membership in the British Medical Association in 1873, she remained the only woman member for nineteen years.

After qualifying, Garrett set up a successful private practice in central London, comparable to her leading male peers. Formally limited to women and children, it set a precedent for British medical women until World War I, after which medical women began to expand their professional roles. She also treated poor women and children, establishing first a dispensary, and in 1871 adding beds to create the New Hospital for Women. The first hospital in Britain with only female medical staff, it would be renamed the Elizabeth Garrett Anderson hospital in 1918. This hospital enabled her to undertake major surgery, including (controversially) in 1872 an ovariotomy, then a risky procedure.

In 1871 she married James George Skelton Anderson (1838–1907), a businessman. They had one son and two daughters, including Louisa Garrett Anderson (1873–1943), later a distinguished doctor. Marriage and motherhood did not seem to hinder her medical career, and she provided a model for medical women who followed, along with this advice: 'the first thing women must learn is to dress like ladies and behave like gentlemen' (quoted in *Oxford DNB*).

Clashes of personality and tactics between Garrett Anderson and Sophia Jex-Blake (1840–1912) marked the campaign for women's entry to the medical profession after the Society of Apothecaries restricted its examination in 1868 to students enrolled at recognized medical schools. Garrett Anderson favored a non-confrontational route, and opposed Jex-Blake's proposal to establish a separate women's medical school. Nevertheless, when the London School of Medicine for Women opened in 1874, largely due to Jex-Blake's efforts, Garrett Anderson supported it and opened the New Hospital for Women to its students. In 1883, despite Jex-Blake's opposition, Garrett Anderson became Dean of the School, serving until 1902 and overseeing its expansion, legal incorporation, and establishment as a college of the University of London.

Garrett Anderson's pioneering activities were not limited to medicine. In 1870, she was elected to the London school board in the first election open to women candidates; and in 1908, she became the first woman mayor (of Aldeburgh) in England.

Although a successful clinician, Garrett Anderson's contribution was as an outstanding administrator and, most of all, as supporter and role model for medical women in Britain in the last quarter of the nineteenth century.

Bibliography

Secondary: Elston, M. A., 1986. 'Women doctors in the British health service: a sociological study of their careers and opportunities.' PhD thesis, University of Leeds; Manton, J., 1965. *Elizabeth Garrett Anderson* (New York); Garrett Anderson, L., 1939. *Elizabeth Garrett Anderson* (London); *Oxford DNB*.

Marguerite Dupree

ANDREAS OF CARYSTUS (fl. after 250 BCE; d. 217 BCE), *pharmacology, surgery, gynecology, medical historiography.*

The son of Chrysareus, coming from Carystus on the island of Euboea (now Greece), Andreas was a doctor of high social status in Ptolemaic Alexandria, acting as court physician to King Ptolemy IV Philopator (c. 244–205 BCE). Mistaken for the king, he was assassinated when sleeping in the king's tent in 217 BCE, on the eve of the battle of Raphia. An early disciple of Herophilus, he was one of the very few Herophileans attached to the Ptolemies and 'one of the few doctors who moved in the two worlds of the professional physician and the Court doctor' (Fraser).

Andreas stood apart in these ways; he was also a controversial figure, praised by some, contested by others. An influential member of the group of Herophileans, he shared with them a solid interest in pharmacy. His recipes were widely known, used by some Empiricist doctors and quoted by Galen, and Dioscorides praised his plant descriptions for their detail. Yet the great Empiricist and rival pharmacologist of the succeeding generation, Heraclides of Tarentum, gave an unflattering account of his methods and contrasted him with Hippocrates: uninterested in the truth, Andreas would have copied from others descriptions of plants he had never himself seen. Galen, in fact, was rather dismissive of Andreas's acceptance of strange folk remedies.

Andreas's expertise covered a much wider range of subjects. One was surgery, where he made an outstanding contribution, according to Oribasius: the invention of an instrument for the treatment of dislocations. The titles of Andreas's lost writings (e.g., *Narthex*, a pharmacopoeia with descriptions of plants, *On Wreaths*, *On Snake-Bites*, *Against Superstitious Beliefs*) betray at least an interest in a great variety of medical topics, ranging from midwifery, physiology, and pathology to historiography and Hippocratic exegesis. For this reason Andreas's books feature among the sources most frequently used by Pliny (he is quoted as a source in fourteen books). But the great contemporary Eratosthenes (c. 275–194 BCE) charged Andreas with plagiarism, much along the line of Heraclides.

The material on Andreas amounts to about fifty possible pieces. However, the identifications of 'Andreas of Carystus', 'Andreas son of Chrysareus', and 'Andreas the Herophilean' remain tentative, so that the story line provided by these ancient references to Andreas must be used with care.

Bibliography

Primary: Staden, Heinrich von, 1989. *Herophilus. The Art of Medicine in Early Alexandria* (New Haven) pp. 475–477 (includes a list of references for fragments).

Secondary: Nutton, V., 2004. *Ancient Medicine* (London) pp. 140–56; Longrigg, J., 1998. *Greek Medicine. From the Heroic to the Hellenistic Age. A Source Book* (London) pp. 164, 167, 189; Staden, Heinrich von, 1989. *Herophilus. The Art of Medicine in Early Alexandria* (New Haven) pp. 472–475; Fraser, P. M., 1972. *Ptolemaic Alexandria* 3 vols. (Oxford) I, pp. 358, 369–371, II, pp. 528, 546; Wellmann, M., 1894. 'Andreas' (11) in Pauly, A., and G. Wissowa, eds., *Real-Encyclopädie der classischen Altertumswissenschaft* (Stuttgart) I. 2, coll. 2136f.

Manuela Tecusan

AL-ANṬĀKĪ, DĀʾUD (aka DAVID OF ANTIOCH, DAVID ANTIOCHENUS, DĀWŪD IBN 'UMAR AL ANṬĀKĪ)

(b. Umar al-Darīr in Antioch, Persia (now Turkey); d. Mecca, Arabia (now Saudi Arabia), 1599) *medicine, pharmacology, lovesickness.*

Blind from birth, the Arab physician Dāʾud al-Anṭākī nonetheless traveled and wrote extensively. By the time of his death in 1599, he had written a 3,000-entry encyclopedia of medicaments, the *Tadhkirat*, as well as treatises on topics as diverse as astrology and love. Al-Anṭākī fit the mold of a natural philosopher and physician in the Greco-Arabic tradition. He was also a bridge-figure between traditional Arabic and modern European medicine.

Many details about al-Anṭākī's life were recorded by his seventeenth-century biographer Muḥammad al-Muḥibbī. As al-Muḥibbī reports, al-Anṭākī was born in Antioch. His father was the *raʾis* (governor or leader) of a nearby town. During his youth, al-Anṭākī met a learned Persian visitor at the shrine of one of Antioch's local saints. Impressed by al-Anṭākī's intelligence, this visitor took him as his student. Al-Anṭākī learned logic, mathematics, and natural philosophy. After receiving this training, al-Anṭākī journeyed across the eastern Mediterranean, going as far as Asia Minor to learn Greek. Having done so, he studied in Cairo and Damascus. In the last one or two years of his life, he completed the *hajj* to Mecca, where he died.

There is consensus in the historiography about al-Anṭākī's legacy to pharmacology. The most important of his works is no doubt the *Tadhkirat*, which is still read by practitioners of unānī medicine. The text is divided into an introduction and four large sections. The introduction to the text explains the sciences discussed in the *Tadhkirat*, and shows their relation to the rest of the book. The first of the large sections deals generally with medicine. In it, al-Anṭākī advised his readers on principles of studying and investigating diseases. The second part dealt specifically with pharmacology. Al-Anṭākī traced the history of pharmacology, describing important figures such as Dioscorides, Galen, Rufus of Ephesus, and Paul of Aegina. In addition to these, al-Anṭākī said a few words about practitioners of Syrian medicine but concentrated mostly on Arabic physicians. As al-Anṭākī noted, his *Tadhkirat* most closely followed the work of Ibn al-Bayṭār, a famous

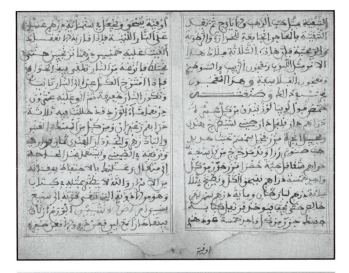

Page of manuscript from *Pleasantness of Oils for Human Health*, folios 21a & b, 18th century. Arabic MS 451, Al-Haddad Collection, Wellcome Library, London.

physician and pharmacologist who studied and catalogued substances with medicinal purposes in the thirteenth century. Like al-Bayṭār, al-Anṭākī was attempting to offer physicians a list of simple and compound medicines even larger than Ibn Sīnā's. The third section, which was ordered according to the Arabic alphabet, contained this list, which describes all manner of *materia medica*, including herbs, plants, minerals, and extracts from animal viscera. The fourth section contained descriptions of diseases and their treatments. Unlike the third section, it was ordered according to the Hebrew alphabet. Some historians have suggested that al-Anṭākī probably did not write all of this section; he seemed to have stopped at the ninth letter of the Hebrew alphabet. His students may have finished this final section.

Although the *Tadhkirat* was widely circulated in the Arabic world, it did not generate nearly the same level of interest in Europe. However, some small portions were translated. Notably, Edward Pococke, an Oxford orientalist, extracted a short description of coffee from the *Tadhkirat* in 1659. Pococke's translation offers a concise description of coffee's attributes, complete with numeric quantification of its degree of hotness, a complexional/humoral quality; he probably did not intend his short translation to have a medical purpose. Indeed, Pococke was much more interested in natural philosophy as a discipline unto itself than he was in medicine, and coffee had only recently been introduced to the English, who may have considered an Arab physician's description of coffee a novelty. This underscores some of the changes in the interface between Western and Eastern medicine around the time al-Anṭākī wrote the *Tadhkirat*. Previously, throughout most of the Middle Ages, medical knowledge flowed almost exclusively from East to West as translations of Arabic texts were completed with great frequency. By the sixteenth century, however, medical knowledge was moving in both directions. Additionally, Europeans sought Arabic medical knowledge less avidly, as Pococke's example illustrates. In some instances, however, the *Tadhkirat* reflects the bidirectional exchange of knowledge. In the section on mercury, al-Anṭākī called syphilis the 'French disease'. As Plessner has noted, al-Anṭākī made this reference because he was using the same description of syphilis as French doctors. One example of Arabic medicine's ongoing, albeit diminished influence on European medicine is al-Anṭākī's recipe for hard soap. A number of Arab scholars—including al-Anṭākī—were able to make hard soap using chemicals such as *al-Qali* (alkali) and *natrūn* (sodium bicarbonate). Their recipes were widely disseminated because hard soaps were more desirable than the viscous liquid soap that was common in Europe.

Al-Anṭākī's other major work is a love story. To many Arabic physicians, love was a topic that demanded exploration; love could lead to sickness, even to the point of causing someone afflicted with a deep, unrequited longing to waste away. Ḥunayn ibn Isḥāq, whose translations of Greek texts formed the core of the Arabic medical curriculum for centuries, had treated it as a psychological disorder; thus, the study of love was long considered an adjunct to medicine. Al-Anṭākī explored love in his *Tazyīn al-aswāq bi-tafṣīl*, an edited and expanded version of a similar story by Muḥammad al-Sarrāj (d. 1106). The story follows the pattern of many Arabic love stories. First, a man falls in love with a slave girl, from whom he is later separated. The slave girl's former owner realizes the profundity of his loss and is pained by it, perhaps even to the point of endangering his own health. Eventually, the new owner recognizes the loss felt by both the former owner and the slave girl and reunites them.

In addition to the *Tazyīn al-aswāq* and the *Tadhkirat*, al-Anṭākī authored several short treatises. These include one on the use of astrology in the study and practice of medicine (*Unmūdhaj fi 'Ilm al-Falak*), which Leclerc suggested was actually taken from the *Tadhkirat*. Other historians have not shared this view. The other is on the philosopher's stone (*Risāla fi 'l-Tā'ir wa'l-Ukāb*). Little is said about these treatises in Western historiography, as they have not had the same lasting influence as the *Tadhkirat*. Consequently, they present a remarkable lacuna in the study of early modern Arabic medicine. Like the *Tadhkirat*, these two treatises might support the thesis that al-Anṭākī was a scholar at the crossroads of medical history. Although he seems a traditional Greco-Arabic medical scholar who was at the end of a long line of medieval physicians and natural philosophers, his *Tadhkirat* reflects the changing interface between Eastern and Western medicine in the early-modern Mediterranean.

Bibliography

Primary: 1669. Selections from *Tadhkirat ūlī al-albāb wa-al-jāmi' lil-'ajab al-ujāb*, 'The nature of the drink Kauhi, or Coffe [sic], and the Berry of which it is made, Described by an Arabian Phisitian' (trans. Pococke, Edward) (Oxford); Al-Mubibbī, Muḥammad Amīn Ibn Fadl Allāh, 1966. *Khuṣāṣat al-athār fi a'yān al-quar al-hādi 'ashar* 4 vols. (Beirut); 1993. (Altūnjī, Muḥammad, ed.) *Tazyīn al-aswāq bi-tafṣīl ashwāq al-'ushshāq* 2 vols. (Beirut); 1996. *Tadhkirat ūlī al-albāb wa-al-jāmi' lil-'ajab al-ujāb* 2 vols. (Beirut).

Secondary: Gelder, G. J. V., 2004. 'Slave-Girl Lost and Regained: Transformations of a Story.' *Marvels and Tales: Journal of Fairy-Tale Studies* 18(2): 201–217; Hassan, Ahmad Y., and Donald R. Hill, 1986. *Islamic Technology: An Illustrated History* (Cambridge); Wustenfeld, Ferdinand, 1963. *Geschichte der arabischen Aertze und Naturforscher* (Hildesheim); Plessner, Martin, 1962. 'Dāwūd al-Antāki's 16th Century Encyclopedia on Medicine, Natural History and Occult Sciences' *Actes du dixième congrès international d'histoire des sciences,* The International Congress on the History of Sciences (Paris) pp. 635–637; Leclerc, Lucien, 1960. *Histoire de la médecine arabe* (New York); Slane, W. M. G. (de), 1883. *Catalogue des manuscrits arabes, Bibliothèque Nationale de France, Departement des manuscrits* (Paris) no. 2625, 8, no. 2357, 7.

Michael J. Neuss

ARANZIO, GIULIO CESARE (b. Bologna, Italy, *c.* 1530; d. Bologna, 7 April 1589), *anatomy, surgery.*

Aranzio was the son of Ottaviano di Jacopo and Maria Maggi, but he so loved and esteemed his maternal uncle, Bartolomeo Maggi, renowned surgeon, anatomist, and lecturer in surgery at the University of Bologna, that he assumed his surname, calling himself Giulio Cesare Aranzio Maggi. His uncle encouraged him to study medicine, and on 20 May 1556 Aranzio received his degree in philosophy and medicine from the University of Bologna. He was then made a lecturer in surgery, a post he held until 1586–87, and it was for him that on 27 September 1570 the chair of anatomy was made independent from the chair of surgery. He held both professorships until 1588, the year in which he was struck down by a serious illness, after which he only lectured on anatomy.

In 1564 Aranzio published his *De humano foetu libellus*, a brief treatise on the physiology of generation and pregnancy, based on his direct anatomical observations and on the practice of obstetrics, in which he made many important contributions to the knowledge of the adnexa and fetal circulation. The third edition (1587) was more accurate and precise in the morphological aspects, which assumed a greater importance than the functional ones expressed according to Galenic doctrine. This was perhaps also due to a more direct contact with Aristotle's biological works, often quoted in the third edition. In 1579 Aranzio published another anatomical work, the *Anatomicarum observationum liber*, in which he put forward original arguments to support the theory of the blood's passage from the right heart to the left, across the lungs (the so-called lesser or pulmonary circulation), which had already been presented by Realdo Colombo. Both works contain important anatomical contributions.

Aranzio produced the first adequate printed account of the gravid uterus, and finally dispelled the idea of a human cotyledonous placenta. He also gave a noteworthy description of the anatomy of the fetus, by far the best up to his time. He made a detailed examination of the fetal heart, and he saw the *ductus arteriosus* and the *foramen ovale*. His name was given to the venous duct (or duct of Arantius), i.e., the terminal branch of the umbilical vein, which in the fetus opens in the inferior vena cava. He also paid particular attention to the vascular system of the adult; he described the little fibrous nodules in the free edge of the aortic semilunar valves to which his name is now attached (nodules of Arantius). Furthermore, he described the hippocampus, the cerebellum with the *arbor vitae*, the fourth ventricle (where the dilatation of the sulcus medianus at the lower ventricular angle was once called 'ventricle of Arantius'), and the coracobrachial and vaginal constrictor muscles; he was also credited with the first description of the elevator of the upper eyelid muscle, which in fact was first described by Gabriele Falloppia (1561).

Aranzio's *De tumoribus secundum locos affectos liber* (1571) was devoted to surgical subjects and demonstrated the high quality of his surgical practice: he dwelt at length on diseases of the head and of the eyes and on the cure of nasal polyps, anal fistulae, and phimosis. He performed rhinoplastic surgery several years before Gaspare Tagliacozzi, but he wrote nothing on these operations. His interest in surgery was confirmed by his comments on Hippocrates' *De vulneribus capitis* (1579).

Bibliography

Primary: 1564. *De humano foetu libellus* (Bologna); 1571. *De tumoribus secundum locos affectos liber* (Bologna); 1579. *Liber anatomicarum observationum* (Basel).

Secondary: Dall'Osso, Eugenio, 1956. 'Giulio Cesare Aranzio e la rinoplastica.' *Annali di medicina navale e tropicale* 61: 617–627; Dall'Osso, Eugenio, 1956. 'Un contributo al pensiero scientifico di Giulio Cesare Aranzio: la sua opera chirurgica.' *Annali di medicina navale e tropicale* 61: 754–767; Medici, Michele, 1857. *Compendio storico della scuola anatomica di Bologna* (Bologna) pp. 78–84; DSB.

Giuseppe Ongaro

ARÁOZ ALFARO, GREGORIO (b. San Miguel de Tucumán, Argentina, 8 June 1870; d. Buenos Aires, Argentina, 26 August 1955), *public health, pediatrics.*

Born in the provincial city of San Miguel de Tucumán, Gregorio Aráoz Alfaro rose to prominence in Argentina's flourishing, turn-of-the-century medical center, Buenos Aires. After graduating from the University of Buenos Aires's medical school in 1892, he taught pathology at his alma mater. He undertook an extended two-year clinical tour of Germany, France, and Italy (a move typical among his peers at the time), and returned to Buenos Aires in 1904, settling down to enjoy his reputation as expert diagnostician and pathologist. For the remainder of his career, he was devoted to preventive medicine and public health, as exemplified by his leading role in the campaigns against tuberculosis at the turn of the century. His most recognized contribution, however, was in pediatrics and preventive medicine.

Part of a circle of reform-minded physicians, like many of his generation, Aráoz Alfaro participated in efforts to centralize, modernize, and expand the federal government's health apparatus. From his position as professor at the University of Buenos Aires in the 1890s, he lobbied the government to consolidate its welfare and sanitary departments. After serving as president of the National Department of Hygiene, he helped to create Argentina's first Ministry of Public Health in the 1910s. Long after his tenure in this post, he continued to serve as an advisor to public health officials. He also took an interest in international work, and in 1924 served as Argentina's representative to the Pan-American Sanitary Code convention.

In addition to achieving renown for his work in public health and sanitation, in the 1890s Aráoz Alfaro made his mark in the nascent field of puericulture—or maternal and infant hygiene, a forerunner of eugenics. Together with colleagues Enrique Feinmann and Cecilia Grierson, Aráoz Alfaro pioneered this new field in Argentina. His main concern was to lower the nation's infant mortality rates, and to diminish such childhood diseases as diphtheria, scarlet fever, tuberculosis, diarrhea, and polio, many of which he considered avoidable. He served as president of the Argentine Pediatrics Society and was viewed as a founder of the specialty in Argentina. Strongly influenced by French approaches to pediatrics, Aráoz Alfaro published on methods of hygiene for children that emphasized fresh air, exercise, nutrition, and education.

Dedicated to preventive medicine and the new field of puericulture, Aráoz Alfaro published a number of training manuals for health professionals who specialized in the treatment of women and children. In addition, his manuals instructed mothers themselves in the latest methods of so-called scientific mothering. His 1899 *El libro de las madres* (*The Mothers' Book*), which dealt with child well-being, from conception and pregnancy on, recommended hygienic reforms in the home and proper ways to feed and clothe children, and made behavioristic recommendations. In furthering puericulture in Argentina, Aráoz Alfaro provided an early intellectual and institutional infrastructure for eugenics in that country. He urged couples considering marriage to choose their partners wisely and on eugenic bases, in order to create normal, 'well developed' offspring. He argued in *The Mothers' Book* that the physician, and only the physician, was able to determine the optimal health of marriage partners.

His emphasis on infant hygiene, fitness, well-being, and the role of heredity in creating healthy children was increasingly taken up in the early twentieth century by organizations devoted to the adoption of punitive and controlling eugenics legislation. Aráoz Alfaro, together with fellow physicians Victor Delfino and Ubaldo Fernández, founded the Argentine Eugenics Society in 1918. Toward the end of his life, onetime social reformer Aráoz Alfaro turned to right-wing causes, including his adherence in 1936 to a pro-German Argentine organization.

Bibliography

Primary: 1899. *El libro de las madres* (Buenos Aires); 1908. *Manual práctico de higiene del niño* (Buenos Aires); 1936. *Por nuestros niños y por las madres* (Buenos Aires).

Secondary: Golero Bacigalupi, Ruben, 1970. 'Gregorio Aráoz Alfaro' *Torax 19*(2): 65–66.

Julia Rodriguez

ARBUTHNOT[T], JOHN   (b. Arbuthnott, Kincardine-shire, Scotland, baptized 29 April 1667; d. London, England, 27 February 1735), *medicine, literature.*

Arbuthnot, eldest son of the Reverend Alexander Arbuthnott, an Anglican clergyman, and Margaret Lammie (or Lamy) Arbuthnott, studied mathematics and natural philosophy at Marischal College, Aberdeen, and received a Masters in Arts in 1685. In 1691 he moved to London and taught mathematics. He became private tutor to Edward Jeffreys, son of a wealthy London merchant and MP, and accompanied him to Oxford from 1694 to 1696, where Arbuthnot studied medicine and made the acquaintance of many natural philosophers, writers, and politicians, including Newton and Pepys. Because Arbuthnot could not receive an MD degree from Oxford (they were granted only to Oxford MA candidates), he enrolled at the University of St Andrews on 11 September 1696 and defended seven theses on the same day, graduating MD.

Arbuthnot returned to London to pursue a medical career that prospered after the accession of Queen Anne to the throne in March 1702. Anne's husband, the prince of Denmark, fell ill at Epsom, and Arbuthnot, who happened to be nearby, successfully treated the prince. This led to Arbuthnot's employment at Court as physician to Prince George. On 30 October 1705 Arbuthnot was appointed Physician Extraordinary to Queen Anne. He became part of the permanent royal household in 1709, when he was appointed fourth Physician in Ordinary. In 1704 Arbuthnot was elected FRS, and on 16 April 1705, during the Queen's visit to Cambridge, Arbuthnot received an MD from that University. In December 1707, he became an honorary fellow of the RCP Edinburgh and, in 1710, was made a FRCP London. In 1713, he was appointed physician at Chelsea Hospital. After Queen Anne's death on 1 August 1714 and the fall of the Tories, Arbuthnot lost his Royal Appointment. He moved to Piccadilly, and maintained a busy private practice in London and in Bath.

Arbuthnot's earliest writings concerned mathematics and were published anonymously. These included *Of the Laws of Chance* (1692, primarily a translation of Christiaan Huygens' *De ratiociniis in ludo Aleae*); *An Essay on the Usefulness of Mathematical Learning* (1701); and 'An Argument for Divine Providence, taken from the Constant Regularity observed in the Births of both Sexes', published in the Royal Society's *Philosophical Transactions* (1710). In 1705, he published a work on ancient coins and measures, which he later revised and expanded in 1727.

Arbuthnot was widely known for his satirical writings, most famously for his John Bull pamphlets published in 1712, in which John Bull stood as a national symbol for England. He became close friends with Alexander Pope, John Gay, and Jonathan Swift, who along with others collectively published *The Memoirs of Martinus Scriblerus*, which satirized learning and pedantry. Arbuthnot also entered into several pamphlet disputes, contributing anonymous satirical works on geology and smallpox.

In 1727 Arbuthnot delivered the Harveian Lecture at the RCP London, where he traced the history of medicine from its early relation to superstition to the emergence of modern medicine in the seventeenth century, highlighting the work of William Harvey (1578–1657). Near the end of his life he published two medical works: *An Essay Concerning the Nature of Aliments* (1731), and *An Essay Concerning the Effects of Air on Human Bodies* (1733). In the first book, Arbuthnot discussed the influence of different foods, climate, and seasons on human health. A second edition contained practical advice on how to tailor diet to specific climates. In his final book, he drew on the contemporary scientific work of (among others) Herman Boerhaave (1668–1738), Robert Boyle (1627–91), and Stephen Hales (1677–1761) on the nature of air. Both books reflected the resurgence of Hippocratic ideas during the eighteenth century.

There are no clear records of Arbuthnot's marriage to Margaret Wemyss. They had ten children, four of whom (two sons and two daughters) survived to adulthood.

Bibliography

Primary: 1731. *An Essay Concerning the Nature of Aliments, and the Choice of Them, According to the different Constitutions of Human Bodies* (London) (2nd edn. 1732); 1733. *An Essay Concerning the Effects of Air on Human Bodies* (London).

Secondary: Steensma, Robert C., 1979. *Dr. John Arbuthnot* (Boston); Beattie, Lester M., 1935. *John Arbuthnot: Mathematician and Satirist* (Cambridge, MA); Aitken, George A., 1892. *The Life and Works of John Arbuthnot* (New York) (reissued, 1968); *DSB*; *Oxford DNB*.

Andrea Rusnock

ARCHAGATHUS   (fl. 219 BCE), *surgery.*

Archagathus, the 'first physician at Rome' according to the sole surviving ancient source, Pliny's *Natural History*, provides one of our few glimpses of medicine in early

Rome. Pliny's evidence comes from the lost *Annals* of Cassius Hemina (fr. 26P), written around 150 BCE. Following a comment that 'thousands of people live without doctors (*medici*)—although not without medicine (*medicina*)—just as the Roman people have done for over 600 years', Pliny described the Greek Archagathus as the son of Lysanias, from the Peloponnese. He came to Rome in the consulship of Lucius Aemilius and Marcus Livius, information that provides us with his date. We are told that Archagathus was given citizen rights, suggesting that he may have been invited by the state, and that public money was used to buy a shop at the crossroads of Acilius for his use. At first he was very popular, and was called 'Wound-Man' (*volnerarius*). Celsus and Caelius Aurelianus mention a wound-plaster allegedly used by a physician called Archagathus. However, this nickname was soon changed to 'Executioner' (*carnifex*) on account of his savage use of the knife and of cautery. Pliny ended by saying that he, and the medical profession more generally, then became the object of loathing. Elsewhere, Pliny associated Greek doctors with savage violence, as well as an undue interest in making money from their patients.

It is far from clear why a Greek physician should travel to the frontier town of Rome at this time, and it is possible that Archagathus arrived on the initiative of an influential Roman patron; both the consuls for the year, and the Acilii, were philhellenes. Whatever Pliny said, the appearance of Greek-style doctors in the plays of Plautus, contemporary with Archagathus, showed that the Roman public was already familiar with the sort of medicine Greeks practiced, but the shift in his nickname may be due to a basic misunderstanding between Greek doctor, and Roman patients, as to what sort of actions made for good medicine. Despite the eventual failure of Archagathus, and subsequent regular expulsions of Greek intellectuals, including physicians, Greek medicine continued to make inroads at Rome. At the same time a vigorously anti-Greek policy was maintained by some public figures, such as the elder Cato (234–149 BCE), who, according to Plutarch, kept his own family healthy by means of a notebook containing remedies. Here we see the tradition of the self-sufficient male head of household (Latin *paterfamilias*) by which nonfamily members were not encouraged to take part in health care.

In the history of medicine, the accident of survival of the story of Archagathus has been used to argue for a Roman past free of disease, and thus of doctors—for an idyllic period of household-based simplicity; for a golden age of self-help; and for an indigenous system of healing based on magic.

Bibliography

Primary: Pliny, *Natural History* 29.5.11–6.13; Plutarch, *Life of Cato*.

Secondary: Von Staden, Heinrich, 1996. 'Liminal Perils: Early Roman Receptions of Greek Medicine' in Ragep, F. J., and S. P. Ragep, eds., *Tradition, Transmission, Transformation* (Leiden) pp. 369–418; Nijhuis, Karen, 1995. 'Greek Doctors and Roman Patients' in van der Eijk, Philip J., H. F. J. Horstmanshoff, and P. I. Schrijvers, eds., *Ancient Medicine in Its Socio-cultural Context* 2 vols. (Amsterdam) pp. 49–67; Nutton, Vivian, 1993. 'Roman Medicine: Tradition, Confrontation, Assimilation.' *Aufstieg und Niedergang der Romanische Welt*, II, 31(2): 49–78; Nutton, Vivian, 1986. 'The Perils of Patriotism: Pliny and Roman Medicine' in French, R., and F. Greenaway, eds., *Science in the Early Roman Empire: Pliny the Elder, His Sources and Influence* (London) pp. 30–58.

Helen King

ARDERNE, JOHN (b. England, 1307/8; d. London, England, *c.* 1380), *surgery*.

The *Practica* of fistula in ano, Arderne's best-known work, begins: 'I, John Arderne, from the first pestilence, which was in the year of our Lord 1349, till the year 1370, lived at Newark, in the county of Nottingham'. Because the name 'Arderne' was extremely common in the fourteenth century, there is no reason to connect him to any of the other John Ardernes encountered in contemporary documents, or to link him to any particular family of Ardernes. He mentioned at four points in his works a Master W. de Hockesworth (otherwise unknown), qualifying him as the 'most noble of surgeons', who practiced in Wiltshire, and may have been Arderne's teacher. In this case Arderne himself may have spent time in Wiltshire before establishing his practice in Newark. He noted that his first patient to be surgically treated for fistula in ano was one Lord Adam of Everingham of Laxton-in-the-Clay near Tukesford. This would likely be the second Baron Everingham, who died in 1378–79 and lived not far from Newark. Lord Adam was on campaign in the entourage of Henry Earl of Derby, later Duke of Lancaster. After consulting unsuccessfully many surgeons at different towns in France, Lord Adam returned to his home in the expectation of imminent death, but Arderne cured him of fistula in ano, and Adam lived a healthy thirty years thereafter. This would seem to chronologically place the cure for fistula in ano before 1349, perhaps in the early 1340s. Arderne may already have been practicing surgery in Newark before the Black Death; he seems to have done his writing in London after 1370. In his *De cura oculorum* (British Library, Sloane MS 75, f.146), Arderne stated he was writing the work in London in the first year of Richard II, and in the seventieth year of his age.

If, as Arderne tells us, he only moved to London in 1370, it is surprising that a number of the case histories he describes evidently involve London patients—surprising because we might not expect Arderne still to be in surgical practice when he was past sixty years of age. The date of publication of the *Practica* of fistula in ano is deduced by Arderne's mention that it was written in the year of the death of the Black Prince, 1376; the *De cura oculi* was written in 1377. All of Arderne's writings, it appears, date to the

1370s, to a stage of his career when he would be expected to have retired from active surgery. The cases of a London fishmonger and other patients indicate continued practice. Arderne's death could not have long followed the writing of *De cura oculi.*

Arderne's *Practica* is exceptional among medieval surgical writings in a number of respects. It deals with a single operation (or two different operations that treat the same complaint), whereas most written surgeries dealt with numerous complaints from head to toe. Arderne listed his successful cures; described and illustrated the instruments he used; gave a step-by-step account of the operations; investigated complications of the operations and ailments related to or confused with fistula in ano; and prescribed the dressings, ointments, and other medicaments given to patients afterward. These are all unusual features in medieval surgical writings and show Arderne at his most original. The remainder of Arderne's writings, sometimes gathered together into a *Liber medicinarum*, are less original, and are often compiled from the writing of others, though spiced throughout with case histories of his own.

Bibliography

Primary: Power, D'Arcy, 1910. *Treatises of fistula in ano haemorrhoids and clysters,* Early English Text Society, O.S. 139 (London); Power, D'Arcy, 1914. 'The Lesser Writings of John Arderne', *XVIIth International Congress of Medicine, 1913,* Section XXIII History of Medicine (London) pp. 107–33.

Secondary: Jones, Peter Murray, 1994. 'John of Arderne and the Mediterranean Tradition of Scholastic Surgery' in Garcia-Ballester, L., R. French, J. Arrizabalaga, and A. Cunningham, eds., *Practical Medicine from Salerno to the Black Death* (Cambridge) pp. 289–321; Jones, Peter Murray, 1989. 'Four Middle English Translations of John of Arderne' in Minnis, A., ed., *Latin and Vernacular: Studies in Late Medieval Manuscripts* (Cambridge) pp. 61–89.

Peter Jones

ARETAEUS OF CAPPADOCIA (fl. ?50–100/150–200), *anatomy, medicine, nosology, pathology.*

Aretaeus of Cappadocia has usually been dated as Galen's near contemporary, although it is now the practice to place him about a century earlier. It is also possible that he flourished in the second half of the second century, if not even later. Galen did not mention Aretaeus by name; but it may have been policy not to call attention to a rival, especially if that person was his contemporary. There was no mention of Aretaeus in later writers such as Caelius Aurelianus and in the extant works of Oribasius, which may indicate either that the diffusion of Aretaeus's writings was limited or that these, and other, compilers felt his work had been superseded. Nothing of Aretaeus's

education is known, and whether he came from Cappadocia or practiced there is uncertain. Aretaeus has been labeled a Pneumatist because his theory of health and disease was based on *pneuma*, a special form of air. Health was the state of *eukrasia*, defined as the correct balance of pneuma and the four elements. An imbalance (*dyskrasia*) resulted in an ill or diseased state. To maintain health, it was essential that pneuma, which was carried in the blood vessels, move through the body and not be impeded or subject to variations in temperature (usually chilling) in any way.

Aretaeus's lost works include *On Fevers, On Diseases of Women, On Surgery,* and *On Drugs.* What has survived, written in Ionic Greek to deliberately invoke Aretaeus's place in the Hippocratic tradition (and, perhaps, if he was Galen's contemporary, to distinguish himself from Galen), are two treatises in eight books that comprised the most comprehensive classification and description of diseases extant in antiquity. These nosological masterworks consisted of four books collectively entitled *On Causes and Symptoms of Acute and Chronic Diseases,* and *On Therapy of Acute and Chronic Diseases,* also in four books. In these texts the earliest accurate description of migraine ('heterocrania') is found, describing its unilateral focus, periodicity, nausea, sweating, eye pain, and photophobia. Leprosy (Hansen's disease) was graphically depicted, and gastrointestinal diseases discussed, including accounts of celiac disease ('celiac diathesis'), cholera, and ileus.

The accuracy of some of the descriptions of diseases given by Aretaeus suggests that a form of pathological examination took place, either by Aretaeus himself (as was the opinion of Morgagni) or by another, unknown source. A profound knowledge of anatomy was displayed concerning the lungs, pleura, heart, aorta, liver, vena cava, kidneys, urinary tract, and bladder (that of the uterus, with its alleged wanderings throughout the abdomen, seems a throwback to Hippocratic notions). His account of spinal cord paralysis not only exhibited a high degree of anatomical knowledge, but also showcased his skills as a clinician. Aretaeus's nosological ability was perfectly encapsulated in his account of asthma, noting the terrible effects of an acute attack and how it was also called *orthopnea* because the patient gains relief only by sitting upright. Aretaeus also gave an outstandingly detailed account of the clinical picture of diabetes, describing with great accuracy the polyuria and polydipsia that are the hallmarks of this disease. Aretaeus noted that it derived its name from the Greek for siphon, since fluid did not remain in the body, and that the flesh seemed to pass out with the urine, for he noted the emaciation encountered in the progression of the disease.

Although cited in the Byzantine tradition, Aretaeus's work was not rediscovered in the West until 1552. His writings were still being used in the eighteenth and nineteenth centuries. Francis Adams's 1856 translation is the most recent in English.

Bibliography

Primary: Adams, Francis, 1856. *The Extant Works of Aretaeus, the Cappadocian* (London) [reprinted 1978, Boston]; Hude, Carl, 1958. *Aretaeus.* Corpus Medicorum Graecorum II (Berlin).

Secondary: Weber, Giorgio, 1996. *Areteo di Cappadocia: Interpretazioni e aspetti della formazione anatomo-patologica del Morgagni* (Florence); Oberhelman, Steven, 1994. 'Aretaeus of Cappadocia—the Pneumatic Physician of the First Century AD.' *Aufstieg und Niedergang der Römischen Welt*, II, 37.2, 941–966; *DSB*.

Julius Rocca

ARGYLE, STANLEY SEYMOUR   (b. Kyneton, Victoria, Australia, 4 December 1867; d. Melbourne, Victoria, Australia, 23 November 1940), *radiology, hospital administration.*

Stanley Argyle, the son of Mary Clark and wealthy pastoralist Edward Argyle, received his medical education at the University of Melbourne, graduating MB (1890) and ChB (1891). He moved to London and studied bacteriology at King's College. The financial crash of the early 1890s destroyed the family fortune and Argyle returned to Melbourne, setting up in general practice in the affluent suburb of Kew. Argyle threw himself into the campaign for improvements in the milk supply, and launched his own proprietary milk company with some commercial success. To break the routine of general practice, Argyle indulged his aptitude for electrical machinery. Although it started out as backyard tinkering, radiology soon became a serious part of Argyle's medical practice. In 1908 he was appointed Medical Electrician and Skiagraphist at Melbourne's Alfred Hospital. He experimented with the use of electrical currents to treat rheumatism and radium to treat skin diseases.

When World War I broke out, Argyle joined the Australian Imperial Force as skiagrapher at the 1st Australian General Hospital in Cairo. He clashed bitterly with Lt. Col. James Barrett, in civilian life a professor of medicine at the University of Melbourne. This conflict over the control of radiology caused a great scandal, but Argyle was vindicated and went on to command Australian radiology units on the Greek island of Lemnos and in France.

The feud sparked a career change. In 1920 Argyle successfully challenged Barrett (now Sir James) for the safe district seat of Toorak in Victoria's Legislative Assembly. From 1923 to 1929 he served as Minister for Health and as chief secretary in conservative state governments. He played a role in crushing the 1923 police strike. Argyle continued his medical practice while meeting the demands of ministerial rank. He was appointed Director of Radiology at the Alfred Hospital (1924–29); the hospital benefited from the ministerial connection. He remained active in the Victorian branch of the British Medical Association, serving as president in 1925.

Argyle's achievement as a policymaker lay in reforms to the public hospital system. Based on the British charitable model, with strict means testing, Melbourne's public hospitals were facing financial crisis while the middle classes demanded access to their equipment and expertise. Argyle arranged increased subsidies while successfully blocking greater government control: 'I dread to think . . . of the day when hospitals will become Government institutions subject to Government control'. In 1926 he invited Malcolm MacEachern from the American College of Surgeons to report on the future of the hospital system. MacEachern advised a shift to the American model of fee-paying community hospitals. This message was reinforced when Argyle visited the United States in 1927 as the guest of the Rockefeller Foundation and was smitten with the American vision of private and intermediate fee-paying hospitals.

Argyle's ambitious plans for hospital rebuilding were destroyed by the Great Depression and new bouts of political instability. He returned to office as state premier (1932) and gave steady but unimaginative leadership as Victoria emerged from the Depression. Conflicts between metropolitan and rural interests brought down his government in 1935. Argyle's lasting achievement was that Melbourne's teaching hospitals led a slow move from British to American models of hospital administration—a major cultural shift in a society that still defined itself by the British connection.

Argyle remained leader of the Opposition in Victoria's state parliament until his death from emphysema in 1940. He was knighted in 1930.

Bibliography

Secondary: Ryan, J., K. Sutton, and M. Baigent, 1996. *Australasian Radiology: A History* (Sydney); Mitchell, Ann, 1977. *The Hospital South of the Yarra: A History of the Alfred Hospital* (Melbourne); *AuDB*.

James Gillespie

ARIAS DE BENAVIDES, PEDRO   (b. Toro, Zamora, Spain, 1505; d. Toro, Zamora, ?), *surgery.*

Little is known of Pedro Arias de Benavides, although his 1567 book, *Secretos de chirurgia*, was the first to examine Mexican medicine and was ahead of its time in regard to topics of surgery. There is no evidence that he graduated from medical school as a physician, but what we do know suggests he was a well-trained surgeon. Arias de Benavides was an academic and can be considered emblematic of the development of Spanish surgery in the sixteenth century. From 1545 to 1550—the period of early colonization—he traveled to America with a Spanish colonial authority; the *oidor* Alonso de Zurita. The reason for his journey is unknown, and he did not participate in campaigns of the conquest. He was a man of the times, aware of the great changes of the Renaissance that had awoken the curiosity of humankind with respect to the unknown. His desire for new experiences, knowledge, and professional perspectives may have motivated Arias de

Benavides to travel to the New World—to lands that represented danger and privation.

His book contains the only references to his personal life, which are retold entertainingly and with passion and naturalism. He landed in what is now Honduras with seventy-seven other passengers, some seventy of whom died, apparently from dysentery. He practiced medicine in Guatemala for four years before continuing on to Mexico. According to his writings, he directed the *Hospital del Amor de Díos* for syphilitics, where for eight years he led the institution that cured syphilis, the so-called *morbo gálico.*

It is believed he returned to Spain in 1564, again with Zurita; settled in his hometown; and began to prepare *Secretos de chirurgia.* He lived prosperously until his death in Toro, Spain, on an unknown date.

His motivation for writing was to publicize the therapeutic properties of the plants, roots, and fruits of the Americas that were unknown in Europe, and to transmit the secrets of surgery that the ancients could not have known. He respected the classics, but felt they were not everything. These two facets well represent the main interests of the period: fascination with the novel paired with the questioning of tradition.

Secretos de chirurgia approached the medical knowledge of two cultures with intelligence, a clear sign that the writer did not follow orthodox medicine, although he did apply the theory of humors. He was practical: Arias de Benavides did not attempt to justify theoretically that which functioned, and never disdained autochthonous practices.

He described the geography of new places; the attitudes, customs, and physical appearance of the people, both indigenous and Spanish; food; and diverse diseases. He narrated specific cases in an agreeable way and established the use of mercury to treat syphilis.

His work reveals clearly that Arias de Benavides acted with common sense, improvising in unexpected situations and putting experience before the judgments of authority. Surgery in the New World was complex, having to deal with local medicine in the face of shortages of European books and other materials. Indigenous and Spanish realities were intertwined in some respects but were contradictory in others; for example, the indigenous depended upon observation and empiricism, whereas the Spanish were more concerned with tradition and academic knowledge.

Secretos de chirurgia examines many American plants and their therapeutic use, devotes several chapters to syphilis, and deals with a variety of diseases that required surgical treatment.

Bibliography

Primary: 1567. *Secretos de chirurgia* (Valladolid, Spain).

Secondary: Fresquet Febrer, José Luis, 1993. *La experiencia americana y la terapéutica en los Secretos de chirurgia (1567) de Pedro Arias de Benavides* (Valencia, Spain); Somolinos Palencia, Juan, 1992. *Secretos de chirurgia.* Academia Nacional de Medicina (Mexico); Martínez, M., 1987. *Catálogo de nombres vulgares y científicos de plantas mexicanas* (Mexico).

Ana Cecilia Rodríguez de Romo

ARISTOTLE (b. Stagira, Thrace (now in Khalkidhikí, Greece), 384 BCE; d. Chalcis, Euboea (now Khalkís, Greece), 322 BCE), *ethics, medicine, philosophy, science.*

One of the greatest and most influential thinkers the world has ever produced, Aristotle was born in Stagira (Stagirus), a town situated on the Macedonian peninsula of Chalcidice in Thrace. According to one traditional account, his birthplace was destroyed by Philip II of Macedon, the father of Alexander the Great. At Aristotle's urging, either Philip (or Alexander) rebuilt it. Aristotle's connection with the Macedonian court had been established by his father Nicomachus, personal physician to King Amyntas II, grandfather of Alexander the Great. The position may have been hereditary; in any case, Nicomachus was an Asclepiad, and, together with Aristotle's mother, Phaestis, claimed descent from Asclepius himself. Aristotle was about ten years old when his parents died, and any hopes of their son's following the family tradition probably died with them. Nevertheless, the medical background in Aristotle's upbringing was clearly influential, and goes some way to explaining Aristotle's keen interest in natural phenomena of all kinds, as well as the use of medical analogies throughout his philosophical works. Aristotle's guardian, Proxenus, continued his education, and at the age of seventeen Aristotle arrived in Athens to complete it by becoming a student of Plato's Academy. Aristotle's first contact was not with Plato but with his younger colleague Eudoxus, as Plato was in Sicily vainly trying to make its king, Dionysius, into a philosopher-ruler. Aristotle would remain at the Academy for almost twenty years. Plato clearly influenced Aristotle in a variety of ways, but it seems that the transcendental nature of the Theory of Forms struck Aristotle as inimical to a study of the natural world, one to which he had been exposed at an early age. But the fact that Aristotle remained there, first as a student and then as a teacher, shows that there was never any open breach with Plato, and Aristotle's own early works were in the form of Platonic dialogues.

After Plato's death (347 BCE), Aristotle left Athens. He may have resented the fact that Speusippus, not himself, was Plato's successor. However, as a Macedonian, Aristotle was a *metic*, or resident alien, and doubtless aware of living in a city where ill feeling against the predatory nature of Philip of Macedon was already being expressed, not least by the Athenian orator Demosthenes. Aristotle, in company with Xenocrates (who would succeed Speusippus as head of the Academy), left for Assos in Asia Minor, taking up an offer from Hermias, ruler of Atarneus, capital of a small Anatolian kingdom, and who might have been a fellow pupil of the Academy. Hermias certainly visited the

Academy, but he never met Plato, even though he was the recipient of Plato's sixth letter. Aristotle, in company with Xenocrates and the Platonists Erastus and Coriscus, formed a philosophical community at Assos, and Aristotle stayed there for almost three years, during which time he married Pythias, adopted daughter (or niece) of Hermias. (After Pythias's death, Aristotle lived with Herpyllis, a slave woman, by whom he had a son, Nicomachus. Aristotle freed her in his will.) The marriage to Pythias formed a background to a deep friendship that developed between Aristotle and Hermias, and after the death of Hermias at the hands of the Persians in 341 BCE, Aristotle wrote a moving encomium, in the style of a hymn to Virtue (*Arete*), the only example of his early output to have survived. It is no accident that, in his later ethical works, Aristotle examined friendship in detail and pronounced it indispensable to the 'good life'. It was at Assos that Aristotle began his biological investigations, and these were continued in Mytilene, on the island of Lesbos (345–43 BCE). There, Aristotle worked with his younger colleague Theophrastus, and a great deal of their biological work undoubtedly took place in the town of Pyrrha, which boasted a large landlocked lagoon, the chief feature of Lesbos.

In 343 BCE Aristotle was invited to Pella by Philip of Macedon, where he became tutor to Philip's son, Alexander, for the next three years. Aristotle likely viewed this as an opportunity to mold a future philosopher-ruler, and it seemed that he and his colleagues had exercised a beneficial effect on Hermias. Aristotle can hardly be censured for his failure with Alexander, and there is evidence in his writings of his criticism of the concept of absolute rule. There is also the fact that Alexander put to death Aristotle's nephew, Callisthenes, allegedly for conspiracy; this can only have confirmed Aristotle in his judgment. Alexander had appointed Antipater, with whom Aristotle was on friendly terms, to be regent of Greece, and in 335 BCE Aristotle returned to Athens. His colleague Xenocrates was now head of the Academy, but Aristotle set up his own school, outside the city in an area called the Lyceum. The school later became known as the *Peripatos*, because of a public walk there, and Aristotle's later followers were called Peripatetics. Aristotle's school functioned as a place where lectures were given, and as a sort of institute of advanced study, where research in the natural sciences and politics was carried out. The school enjoyed a large library, which may have been the model for subsequent ones in antiquity. In 323 BCE, following the death of Alexander, Aristotle, allegedly fearing for his life, left Athens, famously stating that he did not wish the city that had put Socrates to death to sin twice against philosophy. More prosaically, his status as a Macedonian in a city now free of Alexander's yoke meant that his continued residence was untenable. He fled to Chalcis, where he died the following year of a gastric complaint, possibly carcinoma of the stomach or perhaps complications of cholecystitis.

Aristotle's output was prodigious, including works on ethics, politics, logic, metaphysics, rhetoric and poetry, the

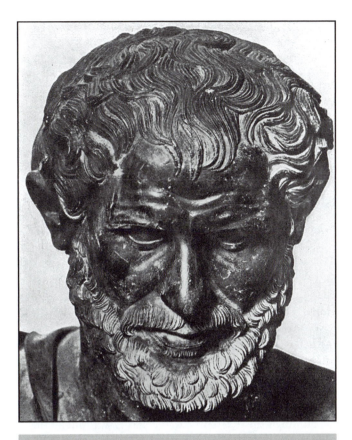

Bust of Aristotle from Herculaneum. Half-tone reproduction from R. W. Livingstone, *The Legacy of Greece*, Oxford, 1923. Wellcome Library, London.

natural sciences, and medicine. Unfortunately, virtually all his works have been lost, and what survives is a series of what have been described as sets of lecture notes, together with memoranda on various subjects. Aristotle's biological works revealed for the first time in antiquity a clearly defined and systematic approach to the subject, as well as the recognition that such a subject was worthy of investigation. In his remarks on dissection of animals, Aristotle noted that it was unpleasant, but it allowed us to know nature's purpose. As a result of his researches, Aristotle maintained that the heart was at the center of the body and that all blood vessels arose from it. Sensation was dependent on a system of blood vessels, and since they arose from the heart, then that organ must be the site of the common sensorium of the body. Although Aristotle never explicitly stated that the heart was a hegemonic or ruling organ of the body, the inference was clearly there, and would be taken up by his immediate successors and in the centuries to come. Even Galen, whose own detailed researches determined that the brain was the central organ of the body, could not entirely overcome this Aristotelian legacy.

Aristotle's works on ethics have also been influential, if at times controversial, but they remain the starting point for any inquiry in this field. Happiness, as the Greek *eudaimonia* was traditionally rendered, was the supreme and ultimate good for human life. It was happiness for the individual, not the group, and it did not lie in seeking pleasure but was an 'activity of the soul in accordance with virtue'. Virtue (or excellence) was acquired by possession of *phronesis*, practical wisdom, and the pursuit of a virtue, such as justice and courage, engendered *phronesis*. An intelligent person would thus seek the eudaimonistic life because this offered the best possibility of flourishing fully as an individual who performed, and wished to perform, the right actions in an excellent way. This is not to say that Aristotelian ethics was unproblematic, for, in order to function properly, such an ethical system had to be set in a good society (something that Aristotle also addressed). Further, it held a perhaps overly optimistic and rational view of human action. Nevertheless, the attraction of Aristotelian virtue-based ethics, which dealt with the person as an individual (and Aristotle used the model of a doctor whose concern lay not so much with the theoretical edifice of medicine but with the needs of a particular patient), lay in offering a set of alternative arguments to utilitarian or rules-based medical ethics, which irreducibly tended to universal rules and judgments.

Medieval scholarship was heavily dependent on Aristotle, although the deferential way his work was often taught unfairly tarnished his reputation. However, such dependency was not entirely unjustified. When Dante referred to him as the 'Master of those who know', it was with good reason. Aristotle succeeded in asking intelligent questions that are still as worthy of consideration as when they were first posed.

Bibliography

Primary: 1831. (ed., Bekker, Immanuel) *Aristotelis Opera*, 5 vols. (Berlin); 1984. (ed., Barnes, Jonathan) *The Complete Works of Aristotle. The Revised Oxford Translation* 2 vols. (Princeton).

Secondary: Gotthelf, Allan, 1985. *Aristotle on Nature and Living Things* (Pittsburgh and Bristol); Lloyd, Geoffrey, 1968. *Aristotle, the Growth and Structure of His Thought* (Cambridge); Durling, Ingemar, 1957. *Aristotle in the Ancient Biographical Tradition* (Göteborg); *DSB*.

Julius Rocca

ARMSTRONG, GEORGE (b. Castleton, Liddesdale, Roxburghshire, Scotland, *c.* 1719–20; d. London, England, 21 January 1789), *pediatrics*.

Son of the local Presbyterian minister and brother of the physician-poet John Armstrong (1708–1779), Armstrong studied anatomy under Alexander Monro in Edinburgh. Later he followed his brother to London and assisted him in his practice. He was married in 1755 to Ann Rawlins or Rawlings, and they moved to Haverstock Hill, Hampstead, where he practiced as a surgeon/apothecary, despite not

having a legal right to practice in London. Armstrong's brother had published anonymously the first anthology of diseases in children in 1742, entitled *A Full View of All the Diseases Incident to Children*. George followed John's example by publishing in 1767 *An Essay on the Diseases most fatal to Infants to which is added Rules to be observed in the Nursing of Children, with a particular View to those who are brought up by Hand*. He dedicated this book to the distinguished physician and fellow Scot, Sir John Pringle. Three further editions (1771, 1777, 1783) appeared, with a posthumous edition edited by Alexander Buchan in 1808.

Armstrong's interest in artificial feeding of infants resulted from the successful rearing of his baby daughter largely using cow's milk. When his wife had insufficient breast milk, he eschewed wet nursing. He wrote, 'There are two ways of feeding children who are bred up by the hand: the one is by means of a horn, and the other is with a boat or spoon. They both have their advocates but the latter in my humble opinion is preferable'. He then described his wife's experience, there being 'danger into falling into watery gripes as was the case with two of mine which were fed for some time in this way. . . . The horn having succeeded so ill, I made no further trial of it, and the last child was fed with the boat.'

Armstrong's greatest contribution to the care of sick children was his establishment of a dispensary for the infant poor on 24 April 1769, in the home of his fellow Scot, the physician John Monro, at 7 Red Lion Square, Holborn, London. This was the first outpatient clinic in the world specifically for children. Clearly there was a great need; it is recorded that between April 1769 and December 1781, nearly 35,000 children were treated. Some children up to the age of '10 or 12 years' were seen, as well as infants.

The creation of dispensaries for infants and children led the way to the establishment of the first hospitals for children in the nineteenth century. G. F. Still, in his *History of Paediatrics*, saw the opening of Armstrong's dispensary as 'the most important step ever taken in this country towards the care of sick children'. Still credited the dispensary as 'the beginning of a great movement which was to lift the study of diseases of children on to a different plain by the accumulation of special experience which could not be obtained in another way'.

However, Armstrong himself argued powerfully against hospital admission for children. He wrote the following in his pamphlet of 1772: 'Several Friends to the Charity have thought it necessary to have a House fitted up for the Reception of such Infants as are very ill, where they might be accommodated in the same Manner as Adults are in other Hospitals. But a very little Refection will convince any thinking Person that such a scheme can never be executed. If you take away a sick Child from its Parent or Nurse you break its heart immediately: and if there must be a Nurse to each Child what kind of an Hospital must there be to contain any Number of them? Besides, as in this case the Wards must be crowded with grown persons as well as with Children must not the Air of the Hospital be thereby much contaminated?' These were powerful arguments against hospital admission for children; nevertheless, Armstrong's dispensary for children is seen as a progenitor of children's hospitals.

His dispensary later moved to other addresses in London yet sadly did not survive Armstrong's death in 1789.

Although his brother who died in 1779, had left him a substantial bequest, Armstrong's last years were plagued by financial problems, borrowing money and incurring debts that could not be repaid. He died in obscurity.

Armstrong's reputation suffered eclipse in the nineteenth century, only to be rediscovered in the twentieth century. W. J. Maloney did much to revive his reputation in his book about the Armstrong brothers. He regarded George Armstrong as the father of modern pediatrics, but he also saw him as 'the medical pioneer of social welfare for children'. He stated that, with publication of Armstrong's book in 1767, 'authority began to yield to observation, conjecture give way to facts, the study of disease in children to be extended from the living to the dead, and paediatrics to take on the form of a science which he rapidly developed in subsequent editions'.

Bibliography

Primary: 1767. *An Essay on the Diseases Most Fatal to Infants to Which Are Added Rules to Be Observed in the Nursing of Children: With a Particular View to Those Who Are Brought up by Hand* (London); 1769. *Proposals for Administering Advice and Medicines to the Children of the Poor* (London); 1772. *A General Account of the Dispensary for the Relief of the Infant Poor* (London).

Secondary: Maloney, W. J., 1931. *George and John Armstrong of Castleton, Two Eighteenth-century Medical Pioneers* (Edinburgh); Still, G. F., 1931. *The History of Paediatrics* (London) [Reprinted, 1965]; *Oxford DNB*.

John Walker-Smith

ARMSTRONG, WILLIAM GEORGE (b. Essex, England, 29 May 1859; d. Vaucluse, Australia, 27 December 1941), *public health, infant welfare.*

Armstrong, eldest son of Eliza Susannah Mallet of Jersey and Lt. Richard Ramsay Armstrong, RN, started his education at King's School, Canterbury. He later moved to New Zealand with his mother, after which the family settled in New South Wales where young Armstrong completed his schooling. He worked as a journalist and later a schoolteacher while completing a BA at the University of Sydney. He enrolled in medicine, graduating MB ChM with honors in 1888. By accident of nominative determinism, Armstrong became the first graduate of the Sydney medical school.

For the next six years Armstrong practiced medicine in several small rural towns, where he became interested in public health. With no opportunities for postgraduate medical study in Australia, he returned to England to complete the Diploma in Public Health at Cambridge. The practical experience he gained in the slums of London's Whitechapel stimulated his interest in the relationship between disease and the environment, and led him to become a Fellow of the (Royal) Sanitary Institute, London.

During his time overseas, Armstrong visited the Charité Hospital in Paris to study Pierre Budin's work on infant nourishment. This demonstrated to him the importance of teaching mothers about the feeding and care of their children. His future career was set by these experiences in London and Paris.

Returning to Sydney in 1898, Armstrong was appointed Medical Officer of Health for metropolitan Sydney. He became city health officer in 1900, just as an epidemic of bubonic plague hit Sydney. He worked closely with the preeminent Australian epidemiologist J. Ashburton Thompson in preventing the spread of plague through systematic eradication of rats. Armstrong's experience in managing epidemics proved valuable during subsequent outbreaks of smallpox and the 1919–20 influenza pandemic, to which he contributed noteworthy insight.

Armstrong was distressed by the high mortality due to enteric diseases among infants in the working-class inner suburbs of Sydney; he argued that close to half of these deaths resulted from inappropriate feeding. He campaigned vigorously for breast-feeding in place of the then-fashionable feeding of prepared baby foods. To make mothers aware of the benefits of breast-feeding, in 1904 he convinced the city council to appoint health visitors—qualified nurses who would visit every new mother within days of childbirth to advise on baby care, feeding, and domestic hygiene. Mortality rates dropped immediately. This initiative led to the formation in 1914 of the first Baby Health Center. By 1918 there were twenty-eight of these so-called baby clinics throughout New South Wales, and soon they could be found in every suburb and country town.

Armstrong's early experience as journalist and schoolteacher served him well in his subsequent medical career. He was a good communicator, able to convey his knowledge and enthusiasm to others. He lectured in public health at the University of Sydney concurrently with serving in his other official positions, becoming one of the first medical graduates to be offered a teaching position at his old university. One of his passions was to raise the standards of health inspectors employed in local government. Few had any formal training, so Armstrong organized lectures in his own home to give the inspectors a basic understanding of environmental health principles.

Armstrong had been appointed Deputy Director-General of Public Health in 1913. Nearing retirement age, he was promoted to Director-General of Public Health and President of the New South Wales Board of Health in 1922. After leaving the Department of Public Health three years later, he retained his membership on the New South Wales Board. He then began a new, and final, career as medical superintendent for a major retail store, which occupied him until 1935.

Bibliography

Primary: 1939. 'The Infant Welfare Movement in Australia' *Medical Journal of Australia* 2: 641–648.

Secondary: 1942. 'Obituary.' *Medical Journal of Australia* 28 February 1942, 272–274; *AuDB.*

Peter J. Tyler

ARNALD OF VILANOVA   (b. Crown of Aragon, Spain, *c.* 1240; d. at sea off Genoa, Italy, 1311), *medicine, Latin Galenism.*

By 1300 medicine had become one of the four branches of institutional knowledge taught and learned at the European *Studia*—and a successful one. University medicine's main representatives became rich and famous, and various strategies were developed to secure for them control over a particular way of understanding health and disease. In addition, a new professional was needed to convince the powerful and the general public of the individual and social usefulness of university medicine, and of the need for university-trained physicians to be granted a monopoly over the healing market. In the attempt to define a space of its own at a theoretical level, university medicine needed to detach itself from natural philosophy. In a professional arena it needed to distinguish its promise from that of non–university-trained healers.

In order to achieve these aims, it was necessary for medicine to create, through the selection and adaptation of Greek and Arabic medical works, a theoretical corpus of its own, and to incorporate a specific method—one characteristic of scholasticism. As a scholastic enterprise, medicine would be grounded in the twin pillars that sustained scholastic knowledge: the authority of the ancients and a logical apparatus based on Aristotelian principles. This would allow university-trained physicians to use the same language as theologians and philosophers when referring to nature and humankind, together with a logic that would provide a sound explanation for the ailments of their potential patients. But because medicine was also a very practical business, the recourse to experience was not left behind, albeit supported by this highly sophisticated scaffolding.

Three main centers and several of their masters were pivotal in developing medicine along these lines: Arnald of Vilanova and Bernard of Gordon at Montpellier, France; John of Saint-Amand at Paris; and Taddeo Alderotti and his pupils at Bologna, Italy. The figure and work of Arnald of Vilanova must be understood within the context of this collective picture. However, a long tradition that started during his lifetime has adorned Arnald with more striking

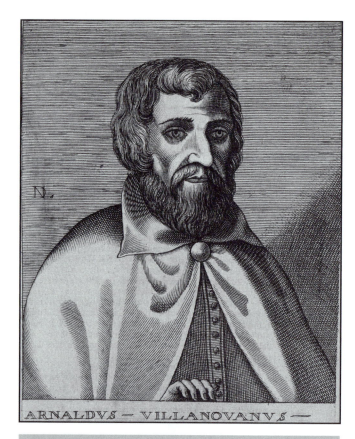

Arnald of Vilanova. Line engraving by Nicolas de Larmessin, 1682. Iconographic Collection, Wellcome Library, London.

features than his colleagues, creating the historical figure of a legendary outcast. From the second half of the twentieth century, historiography has been keen to separate the genuine from the Arnaldian myths and their uses.

Life

Arnald of Vilanova's early biography is full of uncertainties. It is commonly agreed that he was born around 1240, but the place of his birth is not known. His origin was the Crown of Aragon, but it is debated exactly where, and the notion of a Provencal birth seems now discarded. His family background is no easier to ascertain because we lack documentary evidence; a Jewish origin is no more than a conjectural hypothesis. Some have pointed out an early familial setting at Valencia soon after its conquest in 1238; in fact, as a child, Arnald was tonsured in this city. By the 1260s, Arnald was studying medicine at Montpellier, where he earned his degree. He married Agnès Blasi and established himself in Valencia. In 1281 Arnald moved to Barcelona to serve King Pere III as his personal physician. Despite this move and his many later travels, Arnald and his family retained strong personal and economic links to Valencia throughout their lives. On Pere's death in 1285, Arnald continued as royal physician to the king's sons: first to Alfons II and, after the death of Alfons in 1290, to his brother and successor Jaume II, and finally to the youngest brother, Frederic III, who became King of Sicily in 1296. As was the case with many of his colleagues at the royal courts, Arnald's close relationship with the monarchs meant his involvement went beyond matters strictly medical. A personal friend of the monarchs, he served them informally as a political and spiritual advisor, and more formally as representative of the Crown in diplomatic negotiations. His life was not limited to royal duties. From 1289 onward, he was attached to the medical school at Montpellier, where he continued his career as a teacher and author of medical works. The value of his presence at the *Studium* was recognized in 1309 by the papal bull that regulated its medical syllabus. In Montpellier, the flourishing of Arnald's medical production paralleled his growing interest in spiritual matters in line with the reformist views of certain Franciscan groups, although his acquaintance with the Joachimite Peter John Olivi is uncertain. By 1300 he had already completed a number of religious works of a didactic nature, biblical exegeses, anti-Jewish apologetics, and prophetic and reform writings. One of these works—his eschatological treatise, *De tempore adventus Antichristi* [Concerning the time of the arrival of Christ], in which he prophesied the end of the world and the need for a rigorous reform of the Church—would soon cause him serious difficulties. In July 1300 Arnald was sent to Paris by Jaume II on a diplomatic mission to King Philip IV of France. There he took the opportunity to expose the religious thesis contained in this treatise to the Paris theologians. He and his views were condemned. Thereafter, he did not continue to occupy his chair at the medical school, devoting the bulk of his energies instead to diffusing his eschatological views and to defending himself in various conflicts against elements within the Church. These new interests and problems did not require Arnald to curtail his medical activities, however, and he continued his service as physician to the Aragonese royal family and the papal court, first to Pope Boniface VIII and later to his successor, Benedict XI. Arnald's healing abilities must have been rated very highly by the popes because, despite their disagreement with Arnald's spiritual propaganda, both helped him in the conflicts thrown up by his religious views. After Benedict's death in 1304, Clement V was elected as his successor. The new pope was a longtime friend of Arnald and more sympathetic to his ideas than his predecessors had been: 1305 marked the beginning of a period of relative calm in Arnald's life. Enjoying papal patronage and the patronage of the kings of Aragon and Sicily, Arnald envisaged the possibility of realizing his proposals for the social and religious reform of Christendom. The ideals of poverty and charity, and the need to preach evangelical truth to the poor, led Arnald during these years to write a number of religious works in the vernacular that reflected and reinforced the ideals and practices of various groups of lay spirituals. Some of these works were addressed specifically to the Beguin communities (*Informatio beguinorum seu lectio narbone* [Letter to the Beguins] and *Alia informatio beguinorum* [Further letter to the Beguins]). However, the patronage of the King of Aragon that had been so important to Arnald, providing protection and a means for achieving his goals, was soon to be withdrawn. In 1309 the disclosure and prophetic interpretation of the dreams of monarchs Jaume and Frederic to the papal curia in Avignon caused a serious problem for Arnald when the King of Aragon, knowing about Arnald's intervention, asked him to draw up a detailed report of what was said. What the king received from Arnald was an abridged and heavily censored version of the affair written in Catalan and known as the *Raonament d'Avinyó* [The argument of Avignon]. When the king learned the real content of what had been communicated by Arnald to the pope, he was able to discover the scope of Arnald's indiscretion and his actual fraud. Consequently, he broke with Arnald and advised his brother, the King of Sicily, to do the same. Despite this recommendation, Arnald retained the support of the younger brother, Frederic, who was the recipient in 1310 of the *Informaciò espiritual per al rey Frederic* [Spiritual address to King Frederic], in which Arnald set out guidelines on how to be the perfect Christian king. While traveling by sea in the service of this monarch, Arnald died off the coast of Genoa in 1311.

Work and Aftermath

Despite his religious interests and their public impact, Arnald was regarded by his contemporaries first and foremost as a physician. And it was as a physician that he was able to build his influential connections at the royal and papal courts. About his actual healing activities there is not much information, although his success and his patrons' appreciation of his application of the art are well documented. Well-known, for example, is the satisfaction expressed by Pope Boniface VIII when, following Arnald's recommendations, he was freed from the pain caused by a bladder stone by use of an astrological seal. The trust shown by King Jaume II in Arnald's technical abilities and in his medical advice for the maintenance of his and his family's health is documented on various occasions. The king's wearisome insistence on receiving from Arnald a promised work for the maintenance of his health (*pro conservatione salutis nostra*), which Arnald was not ready to deliver, signals the same kind of appreciation. A very positive evaluation about Arnald's medical advice would also explain the use of the threat of excommunication launched by Pope Clement V in 1312 for those who kept out of his reach the practical treatise (*practica medica*) that, according to the pope, Arnald had written for him and which could not be found after Arnald's death.

In fact, some of Arnald's writing was an answer to the demands, intellectual and practical, of his illustrious clientele.

The detailed regimen of health (*Regimen sanitatis ad regem aragonum*) composed *c.* 1305–1308 for King Jaume II is a good example of the necessary adaptation of general medical principles to the actual needs of a particular client. Even more attention to circumstantial events can be seen in the composition of another regimen of health (*Regimen Almarie*) for the same king. Composed to tame the king's anger about the *Avinyó* affair, it was addressed specifically to the circumstances imposed by war on the health of men and animals during the siege of Almería. Other practical treatises in the popular form of *consilia* were composed for anonymous patients or with a wider audience in mind, such as a regimen on gout (*Regimen de podagra*)—this is the only *consilium* of those attributed to Arnald that can be said with certainty to be Arnaldian.

More knowledge of Arnald's medical thought than of his actual practice can be obtained from the wide number of medical writings he produced that are in manuscript form or in sixteenth-century printed editions (Lyons, 1504, 1509, 1520, 1532; Venice, 1505, 1527; Basel, 1585).

Unfortunately, there is no list of his medical works equivalent to that of his spiritual writings prepared in 1305 by Arnald himself. Nor can many references be found in Arnald's medical writings about their dates and places of composition that would help to establish a genuine Arnaldian corpus and an accurate chronology. Manuscript tradition, cross-references, theoretical consistency, data from archival material, and the inventory of his possessions made after his death are the main tools that allow us to draw Arnald's professional profile. From the early 1280s to the date of his death, Arnald touched upon almost all medical genres and subjects: commentaries on medical authorities; monographs on particular diseases in the form of *consilia*, or epistles; aphorisms; medical compendia; and pharmacological treatises.

He made translations as well. Arnald confessed that he knew no Greek, but he mastered Arabic. Probably from Barcelona and in the early 1280s he translated from Arabic into Latin several medical treatises: Avicenna's (Ibn Sīnā,) *On the powers of the heart*, Galen's *On rigor*, and a pharmacological work by Abū-Ṣalt, *On simple medicines*.

No doubt Arnald's main written production must be related to his position as master at the Montpellier medical school. There is no accurate date for either the start or the end of his teaching activities at this *Studium*. García Ballester has proposed the earliest date of 1288 as the beginning of Arnald's involvement at Montpellier, Paniagua preferred 1289, and McVaugh has postponed it to 1291 or 1292.

There is agreement in considering 1301 as the end of a prolific period of production of medical works that would reflect the profile of Arnald's teaching activities and his involvement in the renovation of the medical syllabus. McVaugh has defended a second period of work at Montpellier between 1305 and 1308 and, following archival evi-

dence, he has placed the composition of Arnald's last complete work, the *Speculum medicine* [Mirror of medicine] in these years. For others, this second period could barely be termed as such because it was more a collection of discontinuous moments in which Arnald's attachment to the *Studium* is not clear. For this reason, they argue that the *Speculum*, an ambitious medical compendium that was composed as an introduction to the principles of medicine following the scheme of Johannitius's *Isagoge*, showed an unhurried style and maturity of thought that pointed to a period of more stability in Arnald's dedication to medical matters: they have suggested 1301 as the likely date of composition. Because the *Speculum*, according to Arnald, was composed as a theoretical part of medicine, it has been assumed that the unfinished *De parte operativa* [On the operative part] was the practical sequel of Arnald's projected summa and his final work.

Irrespective of the date in which Arnald ended his teaching activities, 1301 or 1308, there is agreement on placing the bulk of his medical production in the decade of the 1290s at Montpellier. Before this date Arnald seems to have composed only a short treatise devoted to love-sickness—a kind of mental alteration (*Tractatus de amore heroico*, composed before 1285)—and an epistle condemning necromantic practices while analyzing the mental alterations of those who believed that they mastered the devil (*De reprobacione nigromantice ficcionis*, composed *c.* 1276–88).

The first work produced at Montpellier was *De intentione medicorum* [On the intention of the physicians], which set the ground for Arnald's medical epistemology. What is medicine, *scientia* or *ars*? What are the nature and the aim of medical knowledge? What role must be performed by the university physician? And accordingly, what training will best suit the physician for this role? All these questions were contained in this programmatic text, in which Arnald explored the limits between medical and philosophical knowledge and proposing a duality of objectives and two levels of epistemological evaluation. The physician, according to Arnald, is an *artifex sensualis et operativus* [a practical craftsman guided by the senses] and thus, at least rhetorically, his theoretical interests must be limited by their practical usefulness. This stance, which Michael McVaugh has called 'medical instrumentalism', allowed Arnald to establish an intermediary space between the idea of medicine as science that would fulfill itself in theoretical speculation and an anti-intellectual empiricism. Throughout his career, Arnald was very fond of this early treatise, as witnessed by its quotation in later works.

The idea of medicine as *scientia* was identified by Arnald with medical Averroism. In the *Aphorismi de gradibus* [Aphorisms on medicinal degrees], a pharmacological work composed between 1295 and 1300, Arnald confessed that in addition to the *Aphorismi*, he wrote another three pieces against the Averroists: *De intentione medicorum*, the

Epistola de dosi tyriacalium [Letter on the dose of tyriac] (*c.* 1290–99), an epistle on the effect of antidotes designed to refute Averroes's *De tyriaca*, and a work on phlebotomy, *De considerationibus operis medicine sive de flebotomia* [On considerations of medical practice or On phlebotomy] (*c.* 1298–1300). It is a commonplace in historiography to highlight Arnald's violent feelings against Averroists. It is true that Arnald's medical instrumentalism of Avicenic origin would mingle badly with the idea, held by Averroists, of medicine as a branch of natural philosophy. However, theoretical divergences in medical matters could not justify Arnald's attacks, and Paniagua has suggested a religious reason behind them. There is also a chronological problem that has not been explored in depth. If Arnald's doctrinal coherence during this decade can be detected without difficulty, the consistency of his anti-Averroistic positions is not that evident. In fact, despite Arnald's later claims, his work *De intentione* is not at all polemical, and instead has a clear conciliatory tone. Some years later, the *Aphorismi* and the *Epistola de dosi tyriacalium* were fiercely anti-Averroistic, but again, in *De consideratione,* written between 1298 and 1300, the reader can hardly recognize Averroist groups as targets of Arnald's criticisms. Here he ridiculed those who bore the title of physician but were ignorant of Hippocrates and Galen and were unable to base their practice on knowledge of the causes of disease. These charges were the same usually employed to condemn the activities of the empirics, and they do not describe any of the positions of those who follow the magisterium of Averroes. Historiography has highlighted Arnald's supposed anti-intellectualism and has connected it with his religious views. However, this has been based mostly on the erroneous ascription to Arnald of the *Breviarium practice* [Breviary of practice], but Arnald's position toward medieval empirics, as stated in the *De considerationibus* and elsewhere, is by no means a positive one.

The polemical tone employed by Arnald in some of his medical writings depicted a tense intellectual and professional environment at Montpellier, both inside and outside the academic walls. As other medical masters, Arnald exposed in the classroom several texts, some of them on canonical works of the teaching syllabus, such as the *Aphorismi* [Aphorisms], the *Regimen acutorum* [Regimen on acute diseases], and the *Tegni* [Art of medicine]. Others were lectures on less common works such as Galen's *De morbo et accidenti* [On disease and its symptoms], the *De malicia complexionis diverse* [On the evils of an unbalanced complexion], the *De ingenio sanitatis* [On the technique of healing], and the *De elementis* [On the elements]. From those commentaries to which Arnald referred in several of his works, only his lecture (*c.* 1292–95) on the *De malicia complexionis* survived with certainty in a hurried and careless *reportatio*. The rest are lost or their attribution is not yet clear, as with the commentary on *De morbo*

et accidenti and the *Lectura super regimentis acutorum* [Lecture on the regimen on acute diseases]. Extant also are the expositions on some Hippocratic aphorisms, particularly to *In morbis minus* [In disease, less] and to the first aphorism, the *Repetitio super canone Vita Brevis* [Repetition on the canon, Life is short], probably from 1301. Arnald wrote a commentary on the long Galenic book on therapy, *De ingenio sanitatis* [On the technique of healing]; however, the work that has survived under the name of *Aphorismi de ingenio sanitatis*, also known as *Medicationis parabole* [Parables of treatment], was not based on fragments of those lectures but is an independent work composed in 1300 as an aphoristic collection. The reason for the scarce manuscript tradition of Arnald's lectures is unclear. However, Arnald himself gave some hints by explaining that he did not publicize the commentaries he wrote on Hippocrates and Galen in order to deprive his enemies of weapons.

But who was the enemy? Colleagues at the medical school? We do not know yet. What is clearer is Arnald's involvement in the reform of medical studies at Montpellier. The 1309 bull of Pope Clement V regulating those studies gratefully acknowledged Arnald's past involvement with the *Studium* and his present advice in its regulation. As other masters at Paris, Bologna, and Montpellier, Arnald had been pivotal in developing a wider intellectual frame at the medical school that overshadowed the one focused on the canonical texts of the so-called *Articella*. The change, termed by García Ballester the introduction of 'the new Galen' in medical teaching and research, involved paying attention to more than thirty works of Galen that had not been used by previous generations, as well as revisiting Arabic works. Without a doubt, this helped to pose new questions and to offer new answers, at both a theoretical and a practical level. The rhetorical aspect of this movement is clear in giving to university medicine a more attractive packaging, but there is also evidence of actual changes in diagnosis, prognosis, and therapy as a result of this new reading of Galenic works. Apart from works devoted to a practical use such as the *regimina* and *consilia* or the *Practica summaria*, some of the therapeutic indications contained both in *De considerationibus* and in the more complex *Aphorismi de gradibus* could have influenced actual practice not only in the mechanical handling of disease but also in the explanations that justified its implementation.

But Arnald's social influence went far beyond the sphere of health and disease, and conversely the reception of his medical works and the appreciation of his healing activities must have been influenced by his worldly fame and legend. Arnald the successful physician and professor of medicine was also a religious reformer and soon became labeled as a necromancer, a magician, and an alchemist. Arnald himself was conscious of these distortions, and in 1310 he expressed in *Raonament d'Avinyó* his sadness about what he considered false accusations of heresy, necromancy, and magic that ran against him in the court circles. There is no doubt that Arnald's presence at the royal and papal courts, and his deep involvement in political and religious matters far from the strictly medical or academic, provided a suitable rack from which to hang many different coats. As a public persona protected by monarchs and popes, his fame was fed by court gossip during his lifetime, and it was subjected to various distortions immediately after his death. Arnald's name came historically to be used in an antagonistic sense to protect and to accuse: as guarantor of unorthodox intellectual or spiritual positions and as proof of the heretical nature of those positions. Historical falsification and ascription to him of writings of different origin contributed to partially justifying these uses. However, not everything belongs to the legend, and some of Arnald's attitudes and ideas helped to forge the myth. The deep concern with mystical, prophetic, and eschatological views is genuinely Arnaldian, as was the turmoil of conflicts with the Church and the posthumous condemnation and public burning of most of his spiritual works. More puzzling is the origin of a wide textual tradition, both in manuscript and in print, that praised Arnald as an alchemist and leading author on this subject when there is no historical evidence of his involvement in alchemy.

The effort of medical historiography has been devoted to delineating the historical character from its subsequent development. But Arnald's mystification has too often been replaced by another equally distorted view, which has approached his work as an example of an avant-garde scientist opposed to medical and natural philosophical scholasticism. The value of practical knowledge over pure speculation held by Arnald has been stressed anachronistically in order to mirror the needs and desires of modern physicians. It is true that Arnald despised highly theoretical speculation and praised empirical findings, but this position was presented in intellectually complex treatises that faithfully followed the rules of the scholastic method and not in easily read handbooks or spiritual pamphlets. On the other hand, his position on spiritual matters praising the lay understanding of the evangelical truth over complex theological disquisitions has been uncritically taken as proof of Arnald's antischolasticism in medical matters. However, to what extent his religious commitment influenced his medical thought and practice is still a matter of discussion. Some historians have made an effort to show the crossing of boundaries between spiritual intuition and scholastic rationality in Arnald; others have been more ready to defend the independent development of his interests. The presence of some magical concepts in his scholastic rationality is a fact that has usually been overlooked in the task of cleansing the legend, but it is a feature that needs to be analyzed and placed in the wider framework of medical thought in his time.

The project of critically editing the Arnaldian medical corpus accompanied by historical studies (*Arnaldi de Vilanova Opera Medica Omnia*) has been underway since 1975. The same approach has been taken toward his spiritual works, and the first volume of the series appeared in 2004 (*Arnaldi de Vilanova Opera Theologica Omnia*). Scholarly research has shown a renewed interest in the alchemical question in recent years. There is no doubt that this collective effort is setting the basis for a more balanced understanding of Arnald's thought and activities.

Bibliography

Primary: García Ballester, Luis, Michael McVaugh, and Juan A. Paniagua, general eds., 1975–. *Arnaldi de Vilanova Opera Medica Omnia* (Barcelona). Already published: vol. II, *Aphorismi de gradibus*; vol. III, *De amore heroico*; *De dosi tyriacalium medicinarum*; vol. IV, *Tract. de consideracionibus operis medicine sive de flebotomia*; vol. V.1, *Tract. de intentione medicorum*; vol. VI.1, *Medicationis parabole* & *Pirqé*; vol. VI.2, *Comm. in quasdam parabolas et alias aphorismorum series*; vol. X.1, *Regimen sanitatis ad regem Aragonum*; vol. X.2, *Regimen Almarie*; vol. XI, *De esu carnium*; vol. XV, *Commentum supra tractatum Galieni de malicia complexionis diverse* & *Doctrina Galieni de interioribus*; vol. XVI, *Translatio libri Galieni de rigore et tremore et iectigatione et spasmo*.

Secondary: García Ballester, Luis, 2003. *Galen and Galenism. Theory and Medical Practice from Antiquity to the European Renaissance* (Aldershot); Mensa i Valls, J., and S. Giralt, 2003. 'Bibliografía Arnaldiana (1994–2003).' *Arxiu de Textos Catalans Antics* 22: 665–734; Ziegler, Joseph, 1998. *Medicine and Religion c. 1300. The Case of Arnau de Vilanova* (Oxford); Perarnau, Josep, ed., 1995. *Actes de la I Trobada Internacional d'Estudis sobre Arnau de Vilanova* (Barcelona); Paniagua, Juan A., 1994. *Studia Arnaldiana. Trabajos en torno a la obra médica de Arnau de Vilanova, c. 1240–1311* (Barcelona); McVaugh, Michael, 1993. *Medicine before the Plague. Practitioners and Their Patients in the Crown of Aragon, 1285–1345* (Cambridge); *DSB*.

Fernando Salmón

ARROYO VILLAVERDE, TRINIDAD (b. Palencia, Spain, 26 May 1872; d. Mexico City, Mexico, 28 September 1959), *ophthalmology.*

Trinidad Arroyo Villaverde read medicine as a free student at the University of Valladolid (1889–95). She started her medical studies seventeen years after the first Spanish woman had entered university (Elena Maseras, b. 1853, MD, University of Barcelona); in the intervening period only fourteen women had obtained university degrees in Spain, half of them in medicine.

Her university studies were facilitated by the support of her family and by new legislation in June 1888 that recognized the right of women to study at university, although they had to apply for a specific permission not required of men. Her father, owner of a laundry, successfully steered through the administrative obstacles that

Trinidad faced as a woman. Her brother Benito was a fellow student at the School of Medicine and in Madrid, where they went in 1895 for their PhD studies and to start their specialization.

She defended her doctoral thesis in 1896 and trained in ophthalmology with Dr Santiago de los Albitos (1845–1908), director from 1877 of the *Asilo de Santa Lucía,* where he also gave courses in the specialty. Surgery had always attracted her, but she believed that social conventions would prevent her from practicing and obtaining a good clientele. Ophthalmology, however, allowed her to, in her own words, combine 'medicine with meticulous, delicate, precise surgery, "lady's surgery"; and I devote all my enthusiasm to it' (de Juan, 1998, p. 33).

Her thesis, on the effect of certain drugs on the normal functioning of the eye musculature, had a subject very different from those of her predecessors Dolores Aleu (b. 1857) and Martina Castells (1852–88), who researched women's education, and those of many of her immediate successors, who addressed women's health issues. She initiated her own research line on the analgesic effects of codeine chlorhydrate and dionin, publishing the results in specialist journals and congress papers.

In 1898 she returned to Palencia, where she opened an office with her brother and started a successful practice that included nearby locations, which she regularly visited to conduct operations. In 1902, she married Manuel Márquez (1872–1962), a fellow student who entered ophthalmology thanks to her influence and went on to become the first Full Professor in the specialty at the University of Madrid in 1911. The couple maintained a flourishing private office in Madrid (1911–36), also sharing their university and health care activities. Arroyo was Assistant Professor and became the first woman member of the Board of the School of Medicine.

Arroyo was one of the first women in Spain to enjoy a long and recognized medical practice. She lived up to her role as a pioneer by supporting numerous initiatives for the social improvement and health education of women. She was a member of the Lyceum Club of Madrid and Honorary President of the Spanish Women's Medical Association, and she contributed to the journal *Medicina Social Española* (1916–20) in its section 'Feminist Notes. From Woman to Woman.'

In June 1936 she and her husband embarked on an exodus that led them to Valencia and Barcelona and finally to Mexico in 1939. Arroyo continued practicing her specialty there and returned only once to Spain, in 1955, to create from her own funds a foundation to provide grants to baccalaureate students in Palencia and medical students in Valladolid.

Bibliography

Primary: 1896. *Músculos intrínsecos del ojo en estado normal y patológico: acción de los medicamentos* (Madrid); 1910. 'Sobre la anal-gesia ocular local producida por el clorhidrato de codeína sobre el ojo.' *Archivos de Oftalmología Hispano Americanos* 10: 142–143.

Secondary: de Juan, Albano, 1998. *La colegiación femenina* (Palencia); Flecha, Consuelo, 1996. *Las primeras universitarias en España: 1872–1910* (Madrid); García del Carrizo, M. Gloria, 1990. 'Aproximación a una palentina ilustre: doctora Trinidad Arroyo de Márquez' in *Actas del II Congreso de Historia de Palencia* (Palencia) pp. 71–80.

Teresa Ortiz-Gómez

ASADA, SŌHAKU

ASADA, SŌHAKU (b. Kuribayashi, Shinano domain (now Nagano prefecture), Japan, 19 June 1815; d. Tokyo, Japan, 16 March 1894), *Chinese-Japanese medicine.*

Asada Sōhaku was born in 1815 to a family who practiced medicine in Kuribayashi village in Shinano domain, now Nagano prefecture. As the only surviving son, he was destined to a career in medicine and was familiar with medical practice from childhood. Having learned elementary classical Chinese texts, he first studied medicine under a medical practitioner in nearby Takatō province. At eighteen, he headed for Kyoto, where he studied under eminent practitioners in the city, paying particular attention to *Shōkan-ron,* the key classical text of Chinese medicine. He also gained humanistic learning under Rai San'yō (1780–1832), one of the most famous literati and influential thinkers at that time. His education was thus a typical combination of bookish medicine and Chinese classical humanities.

In 1836, when Asada was twenty-two years old, he started practice in Edo. The first step to his success in this most competitive medical market was his introduction to Motoyasu Sōen, one of the physicians at the court of the Shōgunate. Through Motoyasu, he was introduced to other eminent medical practitioners and court physicians in Edo. From 1855 he was involved in the *Bakufu*'s project of revising *Ishinpō,* a voluminous compilation of Chinese medical texts initially completed by Tanba Yasuyori (912–995). In 1866 he treated the fourteenth Shōgun Tokugawa Iemochi (1846–66), who had suffered from beriberi. The appointment earned him the title of *hogan,* the highest honor for court physicians. In the capacity of a court physician, he made friends with influential figures and involved himself in the highly volatile politics of that time. Boosted by successful treatment of the Shōgun, a French consul, and other eminent public figures, his practice flourished: in 1863 he was reputed to have treated in total more than 4,000 patients and earned the fabulous amount of 2,300 *ryōs,* twice as much as the most fashionable doctors' annual earnings. Despite his close connection with the Shōgunate, Asada's career survived the Meiji Revolution. His practice continued to flourish: his house in Yokodera-machi in Tokyo was reputed to have been visited by 500 patients daily. In 1879 he was appointed as a physician to a newborn prince (who later became Emperor Taishō). When he retired from the job, he was given a pension for the service.

The continuing success of Asada's career after the Meiji Revolution, whose government decidedly favored Western medicine, is an eloquent testimony to the enduring popularity of at least some Kanpō (Chinese-Japanese) doctors.

Asada was not, however, successful in stopping the tide of the westernization of medicine. In 1879 Asada and some other major Japanese-Chinese doctors formed Onchi-sha, which vigorously lobbied for the inclusion of Japanese-Chinese medical subjects in the medical examination for a license. In 1881 Asada assumed the leadership of Onchi-sha. After his death in 1894, the bill for amendment of the law regulating medical licenses was proposed to the Diet by those sympathetic toward traditional doctors. The amendment was defeated by a vote of seventy-eight to one hundred, which finally sealed Western medicine's monopoly of Japanese medical education. Asada's failure to secure a place for Kanpō medicine testified to the structural transformation of Japanese medical practice: in the new world of the Meiji medicine, the state decided the fabric of medical practice, while the patronage of the powerful and the rich was of only secondary importance. Asada had virtually no rival in the latter, but was sadly deficient in developing connections in the former.

Bibliography

Primary: 1987–1992. *Asada Sōhaku senshū* [Selected Works of Asada Sōhaku] (Hasegawa, Mitsuto, ed.) 8 vols. (Tokyo); 1986. *Asada Sōhaku shokan-shū* [Collected Letters of Asada Sōhaku] (Tokyo); 1933. *Asada Sōhaku shohō-shū* [Collected Prescriptions of Asada Sōhaku] (Asada, Tasuo, ed.) 2 vols. (Tokyo).

Secondary: Kinzaburo, Asanuma, 1895. *Asada Sōhaku-ō den* [The Life of Asada Sōhaku] 3 vols. (Tokyo); Yakazu, Dōmei, 1982. 'Kaisetsu' [Introduction] to *Kinse Kanpō igakusho shūsei*, vol. 95 (Yoshinori, Ōtsuka, and Dōmei Yakazu, eds.) (Tokyo).

Akihito Suzuki

ASAPH HA-ROFĒH (aka ASAPH BEN BERACHYAHŪ THE PHYSICIAN or ASAPH THE WISE) (fl. Persia, *c.* second century), *medicine.*

Exact biographical data for Asaph have not been preserved. He probably lived either in Persia (Melzer) or in Palestine (Muntner) in the second, seventh, or even the tenth century (Steinschneider). He mastered Greek and Hebrew and was an influential author: his writings widely promoted medical knowledge and deeply influenced medieval works composed in both Hebrew and Arabic languages. Asaph rendered the Greek medical doctrine in the Biblical Hebrew. By doing so, he coined many new medical Hebrew terms. His pupils probably edited the final version of Asaph's writings after his death.

Asaph's writings comprise a book, first mentioned in the tenth century, which begins with a legendary historical introduction to the origins of medicine. He quotes Hippocrates, Dioscorides, and Galen as his predecessors. The whole narration is well organized. The book deals with the microcosm and macrocosm of a human and explains the causation of disease from the basis of humoral theory. Inevitably, it deals with classification of the aliments, and it has significant sections on anatomy and physiology. Asaph writes about various illnesses of different parts of the body and their respective treatments in a chapter that includes a description of 123 medicinal herbs (after Dioscorides) and a section on the antidotes.

The book also contains a Hebrew paraphrase of the *Aphorisms* and *Prognosticon* by Hippocrates, a list of symptoms for various fevers, and formulas for the uroscopy. It closes with a text of an oath, which was probably a part of the graduation ceremony.

The book has been preserved complete in the libraries of Munich, Florence, and Oxford. Apart from these three complete copies, several fragments are known.

Bibliography

Primary: Steinschneider, M., 1875. *Die Hebräischen Handschriften der K. Hof- und Staatsbibliothek in München* (Munich,), NR. 231; Neubauer, A., *Catalogue of the Hebrew Manuscripts in the Bodleian Library and in the College Libraries of Oxford.* Cod. 2138. 2 vols. (Oxford).

Secondary: Newmyer, T. S., 1992. 'Asaph's "Book of Remedies": Greek Science and Jewish Apologetics.' *Sudhoffs Archiv* 76(1): 28–36; Lieber, E., 1991. 'An Ongoing Mystery: The So-called 'Book of Medicine' Attributed to Asaph the Sage.' *Bulletin of Judaeo-Greek Studies* 8: 18–25; Melzer, A., 1972. 'Asaph the Physician—the man and his book: A historical-philological study of the medical treatise, The Book of Drugs.' PhD thesis, Hebrew and Semitic Studies, University of Wisconsin; Muntner, S. 'Assaph (Harofe) the Physician, "Sefer Refuoth".' *Korot* 1965, 3: 396–422, 533–560; 1967–1969, 4: 11–40, 170–207, 389–443, 531–572; 1970, 5(1): 27–68, 160–187, 295–330; 1971–1972, 5(2): 435–473, 603–649, 773–807 (in Hebrew); Venetianer, L., 1916. *Asaf Judaeus: Di aelteste medizinische Schriftsteller in hebraeischer Sprache* (Strassburg); Steinschneider, M. 'Asaph Judeaus' *Hebraische Bibliographie.* 1872, XII: 85; 1877, XVII: 114; 1879, IXX: 35, 64, 84, 105.

Efraim Lev

ASCHOFF, KARL ALBERT LUDWIG (b. Berlin, Germany, 10 January 1866; d. Freiburg im Breisgau, Germany, 24 June 1942), *pathology.*

Aschoff was the son of a Berlin physician. Between 1885 and 1890, he studied medicine in Bonn, Strasbourg, and again Bonn, where he graduated MD in 1889 under the supervision of the pathologist Hugo Ribbert (1855–1920). During 1890–91, Aschoff worked at Robert Koch's (1843–1910) Institute for Hygiene in Berlin and in Würzburg with the anatomist Albert Ritter von Koelliker (1817–1905). In the following years, he was an assistant of the pathologists and Virchow students Friedrich Daniel von Recklinghausen (1833–1910) in Strasbourg (1891–93) and

Johannes Orth (1847–1923) in Göttingen (1893–1903). Under Orth, Aschoff received his teaching license (Habilitation) in 1894 and also became assistant professor (Professor Extraordinarius). Between 1901 and 1902, he worked at the Jenner Institute in London, at the Schools of Tropical Medicine in London and Liverpool, and at the Pasteur Institute in Paris under Elie Mechnikov (1845–1916). In 1903 Aschoff was appointed professor of pathology at the University of Marburg; in 1906 he got the same position at the University of Freiburg im Breisgau, where he retired in 1936.

Aschoff was one of the most influential and well-known German physicians in the first half of the twentieth century. His remarkable international reputation was grounded soundly in pathology's tradition as a basic discipline of nineteenth-century scientific medicine. Aschoff represented this tradition and tried to secure for his discipline a similar position in the troubled waters of twentieth-century medicine. Rudolf Virchow (1821–1902) had concentrated mainly on the investigation of the static condition of morphologically altered cells, tissues, and organs, which had been collected in the morgue. The analysis of disease processes under the auspices of an experimental pathology and the re-establishment of close contacts with clinicians remained as a promise for the future. It was Aschoff's aim to realize these plans. In the years until 1904, he undertook classical morphological investigations. But then in 1906, one of his Japanese scholars, Sunao Tawara (1873–1952) clarified the morphological basis of the electrical stimulation of the mammalian heart. This was a decisive breakthrough, correlating systematically physiological or pathophysiological knowledge about the organism with the respective morphological substrate and combining 'function and structure'. The very same idea influenced—among other subjects—Aschoff's work in the years to come. He undertook research on arteriosclerosis of the vascular system, on the pathogenesis of cholelithiasis (stones of the gall bladder), on thrombosis (obliteration of veins), and on the dynamics of cellular action. Besides (patho) physiology, morphology was related to biochemistry, pathochemistry, and physics. After World War I, Aschoff and many of his students proceeded with this work. In 1924 related efforts led to the theory of the 'reticulo-endothelial system', consisting of a number of specialized defense cells, which are able among other things to ingest foreign particles and microbes. Pathophysiological research could investigate the interplay between different cells, tissues, and organs of the organism and seemed to uncover hidden laws of its general function.

Although effective and quite successful, this was not the only research strand followed by Aschoff. To a certain extent, Aschoff was a child of the nineteenth century. The morgue remained the center of his institute in Freiburg, where he spent most of his research energies. Morphology remained the backbone of his research, and it clearly had importance for Aschoff's work in World War I. In collabo-

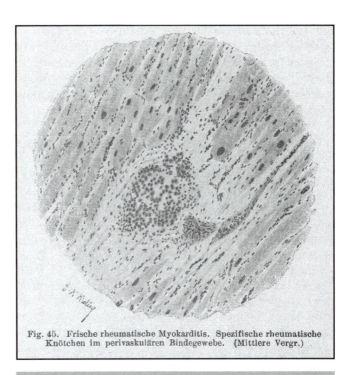

Fig. 45. Frische rheumatische Myokarditis. Spezifische rheumatische Knötchen im perivaskulären Bindegewebe. (Mittlere Vergr.)

Photomicrograph showing Aschoff body in the myocardium, characteristic of rheumatic fever. Halftone reproduction from *Pathologische anatomie . . .*, 5th edn., Jena, 1921. Wellcome Library, London.

ration with the head of the German Army's Medical Service, Otto von Schjerning (1853–1921), he created in his capacity as consulting army pathologist the program, and drew up the syllabus, of 'war pathology' (*Kriegspathologie*). The university pathology institutes had the task of autopsying almost every soldier who was killed in action or who otherwise died in connection with his service. The reason for this program was not restricted to regular duties of pathology, namely to uncover the development of a disease and the ultimate reason of death. The most important reason for the 'war pathology' program was, in Aschoff's view, to provide new insights into 'constitutional pathology' (*Konstitutionspathologie*). This meant making every effort to determine the *habitus* and the overall constitution of the (healthy) individual. Moreover, collected data about the constitution of young (healthy) soldiers were seen as representative for the whole German nation. Aschoff, inspired with enthusiastic nationalism, especially viewed pathological anatomy as a German science and 'war pathology' as a service of the discipline for Imperial Germany. And, as a holistic approach, the program overlapped with and fit well into his broadly designed pathophysiological research.

After 1918 Aschoff entered the political stage more often. Although a supporter of Wilhelmine Germany, as were most of the German professors, Aschoff already before the war had felt uneasy about his country's social encrustation and about the overwhelming influence of materialistic thinking. Similarly to the representatives of the German *Gebildetenreform-bewegung* [German reform movement of educated bourgeois people], Aschoff dreamed of a union of all Germans under the banner of bourgeois moral attitude, mentality, and ideas. Based on this notion, he gave democracy a chance and supported the Weimar Republic. In 1926 he attended a meeting of Republic-friendly docents who wished to support the new government. But Aschoff played no dominant role in the so-called Weimar Circle (*Weimarer Kreis*). In his view the circle was not supportive of science, which should be free of political and ideological ties. Also, Aschoff did not trust democracy. He viewed the state in traditional conservative terms as above all 'party egoism', and therefore only the state could help realize his idea of a unity of German people.

Therefore, Aschoff remained an admirer of Imperial Germany and the monarchy. He saw conservative traditional institutions as student corporations or gymnastics clubs, which promoted physical education, as most usable to install bonds between people and to create the sense of a unified nation. Aschoff's attitudes were fueled by the exclusion of German scientists from the international community after 1918. He tried to revive cooperation between the countries but fought also for a rightful place of 'Germanic Christian culture' within the international concert. One part of this culture was in his view pathological anatomy, which had among others the political role to represent German culture abroad. Aschoff traveled a lot and sought close connections among others, above all with Japan, where he had many students and where he is still well known and admired today.

The connection between his political attitudes and his work made itself felt through the upkeep of the war pathology program even after the defeat of 1918. A vast amount of material had been gathered (Berlin War Pathology Collection: 70,000 autopsy reports and 6,000 preparations), and it awaited exploitation. Results were published in the journal 'Publications from the Fields of War Pathology and Constitutional Pathology' (*Veröffentlichungen aus der Kriegs- und Konstitutionspathologie*), which was newly established in 1920 through the initiative of Aschoff and the Berlin pathologist Walter Koch (1880–1962). Also, the old program fit well into the climate of the inter-war period in Germany, which was characterized by the rejection of materialistic thinking and the propagation of holistic theories, e.g., constitutionalism. Aschoff and Koch used the promotion of occupational medicine to adapt the orientation of the collection and the journal to the new needs of society (occupational pathology as 'war pathology of peace'—Koch). After 1933, again through Aschoff and Koch, both institutions shifted back to military pathology (*Wehrpathologie*). Helpful for Aschoff were Koch's connections with leading National Socialist physicians, e.g., with Leonardo Conti (1900–1945), who in 1939 became Reich Health Leader (*Reichsgesundheitsführer*).

Even before 1914, Aschoff had a certain interest in racial hygiene. This is mirrored to some extent by the war pathology program, which in the last analysis promoted a healthy German nation. Apart from that, Aschoff was reluctant to make any comments on the topic in the years before 1933. He performed research on races as 'pathology of the nations' (*Völkerpathologie*), where he simply investigated the different manifestations of diseases in different geographic regions. This changed after 1933. Now Aschoff frankly developed plans to preserve the purity of the hereditary factors among the German population. He welcomed National Socialism, hoping for the realization of a unified Germany under bourgeois, educated 'leaders'. His ideas to cleanse Germany from Jews and his help for Jewish colleagues to emigrate and to start a new life elsewhere in this sense were not contradictions for him. Aschoff was never a National Socialist, and he was not aware of the atrocities and cruelties of the new government and the impact of the changes after 1933. He was astonished and annoyed that colleagues appeared with brown shirts at academic celebrations.

During his life, Aschoff received many honors. Until his retirement in 1936, he was one of the pillars and leading figures of the Medical Faculty of the University of Freiburg. And after his death in 1942, he was nationally and internationally honored as a great scientist. With hindsight, Aschoff appears to be a dazzling but dubious character. On the one hand, he was a modernizer of pathology in a period of transition of scientific medicine, on the other hand he supported approaches that clearly prepared the ground for the seizure of power of the Nazi Party after 1933 and which served to legitimate Nazi atrocities. In the words of one of his obituary-writers, the pathologist Edward Bell Krumbhaar (1882–1966), Aschoff was 'a leading figure of the twilight period of modern German medical science'.

Bibliography

Primary: 1906. Preface to Tawara, Sunao, *Das Reizleitungssystem des Säugetierherzens* (Jena); 1909 (2nd edn. 1911, 8th edn. 1936). *Pathologische Anatomie* (Jena); 1922 (ed.). *Pathologische Anatomie* (*Handbuch der ärztlichen Erfahrungen im Weltkriege 1914/1918*, Vol. VIII) (Leipzig); 1924. 'Das reticuloendotheliale System.' *Ergebnisse der Inneren Medizin und der Kinderheilkunde* 26: 1–117; 1966. *Ein Gelehrtenleben in Briefen an die Familie* (Freiburg im Breisgau).

Secondary: Prüll, Cay-Rüdiger, 1999. 'Pathology at War 1914–1918—Germany and Britain in Comparison' in Cooter, Roger, Mark Harrison, and Steve Sturdy, eds., *Medicine and Modern Warfare* (Amsterdam and Atlanta) pp. 131–161; Prüll, Cay-Rüdiger, 1998. 'Holism and German Pathology (1914–1933)' in Lawrence, Christopher, and George Weisz, eds., *Greater than the Parts: Holism in Biomedicine, 1920–1950* (Oxford) pp. 46–67; Prüll, Cay-Rüdiger, 1997. 'Pathologie und Politik—Ludwig Aschoff (1866–1942) und Deutschlands Weg ins Dritte Reich.' *History and Philosophy of the*

Life Sciences 19: 331–368; Seidler, Eduard, 1991. *Die Medizinische Fakultät der Universität Freiburg i.Br.* (Berlin); Buscher, Dorothea, 1980. 'Die wissenschaftstheoretischen, medizinhistorischen und zeitkritischen Arbeiten von Ludwig Aschoff.' Thesis, University of Freiburg i.Br.; Büchner, Franz, 1966. 'Ludwig Aschoff zum Gedenken an seinen 100. Geburtstag (10.1.1866–24.6.1942).' *Verhandlungen der Deutschen Gesellschaft für Pathologie* 50: 475–489; Krumbhaar, Edward Bell, 1943. 'Ludwig Aschoff, 1866–1942.' *Archives of Pathology* 35: 198–201.

Cay-Ruediger Pruell

ASCLEPIADES OF BITHYNIA

(b. Cius or Prusias-on-sea, Bithynia, northwest Asia Minor (now Turkey), fl. first century BCE; d. Rome), *dietetics, medicine, physiology.*

Asclepiades, a Greek from Bithynia, which was then a client kingdom of Rome, won renown in Rome by the skill of his medical art. His death has been placed from 91 BCE to some twenty to thirty years later. What is unquestioned is his fame: he attracted students from as far away as Asia, including M. Artorius, later physician to Augustus, and Themison, whose student Thessalus of Tralles would found the Methodist medical sect (to what extent Asclepiades was intellectual godfather to Methodism is debatable). Asclepiades' position was such that he refused an invitation from King Mithridates of Pontus (but for whom he composed several pharmacological works). Asclepiades' renown in Rome rested on a system based on attention to diet, gentle exercise and massage, bathing, the drinking of water, and the drinking of wine in moderation. None of Asclepiades' writings have survived, and he has been largely viewed through a prism of indifferent or hostile sources. Pliny the Elder labeled Asclepiades a failed teacher of rhetoric who turned to medicine only to make a living. To Celsus, Asclepiades' popularity was based on his promise of being able to heal 'safely, quickly, and pleasantly'. Scribonius Largus referred to Asclepiades as the 'greatest medical authority' (*maximus auctor medicinae*), and defended him from the charge that he prescribed no drugs. Largus referred to Asclepiades' (lost) pharmacological work, where it was stated that every doctor should have at least two or three basic preparations at hand.

Asclepiades maintained that the body was composed of miniscule corpuscular lumps ('jointless masses'). They were not 'atoms' or their equivalent, for, unlike atoms, these 'lumps' were breakable. These discrete masses, when bound together, formed composites from which the body was made. In between these masses were pores, blockage of which resulted in a range of effects, including pain, ill health, disease, and death. The origins of Asclepiades' corpuscular theory is disputed, although the term for his breakable lumps was one shared with the philosopher Heraclides of Pontus (fourth century BCE), and his pore theory may have originated with Erasistratus.

Since both male and female bodies were constructed from the same matter, there was no need for a separate gynecology (although males were 'hotter' than females). To Galen, Asclepiades' chief critic, these masses were like atoms in that they acted randomly and therefore were without purpose. For Galen, this was opposed to his own teleological view of the body, functioning in accord with a purposeful nature. Asclepiades' mechanistic, matter-based theory had no place for the doctrine of the humors. To Galen, this rejection of what for him was a central Hippocratic precept (and, again according to Galen, Asclepiades referred to Hippocratic medicine as 'the practice of death') ensured the condemnation of Asclepiades and his followers. For Galen, health was absolutely dependent on the correct balance of the four humors, while physiological function required the presence of pneuma, a substance derived from air and which was qualitatively changed by the lungs, heart, and brain.

Beneath Asclepiades' undoubtedly carefully crafted self-promotion lay a system that recognized the futility or dubious value of many current forms of treatment. His holistic system, as much as can be reconstructed, had much to commend it, relying as it did on a prescription of moderation in food and drink, sensible exercise, and a restricted, judicious use of drugs. Asclepiades' success helped ensure that Greek medical practitioners in Rome would henceforth not only be tolerated, but also accepted.

Bibliography

Primary: Gumpert, Ch., 1794. *Asclepiadis Bithyni fragmenta* (Weimar); Green, Richard, 1955. *Asclepiades: His Life and Writings. A Translation of Cocchi's* Life of Asclepiades *and Gumpert's* Fragments of Asclepiades (New Haven, CT).

Secondary: Asmis, Elizabeth, 1993. 'Asclepiades of Bithynia Rediscovered?' *Classical Philology* 88(2): 145–156; Vallance, John, 1990. *The Lost Theory of Asclepiades of Bithynia* (Oxford); Rawson, Elizabeth, 1982. 'The Life and Death of Asclepiades of Bithynia.' *Classical Quarterly* 32: 358–370.

Julius Rocca

ASELLI, GASPARE

(b. Cremona, Italy, 1581; d. Milan, Italy, 9 September 1625), *anatomy.*

Born of noble descent, Aselli from a very early age showed a keen interest in natural sciences. He studied medicine at the University of Pavia, and after graduating moved to Milan, where he had the opportunity to continue his anatomical researches and later became an honorary citizen. His profound knowledge of anatomy won him the nomination for chief surgeon of the Spanish army in Italy, a position he held from 1612 to 1620. In 1624 he was offered the position of professor of anatomy at the University of Pavia.

Aselli discovered the chylous vessels on 23 July 1622 while carrying out the vivisection of a dog, which had recently eaten, in the presence of several of his friends, all distinguished Milanese physicians, including Alessandro

Tadino, Senatore Settala, and Ludovico Settala. Even though these vessels had been noted in ancient times, their existence had been completely forgotten. After having pointed out the recurrent nerves, he moved the intestine to reveal the movements of the diaphragm; he then noticed numerous thin white cords, which branched out into the mesentery and intestines. On cutting one of these cords, a milky-white liquid was released. Therefore, Aselli believed these formations of cords were small vessels, that transported chyle, and he thus called them 'lacteal veins'.

Aselli studied these vascular structures systematically, recognizing the relationship between their turgidity and the animal's recent meal, and demonstrating their existence in other animal species. The results of his researches were reported in *De lactibus sive lacteis venis quarto vasorum mesaraicorum genere novo invento*, published posthumously in 1627. In this work Aselli documented the fact that the 'lacteal veins' served to absorb the chyle, whose centripetal movement was ensured by the numerous valves he meticulously described, from the departure of the chylous vessels from the intestine and along their successive course. He considered these vessels as a new type of mesenteric vessel—a fourth type, as he added them to the three types of vessels previously supposed (in addition to the arteries and veins, there were also nerves, which at that time were believed to be hollow to transport the nervous fluid). The work contains four large colored woodcuts illustrating the fourth type of vessel he had discovered. These engravings were in fact the first anatomical illustrations to be printed in color.

Following the Galenic doctrine, Aselli had the chylous vessels arrive in the liver, where the chyle was elaborated into blood, entering the pancreas during its course from the intestines to the liver. This error derives from his having confused the large group of lymph nodes at the root of the mesentery (the 'pancreas of Aselli') for the real pancreas. Aselli's findings were confirmed by various anatomists, including Johann Wesling, who produced the first representation of the chylous vessels in man (1647), and who also had them flow into the pancreas and thence into the liver.

Aselli's error concerning the final destination of the 'lacteal veins' was corrected in 1647 by Jean Pecquet (1622–74), who showed that chyle collected by the 'lacteal veins' did not go to the liver, but was directly introduced into the blood through the thoracic duct (discovered by him in a dog), which received the chyle by the ampullar dilatation nowadays known as the cistern of Pecquet, into which the chylous vessels flow.

Bibliography

Primary: 1627. *De lactibus sive lacteis venis quarto vasorum mesaraicorum genere novo invento* (Milan) (1972 reprint by Franceschini, Pietro (Milan)).

Secondary: Belloni, Luigi, 1958. 'Gaspare Aselli e la scoperta dei vasi chiliferi' in *Storia di Milano*, XI (Milan) pp. 678–682; Capparoni, Pietro, 1933. 'Il manoscritto di Gaspare Aselli sulla scoperta dei vasi chiliferi.' *Bollettino dell'Istituto storico italiano dell'arte sanitaria* 13: 298–313; Ducceschi, Virgilio, 1922. 'I manoscritti di Gaspare Aselli (1581–1625).' *Archivio di storia della scienza* 3: 125–134; *DSB*.

Giuseppe Ongaro

ASTRUC, JEAN (b. Sauves, France, 19 March 1684; d. Paris, France, 5 May 1766), *medicine, history, biblical criticism.*

Astruc was born in lower Languedoc, in the south of France, to Pierre Astruc, a Protestant pastor. The latter, however, converted shortly afterward to Catholicism, probably in response to the revocation of the Edict of Nantes (1685). The name Astruc was rather common among Jews in Provence and Languedoc throughout the Middle Ages. No traces could, however, be documented of any Jewish parentage (there are no documents on the birth of Pierre Astruc at the Sauves townhall). Jean Astruc studied medicine in Montpellier; he became a licentiate in 1702 and a doctor in medicine in 1703. He was soon chosen as a substitute by his teacher, Pierre Chirac (1650–1732), and in 1710 he was called to the chair of anatomy at Toulouse University. Seven years later, Astruc was back in Montpellier, having been appointed there to the prestigious chair of medicine. In 1728 he became Physician-in-Ordinary to the Duke of Orleans, which was well in tune with his attraction to Paris. One year later the King of Poland, Augustus II, chose him as his First Physician, but in 1730 the French King Louis XV appointed him Consulting Physician, an honor he could hardly reject. This nomination most probably opened for him the door to the Collège Royal, where he obtained the chair of medicine. Astruc had thus reached his highest ambitions. He taught there with great applause from February 1731 until May 1766. He died 'at his desk with his pen in his hands' (Doe, 1960, p. 191).

Astruc's erudition and memory were quite remarkable. He had read and memorized an enormous amount of literature. His teaching program covered the medical art in its entirety and was distributed over a period of six or seven years. A number of manuscript copies of these lectures, written down by diligent students, have survived in various French libraries and in private collections. Some of these courses were translated and published abroad, particularly in England, as pirate editions. His most acclaimed works were those on venereal diseases, in which he included a well-documented history of syphilis, and those on gynecology and obstetrics.

Astruc participated actively in the legal battles between the surgeons of Paris and the Faculty of Medicine. His advocacy on the side of the physicians earned him admission to the Faculty without the usual examinations and fees.

Last, but not least, Astruc published in 1753 his *Conjectures sur la Genèse*, which established his pioneering expertise in biblical criticism.

Astruc's historical work on the University of Montpellier was edited by his disciple Lorry in 1767. Astruc had worked on this scholarly research for many years, and it remains a valuable work to this day.

Astruc's library counted no less than 3,544 volumes, according to a catalog that was printed in 1766 after his death.

It has been said of Astruc that 'He knew everything—even medicine.' In a satirical essay, La Mettrie called him *Savantasse* (Huard, 1972, p. 11). To hold the scales even, we can follow Janet Doe in regarding Astruc as 'a characteristic exponent of his era, rather than a figure standing out of it' (Doe, 1960, p. 184).

Bibliography

Primary: 1736. *De Morbis Venereis Libri Sex* (Paris); 1753. *Conjectures sur les mémoires originaux dont il paraît que Moyse s'est servi pour composer le Livre de la Genèse* (Bruxelles [actually Paris]); 1761–65. *Traité des maladies des femmes* 6 vols. (Paris); 1767. *Mémoires pour servir à l'histoire de la Faculté de Médecine de Montpellier* (Paris).

Secondary: Kottek, Samuel (edited and introduction by), 1980. *Jean Astruc: Traité des Maladies des Enfants—Fac-simile du manuscrit inédit de 1747* (Geneva); Kottek, Samuel, 1978. 'Jean Astruc et les chirurgiens: Une polémique acerbe.' *Revue d'Histoire de la Médecine Hébraïque* 125: 29–32; Huard, Pierre, 1972. 'Jean Astruc (1684–1766)' in Huard, Pierre, ed., *Biographies médicales et scientifiques, XVIIIe siècle* (Paris) pp. 7–30; Doe, Janet, 1960. 'Jean Astruc (1684–1766): A Biographical and Bibliographical Study.' *Journal of the History of Medicine* 15: 184–197.

Samuel Kottek

ATIMAN, ADRIEN   (b. Toundourma, French Sudan (now Mali), *c.* 1866; d. Karema, Tanganyika (now Tanzania), 24 April 1956), *missionary medicine.*

Atiman was a doctor-catechist who worked for the majority of his life in Karema, Western Tanzania. He was born at Toundourma on the River Niger near Timbuktu, which was at that time a stronghold of the Tuareg tribe, renowned for their close interest in slave trading. Very little is known about Atiman's early life, other than that his mother, Tandumosa, and his father, Jucda, were probably Muslims.

At around ten years of age Atiman was abducted from his family by raiding Tuareg slave traders, who sold him to an Arab in Timbuktu. After being taken by camel on an arduous journey across the Sahara to Algeria, he was put up for sale at a slave market in Metlili in the northern part of the country. He was sold along with five other African children in 1876 for three hundred francs to two members of the White Fathers, who had been instructed by Archbishop Lavigerie to buy slave boys in order to free them, educate them, and hopefully encourage them to become missionaries to Africa. He was then taken to Algiers, where he met Lavigerie, who arranged for his education as a doctor-catechist. After a brief period in an orphanage for ex-slaves, he was sent to Malta in 1881 to study medicine at the University of Knights Hospitallers at St John, where he qualified in Italian. Atiman spent a total of seven years training in Malta, during which time he was also baptized (1882). During the celebration of Pope Leo XIII's golden jubilee in 1888, Cardinal Lavigerie led a pilgrimage from Africa to Rome, taking Adrien and his companions along. It was said to be during this Roman visit that Adrien fully committed his life to the service of God and mankind.

In July 1888 Atiman sailed for Africa with a group of other doctor-catechists to join the White Fathers, arriving in Zanzibar, where he stayed for a year studying tropical diseases. He was posted thereafter first briefly to Mpala and then Karema, both forts established by the Belgians on the shore of Lake Tanganyika. This was a war-ravaged region with severe health problems, and Atiman's chief tasks were to provide basic medical care in the day and the teaching of catechism in the evenings. In 1889 Atiman married Agnes Wansahira, daughter of Mwami Mrundi, Chief of the Bende tribe, in order to improve relationships with the Bende and thereby find a route to securing greater numbers of conversions. This marriage was seen as an important political alliance, but it was not a happy one, although Atiman did experience great joy when his only child, Joseph, was ordained a Catholic priest in 1923.

During World War I Atiman's medical care provided to Belgian soldiers won wide acclaim, although he refused to accept payment for his services and was never enticed by the offer of well-paid government positions. Despite the fact that he was not a specialist surgeon, he learned a variety of surgical techniques from medical journals and became skilled in the art. He also, unusually, combined the use of indigenous African medicines with new findings within the Western medical tradition.

In old age, Atiman was much decorated. He was awarded the papal medal *Pro ecclesia et Pontifice* (1912), received the Legion d'Honneur from the French government, the papal *Bene Merenti* medal, and several British awards, among them the Wellcome Bronze Medal of the Royal African Society in 1955. He was ninety years old and the first African to be so honored.

Bibliography

Primary: 1946. 'An Autobiography.' *Tanganyika Notes and Records* 21: 46–76.

Secondary: Kabeya, John, 1978. *Daktari Adriano Atiman* (Tabora, Tanzania); Breedveld, Walter, 1965. *Atiman, de Negerdoktor Bij Het Tanganyikameer* (Nijmegen, the Netherlands); Fouquer, Roger, 1964. *Le Docteur Adrien Atiman, Médecin-catéchiste au Tanganyika* (Paris).

Anna Crozier

AUENBRUGGER, JOSEPH LEOPOLD   (b. Graz, Austria, 19 November 1722, d. Vienna, Austria, 18 May 1809), *medicine.*

Auenbrugger's father, an innkeeper, gave his son every opportunity for a solid preliminary education in his native town and later sent him to Vienna to study medicine. Auenbrugger graduated on November 18, 1752. He was so strongly influenced by his teacher Gerhard van Swieten that he dedicated one of his books to his much admired mentor.

In this medical treatise published in 1776, Auenbrugger suggests camphor as a treatment for a special form of mania. From 1751 to 1758 Auenbrugger worked as assistant physician at the Spanish Military Hospital but did not receive a salary until 1755. Because of his work in the hospital, Empress Maria Theresa ordered the Faculty of Medicine in 1757 to admit him as a member without charging him any fees. From 1758 to 1762 he was chief physician at the Spanish Hospital, obtaining experience in the diagnosis of chest diseases. After leaving the Spanish Hospital, Auenbrugger became one of Vienna's most distinguished physicians.

It was in 1754, while he was still working as a volunteer in the hospital, that Auenbrugger (who also wrote an opera libretto) discovered the method of percussion of the chest in order to judge the condition of the inner organs on the basis of the sound. The popular story goes that this new technique was rooted in two unrelated strains in Auenbrugger's biography: as the son of an innkeeper, he used to tap wine casks to determine their relative fullness, providing him with an analogy for the hollow cavity of the chest. And because he was highly musical, he noticed that the sounds produced by diseased and healthy chests varied considerably. Auenbrugger found out, for example, that the area over the heart gave a modified, dull sound, and that in this way the limits of heart-dullness could be determined. This gave the first definite information as to pathological changes in the heart. During the following years, Auenbrugger confirmed his initial observations by comparison with postmortem specimens, doing a number of experimental researches on dead bodies. He injected fluid into the pleural cavity and showed that it was perfectly possible by percussion to tell exactly the limits of the fluid present and thus to decide when and where efforts should be made for its removal.

Auenbrugger published his important discovery in a book entitled (in an English translation) *A New Discovery that Enables the Physician from the Percussion of the Human Thorax to Detect the Diseases Hidden Within the Chest* (1761). This seminal work is today reckoned as one of the classics in medical literature. Half a year later he published a book on lung diseases of workers in stone quarries. Although his discovery was extremely important and today still is a basic diagnostic method, it received little attention in the medical world during Auenbrugger's lifetime, although as early as 1762 Albrecht von Haller had drawn attention to 'this important work' in his lengthy review in the *Göttingische Anzeigen von Gelehrten Sachen*. Interestingly, not even his teacher Gerhard van Swieten mentioned Auenbrugger's discovery when discussing diseases of the chest. On 12 November 1783 Auenbrugger was knighted for his contributions to medicine by the Emperor Joseph II. From then on his full name was Joseph Leopold Auenbrugger, Edler von Auenbrugg. Auenbrugger died from a fatal pneumonia. Legend has it that he predicted his own death: shortly before noon of the day of his death, he surveyed his condition and, looking at the clock, stated that when 2 P.M. arrived he would have passed on. He was eighty-seven years old.

Bibliography

Primary: 1761. *Inventum novum ex percussione thoracis humani ut signo abstrusos interni pectoris morbos detegendi* (Vienna) [English translation, 1824]; 1776. *Experimentum nascens de remedio specifico sub signo specifico in mania virorum* (Vienna); 1783. *Von der stillen Wuth oder dem Triebe zum Selbstmorde als einer wirklichen Krankheit, mit Original-Beobachtungen und Anmerkungen* (Dessau).

Secondary: Smith, J. J., 1962. 'The "Inventum novum" of Joseph Leopold Auenbrugger.' *Bulletin of the New York Academy of Medicine* 38: 691–701; Bishop, P. James, 1961. 'A List of Papers, etc., on Leopold Auenbrugger (1722–1809) and the History of Percussion.' *Medical History* 5: 192–196; Ducret, Joseph, 1955. *Auenbrugger als Psychiater.* (Medical Dissertation, University of Zurich); Neuburger, Max, 1922. *Leopold Auenbrugger und sein Inventum novum.* (Vienna); Noltenius, Bernhard, 1908. *Zu der Geschichte der Perkussion von ihrer Bekanntgabe durch Auenbrugger 1761 bis zu ihrer Wiederbelebung durch Corvisart 1808.* (Leipzig).

Robert Jütte

AUTENRIETH, JOHANN HEINRICH FERDINAND VON

(b. Stuttgart, Germany, 20 October 1772; d. Tübingen, Germany, 2 May 1835), *physiology, medicine.*

Autenrieth was the son of the senior civil servant and professor of public administration Jakob Friedrich Autenrieth. Aged only thirteen, he attended lectures (1785) on natural sciences and medicine at the famous Karls-Akademie in Stuttgart, where his father gave courses as did Carl Friedrich Kielmeyer (1765–1844), whose lecture 'Ueber das Verhältnis der organischen Kräfte' [On the connection of organic forces] (1793) exerted a lasting influence on the new generation of life scientists. During Autenrieth's time at the Academy several young intellectuals also studied who would later introduce the mental transition to the romantic movement in Germany—the philosophers Friedrich Wilhelm Joseph Schelling (1775–1854) and Georg Friedrich Wilhelm Hegel (1770–1831), the lyric poet Friedrich Hölderlin (1770–1843)—as did the physiologist Christoph Heinrich Pfaff (1773–1852) and the zoologist Baron Georges Cuvier (1769–1832). Autenrieth became a member of the circle of natural scientists at the Academy and was conferred a doctorate in medicine in 1792. He then immediately went on a scientific journey to Pavia—at that time part of the Austrian-Hungarian Monarchy—to further substantiate his knowledge by studying under the Italian anatomist Antonio Scarpa (1752–1832) and the physician and head of the so-called School of Vienna, Johann Peter Frank (1745–1821). From Frank he became acquainted with the new method of bedside teaching and his ideas of public health. Two years later he returned to Stuttgart and published some of the results and experiences gathered during his scientific journeys.

In the same year Autenrieth accompanied his father to Pennsylvania. He practiced medicine for half a year in Lancaster. He survived a yellow fever infection, which encouraged his translation of Benjamin Rush's book on the 1793 yellow fever outbreak in Philadelphia. After an absence of more than a year, he returned to Stuttgart, where he received the title of Hofmedicus and, along with several other appointments, became inspector of the zoological part of the natural collection of the grand duke of Württemberg. Some years later he was appointed full professor of anatomy, physiology, surgery, and obstetrics at the University of Tübingen (1797), where he was also entrusted with the medical clinic. During the first eight years of his professorship he taught, besides anatomy and physiology, surgery, operative surgery, dietetics, and obstetrics. He planned and organized a new clinical building (1805) and was public health officer of Württemberg (1813). In this period Autenrieth excelled as a teacher of comparative anatomy and general medicine. As a clinician he distinguished himself by his unsurpassed ability to elucidate complicated cases. His main contribution may well have been that he favored a physiological approach rather than often fruitless theorizing about clinical observations. Later on, he concentrated his efforts on general pathology and therapy. Autenrieth particularly taught forensic medicine, a field in which his broad knowledge of anatomy, physiology, chemistry, and obstetrics fully proved itself. He headed the health system of a large part of Württemberg and gave numerous expert opinions in courts. He played an important part in the reorganization of the entire Württemberg health system.

Autenrieth was renowned and influential not only in Germany; his advice was much sought by foreigners, too. Autenrieth rejected several academic appointments but received many honors. Following the retirement of a former chancellor, Autenrieth became chancellor of the University of Tübingen (1822). This position too often interfered with his teaching, so he left this work to his son Hermann Friedrich Autenrieth (1799–1874), who became a distinguished physician in his own right.

Bibliography

Primary: Rush, B., 1796. *Beschreibung des gelben Fiebers, das 1793 in Philadelphia herrschte.* trans. by Johann Heinrich Ferdinand Autenrieth and Philipp Friedrich Hopfengärtner (Tübingen); 1801–02. *Handbuch der empirischen menschlichen Physiologie* 3 vols. (Tübingen); 1825. 'Wissenschaft des Menschen und seine angeborenen Beschränktheit hierin' in Autenrieth, Hermann Friedrich, ed., 1836. *Ansichten über Natur- und Seelenleben* (Stuttgart).

Secondary: Neumann, Joseph, 1985. 'Theorie und Praxis der Kinderheilkunde bei Johann Heinrich Ferdinand von Autenrieth.' *Medizinhistorisches Journal* 20: 66–82; *ADB*.

Brigitte Lohff

AZIZ, HAKIM MUHAMMAD ABDUL (b. Lucknow, India, 1855; d. Lucknow, 1911), *hakim, physician of unani.*

Hakim Abdul Aziz was the eldest son of Hakim Muhammad Ismail, a noted hakim of Lucknow (Awadh province, North India). Aziz followed the family profession of unani medicine and is remembered for establishing the first unani institution of learning in Lucknow (1902). He is also known as the founder of the Azizi family of Lucknow hakims.

Like most hakims of his time Aziz was educated at the famous Sunni Muslim seminary at Lucknow, the Firangi Mahal, where he studied religious and rational sciences. His grandfather, Hakim Muhammad Yaqub, and uncle Hakim Muhammad Ibrahim, were particularly influential in his education in unani medicine.

At a very young age, he started his own clinic, where he taught and practiced unani medicine. As a teacher, he was exemplary in his oration and memory skills. He reputedly mastered Ibn Sīnā's monumental text, the *Qanun*. He emphasized the philosophical dimension of unani and his lectures were widely attended by local students, philosophers, and leading religious scholars from Central Asia.

Aziz was a crusader for reforms in unani learning. He believed the need for reforms in the late nineteenth century was particularly pressing because of the threat unani encountered from British medicine. As the infrastructure of British medicine (in the form of dispensaries and hospitals) fanned out and British trained doctors became locally available, hakims felt threatened as never before. As colonial medicine spread, survival was possible only through adapting and changing. Aziz campaigned for two major reforms. The first was to introduce surgery in the curriculum of unani. The second was to formalize and institutionalize unani learning so that it moved from a family-based tradition to a wider public arena. Both these reforms were meant to bring unani in line and on a par with Western medicine, which was organized around these principles. Unani-trained physicians would then be competent to gain employment in the dispensaries and hospitals established by the British government in India.

Unexpectedly, Aziz received encouragement and support from the British administration in Lucknow for his reformist agenda. Lt. Col. J. Anderson, the Civil Surgeon in Lucknow, became his greatest supporter, champion, and friend. He accepted Aziz's proposal for sending hakims to the Agra Medical College for surgical training. Among the first students sent to Agra were Aziz's two sons: Abdul Rashid and Abdul Hamid. These two worked hard, learned anatomy and physiology, and mastered the art of surgery. Returning to Lucknow, they emerged as two of the earliest hakim-surgeons. Their example inspired many others to go for such training.

Hakim Aziz also received full government support for his second reform endeavor, the establishment of a unani teaching institution at Lucknow. A consultative committee comprising administrators, prominent citizens of the city, religious leaders, and talluqdars decided at its first meeting

(2 March 1902) to lay the foundations for the proposed institution. Anderson was delighted with this decision and pledged full British support. Hakim Abdul Aziz used his own resources for the initial infrastructure, the hakims of his family volunteering to teach without remuneration. Financial donations soon poured in from leading talluqdars, prominent citizens, and British surgeons. In July 1902, the 'Madrasa Takmil ut Tibb' [a school for the completion of medical education] opened in Jhawai Tola, Lucknow.

The institution offered formalized unani education during a three-year course. Ibn Sīnā's *Qanun* remained the authoritative text for the curriculum, but students received clinical and surgery lessons in the new facilities. Surgery was an important part of the curriculum. Anatomy, physiology, and chemistry were compulsory. Merit was the sole criterion for admission. Students needed a certificate from a madrasa indicating their proficiency in logic and philosophy.

Hakim Abdul Aziz thus revolutionized unani learning in colonial India. He is remembered as a renowned healer, a crusader for reform, and an able scholar. Many of his texts, e.g., *Risala Tuhafa I Azizi*, are still considered masterpieces for unani learning.

Bibliography

Primary: (reprint n. d.). Ibn Sīnā, *Al-Qanun fil Tibb* [Canon of Medicine] (Lucknow); 1888. *Risala Tuhafa I Azizi* [The Azizi Journal of Medicine] (Lucknow).

Secondary: Rahman, Hakim Syed Zillur, 1978. *Tazkira-I-Khandan-I-Azizi* [Description of the Azizi family] (Aligarh).

Seema Alavi

AZÚA Y SUÁREZ, JUAN DE (b. Madrid, Spain, 1 September 1858; d. Madrid, 5 May 1922), *dermatology, venereology.*

Azúa, son of Francisco de Azúa, a white collar worker, and of Teresa Suárez, was nephew of the homeopathic physician Juan Suárez Monge, who supported his education until his death. He finished high school in June 1873, and the same year began his studies at the Faculty of Medicine in Madrid. He was an intern pupil in the San Carlos Hospital from 1876 and graduated as MD in March 1879.

In 1886 he was admitted to the ranks of the province of Madrid's Poor Law medical services (*Beneficencia provincial*), where he worked until his death. His medical activity was closely associated with the San Juan de Dios Hospital, one of the centers belonging to the service. There, from 1860, José Eugenio Olavide (1836–1901), a prominent Spanish dermatologist, took charge of 120 beds exclusively dedicated to dermatoses. Even though Olavide backed the nosological theses held by Pierre Bazin, Azúa adopted the principles of the pathological anatomy school created by Ferdinand von Hebra in Vienna.

In 1889 he took charge of one of the two outpatient departments the hospital provided for dermatological and venereal diseases. He combined his clinical activity in the hospital with his private practice.

In 1902 Azúa started teaching the compulsory course on dermatology and syphilology at the Faculty of Medicine in Madrid. There, in 1911, he won the first chair of dermatology that was created in Spain.

It is important to emphasize his health educational activities at the public consultation room in the San Juan de Dios Hospital. He distributed 'sanitary information' consisting of printed material that included information about syphilis, gonorrhea, scabies, and ringworm; their modes of transmission; and the preventive measures recommended against them. These 'sanitary advices' were presented at the Ninth International Congress of Hygiene and Demography, which took place in Madrid in 1898, as well as at the Second International Conference for the Prophylaxis of Syphilis and Venereal Diseases (Brussels, 1902), where they were included in the conclusions. Azúa defended the benefits of disseminating notions about venereal diseases and their prevention among male adolescents and adults.

He was the driving force behind the creation, on 6 May 1909, of the Spanish Society of Dermatology and Syphilology, which was constituted in Madrid and which named him as its first President. The society's journal, *Actas Dermo-Sifiliográficas*, is still the most prestigious scientific review of Spanish dermatology.

In 1910 Azúa traveled to Frankfurt, commissioned by the Spanish government to make an on-the-spot assessment of Ehrlich's Salvarsan. His support for the treatment of syphilis with the '606', as expressed in his 1911 monograph, was decisive in the subsequent diffusion of Salvarsan in Spain. Although suffering from a hemiplegia that left him unfit to write after 1918, he presented in 1919, at the occasion of First Spanish National Congress of Medicine, a report with his results of a series of 1,838 patients treated with Salvarsan and Neosalvarsan.

His contributions to the dermatological literature include information on the 'washing dermatitis', a contact dermatitis, and on the 'cutaneous pseudoepithelioma'. In the first case, he opposed Bazin's theory of diathesis and defined 'washing dermatitis' from the point of view of external etiology.

Bibliography

Primary: 1898. 'Enfermedades de la piel' in Gayarre, M., *Vademecum clínico-terapéutico* (Madrid) pp. 289–395; 1911. *Ensayo clínico del 606* (Madrid); 1919. 'Salvarsanterapia.' *Actas Dermosifiliográficas* 11: 227–245.

Secondary: Sierra, Xavier, 1999. *Juan de Azúa y su tiempo* (Madrid); García, Antonio, and Emilio del Río, 1997. 'Los orígenes de la enseñanza de la dermatología en España.' *Actas Dermosifiliográficas* 88: 421–433; Río, Emilio del, 1996. *Los orígenes de la escuela madrileña de dermatología* (Madrid).

Ramón Castejón-Bolea

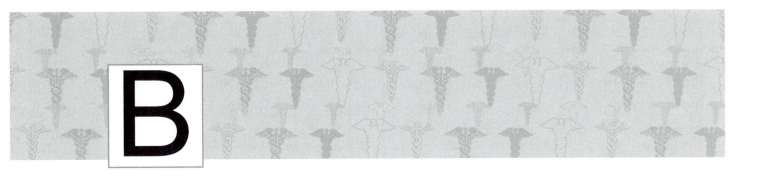

B

BABEŞ, VICTOR   (b. Vienna, Austria, 4 July 1854; d. Bucharest, Romania, 19 October 1926), *bacteriology.*

Babeş, son of Viceniu Babeş (1821–1907), one of the leaders of the Romanian national movement in Austria-Hungary, attended the lyceum in Lugoj, Budapest, and Vienna. In 1874, he was appointed assistant lecturer at the Institute of Pathological Anatomy of the Faculty of Medicine in Budapest. In 1878, he obtained his doctorate in medicine. Between 1883 and 1885, Babeş studied in Germany with Otto von Bollinger (1843–1909), Rudolf Virchow (1821–1902), and Robert Koch (1843–1910) and published his first research studies on pathological anatomy and bacteriology.

In 1884 Babeş was appointed professor agrégé in the Chair of Histopathology and Bacteriology at the Faculty of Medicine in Budapest. In 1885, together with Andre-Victor Cornil (1837–1908), he published *Les bactéries et leur role dans l'anatomie et l'histologie pathologiques des maladies infectieuses*, which is considered to be the first treatise on bacteriology. In 1887, Babeş was appointed professor of pathology and bacteriology at the Faculty of Medicine in Bucharest. In the same year, he founded the Institute of Pathology and Bacteriology, the first institute of medicine in Romania. In 1889, Babeş became a corresponding member of the Romanian Academy and was elected an active member in 1893.

Babeş synthesized many of the physiological and bacteriological theories of the time in his research. In microbiol-

ogy, for instance, he focused on the mode of infection and the ways microbes spread in organisms. He analyzed their manifestations at the level of different tissues and organs, and then illustrated the body's defense and compensation mechanisms. In 1885, Babeş demonstrated the existence of microorganisms that could create a substance capable of obstructing the growth, development, and multiplication of other microorganisms. The process of producing such a substance is known as 'antibiosis', and in many ways it complemented the principle of bacterial antagonism discovered by Louis Pasteur (1822–95) in 1877.

According to Babeş, diseases are the result of the complex interaction between micro- and macroorganisms. In 1886, while studying the morphology of microbes, he discovered a group of microorganisms (known today as Babeş's and Ernst's metachromatic granules), whose structural peculiarity helped differentiate pseudodiphtheria from diphtheria.

His research on microorganisms led Babeş into the study of parasitology. In 1888, he discovered the endoglobular parasite (*Babesia bigeminum*) responsible for the existence of hemoglobinurea in bovines—named 'Babesia' in his honor. Babeş also discovered the phenomenon of passive immunity and conducted one of the first serotherapy treatments. His research in serotherapy was furthered by the study of other laws of immunity, such as the transmission of immunity from mother to fetus (in the case of diphtheria).

In 1894, Babeş developed an original method to prepare antidiphtheric serum.

Babeş also studied the morphology of leprosy and tuberculosis, disclosing the existence of ramified infections (the actinomycosis type) in various forms of tuberculosis. He suggested that the bacillus of tuberculosis should be placed in the same bacterial group as the actinomycetes. He showed a similar interest in the study of the streptococci that caused scarlet fever. Ultimately, the morphological studies of streptococcal cultures isolated from different diseases led Babeş to conclude that streptococci constitute a wide group of parasitic germs, with marked differences among them.

Babeş is recognized as one of the founders of modern microbiology. He discovered and described more than fifty pathogenic microorganisms and made important contributions to the study of rabies, diphtheria, leprosy, serotherapy, and immunology. Babeş also exerted a decisive influence on the formation of modern Romanian biomedical thought.

Bibliography

Primary: 1885. (with Cornil, V. A.) *Les bactéries et leur role dans l'anatomie et l'histologie pathologiques des maladies infectieuses* (Paris); 1889. *Bacteriologische Untersuchungen über septische Processe des Kindesalters* (Leipzig); 1906. *Histologie des lésions experimentelles et pathologiques des cellules nerveuses, surtout des ganglions spinaux* (Berlin).

Secondary: 1979, 1980, 1982. *Opere alese* 3 vols. (Bucharest); 1954. *Bibliografia lucrărilor lui Victor Babeş* (Bucharest).

Marius Turda

BABINSKI, JOSEPH-FÉLIX-FRANÇOIS   (b. Paris, France, 17 November 1857; d. Paris, 29 October 1932), *neurology.*

Babinski's father was a Polish emigrant who left his native country for Paris in 1848 and married his compatriot, Henriette Weren. Joseph's older brother, Henri, was born in 1855. Henri would be an important person in his life. During Joseph's medical training, Henri worked abroad as a mining engineer and subsequently became Joseph's housekeeper, cook, and personal secretary. He became well-known by publishing an important book on gastronomy under the pseudonym Ali-Bab.

Babinski studied medicine, became interne des hôpitaux in 1879, and wrote a thesis on multiple sclerosis in 1885, under the supervision of Edmé-Félix Vulpian (1826–87) and André-Victor Cornil (1837–98). Subsequently, he became chef-de-clinique to Jean-Martin Charcot (1825–93). At the time, Charcot's main research subject was hysteria. In Brouillet's famous painting *Leçon clinique à la Salpêtrière*, Babinski is depicted holding the patient, Blanche Wittman.

The Babinski family moved to Boulevard Hausmann (Paris). After the death of their parents, the brothers lived there as bachelors for about thirty years. Babinski became *médecin des hôpitaux* in 1890, but failed in the competition to become *professeur agrégé*, probably due to intrigue and rivalry between the school of Charcot and that of Charcot's former pupil, Charles Bouchard (1837–1915), who was chairman of the jury. This setback blocked an academic career, and starting in 1890 Babinski worked at the *Pitié* hospital, where he stayed until his retirement in 1922. He was one of the founding members of the *Société de Neurologie* (1899), serving as a president in 1907. During World War I, he was an advisor to the French army medical corps.

Babinski performed a meticulous neurological examination after asking only a few questions. He discovered several useful tests to distinguish organic from hysterical signs, including one to distinguish organic from hysterical contracture of the hand. He also described the involuntary hip flexion on the paralyzed side when organic hemiplegic patients attempt to rise from a recumbent position ('trunk-thigh test', 1900). The best-known test is the extensor plantar response (1896), later named 'Babinski's sign' by the Belgian neurologist Arthur van Gehuchten (1861–1914). Pricking the sole of the foot on the paralyzed side elicits extension of the big toe, whereas pricking on the healthy side causes flexion. This test continues to be an important part of the present-day neurological examination, indicating a lesion of the pyramidal tract. The extensor plantar response is physiological during the first year of life and disappears as the tract becomes myelinated.

Babinski revised and greatly limited the scope of Charcot's conception of hysteria after his mentor's death. He redefined hysteria in reference to symptoms and signs that could be induced by suggestion and made to disappear by counter-suggestion. He applied the term 'pithiatism' (from Greek, cure by suggestion) instead of hysteria.

Babinski's influence on his pupils Clovis Vincent (1879–1947) and Thierry de Martel (1875–1940) was essential to the origin of French neurosurgery. As a physician interested in clinical neurology, Babinski published a large number of papers on several subjects, including brain tumors, hysteria, involuntary movements, and diseases of the spinal cord. The bibliography of his papers, collected and published two years after his death, lists 288 publications, including letters, discussions, and abstracts (1934).

Bibliography

Primary: 1896. 'Sur le réflexe cutané plantaire dans certaines affections du système nerveux central'. *CR Soc. Biol.* 48: 207–208; 1900. 'Diagnostic différentiel de l'hémiplégie organique et de l'hémiplégie hystérique'. *Gazette des Hôpitaux* 73: 521–527, 533–537; 1934. (Barré, J.-A., et al., eds.) *Oeuvres scientifiques: recueil des principaux travaux* (Paris).

Secondary: van Gijn, Jan, 1996. *The Babinski Sign—a Centenary* (Utrecht); Wartenberg, Robert, 1970. 'Joseph François Félix Babinski' in Haymaker, Webb, and Francis Schiller, eds., *The Founders of Neurology*, 2nd edn. (Springfield, IL); Alajouanine, Théophile,

1959. 'Joseph Babinski' in Kolle, K., ed., *Grosse Nervenärzte*, vol. 2 (Stuttgart) pp. 162–171.

Peter Koehler

BAELZ, ERWIN OTTO EDUARD VON (b. Bietigheim, Schwaben, Germany, 13 January 1849; d. Stuttgart, Germany, 31 August 1913), *medical education, parasitology, anthropology.*

Baelz was the second son of the nine children of Karl Baelz, a builder, and his wife Karoline. After the early death of his father and elder brother, he was expected to bear the burden of supporting the large family. Baelz (as he was called in Japan) studied at a gymnasium in Stuttgart, entered medical school at the University of Tübingen at the age of seventeen, and then moved to the University of Leipzig in 1869, where he studied under Carl A. Wunderlich (1815–77). Hard-working and competent, he became an assistant to Wunderlich and other professors at Leipzig, ready to pursue an academic career at one of the leading medical institutions in Germany.

In 1875, Baelz encountered a patient who was to change his life course entirely. He treated a Japanese public servant who had fallen ill at Leipzig. On the patient's recommendation, the Japanese government offered Baelz a professorship at the University of Tokyo, with an astonishingly competitive salary of 16,200 Deutschmarks in gold. Baelz accepted the offer, no doubt planning to come back to Germany relatively quickly. The intended short sojourn in Japan, however, turned out to be the work of a lifetime: Baelz worked for the University of Tokyo until 1902.

Building on the hard work and tough negotiation of earlier foreigner-professors such as Leopold Müller (1824–93) and Albrecht L. A. Wernich (1843–96), Baelz found it relatively easy and enjoyable to teach at the University of Tokyo. He was active also beyond the narrow confines of the medical school. Observing cholera in Tokyo in 1877, he published a pamphlet on treatment of the disease. He became a member of the Central Hygiene Board in 1879 and dealt with the Tokyo beriberi outbreak of 1881.

Baelz traveled widely in Japan, researching medical geography and anthropology. In the late 1870s and early 1880s he published dozens of important works, such as studies of indigenous varieties of *distomiasis* (liver fluke), *paragonimiasis* (lung fluke), *schistosomiasis* japonica (Oriental *schistosomiasis*), and scrub typhus (tsutsugamushi disease). He examined the medical virtues of hot spring baths and accounts of Japanese lycanthropy (possession thought to be caused by fox demons).

Baelz maintained a keen interest in anthropology, publishing extensively on the physical and cultural characteristics of people in Japan and other regions of Asia, including the *ainu* people of Hokkaido and other northern islands of Japan. He involved himself in two major disputes among Japanese intellectuals, one involving criticism of the eugenic improvement of the Japanese race (1886), and the other a defense of medical inspection of prostitutes. While engaged in intellectual pursuits, he maintained an extensive private practice among elites in Tokyo, the most important of whom was Prince Yoshihito, who later ascended to the throne as Emperor Taisho. Baelz was paid handsomely for such services, and during his stay in Japan he amassed a large collection of Japanese art that is now at the Linden Museum of Stuttgart.

While in Japan, Baelz cohabited for years with Hana, whom he married shortly before they went back to Germany in 1905. Baelz did not practice medicine after he returned home. Instead, he traveled widely and worked on a comparative anthropology project.

Baelz died in 1913. His only surviving child, Toku, edited his father's voluminous diaries and published them in 1931, heavily censoring accounts of Baelz's private life and political views. A bronze bust of Baelz adorns the Medical School of the University of Tokyo, and a medicine that bears his name (Baelz water) is still sold today.

Bibliography

Primary: 1979. (Baelz, Toku, ed.) *Berutsu no nikki* [Diaries of Baelz] trans. Suganuma Ryūtaō (Tokyo). [Originally in German (1931), *Das Leben eines deutschen Arztes im erwachenden Japan*; in English (1932), *Awakening Japan: the Diary of a German Doctor Erwin Baelz*]; 2000. *Berutsu Nihon saihō* [Revisiting Baelz's Japan] trans. Hiroko Ikegami (Tokyo); 2001. *Berutsu Nihon bunka ronshū* [Collected Papers of Baelz on Japanese Culture] trans. Misako Wakabayashi and Sei-ichi Yamaguchi (Tokyo).

Secondary: Yasui, Hiroshi, 1995. *Berutsu no shōgai* [The Life of Baelz] (Kyoto).

Akihito Suzuki

BAER, KARL ERNST VON (b. Piep, near Jerwen, Estonia, 29 February 1792; d. Dorpat, Estonia, 28 November 1876), *biology, embryology, anthropology, geography.*

Von Baer was one of ten children born to Magnus Johann von Baer, an Estonian landholder and head of a district authority, and his cousin Louise von Baer. Because of the large size of the family, Karl lived for his first seven years with Magnus Johann's brother and his wife, Baroness Ernestine von Canne, who were childless. There he acquired the love for plants that would lead to his lifelong interest in botany and natural history.

After finishing his schooling in Reval (Tallinn), Baer studied medicine at the University of Dorpat. He was particularly impressed by the physiology lectures of Karl Friedrich Burdach (1776–1847) and those in geography by Georg Friedrich Parrot (1767–1852). After writing his medical thesis on endemic diseases in Estonians (1814), he left Dorpat for further studies in Germany and Austria. In 1815 and 1816 he trained in comparative anatomy at the University of Würzburg with Ignaz Döllinger (1770–1841), who introduced him to the new world of developmental problems and embryology. His teacher, Burdach, invited him to

Königsberg in 1816. Three years later Baer was elected extraordinary professor of anatomy at the University of Königsberg, where he later became full professor of zoology (1821) and anatomy (1826). He founded a zoological museum there and served several times as director of the botanical gardens. In 1820, Baer married Auguste von Medem of Königsberg, by whom he had six children.

Baer taught for twelve years at the University of Königsberg (1821–33), and the whole time he hesitated to accept an academic position at the Academy of Sciences in St Petersburg. After receiving a second invitation, Baer became a full member in zoology of the St Petersburg Academy of Sciences (1834). He remained there for the rest of his working life, more than thirty years. Baer received many honors and belonged to several international academies of science. His scientific work was of vital importance to the development of Russian science, and in recognition of his contributions an island in northern Russia was named after him.

In Würzburg, Döllinger had suggested that Baer study chick development by improved methods. He analyzed the blastoderm removed from the egg yolk, working with Christian Heinrich Pander (1794–1864), who described (1817) the early development of the chick in the well-known terms of the primary germ layers. From 1819 to 1834, Baer devoted most of his time to embryology, extending the concept of germ-layer formation to all vertebrates. Baer's discovery that the ovaries of mammals—including humans—contained eggs (1826) was published in *De ovi mammalium et homiinis genesi*. He concluded that 'every animal which springs from the coition of male and female is developed from an ovum, and none from a simple formative liquid' (Baer, 1827, p. 37). This was a unifying doctrine whose scientific importance cannot be overemphasized. He also studied the development of other vertebrates.

In 1828, Baer proposed his law of animal development, which states that embryos of one species can resemble the embryos—but not the adults—of another species, and that the younger the embryo, the greater the resemblance. In pre-Darwinian times the descent of animals was seen as equivalent to embryonic development. Baer established the new science of comparative embryology as a complement to comparative anatomy. His most important work was his treatise *Ueber die Entwicklungsgeschichte der Thiere, Beobachtung und Reflexion*, the publication of which provided the basis for the systematic study of animal development. He was also a pioneer in geography, ethnology, and physical anthropology.

Bibliography

Primary: 1827. *Ueber die Bildung des Eies der Säugetiere und des Menschen.* (Leipzig) [English trans., 1956]; 1828–37. *Ueber Entwicklungsgeschichte der Thiere: Beobachtung und Reflexion* 2 vols. (Königsberg); 1864–1876. *Reden* 3 vols. (St Petersburg).

Secondary: Groeben, Christiane, 1993. 'Karl Ernst Von Baer (1792–1876) und Anton Dohrn (1840–1909): Correspondence'. *Transactions of the American Philosophical Society* 83 (part 3); Conradi, Paul, ed., 1912. *Dr. Karl Ernst von Baer. Eine Selbstbiographie* (Leipzig); Stieda, Ludwig, 1886. *Karl Ernst von Baer*, 2nd edn. (Königsberg) [English edn., 1986, Canton, MA], *DSB.*

Brigitte Lohff

BAGLIVI, GIORGIO (b. Republic of Dubrovnick [now Dubrovnick, Croatia], 8 September 1668; d. Rome, Italy, 15 June 1707), *medicine, physiology.*

Baglivi's father, Vlaho Armen, was a merchant of Armenian origin (hence his name) who lived in Dubrovnik. His mother, Anica Vukovic, died during the delivery of her second son, Jakov, when Giorgio was two years old, and their father died soon afterwards. The two brothers were first brought up by their uncles and then entered the Jesuit College.

When Giorgio was fifteen, a request came to the Jesuit school from Pietro Angelo Baglivi (1624–1704), a physician from Lecce who had no son and wished to adopt a boy of talent. The physician adopted the two brothers officially in 1687, giving them his family name. Jakov (Giacomo) pursued an ecclesiastic career, and Giorgio, after a preliminary training in practical medicine with his adoptive father, went to study medicine in Naples and Salerno, receiving his MD and PhD in 1686.

After receiving his degrees, Baglivi visited the most prestigious Italian universities, namely Ferrara, Padua, and Florence, where he studied with Lorenzo Bellini (1643–1704), working also in the hospitals of those cities. He came into contact with several leading physicians and scientists and started an extensive correspondence, most of which survives.

In 1691 Baglivi settled in Bologna. He studied with Marcello Malpighi (1628–94), who pushed him to continue his research in physiology and microscopic anatomy. When Pope Innocent XII appointed Malpighi as his personal physician, the latter moved to Rome. Baglivi followed him as his secretary, living in his house. In Rome Baglivi also became Giovanni Lancisi's (1654–1720) assistant.

After Malpighi's death in 1694, Baglivi performed the autopsy, showing that the cause of the death had been a cerebral hemorrhage. Baglivi became the second physician to Pope Innocent XII in 1695, and later Pope Clement XI confirmed his position at court. In 1696 he was appointed professor of anatomy at the University of Rome 'La Sapienza', where in 1701 he became professor of theoretical medicine. Baglivi was a member of many academies, including the Royal Society of London (1698), the German academy Caesareo-Leopoldina Natura Curiosorum (1696), and the Accademia dei Fisiocratici (1700).

Baglivi's works center on two main domains, clinical medicine and experimental physiology. In the first field, he produced a classic work, *De praxi medica* (1696), in which he suggested a new Hippocratism: a return to the Hippocratic method, based on clinical and empirical observations. This book had a large impact and was translated into English eight years later.

The return to Hippocratic empiricism was combined in *De praxi medica* with an explicit adhesion to a Baconian scientific methodology. On the first page of the book he wrote: 'a physician is the minister and the interpreter of nature; whatever he thinks and does, if he does not obey nature, he will not command nature.' The starting point of medical knowledge was the *Historiae morborum*, i.e., bedside observations of pathological phenomena, considered to be the *Medicina prima*, with the treatment of diseases being only the *Medicina secunda*. The first chapter was titled 'Of the absolute necessity of Observations in the way of Physick', and in several places he condemned 'the preposterous interpretation of books' and refuted 'the pernicious custom of making systems'. Baglivi referred frequently to the ideas of Thomas Sydenham (1624–89) as a model for a medicine based on direct observation of clinical cases. He agreed with Sydenham that a disease was a specific entity, which exists independently, and that each disease had an essential nature, which remains identical in different individuals, thus allowing the definition of the essence of disease and its classification.

Baglivi, however, went further. He opposed the traditional medical systems and considered isolation of the specific cause of each disease imperative. This was possible only through experimentation; microscopy, comparative physiology, and anatomy were the experimental tools needed. He proposed a Galilean method based on physical analyses—numbering, weighing, and measuring—and on this basis he edited Santorio Santorio's book *De statica medicina* (1614) in 1704.

There was therefore a strict continuity between clinical observation on one hand and anatomical, physiological, and pathological observations and experiments in the other. Baglivi included several descriptions of vivisections and experiments he had performed. For example, he took out the heart of a frog and put it upon a table, observing that the isolated organ continued to beat with a regular systole and diastole for half an hour after. This suggested that the heartbeat was independent of innervations and resulted from a myogenic force.

The same effort to counsel observation and experimentation was evident in Baglivi's proposal to the Roman authorities to create a new kind of medical academy. In his *De praxi medica* he suggested the creation of a *Medicorum collegium*, composed of two kinds of members, one to consist of 'commentators' devoted to 'reading the Books that contain Observations' and the other, the 'collectors', charged with daily 'making and setting down new Observations'. The collection of clinical observations through the critical reading of texts produced *experientia*, and the direct clinical observation and laboratory work were defined as *experimentum*. The rational combination of experientia with experimentum was the only valid *Methodus medendi* according to Baglivi.

The second center of interest for Baglivi was the search for the mechanical causes of disease. The book *De fibra mot-*rice expounded his solidistic physiopathology, in which diseases were explained as clinical syndromes due to a lesion of a specific organ or tissue. Baglivi's two major works were directly continuous and actually written in parallel, starting in 1692, but the two books had different destinies. *De praxi medica* was published in a complete form and had a magnificent linguistic and stylistic accuracy and a clear and rational aphoristic structure. *De fibra motrice* in contrast was never finished, first published in 1700 as a letter to the doctor Alessandro Pascoli and then printed in Rome in 1702 as *Specimen quatuor librorum de fibra motrice et morbosa, in quibus de solidorum structura, vi, elatere, aequilibrio, usu potestate, et morbis disseretur*. The title was repeated when the same provisional version was integrated into the 1704 *Opera omnia*.

The two books, with their differing form and content, together constituted the expression of Baglivi's efforts to realize a 'rational medicine', a synthesis of the clinical activity of bedside observation and the theoretical and systematic search for the cause of natural phenomena, normal and pathological. He was against the use in medicine of principles and explanations drawn from other sciences or from philosophical postulates, but at the same time he insisted on the need for a theoretical analysis of laws and principles used to find the causes of disease. For that reason, a century later, Philippe Pinel (1745–1826) considered Baglivi to be the author of the new project for a general pathology, i.e., a general medical science 'based on the descriptive observation of acute diseases' (1819).

Baglivi defined fibers as the fundamental component of the living organism. To Baglivi, fibers were more important than the traditional liquids suggested by the humoral pathology. They were composed of atoms and possessed a *vis innata*, an innate irritability and spontaneous contractility, in addition to the passive movement of the solid parts. Living fibers were the seat of vital functions and the seat also of diseases.

Baglivi divided fibers into two types: fleshy and membranous, the first being a component of muscles, tendons, and bones. With the help of a compound microscope, he studied isolated muscle fibers, obtained by soaking muscle in a solution of water, alcohol, and vinegar, and established the difference between smooth and striated muscles. Membranous fibers were finer and formed from the nervous fluid and lymph: they were the constituents of nerves, glands, and sensory and visceral organs. Muscles were also wrapped in a membrane originating from the nerves, which explained the brain's ability to influence the muscles. Baglivi also suggested a difference between the autonomous and voluntary nervous systems: the differences between innate (vegetative) and voluntary (animal) movements resulted from 'the different constitution of the parts that are moved naturally and without a voluntary decision, such as heart, vessels, intestines, and sphincters'.

Fibers were the structural elements of bodily parts, but they were also the basis of their dynamic behavior. Giovanni Borelli (1608–79) had already suggested an oscillatory movement of the organism's solid parts. Baglivi developed this idea, attributing to each fiber an essential oscillatory movement, with the whole forming a pulsating structure. The body was thus an oscillating machine—a *horologium oscillatorium*—continuously controlled by the soul. The soul was located in the brain, which he considered a sort of 'control center', which ensured the coordination of the movements of the parts.

On this basis, Baglivi suggested in a famous work, written at the request of J. J. Manget and published in 1698 in his medical encyclopedia, a mechanical explanation of the therapeutic effect of music in the cases of tarantulism. The bite of the tarantula produced a total disharmony of body's vibrations. The body's order could be reestablished by the order imposed by music and continuous dancing. Music and dance had a positive effect because they reestablished the natural oscillations of the fibers, equilibrating their excess or absence and also eliminating the pathological particles inoculated.

Baglivi tried to establish a great synthesis between clinical medicine and its theoretical basis, transforming both to produce a rational medicine based on a critical and informed reading of classical texts, the collection of evidence at the bedside, and the production of results in the laboratory with the new experimental method and through comparative microscopy. The result was to be a rational therapeutics. It was a very ambitious program, and Baglivi would not have the time to try to realize his ambitions. He died in 1707, aged thirty-nine, probably from the consequences of a severe malarial attack, common in the Roman Campagna.

Bibliography

Primary: 1704. *Opera omnia medico-practica et anatomica* (Lugduni); 1696. *De praxi medica ad priscam observandi rationem revocanda. Libri duo. Accedunt dissertationes novae.* (Rome) (English trans., 1704. *The Practice of Physick,* London); 1698. 'De Anatome, Morsu & Effectibus Tarantulae' in Manget, Johannes Jacobus, ed., *Bibliotheca medico-pratica* vol. 4 (Geneva) pp. 616–645; 1700. *De fibra motrice et morbosa* (Epistola ad Alexandrum Pascolum) (Rome); 1702. *Specimen quatuor librorum de fibra motrice et morbosa, in quibus de solidorum structura, vi, elatere, aequilibrio, usu potestate, et morbis disseretur* (Rome); 1974. (Schullian, Dorothy, ed.) *The Baglivi correspondence from the library of Sir William Osler* (Ithaca and London).

Secondary: Fye, W. B., 2002. 'Giorgio Baglivi.' *Clinical Cardiology* 25: 487–489; Grmek, M. D., 1991. 'La vita e l'opera di Giorgio Baglivi, medico raguseo e leccese (1668–1707)' in Cimino, G., U. Sanzo, and G. Sava, eds., *Il nucleo filosofico della scienza* (Galatina) pp. 93–139; *DSB.*

Bernardino Fantini

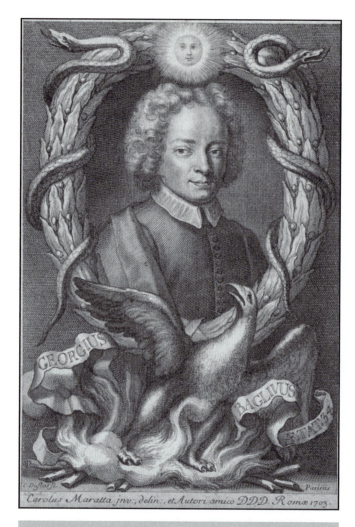

Giorgio Baglivi. Line engraving by Claude Duflos after Carlo Maratta, 1703. Iconographic Collection, Wellcome Library, London.

BAILLIE, MATTHEW (b. Shotts, Lanarkshire, Scotland, 27 October 1761; d. Duntisbourne Abbots, Gloucestershire, England, 23 September 1823), *medicine, pathology.*

Baillie was the second son of James Baillie, clergyman and later Professor of Divinity at the University of Glasgow, and Dorothea Hunter, sister of William and John Hunter. He was educated at schools in Hamilton and then at the University of Glasgow. In 1779 he was nominated for the Snell Exhibition at Balliol College, Oxford, which was in the gift of the Glasgow professors. He lived in Oxford for eighteen months, studying classics and English history, but late in 1780 moved to London to take up residence with William Hunter (1718–83). He kept the terms at Oxford and graduated BA in 1783. Baillie attended the lectures and demonstrations at his uncle's school on Great Windmill Street and began to teach in the dissecting room in the following year. He also took classes in physic, surgery, obstetrics, and chemistry from, among other teachers, John Hunter (1728–93), and walked the wards at St George's Hospital.

In 1783 William Hunter died, leaving the school and its premises to Baillie. Hunter's museum collection was gifted to Glasgow University, but Baillie was granted a lifetime's use of it. Baillie graduated BM from Oxford in 1786 and DM in 1789. He was appointed physician to St George's in 1787 and elected FRCP and FRS in 1790.

On Hunter's death, his second major work, *An Anatomical Description of the Human Gravid Uterus and Its Contents*, remained in manuscript. Baillie prepared a publishable edition, which appeared in 1794. Baillie's historical importance rests, however, with his *The Morbid Anatomy of Some of the Most Important Parts of the Human Body*, which he published in 1793. In the preface, Baillie acknowledged his debt to the earlier work of Giovanni Morgagni (1682–1771), *De sedibus et causis morborum* (1761), but Baillie's approach to his subject matter differed radically from that of the Italian physician and anatomist. In the three volumes of his great compendium, Morgagni labored to record all the details of each case he discussed, from initial presentation to postmortem appearances. His prolix accounts displayed the value of careful description of pathological lesions and of correlating observations made at the bedside with those made at necropsy. But it requires some dedication to read Morgagni's text, and *De sedibus* would certainly not have been easy to use as a work of reference. Baillie, in contrast, provided concise and exact descriptions of a carefully chosen selection of pathological alterations of structure. *Morbid Anatomy* is a neat octavo book, with 314 pages of main text, compared to the three quarto volumes and thousands of leaves of *De sedibus*. The difference between the two books represents not merely a more ruthless editing and pruning of extraneous material from the later publication, but a determination to focus attention more narrowly on pathological change. Baillie's text effectively expressed a novel conception of morbid anatomy as a scientific pursuit in its own right, a form of inquiry that, while remaining relevant to clinical practice, was not wholly encompassed within it, as had been assumed in Morgagni's enterprise.

Baillie drew upon his considerable experience in hospital practice, where he enjoyed a regular supply of postmortem material. He also fruitfully exploited his privileged access to Hunter's substantial collection of pathological specimens. In some instances, Baillie presented unusual cases with the relish of a collector but, overall, he provided matter-of-fact, yet memorable, descriptions of the most common pathological alterations of each organ. For example, his account of emphysema (he did not use that term) was vivid and precise. Baillie's survey was confined to the brain, the organs of the abdominal and thoracic cavities, and the genitalia, but included congenital abnormalities as well as acquired pathological changes. He described several 'defects of formation' of the sexual organs, as well as discussing patent ductus arteriosis and ventricular septal defect. While *Morbid Anatomy* was not organized around specific case histo-

ries, Baillie was sufficiently experienced and acute as a practitioner to be able reliably to distinguish between pathological changes that were clinically significant and structural alterations that were either trivial or within normal variation. He also confidently differentiated between changes that had occurred during life and those that had followed death.

Baillie generally chose not to speculate upon the link between morbid cause and structural effect. For instance, while he tellingly noted the association between the formation of what he termed 'tubercles' in the substance of the liver and heavy drinking, he remarked 'we cannot see any connection between that mode of life and this particular disease'. Baillie was regretfully aware that 'the knowledge of morbid structure does not certainly lead to the knowledge of morbid action', but argued that 'surely it lays the most solid foundation for prosecuting such inquiries with success' in the future. Likewise he chose only occasionally to comment on the clinical significance of the changes he described. Baillie was not insensitive to such matters, however. For instance, he advised caution in surgical management of prostate enlargement and remarked that a gross enlargement of the clitoris is a 'most unfortunate monstrosity, because it depresses the mind, by a consciousness of imperfect function in a very important part of the body'.

In his preface to the first edition, Baillie indicated his intention to revise the text periodically as his knowledge of morbid anatomy increased. That was not, however, the direction taken by the second edition of 1797. Presumably in response to the reactions of the readership of the first edition, Baillie appended a section on symptoms to the end of most of the chapters. This may be seen either as a step back toward Morgagni's exemplar or as paralleling the development of a clinico-anatomical approach by the members of the Paris School. What seems certain is that the new clinical material greatly enhanced the popularity of the text among students and practitioners. Most of the numerous translations and foreign editions of *Morbid Anatomy* were based upon the second edition, and it has been regarded as being the most influential version of Baillie's work.

Baillie qualified and practiced as a physician. But he might be said to have also acquired a surgical outlook, both from the teachings of his celebrated uncles and in the course of his own studies in normal and morbid anatomy. Owsei Temkin famously associated the origins of nineteenth-century clinico-anatomical medicine with the assimilation of surgical modes of thought into the theory and practice of internal medicine. He cited, for instance, the rise of physical examination in the first half of the century as an example of this process of cross-fertilization. In the eighteenth century, by contrast, diagnosis was largely based upon the patient's verbal account of his or her condition. Thus it is interesting to note that in the second edition of *Morbid Anatomy* there are several examples of Baillie laying his hands directly on the bodies of his patients in the course of his consultations:

'An accurate attention to the feeling, which the tumour yields upon pressure, or upon striking it gently with the hand, may also assist in forming a probable conjecture about its nature. When the tumour consists of hydatids, it will generally feel to a certain degree soft; and if the hydatids should be very large, there will be an obscure sense of fluctuation upon striking the tumour with one's hand, while the other is applied to the opposite side of it' (cited in Rodin, 1973, p. 180).

Baillie also described vaginal examination and the palpation of a hydropic testicle. That Baillie was exceptional in this aspect of his practice may be gauged from the reaction of his fellow physicians. His younger contemporary, William MacMichael (1784–1839), for instance, commented upon Baillie's use of physical examination but concluded that the method was problematic and yielded uncertain results.

A new edition of *Morbid Anatomy* was published in ten parts between 1799 and 1802, with the text illustrated by a series of very fine engravings of drawings by William Clift (1775–1849) and with additional commentary by Baillie. This was, however, Baillie's last major publication. His practice as a physician was so successful that in 1799 he gave up both his position at St George's Hospital and his teaching of anatomy. In 1810 he was appointed physician-in-ordinary to George III, and he was one of the medical attendants during the King's 'madness'. Baillie's professional reputation seems to have survived his involvement, as a physician, in the disastrous confinement of Princess Charlotte in 1817. He became a very wealthy man and purchased an estate in Gloucestershire, from which he consulted by correspondence. He enjoyed good health until early 1823, when he began to suffer from a wasting disease, possibly tubercular in nature. He died later that year.

Bibliography

Primary: Wardrop, James, ed., 1825. *The Works of Matthew Baillie: To Which Is Prefixed an Account of His Life* (London); 1793. *The Morbid Anatomy of Some of the Most Important Parts of the Human Body* (London).

Secondary: Rodin, A. E., 1973. *The Influence of Matthew Baillie's Morbid Anatomy: Biography, Evaluation and Reprint* (Springfield, IL); MacMichael, W., 1968. (facsimile of 1827 edition) *The Gold-Headed Cane* (London); *DSB*; *Oxford DNB*.

Malcolm Nicolson

BAKER, SARA JOSEPHINE

BAKER, SARA JOSEPHINE (b. Poughkeepsie, New York, USA, 15 November 1873; d. New York, New York, USA, 22 February 1945), *medicine, public health administration, pediatrics.*

Baker was the daughter of Orlando Daniel Mosher Baker, an attorney, and Jenny Harwood Brown Baker. She received her MD from the Woman's Medical College of the New York

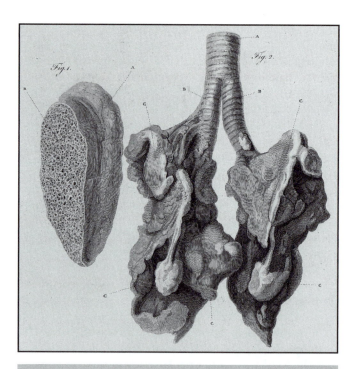

Pathological specimen of Samuel Johnson's emphysematous lungs. Engraving from Baillie's *Morbid Anatomy . . .* London, 1793. Rare Books, Wellcome Library, London.

Infirmary in 1898 and her DPH from New York University's Bellevue Medical College in 1917. She interned at the New England Hospital for Women and Children in Boston in 1898–99. Afterward she returned to Manhattan and opened a private practice. To supplement her income, Baker became a medical inspector for the New York Health Department and eventually an assistant to the commissioner of health. Baker soon devoted her career to public health work and played a vital role in the massive expansion of public health services in the United States at the turn of the century.

In her early years at the health department, Baker surveyed the health of children, tracked contagious diseases in schools, vaccinated against smallpox in the lodging-houses of the Bowery, and observed the treacherous living conditions of the city's working and immigrant poor. She even took part in the search for Mary Mallon, 'Typhoid Mary', and tried to collect specimens from the resistant Irish cook.

Baker witnessed firsthand the serious problems of childhood illness and death that plagued New York City and called for the creation of public health education and preventive medicine programs. She was fundamental in the founding of the first Division of Child Hygiene and served as its chief between 1908 and 1923. She directed the regulation and education of midwives, worked to upgrade conditions in nurseries and hospitals, and expanded health inspections in city schools. Baker implemented a new program for foundlings, removing them from hospitals and boarding them out to private homes, into the personal care of qualified foster mothers. In addition, Baker created Baby Health Stations to provide quality milk to needy mothers and to educate women in 'scientific child care'. She also created 'Little Mothers' Leagues' to teach young immigrant girls how to better care for their younger siblings while their mothers were occupied with work. Baker advocated the adoption of these policies on a national level, and became a supporter of and consultant to the federal Children's Bureau.

Between 1915 and 1930, Baker lectured on child hygiene at Bellevue Hospital Medical School of New York University. As part of her compensation, she demanded admission to the school's Doctor of Public Health program; the administration reluctantly agreed, and she became the program's first female student and graduate. In addition to her teaching, Baker published numerous articles and a series of books on infant, child, and maternal health; she also published her autobiography, *Fighting for Life* (1939). Between 1922 and 1924, she was the U.S. representative to the Health Committee of the League of Nations. She was a strong advocate for women physicians, serving as President of the American Medical Women's Association in 1935. Baker was also active in the last phase of the American woman suffrage movement, delivering lectures and taking part in Fifth Avenue parades.

Baker is remembered for her vital contributions to the sharp decline in New York City's infant mortality rate. She believed in the power of government agencies to secure the health of children and families, and her programs served as national models for public health departments. Baker also carved out new space for women in medicine by helping to expand their role as public health workers in the Progressive era.

Bibliography

Primary: 1920. *Healthy Mothers* (Boston); 1923. *Healthy Babies* (Boston); 1925. *Child Hygiene* (New York); 1939. *Fighting for Life* (New York).

Secondary: More, Ellen S., 1999. *Restoring the Balance: Women Physicians and the Profession of Medicine, 1850–1995* (Cambridge, MA); Morantz-Sanchez, Regina, 1985. *Sympathy and Science: Women Physicians in American Medicine* (New York); Baumgartner, Leona, 1971. 'Sara Josephine Baker.' *Notable American Women* (Cambridge, MA) 1: 85–86; *DAMB*.

Carla Bittel

BALASSA, JÁNOS VON   (b. Sárszentlőrinc, Hungary, 5 May 1814; d. Pest, Hungary, 9 December 1868), *surgery, medical education, medical publishing.*

The son of a Protestant minister serving a rural parish, Balassa studied in Vienna, as did other promising prospective Hungarian physicians of the day. There he earned his doctor's credentials (he was said to have a natural talent for the study of medicine) and came under the influence of the reform-minded members of the faculty, notably Joseph Skoda (1805–81) and Karl Rokitansky (1804–78). Balassa found one hallmark of this so-called Vienna School—the use of pathological anatomy as a diagnostic tool—particularly exciting, though his surgical mentor, Joseph Wattmann, did not wholly share his enthusiasm.

When another faculty member (Franz Schuh) was appointed to a second surgical chair, he chose Balassa as his assistant and gave his young protégé free rein to develop his scientific understanding of pathology and anatomy. With his medical degree only four years old, Balassa was offered the chair in surgery at the Pest university in 1842. Working in a Catholic institution, he insisted that both Protestants and Catholics be permitted to study science and that medicine be scientifically based. Balassa is generally considered responsible for raising medical education standards in Budapest and for modernizing surgery in Hungary. Despite initial skepticism from older colleagues, his message that science should prevail over dogma was accepted in due course.

Balassa had exemplary surgical skills. Famous for his steady hand and bold approach, he carried out a wide variety of operations and is credited with several surgical firsts in Hungary. He performed some of the earliest laparotomies and operated successfully on ovarian cysts. He was a master at 'cutting for the stone', and he had remarkable success in reconstructive surgery. Balassa also performed one of the first operations in Europe using ether anesthesia, just after John Collins Warren had done so in Boston.

At the stirrings of revolutionary activity in Hungary in 1848, Balassa was appointed surgeon general of the Hungarian army (he directed that all field surgery be performed under general anesthesia). His prominence in that position led to his being imprisoned after the revolution, but his early release, in response to widespread pleas for mercy, is a measure of the public esteem in which he was held. This esteem was evident again, when—shortly before his death—the twenty-fifth anniversary of his university appointment was celebrated by ordinary citizens and the academic world alike.

Though Balassa published no major original works, he wrote numerous journal articles in Latin, German, and Hungarian. He made a valuable and well-received contribution when he edited, in Hungarian, two volumes of monographs on surgery. He was instrumental in establishing a medical publishing company that gave Hungarian physicians an incentive to publish their own work and helped them stay abreast of what their Hungarian colleagues were writing. Balassa was involved also in the founding of *Orvosi Hetilap* [Medical Weekly] and was the founding president of the Hungarian Public Health Commission.

Only fifty-six when he died, Balassa had been honored with the Austrian title of *Hofrat*, made personal physician to the Empress of Austria-Hungary and knighted. He had been made an honored member of the Hungarian Academy of Sciences in 1858. Mourned as Hungary's greatest medical teacher and most-loved physician, he received numerous tributes.

Balassa's death was deemed a national tragedy. A black flag was hung from the window of the surgical clinic in Pest, and Hungarian medical students in Vienna rushed home to pay final tribute. In Budapest, thousands followed his coffin.

Bibliography

Primary: 1851. 'Andeutung zur zweckmässigen Einrichtung des chirurgischen Studiums.' *Wiener med. Wochenschr.* 1: 241; 1856. *Unterleibs-Hernien. Vom klinischen Standpunkte mit topographisch-u. pathologisch-anatomischen Daten beleuchtet* (Vienna); 1858. 'Über Harnsteine in Ungarn.' *Wiener med. Wochenschr.* 8: 441, 465.

Secondary: Albert, E. et al., eds., 1929–34. *Biographisches Lexikon der hervorragenden Ärzte aller Zeiten und Völker*, vol. 1: 298–299 (Berlin). [Obituary], 1868. *Allg. Wiener med. Zeitung* 13: 412–413.

Constance Putnam

BALINT, MICHAEL MAURICE   (b. Budapest, Hungary, 3 December 1896; d. London, England, 31 December 1970), *psychoanalysis, general practice.*

The son of a Budapest Jewish general practitioner (GP), Mihaly Maurice Bergman changed his name early to Michael Balint. His medical training in Budapest was interrupted by World War I; he served on the Russian front and the Italian Dolomites until a grenade accident invalided him back home. He married Alice Székely-Kovács in 1918 and gained his MD in 1920. The couple moved to Berlin, where Balint obtained his PhD in biochemistry in 1924 but was increasingly occupied by his other passion, psychoanalysis. In Berlin he had studied part-time under the psychoanalyst Hanns Sachs, and after returning to Budapest in 1924, he trained under Sandor Ferenczi—both former pupils of Sigmund Freud. He entered psychoanalytic practice in Budapest and during the late 1920s began to run psychoanalysis seminars for GPs.

A decade later, Hungary's reactionary Horthy regime was sympathetic neither to psychoanalysis nor to Jews; in 1939 Balint emigrated to England with Alice, who died a few months later. Balint remarried, to Edna Hernshaw in 1943, but separated from her shortly after. Facing execution by the Nazis, Balint's parents committed suicide in 1945. Balint requalified in order to practice medicine in Britain, and worked as a psychiatrist first in Manchester, where he obtained his MSc in 1948 studying infant behavior, then at the Tavistock clinic in London, where he moved in 1949. His interest in psychodynamic techniques in general practice was rekindled by his involvement with the Family Discussion Bureau, a group training social workers

in managing marriage problems; in 1953 the group leader, Enid Flora Eicholtz (later Balint-Edmonds after remarriage following Balint's death) became his third wife. Balint ran seminars for GPs at the Tavistock clinic from 1950, and developed his own concepts and teaching methods. His ideas became codified, notably in his 1956 publication *The Doctor, His Patient and the Illness.* He and Enid disseminated his methods in Britain and abroad, where interested practitioners formed 'Balint groups' to employ his techniques. Retiring from the Tavistock clinic at sixty-five, Balint continued his work with GPs in the psychological medicine department at London's University College Hospital. He was made president of the British Psychoanalytical Society in 1970; suffering poor health and deteriorating vision due to diabetes and glaucoma, he died at the end of that year.

Balint's contribution to psychotherapeutics is significant and derives from the implications of the early mother-infant relationship for psychoanalytical technique. But it is his insights into the work of the GP that form his enduring legacy. Balint placed the doctor-patient relationship center stage as a valid object for study. Central to his ideas was the therapeutic potential of the doctor-patient interaction—characterized in the phrase 'the doctor as drug'. Like any other drug, this one had to be employed judiciously and had a potential for side effects or inappropriate use. His GP seminars involved discussion of individual cases, exploring the doctor's emotional responses to the patient's presentation. The 'doctor as drug', Balint reasoned, was a reflection of the physician's own personality, and therefore to employ it optimally required subtle changes in personality—the aim of Balint's sessions. Many British GPs felt demoralized during the 1950s and early 1960s, when they were in the shadow of their more glamorous hospital colleagues, poorly paid, working in inadequate conditions, and overwhelmed by patients with 'trivial' or neurotic illnesses for which medical school training had ill prepared them. Balint's work represented an important part of a movement to reclaim a unique and privileged status for general practice, and enabled the renaissance in GPs' confidence and status beginning in the late 1960s.

Bibliography

Primary: 1956. *The Doctor, His Patient and the Illness* (London); 1961. (with Balint, E.) *Psychotherapeutic Techniques in Medicine* (London).

Secondary: Osborne, Thomas, 1993. 'Mobilizing Psychoanalysis: Michael Balint and the General Practitioners.' *Social Studies of Science* 23: 175–200; Balint-Edmonds, Enid, 1984. 'The history of training and research in Balint-groups.' *Journal of the Balint Society* 12: 3–7; [Obituary], 1971. 'Michael Balint.' *British Medical Journal* i: 179; [Obituary], 1971. 'Michael Balint.' *Lancet* i: 144–145; *Oxford DNB.*

Martin Edwards

BALLINGALL, GEORGE

BALLINGALL, GEORGE   (b. Forglen, Banffshire, Scotland, 2 May 1786; d. Altamont, Blairgowrie, Perthshire, Scotland, 4 December 1855), *surgery, military surgery.*

Ballingall was the eldest son of the Rev Robert Ballingall, minister of Forglen, Banffshire, and his wife Elizabeth, daughter of James Simpson of Edenhead. He attended the Parish School of Falkland, Fifeshire, then St Andrews University, and was apprenticed to Dr Melville. He commenced his medical studies in the University of Edinburgh in 1803. He also attended the extramural classes in anatomy of John Barclay (1758–1826), to complement the uninspiring classes of the University's professor of anatomy and surgery, Alexander Monro *tertius* (1773–1859), and later became Barclay's assistant. Ballingall gained the LRCSEd diploma in December 1805.

Ballingall entered the 2nd Battalion of the 1st (Royal) Regiment of Foot in May 1806 as a Hospital Mate, but was soon promoted to the rank of Assistant Surgeon. His commanding officer was the Duke of Kent, who later became one of Ballingall's principal patrons. Ballingall initially went with this regiment to Madras, but in 1811 transferred to the 22nd Dragoons and accompanied them on an expedition to Java. He returned to India, where he spent most of the rest of his military career. In October 1815, after his appointment as Surgeon to the 33rd Regiment of Foot, he attended the occupation of Paris following the Allied victory at Waterloo. He returned to Edinburgh on half pay from the army in 1818, and was eventually put on the retired list in 1831. He returned to the University of Edinburgh in 1816–17 and obtained his MD degree in 1819. In 1818 he married the daughter of a distant cousin, James Ballingall of Perth. In 1821 he obtained his FRCSEd diploma, having the previous year been elected FRS Ed.

Ballingall's Commission of Appointment to the Regius Chair of Military Surgery in the University of Edinburgh was dated 21 November 1822. He succeeded John Thomson, who from 1804 had been the first Professor of Surgery to the Royal College of Surgeons of Edinburgh and from 1806 the first holder of this Regius Chair. This was then the only chair in the subject in Britain, although later a lectureship from 1851 and a chair from 1854 would also exist, in Dublin, for a few years. Throughout his career at the University, Ballingall taught large numbers of undergraduates as well as medical officers in the army, navy, and Honourable East India Company. Many of the undergraduates who intended to enter one of the public services were actively encouraged to attend his course, as it covered a wide range of subjects not considered elsewhere in the medical curriculum.

To supplement the salary of his Regius Chair from the Crown, of one hundred pounds sterling per year, and his half pay from the army, Ballingall held various surgical appointments in Edinburgh, at James Syme's Minto House Surgical Hospital, and at the Royal Infirmary of Edinburgh. He was knighted on the accession of William IV (1830), and later appointed Surgeon to Queen Victoria and the Duchess of Kent in Scotland. Because of recurring bouts of bronchitis during his final years, he was forced to lecture only during the summer months. Due to the influence of Professor Syme (1799–1870), Ballingall's chair was withdrawn in 1855, on the suggestion that it should be relocated at Chatham. This never occurred.

Bibliography

Primary: 1833. *Outlines of the Course of Lectures on Military Surgery* (subsequently *Outlines of Military Surgery*: 2nd edn., 1838; 3rd, 1844; 4th, 1852; 5th, 1855) (Edinburgh).

Secondary: Kaufman, M. H., 2003. *Musket-Ball and Sabre Injuries* (Edinburgh); Kaufman, M. H., 2003. *Surgeons at War* (Westport, CT); Kaufman, M. H., 2003. *The Regius Chair of Military Surgery in the University of Edinburgh* (Amsterdam); Ballingall, G. A., 1906. 'A Memoir of the late Sir George Ballingall.' *Journal of the Royal Army Medical Corps* 6: 59–63; *Oxford DNB*.

Matthew Howard Kaufman

BALLS-HEADLEY, WALTER

BALLS-HEADLEY, WALTER   (b. Stapleford, Cambridgeshire, England, 27 August 1841; d. Miramichi, Procter, British Columbia, Canada, 7 March 1918), *gynecology.*

Balls-Headley was the son of William Balls and his wife Rebecca, née Emson. In his early professional life he assumed the additional surname of Headley, and his gentlemanly origins later earned an entry in Burke's dubious *Colonial Gentry*. He went to Clapham Grammar School under Rev. Charles Pritchard, later an eminent astronomer. In 1858 he was admitted to Peterhouse, Cambridge (BA, 1862; MB, 1864; MA, 1865; ChM, 1865; MD, 1868). He studied medicine at Addenbrooke's Hospital, Cambridge, and St. Bartholomew's, London (MRCP, 1866; FRCP, 1888). He held resident appointments at St. Bartholomew's and Great Ormond Street Children's Hospital, London. In 1866, while serving as traveling physician to the Marquess of Bute, he developed pulmonary tuberculosis during a tour of the Middle East and became one of many British consumptives forced to emigrate to Australia, arriving in 1869.

Balls-Headley first settled in Warwick, Queensland. In 1875 he moved to Melbourne, where he practiced in Collins Street East and was admitted to the University of Melbourne (MD *ad eund.*, 1876). In 1878 he was a physician at the Alfred Hospital, but he made his mark as a physician and surgeon at the Women's Hospital, Melbourne, from 1878 to 1900. He soon exhibited what appeared to be natural leadership at the Women's Hospital and in the Melbourne medical profession, and he was recognized to be a neat and safe surgeon. He was the first of the medical staff to use a hospital case book (from 1883), and he became chairman of the medical staff. His ascendancy did not go unchallenged, however; his slowness to comprehend germ theory and antisepsis infuriated the gifted Scot, James Jamieson, who was lecturer in obstetrics at the University of Melbourne.

As the hospital's maternal death rate rose in 1884, Balls-Headley advised the construction of a new building with more ventilation and the admission of a better class of patient, women less likely to die in childbirth. The adoption of antiseptic midwifery in the hospital was initiated by junior residents during his absence on an overseas tour, but he returned from Europe a convert to antisepsis, bringing with him the first device for special care of premature babies.

In 1889–1900 he was a lecturer in obstetric medicine and diseases of women and children at the University of Melbourne, replacing Jamieson, who went on to a distinguished incumbency as the lecturer in medicine. In 1891 Balls-Headley, who considered himself to be above the vulgar lobbying required for public election to the hospital staff, failed to be elected. That led to the hospital's acceptance of the university lecturer as an *ex officio* member of the staff with clinical rights. He was also an examiner in his specialties in the University of Adelaide.

In the 1890s Balls-Headley occupied an important position in Australian medicine. He was president of the Medical Society of Victoria in 1889; president of the obstetrics and gynecology section at the Intercolonial Medical Congress in Sydney in 1892; and a vice-president of the British Gynaecological Society of London in 1897 and 1898. He was a prominent Freemason and read widely. In 1876 he published *Dress, with Reference to Heat*, a lecture to the Australian Health Society. He also wrote two medical works. *On Internal Tumours: Their Characteristic Distinctions and Diagnosis* (1876) was the first major gynecological study published in Australia. In *The Evolution of the Diseases of Women* (1894), Balls-Headley drew on his reading of Charles Darwin, Herbert Spencer, and continental thinkers on marriage and criminality to develop a case for reproductive health as an evolutionary symbiosis between culture and biology. The originality of this second work led to an invitation to write the article, 'The Etiology of Diseases of the Female Genital Organs', in *A System of Gynaecology* (1896), edited by T. C. Allbutt and W. S. Playfair. His contributions to gynecological literature were well received by senior members of the profession in Britain and Australia. In 1886 he performed the Women's Hospital's first successful cesarean section.

Balls-Headley was married to Helen Elizabeth Mary, née Young. In 1907 he practiced for a short time in Tavistock Square, London, and after two years at Bideford, Devon, he settled in British Columbia. He died there on 7 March 1918, leaving no children.

Bibliography

Primary: 1894. *The Evolution of the Diseases of Women* (London).

Secondary: McCalman, Janet, 1999. *Sex and Suffering: Women's Health and a Women's Hospital, the Royal Women's Hospital, Melbourne, 1856–1996* (Baltimore); *AuDB*; *Munk's Roll*.

Janet McCalman

BALMIS, FRANCISCO XAVIER DE (b. Alicante, Spain, 2 December 1753; d. Madrid, Spain, 12 February 1819), *smallpox vaccination.*

Little is known about Balmis's family background and early schooling, but it appears that he came from a family of surgeons (his father, uncle and grandfather were highly reputed surgeons in Alicante). He was trained and served as a military surgeon in the Spanish Royal Navy during a period when the Spanish Bourbon monarchs, who had ruled the country from the early eighteenth century, were influenced by the European Enlightenment to increase the training and use of military surgeons, physicians, and engineers. During the second half of the century, those monarchs promoted political and economic changes (the 'Bourbon Reforms') to achieve greater control over and profit from their colonies. The renewed interest in their possessions overseas brought some improvement of sanitary conditions in the main urban areas, as well as scientific expeditions intended to identify primary products that could augment Spain's store of knowledge and ability to compete in the world market. In short, Balmis grew up in a context that considered science, technology, and medicine to be crucial for achieving the political goals, economic system, and cultural hegemony of the Spanish crown.

First Experiences Abroad

After finishing his studies as a surgeon, Balmis served as a military physician on a Spanish expedition to Algiers (1775). Afterward he lived in Havana and Mexico City (as well as other Mexican cities) from 1778 to 1790. He worked in Mexican hospitals and became interested in collecting indigenous plants to treat syphilis and other illnesses. Balmis was in western Venezuela briefly during this period, working against an epidemic fever. He returned to Spain in 1792 and held various positions in the official medical bureaucracy, including membership of the Royal Board of Surgery and general inspector for smallpox vaccination in Spain and in the Spanish Indies. Balmis also made a reputation as an efficient vaccinator in Madrid and as the translator into Spanish of the French manual on vaccination, *Traité historique et practique de la vaccine* (1801). It had been written by Jacques Louis Moreau de la Sarthe (1771–1826), one of the strongest advocates of Jenner's technique in continental Europe.

A Memorable Expedition

In 1803, King Charles IV of Spain—whose daughter had suffered from smallpox and who lived in a political atmosphere in which Jenner's ideas were enthusiastically validated by Spanish physicians—issued an order to extend smallpox vaccination throughout his dominions. Smallpox, considered to be a major factor in the collapse of the Aztec and Inca empires, had been one of the major killers of the Amerindian population since the sixteenth-century Spanish conquest, and in 1802 an epidemic struck Lima, the capital of the Vice-

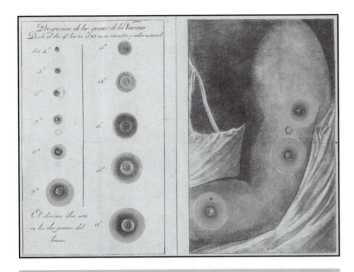

Smallpox vaccination reactions from days four to fifteen (left) and showing the strongest reaction, on day eleven (right). From *Tratado histórico y práctico de la vacuna . . .* Madrid, 1803. Rare Books, Wellcome Library, London.

royalty of Peru. Balmis's plan was to use the lymph in a chain of arm-to-arm vaccinations of foundlings. This so-called Royal Philanthropic Vaccine Expedition directed by Balmis also included José Salvany (1776–1810), who was second in command, as well as a few physicians, assistants, nurses, and twenty-two children from an orphanage. Equipped with barometers, thermometers, and glass plates containing samples of the vaccine, they set sail on 30 November 1803 from the Spanish port of La Coruña, on a voyage that would last more than three years. Circulars were distributed to the main cities beforehand so that arrangements could be made for the positive reception of the expedition's team and valuable cargo (but as the expeditionaries would find later, these instructions were not always followed).

After vaccinating in Tenerife and Puerto Rico, the expedition arrived in Puerto Cabello, which was at that time part of the Capitanía General de Venezuela, in March 1804. From there the party divided and followed different paths. Balmis proceeded to Cuba and Mexico, while Salvany went south to New Granada (now Colombia), Ecuador, and Peru. Salvany carried out a heroic effort for smallpox vaccination in several Andean provinces of Peru over several years. His assistant, Grajales, took the vaccine farther south to the Chilean Patagonia in 1811.

In Caracas, Balmis received a warm welcome, and thanks to the governor's help he started a true vaccination program. As a result, 2,000 people were vaccinated during his stay in the city, whose government covered all expenses of the expedition during this period. In Caracas, Balmis created the Central Board of Directors for the Vaccine, which became a model for the organization of vaccination services elsewhere. It was composed of ecclesiastical authorities, officers of the town council, and prominent physicians who were entrusted with the mission of making vaccination a regular practice in the city. Balmis instructed local physicians and members of the Board on how to prepare, preserve, and apply the vaccine. He also required school teachers and parish priests to cooperate in keeping records of those who were vaccinated (eventually, much of the local work relied on priests).

Similar central and provincial boards would be established in other cities of Spanish America, using up to 500 copies of the Spanish version of Moreau de la Sarthe's manual on vaccination, as translated by Balmis. Under adverse conditions and with scarce resources, these boards worked throughout the nineteenth century to produce, conserve, and distribute the lymph. They created the first local health position in Latin American municipal towns: the vaccinator. Moreover, in many of the emergent and fragile Latin American republics this was the main (though clearly insufficient and ephemeral) health intervention that the State supported in the provinces.

A few months after finishing his work in Venezuela, Balmis began to work in the Yucatan, namely in Mexican territory. This was also the beginning of a tense relationship between the authorities of New Spain (now Mexico) and Balmis. In the first place, Viceroy José de Iturrigaray had successfully anticipated the Spanish Crown's intentions, obtaining the vaccine from Cuba and using it locally in Mexico. Apparently, the Viceroy disliked Balmis and his insistent demands for funding, which were made because the expedition was designed to seek complementary financing wherever it operated. In addition, local physicians had been familiar with smallpox inoculation since the late eighteenth century, and some also knew and used Jenner's technique. They resented Balmis's disregard for the inoculations and vaccinations applied before his arrival (which Balmis considered unreliable and unsafe), his insistence that vaccination should be compulsory, and his authoritarian style of command.

Balmis's situation in the Yucatan was not unique. Salvany found in Lima that the vaccine had also preceded the Spanish expedition, having been sent by the Viceroy of the Rio de la Plata in Buenos Aires. Although some doctors, such as Hipolito Unanue, supported Salvany, others made their opinion clear that the expedition was unnecessary in Lima. In Mexico and other major cities of the Spanish Empire, the reception of the Spanish expedition went through a process of sometimes tense negotiation with proud intellectual and medical leaders who had been adapting and recreating the European Enlightenment values from the mid- to late-eighteenth century. Among the goals of these local elites were self-sufficiency in science and technology, and population growth, considered crucial to economic development. Many of these elite individuals would play leading political roles in the independence movements of the 1810s and 1820s.

The difficulties that the expedition found were also caused by the precarious economic situation and political unrest in the viceroyalties and the Spanish Empire during the early nineteenth century. The political context in the peninsula was dominated by the French emperor Napoleon, who dethroned the Spanish king, Charles IV, in 1808 and made his own brother, Joseph Bonaparte, king of Spain for several years. Nevertheless, Balmis's mission in several locations overcame political intrigue, scarce financial resources, and the antagonism of the indigenous population to forced vaccination. In what appears to have been heroic devotion to his medical mission, Salvany traveled through the southern Andes and died in Cochabamba, Bolivia, in 1810.

Despite the tension in the capital of Mexico, Balmis achieved success in his work in other Mexican cities such as Celaya, Oaxaca, and (especially) Puebla, where he was welcomed with the pomp and style indicated in the King's decree. Extensions of the main expedition even reached Texas and Guatemala, which then formed part of the Mexican viceroyalty. The work with a large Indian population in Guatemala was especially important, because it created its own board and kept a careful registry of 200,000 vaccinated individuals.

Return to Spain, and the Legacies

In 1805 Balmis sailed from the port of Acapulco toward another Spanish possession—the Philippine Islands. More than twenty Mexican children accompanied him, carrying the vaccine's fluid. Eventually, Balmis extended his mission to Macao and China and returned to Spain after circumnavigating the globe (with stops in St Helena and Lisbon), to be congratulated by the Spanish king. About three years later he would return to Mexico to continue the vaccination expedition, but political conditions in the viceroyalty and the crisis in the Spanish Empire caused him to return to his home country around 1811.

The expedition directed by Balmis taught the basics of smallpox vaccination, including its advantages over inoculation, and institutionalized Jenner's technology in America, the Philippines, and China. There is no definitive account of the number vaccinated by this ambitious enterprise, but some sources estimate the figure at more than 450,000 individuals. A by-product of the expedition was to enhance the visibility of local physicians and political authorities who embraced and adapted Jenner's technique as part of an emergent nationalism. Balmis's expedition was considered to be both the last of the Spanish scientific expeditions promoted by the Bourbon monarchs and the first international health mission. For decades afterward it inspired major medical interventions in colonial and postcolonial countries around the world and made immunization a symbol and a vanguard of international public health.

Bibliography

Primary: 1791. *Demostración de las eficaces virtudes nuevamente descubiertas en las raíces de dos plantas de Nueva España* (Madrid); 1803. *Prólogo y traducción castellana del Tratado histórico y práctico de la vacuna de J.L. Moreau by Francisco Xavier Balmis.* [1987. Introduction by Emili Balaguer i Perigüell] (Valencia).

Secondary: Rigau-Perez, José G., 2004. 'The Real Philanthropic Expedition of the Smallpox Vaccine: Monarchy and Modernity in 1803.' *Puerto Rico Health Science Journal* 23(3): 223–231; Ramírez Martín, Susana, 2002. *La salud del Imperio: La Real Expedición Filantrópica de la Vacuna* (Madrid); Aceves Pastrana, Patricia, and Alba Morales Cosme, 1997. 'Conflictos y negociaciones en las expediciones de Balmis.' *Estudios de Historia Novohispana* 17: 171–200; Archila, Ricardo, 1969. *La expedición de Balmis a Venezuela* (Caracas); Fernández del Castillo, Francisco. 1960. *Los viajes de Don Francisco Xavier de Balmis; notas para la historia de la expedición vacunal de España a América y Filipinas (1803–06)* (Mexico).

Yajaira Freites and Marcos Cueto
(with thanks to Susana Ramirez)

BANCROFT, JOSEPH (b. Manchester, England, 21 February 1836; d. Brisbane, Australia, 16 June 1894), *medicine, surgery, medical research, public health, natural history, horticulture.*

Bancroft was the son of Mary Lane and her husband, Joseph Bancroft, a farmer of Stretford, near Manchester. As a teenager he completed a five-year apprenticeship with Dr Renshaw at Sale in Cheshire, then studied at the Manchester Royal School of Medicine and Surgery, qualifying MRCS LSA, MD St. Andrews, 1859. He initially practiced in Nottingham (1859–64), where his passion for natural history developed. At age twenty-six he was elected president of the Nottingham Naturalists' Society. He contracted nephritis, and for health reasons emigrated to Brisbane with his wife and two surviving children.

With his alert and inquiring mind, Bancroft soon established himself as the leader of the medical profession in Queensland. He was president of the Philosophical Society of Queensland (1882–83), foundation president of the Royal Society of Queensland (1885), a member of the first two Queensland Medical Societies, and the foundation president (1886) of the third (which became the Queensland Branch of the British Medical Association, and later the Australian Medical Association). He was a member (1876–82) and president (1882–94) of the Medical Board of Queensland.

Bancroft was a prominent clinician in Queensland, and was appointed visiting surgeon (1867) and resident house surgeon (1868–77) at the Brisbane Hospital. He enjoyed a particularly high reputation for his skills in lithotomy and the treatment of urethral stricture. He practiced at Wickham Terrace and later at his second home on the corner of Ann and Wharf Streets. He was the first to describe Hansen's disease in the colony, wrote the first paper on tick paralysis, and was the Australian authority on filariasis and typhoid fever. His international fame rests on his discovery of the adult filarial nematode, named *Filaria bancrofti* (1877) in his honor by the helminthologist Thomas Spencer Cobbold. Bancroft also suggested that a human systemic disease might be caused by insects. His work on the mosquito-filaria nexus, confirmed by Patrick Manson in China, was undertaken twenty years prior to Ronald Ross's demonstration of the mosquito-malaria link.

Intensely interested in botany, especially medical botany, Bancroft wrote the original *Flora of Brisbane* (1882). He was the first to write about *pituri*, the mood-altering preparation made from Australian native corkwood that was known and used extensively by aboriginal Australians for millennia prior to Bancroft's time. Using cats, he experimented with corkwood's mydriatic and other properties. Other experiments involved the use of local 'bitter bark' (*Alstonia constricta*) as a treatment for typhoid and the use of native pepper for the treatment of gonorrhea. Bancroft coordinated and arranged a display of Australian medicinal plants for the Colonial and Indian Exhibition in London (1886). As a horticulturist, he introduced, hybridized, tested for acclimatization, and experimented with different varieties of rice, wheat, grapes, bananas, and strawberries.

Bancroft was elected first president of the Section of Hygiene and Public Health of the Australasian Association for the Advancement of Science, and he was a pioneer in the biological control of introduced pests. He insisted on controlled and contained experiments prior to the proposed release of fowl cholera to control rabbit populations, which resulted in the establishment of the containment laboratory on Rodd Island in Sydney Harbor.

His influence in medical research and natural history was carried on by his son, Thomas Lane Bancroft (1860–1933), and his granddaughter, Josephine Mackerras (1896–1971), who made significant contributions to Australian natural history in their own right. Scores of memorials record the life and works of the Bancroft family. They include the names of trees, parks, streets, and townships, as well as a granite memorial, medals, and prizes. Bancroft Park, the Bancroft Centre for Medical Research, and the Bancroft Oration (of the Queensland Branch of the Australian Medical Association), all in Brisbane, are testimony to the influence of his life and works.

Bibliography

Secondary: Pearn, J. H., and L. Powell, eds., 1991. *The Bancroft Tradition* (Brisbane).

John Pearn

BANTING, FREDERICK GRANT

BANTING, FREDERICK GRANT (b. Alliston, Ontario, Canada, 14 November 1891; d. near Musgrave Harbour, Newfoundland, Canada, 21 February 1941), *physiology, insulin.*

The son of William Thompson Banting and Margaret Grant Banting, Fred was a shy, mediocre student, more comfortable in the fields and woods of rural Ontario than in the classroom. He entered Victoria College at the University of Toronto and, despite a lackluster academic showing, entered medical school. After graduating MB in 1916 he enlisted in the Royal Canadian Medical Corps, and was wounded at the battle of Cambrai in 1918, awarded the Military Cross for gallantry, and discharged in the summer of 1919. Following postgraduate surgical training in Toronto he moved to London, Ontario, to set up practice. The income from the practice was minimal, and his first teaching efforts were poorly received.

On October 30, 1920 (he would later scratch in 31) he was unable to sleep after preparing a lecture on the pancreas, and scribbled an idea: 'Diabetus. [sic] Ligate pancreatic ducts of dogs. Keep dogs alive till acini degenerate leaving islets. Try to isolate the internal secretion of these to relieve glycosuria.'

Armed with only this idea, he approached J. J. R. Macleod (1876–1935), Professor of Physiology at the University of Toronto, who reluctantly provided him access to a small dingy laboratory and some dogs for the summer, as well as the help of a medical student assistant, Charles Best (1899–1978). Work began in May 1921, after Macleod taught them how to do a pancreatectomy on a dog. The first experiments were mostly failures, but a few dogs showed transient lowering of blood and urine sugar. The work in progress was presentation to the Physiological Journal Club on 21 November 1921.

Banting found simpler ways to get an extract, and J. B. Collip joined the team and devised ways to purify the compound, which they initially called *isletin*. The first human administration was given orally to Dr Joe Gilcrest, without effect. Banting's presentation to the American Physiological Society at Yale University was unimpressive, but during the questions Macleod clarified the work and the audience realized the Canadians were onto something important. Their next step was to administer Collip's more purified preparation to a fourteen-year-old, very ill Leonard Thompson on Ward H of the Toronto General Hospital. After an unimpressive first attempt, an increased dose produced remarkable lowering of the blood and urine glucose. They renamed the extract *insulin*, and when Macleod presented the work at the Association of American Physicians in May the world became aware of a great medical discovery. Patients clamored for the new drug, and it was soon in mass production by Connaught Laboratories in Canada and by Eli Lilly in the United States.

During that year Banting had been difficult, argumentative, and suspicious with his collaborators, and the arguments spread to the University's administration, who regarded Banting as difficult. They were reluctant to provide a professorial appointment to an inexperienced, young, and belligerent surgeon, but he was now the most famous person in the nation, hailed as a hero, and so under pressure they appointed him the first research professor and gave him some research space. Banting's rancor continued with the announcement that the Nobel Prize in Medicine would go to him and Macleod. Banting never thought Macleod deserved credit, so he at first considered refusing the prize, but announced he would share his prize equally with Best, and Macleod followed by sharing with Collip. The public, however, would always link two names with the discovery—Banting and Best.

He was given many awards and honorary degrees, including a knighthood, but was uncomfortable with the fame. An adoring public were shocked when newspapers publicized his very embarrassing and difficult divorce. He continued to explore research ideas, and although most of the subsequent work on adrenal secretion and cancer mechanisms was ill conceived and unsuccessful, he worked hard at it. He still fought with the University even when a new building was named The Banting Institute, with a top floor of space set aside for his research.

His only outside interest was painting; he imitated the Group of Seven and went on painting excursions with its best-known member, A. Y. Jackson. He was approached in 1939 to chair the newly formed Associate Committee on Medical Research, a branch of the National Research Council, which would tour Canada to assess the research capacity of the medical schools. He recommended the development of research in aviation medicine, low-pressure physiology, and bacteriological and chemical warfare for the impending war. On a trip to England to assess research activity his plane crashed in Newfoundland. There were rumors of espionage, but it is probable that the plane's engine oil cooler froze. His body lay in state in Convocation Hall at the University of Toronto, and he was buried in Mount Pleasant Cemetery as a great hero to his nation and to medicine.

Bibliography

Primary: 1921–22. (with Best, C. H.) 'The Internal Secretion of the Pancreas.' *J. Lab. Clin. Med.* 7: 251–266; 1922. (with Best, C. H., and J. J. R. Macleod) 'The Internal Secretion of the Pancreas.' *Amer. J. Physiol.* 59: 479; 1922. (with Collip, J. R., W. R. Campbell, and A. A. Fletcher) 'Pancreatic Extracts in the Treatment of Diabetes Mellitus. Preliminary Report.' *J. Can. Med. Assoc.* 12: 141–146.

Secondary: Bliss, Michael, 1992. *Banting: A Biography* (Toronto); Bliss, Michael, 1982. *The Discovery of Insulin* (Toronto); Stephenson, Lloyd, 1946. *Sir Frederick Banting* (Toronto); *DSB*.

Jock Murray

BARKER, LEWELLYS FRANKLIN (b. Milldale, Ontario, Canada, 16 September 1867; d. Baltimore, Maryland, USA, 13 July 1943), *anatomy, medicine.*

Barker was the eldest of three children born to James Frederick Barker, a farmer, and Sarah Jane Taylor, a miller's daughter. The Barkers were strict Quakers until James rejected the Society of Friends and became a Baptist minister. The family moved to Whitby, Ontario, where Barker was

apprenticed to a pharmacist (1884). Two years later he won a scholarship and attended the University of Toronto, completing his Bachelor of Medicine in 1890. (The University would later, 1905, confer an honorary MD upon him.) After an internship at the Toronto General Hospital, Barker went to Baltimore (1891), intent on studying under William Osler at the Johns Hopkins Hospital. When a resident post opened, Osler offered it to the Canadian. Thereafter, Barker enjoyed steady success. He was named fellow in pathology (1892), rising within eight years to associate professor in pathology. Franklin P. Mall soon appointed him his associate in anatomy (1893–97). In 1897 he became associate professor in anatomy.

Barker expanded his medical knowledge with trips abroad. In 1895 he studied in Leipzig. After the Spanish-American War, he and Simon Flexner headed the Johns Hopkins Medical Commission to the Philippines (1899), where they studied 'tropical' diseases in Richard Pearson Strong's laboratory. It was plague that made the strongest impression on Barker. Though absent from Manila, plague was present in Bombay, India, where the Commission visited on its return trip. Barker later commented that the experience helped him understand the 'horrors of the Black Death of Europe in earlier centuries', and he left India 'with a profound sense of gratitude that, after all, the West is not the East' (Barker, 1942, p. 83). Six years later, he was sent to investigate plague in San Francisco.

Barker returned to Baltimore and wrote a book on the nervous system (1899). In 1900 he was appointed Chair of Anatomy at the University of Chicago. While there, he published a translation of Werner Spalteholz's *Hand Atlas of Human Anatomy*. He also married Lilian Halsey (1903), and the pair traveled through Europe, with Lewellys punctuating sightseeing with trips to visit—and to work in—numerous laboratories, particularly in Munich. Though happy in Chicago, Barker welcomed the opportunity to return to Johns Hopkins when, in 1905, he took Osler's place as head of the Department of Medicine.

Barker made several changes to the department. A supporter of psychiatric medicine, he encouraged work on functional nervous disorders and advocated the judicious use of psychotherapy. He created research divisions in biology, physiology, and biochemistry, run by 'pure' scientists who investigated medical problems. Barker also helped realize one of his long-standing ideals: turning clinical departments into 'true' university departments. Teaching clinicians were paid low salaries, which they were expected to supplement by taking private patients. Barker, influenced by the German model, believed the practice took time away from teaching and research. Clinical professors should instead be paid sufficiently to focus their energies on university duties. By the time Johns Hopkins received the necessary funding and approved full-time clinical positions (1913), Barker was conflicted. The salary offered could not match his income from private practice, and family debts discouraged accepting a pay cut. Barker thus resigned his headship (1914) and was appointed clinical professor of medicine, a position he held until he retired (1921). Tellingly, he wrote a textbook on clinical medicine but made no significant contribution to medical research.

Upon retirement, Barker was appointed emeritus professor. He served on a number of committees and continued to write, including his autobiography, published a year before he died.

Bibliography

Primary: 1899. *The Nervous System and Its Constituent Neurones* (New York); 1902. 'Medicine and the Universities.' *American Medicine* 4: 143–147; 1916. *The Clinical Diagnosis of Internal Diseases* 3 vols. (New York); 1942. *Time and the Physician: The Autobiography of Lewellys F. Barker* (New York).

Secondary: Harvey, A. McGee, 1975. 'Creators of Clinical Medicine's Scientific Basis: Franklin Paine Mall, Lewellys Franklin Barker, and Rufus Cole.' *Johns Hopkins Medical Journal* 136: 168–177; Longcope, T. Warfield, 1943. 'Lewellys F. Barker.' *Science* 98: 316–318; *DAMB*.

Kim Pelis

BARNARD, CHRISTIAAN NEETHLING   (b. Beaufort West, South Africa, 8 November 1922; d. Paphos, Cyprus, 2 September 2001), *cardiac surgery.*

The fifth child of a Dutch Reformed Mission Church pastor and his ambitious wife in the Cape country town of Beaufort West, Barnard studied medicine at the University of Cape Town (UCT) from 1941 to 1946, aided by a loan from a fund for the education of poor Afrikaners. This medical training, quite typically, inculcated in him the need to take precise case histories and monitor his patients very closely.

Short spells as a country general practitioner, a medical officer in an infectious diseases hospital, and a registrar in medicine in Cape Town after his MB, ChB (1946) widened his clinical horizons considerably and allowed him to gain the degrees of MD and MMed in 1953 and 1954, respectively. These accomplishments did not dilute his determination to specialize in surgery, which he began to do in 1954 when he became a surgical registrar at the state-run Groote Schuur Hospital (GSH) in Cape Town. There he revealed himself to be a quick and astute learner, meticulous in everything he did in the operating theatre and irascibly intolerant of anything less from those around him.

Barnard's self-confidence and skill grew rapidly, and he was soon known as an up-and-coming surgeon who strove for perfection. This reputation, and especially his painstaking work devising a successful surgical procedure for intestinal atresia in neonates, convinced his seniors that he should be given every opportunity to develop his talents further. On their recommendation, in 1955 he was accepted for advanced training in general surgery at the University of Minnesota's state-of-the-

art surgical training center in Minneapolis. There the exciting possibilities of the emerging field of cardiac surgery rapidly attracted him. Under the supervision of pioneers such as Walton Lillehei and Richard Varco, he steeped himself in the latest techniques of cardio-thoracic surgery while he completed a Master of Surgery thesis on artificial aortic valves, as well as a PhD in his original specialty, intestinal atresia.

On the wave of these successes, Barnard returned to Cape Town in 1958 as both a specialist cardiothoracic surgeon at GSH and director of surgical research at UCT. Using a heart-lung machine donated by America's National Institutes of Health, he started an extensive program of open-heart surgery and experimentation at GSH and the nearby Red Cross Children's Hospital, with generous backing from the state hospital authorities. Relative success in these operations combined with his own ambition and inventiveness spurred him to tackle more complicated surgery. By the early 1960s, having kept well abreast of the most recent advances in cardiac surgery in the United States, he was contemplating transplanting a healthy human heart as the ultimate way to cure terminal heart disease.

For Barnard, the heart was 'just a pump' (Logan, 2003, p. 110). With his characteristic energy and thoroughness, he tackled repeated trial heart transplants into dogs, mastery of the principles of immunosuppressive therapy and tissue typing, and clarification of the legal implications of donation. It all paved the way for him to perform the world's first human heart transplant operation at GSH on 3 December 1967. In this five-hour operation, Barnard and his seventeen-person team transplanted the heart of a twenty-five-year-old woman who had been fatally injured by a car into fifty-four-year-old Louis Washkansky, whose diseased heart was at the point of failure. Washkansky was white, and to avoid political controversy in apartheid South Africa the donor had to be white-skinned, too.

Washkansky survived eighteen days after the operation before succumbing to pneumonia, not to rejection of the transplanted heart. Nevertheless, the media latched onto Barnard's pioneering breakthrough and turned it into an unprecedented event, 'the surgical equivalent', as *Time* put it, 'of the ascent of Everest' (Logan, 2003, p. 154). This flood of attention elevated the articulate and photogenic Barnard to world celebrity status overnight, stoking his vanity and turning him into a high-profile, jet-setting international figure—the object simultaneously of adulation, envy, and scorn by public and peers alike. The sudden exposure to so much limelight and so many honors (including an honorary DSc and professorship from UCT) fanned Barnard's self-importance. The go-getting outsider from a rural Afrikaner backwater had become an acclaimed international icon, and Groote Schuur Hospital became a household name around the globe.

Over the next five years, Barnard performed eight more transplants of this type. Most of the recipients survived for more than a year. Not satisfied with these results, and as resourceful and audacious as ever, he introduced an important variation to heart transplants in 1974 by undertaking a successful piggyback heart operation, in which the donor's heart was inserted alongside the recipient's to help it function. The recipient lived for nineteen weeks. Barnard performed more than forty similar operations over the next nine years, along with hundreds of more routine open-heart procedures.

In the late 1970s his zest for cardiac surgery began to wane, in inverse proportion to the increasing arthritis in his hands; his almost insatiable attraction to conferences and travel abroad; and his growing career as an unofficial ambassador for South Africa. He was also a farmer, a restaurateur, and the coauthor of popular medical texts, newspaper columns, and novels. A combination of all of these interests led him to retire from his dual posts at GSH and UCT in 1983, four years earlier than required of a doctor in the public sector.

Barnard's self-seeking zeal did not flag in his retirement. He traded on his name lucratively, lending it to a number of medical and nonmedical commercial ventures and spending two years as adviser to the new heart transplant unit at the Baptist Medical Center in Oklahoma.

Barnard died of asthma on Cyprus while on yet another overseas trip from his home in South Africa. His personal life had been tumultuous; married and divorced three times, his relationships with his wives and six children were like roller coaster rides. Thanks to his skill and boldness as a surgeon, he had been in the glare of the media spotlight from the age of forty-five. His virtues and vices were magnified many times over, radically polarizing public and professional opinion about him. But despite his considerable achievements, Barnard always proudly emphasized that he had made good against the odds, declaring, 'In my job . . . they [medical experts] don't suffer upstarts easily' (Barnard, 1983, p. 9).

Bibliography

Primary: 1967. 'A Human Cardiac Transplant: an Interim Report of a Successful Operation Performed at the Groote Schuur Hospital, Cape Town.' *South African Medical Journal* 41: 1271–1274; 1969. (with Pepper, C. B.) *Christiaan Barnard—One Life* (Cape Town); 1983. 'Ending a Whole Chapter.' *Cape Times*, 31 January, p. 9. 1993. (Brewer, D., ed.) *The Second Life—Memoirs* (Cape Town).

Secondary: Logan, Chris, 2003. *Celebrity Surgeon: Chris Barnard— A Life* (Johannesburg and Cape Town); Cooper, David, 1992. *Chris Barnard by Those Who Know Him* (Vlaeberg).

Howard Phillips

BARNETT, LOUIS EDWARD (b. Wellington, New Zealand, 24 March 1865; d. Dunedin, New Zealand, 27 October 1946), *surgery.*

Barnett was the son of Alfred Abram Barnett, an auctioneer and merchant of Jewish descent, and Julia Joshua. He distinguished himself from an early age, combining academic achievements with sporting prowess at Wellington College in New Zealand. Awarded a university junior scholarship, Barnett spent two years at Dunedin's University of Otago Medical School before completing his studies at Edinburgh University, where in 1888 he graduated MB CM, with first-class honors.

A position as house surgeon at the Middlesex Hospital, London, followed in 1889, and in 1890 he became the first New Zealander to qualify FRCS. His career in New Zealand began in 1891 with *locum tenens* appointments. Appointed to a lectureship in 1894, Barnett became the University of Otago's first professor of surgery in 1909. Following his retirement in 1924, he endowed a chair of surgery at Otago in memory of his son Ralph, who died in World War I.

Barnett played a pioneering role in New Zealand surgery. Alert to the importance of keeping pace with modern surgical methods, he traveled regularly to Britain and America, and in 1904 was the first New Zealander to visit the Mayo Clinic. Subsequently, he was the first surgeon in New Zealand to habitually wear a gauze mask and rubber gloves while operating.

When he was still a young surgeon, the death of a boy from complications arising from human hydatid disease inspired Barnett to wage a strenuous, often solitary war against hydatids, which were then prevalent in New Zealand at that time. Even in retirement he devoted much time and energy to hydatid research, contributing substantially to the literature on this dreaded disease. Organizing and partly funding a Hydatid Research Committee at the Otago Medical School, Barnett was instrumental in establishing the hydatid registry of the Royal Australasian College of Surgeons. A similar interest in cancer research led him to play a major role in the establishment of both the Radium Institute in Dunedin and the British Empire Cancer Campaign.

Barnett's contribution to surgery was not restricted to New Zealand's shores. During the First World War, Lieutenant-Colonel Barnett acted as consulting surgeon with the New Zealand Expeditionary Force, receiving the CMG in 1918 in recognition of his service.

Impressed by the work of the American College of Surgeons, to which he was admitted as an honorary fellow in 1926, Barnett believed that a similar organization would benefit New Zealand surgeons. His proposal, enlarged to include Australasia, was initially rejected by his more conservative colleagues in 1920. His vision was finally realized in 1927, however, when Barnett was elected a vice-president of the fledgling Australasian College of Surgeons. He became president in 1937.

Barnett's service to medicine, recognized by the award of a Knight Bachelor in 1927, also included editorship of the *New Zealand Medical Journal* from 1893 to 1900. He presided over the surgical section of the Australasian Medical Congress in 1902 and was elected president of that organization in 1924. In 1907 he became president of the New Zealand Branch of the British Medical Association. A past associate and district surgeon for the Order of St John of Jerusalem, Barnett was created a Knight of Grace of that order in 1935.

Philanthropic throughout his life, Barnett gave liberally to a number of causes. He died at the age of eighty-one, survived by his wife, Mabel Violet Fulton, and four children. Described in the *Otago Daily Times* as a 'Great Dominion Surgeon', Barnett's distinguished record and talent for leadership enabled him to play a legendary role in medicine in New Zealand.

Bibliography

Secondary: Cole, David Simpson, 1977. *The First Half Century of the College in New Zealand: Royal Australasian College of Surgeons, 1927–1977* (Auckland); Hercus, Charles, and Gordon Bell, 1964. *The Otago Medical School under the First Three Deans* (Edinburgh and London); [Obituary], 1946. *Otago Daily Times*, 29 October p. 6; [Obituary], 1946. *Lancet* i: p. 773.

Jill Wrapson

BARNOR, MATTHEW ANUM   (b. Accra, British Gold Coast (now Ghana), 1917; d. Accra, Ghana, 20 June 2005), *family planning, public health.*

A chronicler of medical history and African social life, Barnor was crucial to the establishment of the medical profession in Ghana. Barnor was among the ten initial recipients of the Gold Coast Medical Scholarship to the University of Edinburgh (1940). He returned to Accra to lead the creation of African-directed medical and health services, including most notably the Ghana Medical Association and the Planned Parenthood Association of Ghana.

Barnor was born into humble circumstances and dreamed of achieving social stature through higher education. His father had not had the means to finish secondary school and worked as a clerk for the Forestry Department. Barnor passed his early years in Accra and Kumasi, where he became a young enthusiast of modern science and technology after observing the first airplanes, automobiles, and radios to reach the colony. He attended the Government Junior Boys' School in Jamestown and the Senior School on Rowe Road in Accra, then continued his studies at the renowned Mfantsipim School from 1933 to 1937. A Cadbury Fellowship combined with school supplementary funds allowed him to study for the Intermediate BSc at Achimota (formerly Prince of Wales College).

His receipt of the Gold Coast Medical Scholarship to study for his medical degree at the University of Edinburgh effectively opened the second decade of what emerged as a training course for the scientific and political leaders of independent Ghana. His time in Europe was heightened by the continuation of World War II, with the constant threat of submarines and bombings making travel dangerous. After qualifying in 1947, he supplemented his studies with a hospital internship in Sunderland and a course at the London School of Hygiene and Tropical Medicine (1948). He passed through the West African Students' Union, a fertile ground for nationalist activities, and experienced a brief stay in Paris. Barnor also participated in the Student Christian Movement and Cosmopolitan Club.

Barnor was received into the colonial service as a medical officer after returning to the Gold Coast in 1949. Black African and European medical staff enjoyed a degree of equality by this point, after the Watson Commission abolished separate classes of officers in 1948. By 1950, Barnor was one of eighteen African doctors in a service of eighty-five, with fifteen additional African doctors in private practice around the colony. He was posted to disparate areas including Kumasi, Wa, and Cape Coast, where he confronted limited medical resources for large, often impoverished populations. Barnor was a key proponent of the Medical Field Unit system for providing rural services during the 1950s.

After first president Kwame Nkrumah led Ghana to independence in 1957, the development of a new medical system fell to young physicians such as Barnor. He became the first secretary of the Ghana Medical Association (GMA), established in 1958 as an ostensibly black African organization to replace the Gold Coast Branch of the British Medical Association. Barnor and the emerging African physicians worked to create public confidence in their competence, including the founding of Ghana's first medical school. Barnor was also president of the GMA at a critical point during the overthrow of Nkrumah. His leadership continued as a member of the Ghana Medical and Dental Council, a professional regulatory body created by the GMA, when he sought ways to keep medical services afloat during a series of military *coups d'état* in the 1970s.

Confronted with high abortion and pregnancy rates among his female patients, Barnor headed the movement to create family planning services in Ghana and was one of the first physicians to install intrauterine devices. Barnor and his wife, Dorothy Quartey-Papafio, opened their home to interested health workers and community figures, leading to the establishment of the Planned Parenthood Association of Ghana (PPAG) by 1968.

In his later years, Barnor continued work with the PPAG while serving patients in his private practice at Link Road Clinic. He also established himself as a medical historian, publishing (with author Victor A. Osei) a formidable autobiography entitled *A Socio-Medical Adventure in Ghana*.

Bibliography

Primary: 1962. 'A History of Medical Societies in Ghana.' *Ghana Medical Journal* 1: 4–7; 2001. (with Osei, Victor A.) *A Socio-Medical Adventure in Ghana: Autobiography of Dr. M. A. Barnor* (Accra, Ghana).

Secondary: Addae, Steven, 1996. *The Evolution of Modern Medicine in a Developing Country: Ghana 1880–1960* (Durham, NC).

Abena Dove Osseo-Asare

BARROS BARRETO, JOÃO DE (b. Rio de Janeiro, Brazil, 14 December 1890; d. Rio de Janeiro, 20 August 1956), *occupational medicine.*

Barros Barreto graduated in 1912 from Rio de Janeiro's School of Medicine. In 1915, he became sanitary inspector of the national sanitary services, at the same time pursuing a one-year specialization course at the prestigious Oswaldo Cruz Institution. With the creation of a national service of rural prophylaxis in 1918, Barros Barreto worked for about six years in suburban areas of Rio. During that period he also organized rural sanitation services in a number of Brazilian states.

Thanks to Rockefeller Foundation scholarships, he took courses at the Johns Hopkins School of Hygiene and Public Health and at Harvard's School of Public Health during 1924 and 1925. He was deeply influenced by his studies in the United States. Inspired by American models, Barros Barreto would eagerly support the need for well-designed training courses for Brazilian health professionals and the rational administration of public health services. Upon his return to his home country, he was elected a member of the National Academy of Medicine.

Barros Barreto first made his reputation in industrial hygiene by teaching at the university and publishing in that field. His work is considered to be a sound and early contribution to the institutionalization of occupational medicine in Brazil. That process paralleled the country's industrialization, which created anxieties about the safety and proper protection of workers' health. From 1925 to 1936 he taught hygiene at the School of Medicine of Rio de Janeiro. He also taught industrial hygiene at the same school, as part of the training of the first cadre of specialists in occupational medicine. From the late 1930s on he actively participated in the Pan-American Sanitary Conferences and meetings of the Pan-American Sanitary Bureau. He also represented Brazil in the Hygiene Section of the League of Nations and on the Industrial Hygiene Committee of the International Labor Office.

Between 1926 and 1929, Barros Barreto was an assistant to Clementino Fraga, director of the National Department of Public Health. Under the authoritarian government of Getúlio Vargas (1930–45), Barros Barreto was health director in various states. During the periods of 1937–39 and 1941–45, he occupied the highest position in the Brazilian public health service, which was then under the Ministry of Education and Health.

As the National Health Service Director, Barros Barreto oversaw a health reform consonant with the authoritarian, technocratic, and centralist ideology of the Vargas government, which advocated strong state intervention in social policies. He promoted the government's coordination and control of all official health institutions, programs, and activities; a uniform and standard form of sanitary administration; the creation of sanitary districts in the cities; the specialized training of public health professionals; and the creation of a career in the state's bureaucracy for those professionals. His administration was also characterized by an emphasis on the control of rural endemics. In 1941, he designed national services for fighting malaria, leprosy, bubonic plague, tuberculosis, yellow fever, and cancer. Barros Barreto's model of public health interventions from above, as well as the state-supported, disease-oriented services he organized, had a significant impact on Brazilian public health during four decades.

Another important event of his administration was an agreement with the International Health Division of the Rockefeller Foundation for eradication of the malaria-carrying mosquito, *Anopheles gambiae.* In 1942 he also signed an agreement with the U.S. State Department for a special health service in areas of strategic and military interest, but he disagreed with the autonomy of this service that relied on the direction of an American physician. His position was not taken into account, however. With the end of Vargas's presidency, Barros Barreto left his official post and returned to the university, where he published his important and comprehensive book on hygiene (1948).

Bibliography

Primary: 1948. *Tratado de Higiene* (Rio de Janeiro).

Secondary: [Obituary], 1956. 'João de Barros Barreto.' *Revista Brasileira de Malariologia e Doenças Tropicais* 8: 641.

Gilberto Hochman

BARRY, JAMES MIRANDA STEUART (b. Ireland?, 1795?; d. London, England, 25 July 1865), *surgery, public health.*

Although information about his private life is sparse, Barry was probably an intersexual who decided at puberty to present himself as a man, thereby allowing him to pursue a medical career that was then closed to women. Possibly the child of shopkeeping parents who subsequently separated, Barry adopted the name of his famous, recently-deceased artist uncle to help secure the patronage of the dead man's wealthy and progressive-minded circle of friends, whose names he then added as his own middle names. With their financial support, he was able to study at the University of Edinburgh, where he received the MD in 1812. His doctoral thesis investigated femoral hernias, then commonly confused with late-descending testicles in intersexuals. Further training as a pupil-dresser to Astley Cooper in London pointed to a surgical career, but Barry's need for financial security led him to join the army as a regimental surgeon first.

From 1813 to 1816 he served in military hospitals in England, before being promoted to assistant staff surgeon and posted to Britain's newly-conquered Cape Colony in 1816. This was the first of eight colonial appointments in what became a permanent career in the military, ranging from the Cape (1816–28) to Mauritius (1828–29), Jamaica (1831–35), St Helena (1836–38), the West Indies (1839–45), Malta (1846–51), Corfu (1851–57), and Canada (1857–59).

In Cape Town, his skill as an all-round doctor and wit as a conversationalist caused him to readily find favor with the governor, Lord Charles Somerset. Consequently, despite his youth, Barry was soon appointed personal physician to the Somerset family. He was also appointed as a member of the Vaccine Institute and the Quarantine Board, and in 1822 he became the colonial medical inspector, with supreme authority over medical affairs in the colony. His three years in that position gave his progressive, humanitarian zeal full scope. At his initiative, the local medical profession was restructured, the quality and sale of drugs became tightly regulated, and a comprehensive program of public vaccination was organized. Institutions such as the leper colony, the Somerset Hospital, and the prison were overhauled in accordance with a strict regimen of cleanliness, good ventilation and drainage, adequate diet, and caring treatment. 'Want of cleanliness renders most diseases virulent, which by care would be of little consequence' was Barry's firm belief (Rose, 1977, p. 72). This conviction became a hallmark of his public health initiatives in all of his subsequent postings, and it was the key to his success in curbing epidemics there.

Equally characteristic, however, were Barry's thin-skinned personality, sharp tongue, and refusal to compromise. Those traits brought him to being charged in court or court-martialed three times in his long career. Twice they led to demotion, once to being sent home in disgrace, once to a duel, and countless times to clashes with fellow-officers and the military establishment, usually on issues of medical administration or the health of troops. In Somerset's frank opinion, Barry was 'the most skilful of physicians, [the] most wayward of men' (Rose, 1977, p. 43). It is not surprising, therefore, that after he reached the rank of staff surgeon in 1827, it took another twenty-four years before he was promoted again.

Even then, with the ranks of deputy inspector of hospitals and inspector of hospitals in his last two postings—the highest medical positions in the British army—Barry did not abandon his vigorous commitment to his original public health principles. In the words of a biographer, he remained 'a maverick force, insisting that medical innovation was a key weapon in the arsenal of military modernization' (Holmes, 2002, p. 240).

He was no less diligent in his clinical practice, for it is clear that he kept his hands-on surgical and scientific skills well-honed throughout his career. For instance, in 1826 he performed one of the first wholly successful deliveries by cesarean section; a year later he published a pioneering analysis of the medicinal properties of a Cape plant; and his report on cholera on the island of Malta in 1848 is the work of someone well abreast of the latest thinking in Britain.

After his health began to fail in 1859, Barry spent the last six years of his life in cantankerous retirement, mainly in the company of his long-time companions—his dog, Psyche, and his black manservant. His charwoman's insistence that, on his death, she discovered that he was female, is a *cause célèbre* that continues to reverberate today.

Bibliography

Secondary: Holmes, Rachel, 2002. *Scanty Particulars: The Life of Dr James Barry* (London); Rose, June, 1977. *The Perfect Gentleman: The Remarkable Life of Dr James Miranda Barry* (London); Oxford DNB.

Howard Phillips

BARTHOLIN, THOMAS   (b. Copenhagen, Denmark, 20 October 1616; d. Copenhagen, 4 December 1680), *anatomy, pharmacology, physiology.*

Bartholin was a member of the Bartholin-Fincke clan, which completely dominated the Faculty of Medicine and held numerous chairs in the other faculties at the University of Copenhagen in the seventeenth century. Consequently, an academic career was always expected of him. He was the second-eldest son of professor of medicine (and later of theology) Caspar Bartholin the Elder. His grandfather, Thomas Fincke, was also professor of medicine at the University of Copenhagen, and when Bartholin's father died in 1629 his uncle Ole Worm, also professor of medicine, oversaw his education.

Bartholin received his first higher education at the University of Copenhagen (1634–37) and then embarked on the customary grand tour of Europe, with prolonged stays in Leiden (1637–40) and Padua (1641–43, 1644–45). The subjects he studied at home and abroad were not restricted to medicine. Reflecting the academic versatility of his father, he was trained in all the liberal arts as well as medicine and theology, and it was not until his arrival in Leiden that he somewhat hesitatingly decided to focus on a career in medicine. Still, he never lost his interest in philology, natural philosophy, and theology, and he would often seek to combine them with his work in medicine.

In 1640 Bartholin left Leiden for Paris, where he studied at Collège Royal. The following year he briefly stayed in Montpellier before reaching Padua. His four years in Padua were interrupted only by a trip to southern Italy (Rome, Naples, and Sicily) in the winter of 1643–44. He even tried to reach Egypt, but only got as far as Malta. Following in the footsteps of his father and Ole Worm, Bartholin left Padua for Basel, where he received his MD in 1645.

Anatomical Textbook

Bartholin had begun specializing in anatomy while in Leiden, and in 1641 he issued a new edition of his father's anatomical textbook, *Institutiones anatomicae*, which was first published in 1611. Thomas made few alterations to the original text, but he added Vesalian illustrations and included as an appendix two papers by his teacher, the anatomist Jan de Wale (Walaeus). Those papers dealt with two subjects that had particularly caught the attention of the medical profession of the day. One was the movement of chyle, as discussed by Aselli with his discovery of the lacteal vessels, and the other was Harvey's theory of the circulation of the blood. It was the first time that Harvey's theory was mentioned with approval in an anatomical textbook.

Bartholin issued a second edition in 1645, which would soon be translated into French (1647), German (1648), and Italian (1651). The task remained, however, to incorporate the theory of blood circulation into the text proper. That was achieved in 1651 with the publication of *Anatomia reformata*, which was an altered edition of *Institutiones anatomicae*. The 1651 edition also saw new figures by Casserius and Vesling replacing most of the earlier Vesalian illustrations. *Anatomia reformata* was hugely successful; it was reprinted in the Netherlands at least seven times by 1669, and in 1653 a translation into Dutch appeared, with six reprints by 1671. An English translation was published in 1668. Bartholin issued a fourth version of the book, rewritten and updated, in 1673. This edition also was frequently reprinted and translated, and with a total of some thirty editions Bartholin's anatomical textbook was one of the most influential of the seventeenth century.

Lymphatic System

After almost ten years abroad, Bartholin finally returned to Denmark, and in 1647 he accepted a position as professor of mathematics at the University of Copenhagen. The following year he succeeded Simon Paulli in the chair of anatomy. Bartholin's father had already introduced the theories of Paduan anatomy in Copenhagen, but Bartholin found that the newly built anatomical theater (inaugurated in 1645) offered better facilities for conducting dissections (including a steady supply of corpses) than had previously been available. Significant progress in the study of anatomy followed, and Bartholin attracted many students—Niels Stensen (Steno) being the most talented. A large collection of curious anatomical problems stemming from these years can be found in *Historiarum anatomicarum rariorum centuria I–IV* (1654–61).

Alerted by the discoveries of the French anatomist Pecquet, who had dissected animals, Bartholin and Michael Lyser, his gifted German prosector, found the human thoracic duct in 1652. Their discovery proved that the lacteals in man did not convey chyle to the liver, there to be transformed into blood. They found that the chyle ran past the liver through the thoracic duct, before eventually being mixed with blood in the left subclavian vein. Bartholin's findings were published that same year in *De lacteis thoracicis*. Further investigations led him to discover what he named the lymphatic system, an entirely independent system of vessels. He also concluded that the liver did not produce blood, as Galen had suggested. In 1653 Bartholin published his discovery of the lymphatic system in animals (*Vasa lymphatica*), and he self-confidently ended the book with an epitaph for the liver.

By that time Bartholin had attracted the scorn of many a traditional Galenist. One prominent foe in Paris was Jean Riolan the Younger, and a number of polemical exchanges took place between them. This debate allowed Bartholin to eloquently combine flattery with sarcasm. He hailed Riolan as the greatest anatomist in the world, but he also complained that Riolan was too old and stubborn to realize the importance of his (Bartholin's) work. Bartholin's contemporaries admired his baroque style, and a collection of his many orations was published (*Orationes*, 1668), as was his poetry (*Carmina*, 1669).

Publication of the *Vasa lymphatica* also sparked a rivalry with the Swedish medical student Olof Rudbeck. Rudbeck had independently reached the same conclusions as Bartholin, but he now claimed—probably correctly—that he had reached them a few months before Bartholin. Nevertheless, Bartholin was the first to actually publish his findings. The dispute began in 1654 when a new edition of *Vasa lymphatica* was published in Leiden. Bartholin had added some rather unlikely dates, probably to prove that he had made the lymphatic system discovery before Rudbeck, of whom he had now become aware. Rudbeck in turn publicly accused Bartholin of swindle, but Bartholin felt it was beneath him to refute the young man and left the job to his students.

It appears that Bartholin and Rudbeck were reconciled years later. Meanwhile, Bartholin continued to refine the presentation of his discovery of the lymphatic system, and in March 1654 he saw the human lymphatic vessels for the first time. He published the finding with great haste in order to claim the discovery as his own, and *Vasa lymphatica in Homine nuper inventa* appeared in May 1654.

Royal Physician

Despite being a famous anatomist, Bartholin all but stopped performing public dissections in 1654 when he assumed the chair of medicine that had become vacant with the death of his mentor, Ole Worm. When Thomas Fincke died in 1656, Bartholin ascended to the *medicus primus* professorship and became dean of the Faculty of Medicine. On that occasion, he performed his last public dissection in the presence of the king and other notables.

After suffering for years from the renal stones that would ultimately cause his death, Bartholin was appointed *professor honorarius* in 1661, which freed him from his teaching obligations altogether. Retaining his position as dean of the Faculty of Medicine, however, left him in a position to exert great influence on university matters, as well as on the organization of the medical profession in the joint kingdom of Denmark and Norway. In 1658 he was instrumental in the publication of the first Danish pharmacopeia, *Dispensatorium Hafniense*. In 1672 he was jointly responsible for the royal decree on the organization of the medical profession in Denmark, and in 1673 he held the first exams for Danish midwives. He served as vice-chancellor (*Rector magnificus*) of the university for four terms.

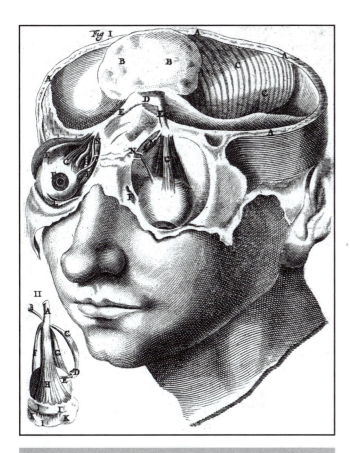

Muscles of the eye and orbit. Engraving from *Anatomia ex Caspar Bartolini . . . reformata,* The Hague, 1655. Rare Books, Wellcome Library, London.

In 1663 Bartholin retired to a manor he bought in Western Sealand, where he devoted himself to the publication of his many manuscripts. These included his extensive correspondence with the learned world of Europe in the *Epistolarum medicinalium I–IV* (1663–67). Other works, such as *De medicina Danorum domestica* (1666), detailed the history and current state of the medical profession in Denmark.

His estate was destroyed by fire in 1670, along with many still-unpublished manuscripts and letters. The fire did not, however, stop Bartholin's quill. As he remarked on one occasion, he was capable of producing a text faster than fungi could shoot up. In 1673 he began publishing *Acta medica et philosophica Hafniensia,* the first scientific periodical in Scandinavia and one of the first in the world. It appeared in five volumes, but ceased publication with the death of Bartholin, who had been a major contributor. In 1674 his treatise on pathological anatomy appeared—*De anatome practica ex cadaveribus morbosis adornanda.*

He was much favored by King Frederik III, who frequently attended his lectures on anatomy and appointed him *archiater honorarius,* personal physician to the king. When King Christian V assumed power in 1670, he retained Bartholin's services, and in 1671 made him head of the university library. In 1675 he was appointed judge of the

Supreme Court of Judicature. The king made Bartholin's estate tax-free for three years after the fire in 1670, which enabled him to rebuild it.

In the mind of Bartholin, ever more sophisticated methods and continuous experimentation gave anatomy a crucial role in the art of medicine and natural philosophy, but it also gave men an unprecedented understanding of God's greatest creature, which would lead them to piety. Accordingly, he advised his students not to neglect theology, and he always accompanied his writings on, say, the lymphatic system (which have won a place in the history of medicine) with a host of writings committed to exploring medicine in a biblical connection. These include a treatise on the abdominal wound of Christ (1646), a collection of disputations on the subject of paralytics in the New Testament (1653), and a general discussion of maladies in the Bible and the Talmud (1672). Bartholin also translated the works of several devotional authors into Danish. It is unlikely that he believed that these writings should be deemed inferior or less important than his other writings on medicine.

A testament to Bartholin's fame was the offer he received in 1675 to take over the chair of anatomy in Padua. Citing his ailing health, the fifty-nine-year-old Bartholin declined the offer. By 1680 his health was rapidly deteriorating, so he sold off his country seat and settled in his Copenhagen mansion, were he died that same year. He had been married twice and had eight children. His eldest, Caspar Bartholin the Younger, also became professor of medicine. He discovered the sublingual duct (Bartholin's duct) and the vulvovaginal gland (Bartholin's gland).

Bibliography

Primary: 1651. *Casp. Bartholini Institutiones anatomicae, novis recentiorum opinionibus et observationibus figurisque auctae a Thoma Bartholino* (Leiden); 1652. *De lacteis thoracicis in homine brutisque nuper observatis historia anatomica* (Copenhagen); 1653. *Vasa lymphatica, nuper Hafniae in animalibus inventa et hepatitis exeqviae* (Copenhagen); 1654. *Vasa lymphatica in homine nuper inventa* (Copenhagen).

Secondary: Bartholin, Thomas, 1994. *On Diseases in the Bible. A Medical Miscellany—1672* [trans. Willis, James] Schioldann-Nielsen, Johan, and Kurt Sørensen, eds. (Copenhagen); Bartholin, Thomas, 1961. *On The Burning of His Library and On Medical Travel* [trans. O'Malley, Charles D.] (Lawrence, KS); Garboe, Axel, 1949–50. *Thomas Bartholin. Et Bidrag til dansk Natur- og Lægevidenskabs Historie i det 17. Aarhundrede I–II* (Copenhagen); Skavlem, John H., 1921. 'The Scientific Life of Thomas Bartholin.' *Annals of Medical History* 3: 67–81; DSB.

Morten Fink-Jensen

BARTISCH, GEORG (b. Gräfenhain, Königsbrück, Germany, *c.* 1535; d. Dresden, Germany, 1606/07), *surgery, ophthalmology.*

Bartisch was born around 1535 in Gräfenhain near Königsbrück, a village not far from Dresden. His parents seem to have been small-scale peasants with few financial means. As a boy he was apprenticed to a barber surgeon, and within only a few years must have acquired considerable operative skills. He became famous at a relatively early age, and in 1558 he was named court oculist in Dresden. Little is known about his family and private life, except that he was based in Döbeln from 1564. He lost his wife and children to the plague in 1567, but he married again in 1568. His son, Tobias, followed in his father's footsteps and also became a surgeon and oculist.

Demand for invasive surgery was very limited at that time because of high fatality rates and the lack of safe and powerful anesthesia. Cataracts, tumors, bladder stones, and hernias made up the bulk of major operations. Consequently, surgeons who specialized in these types of medical services usually found it very difficult to make a living just in one place, even in a major urban center. Bartisch therefore traveled from town to town over many years, working in Magdeburg, Breslau, and Prague, among others. As an itinerant healer, he also had to comply with the rules of marketplace medicine. He provided himself with official certificates that testified to his operative successes. Flyers praising his skills were printed and presumably distributed among the population wherever he arrived, and he even succeeded in enticing priests to announce his arrival in the churches. He promised to cure not only cataracts, bladder stones, and hare lips, but also large tumors, goiters, and cancerous ulcers. He also offered to diagnose and cure internal diseases, inviting the sick to send him samples of their urine.

Bartisch helped shape the new profile of the highly trained and knowledgeable surgeon. He proclaimed that ideally, a surgeon should have studied, but extensive practical experience was even more important. It could not be acquired from studying books at the universities, but only through years of practicing and direct observation. At the same time, however, Bartisch did much to bolster his image as a learned man. He used the privileged medium of academic medicine—the medical treatise—and appropriated the rhetorical strategies of learned physicians. For example, he wrote in German—which had the advantage of making his treatises accessible to less learned surgeons—but he interspersed his texts with Greek and Latin terms and quotations. Presumably he relied on the help of others for this, since he did not know Latin, and like the leading learned physicians he dedicated his works to a ruler.

According to Bartisch's own account, he intended to publish a whole series of medical works. But, apart from a little pamphlet praising the virtues of a theriac medicine, only two of his works have come down to us. Around 1575, he completed the manuscript for his *Kunstbuch*, a comprehensive account of the causes and treatment of bladder stones. In great detail it explained and illustrated how the patient had to be prepared for the operation, how and in

what position he should be tied, and above all, how the surgeon should proceed during the operation and deal with complications. The book did not appear in print, however, until the manuscript was rediscovered some 300 years later; Bartisch apparently had not been able find a publisher.

His fame as one of the greatest early modern surgeons rests almost entirely on his *Ophthalmodouleia* (eye service), published in 1583. The book offers an excellent, comprehensive survey of the contemporary state of the art in ophthalmology. A brief section on ocular anatomy is followed by an in-depth account of the most important eye diseases and their treatment. In addition to various surgical techniques, the book devotes considerable space to medical therapies, such as eye waters for external use and drugs to prepare the body for an eye operation. The book was adorned with many large illustrations that showed the various eye diseases, as well as therapeutic methods and surgical tools. Examples ranged from the use of a special face mask for the treatment of strabismus, to the outward appearance of an eye with a cataract, to surgical methods to remove tumors.

Bartisch's conceptual framework was largely traditional and borrowed from humoral pathology. For example, eye diseases were believed to be caused most frequently by morbid humors in the body and the local deposits they formed, in particular in the area of the eye. Innovations were to be found only occasionally. One of the best known is a special surgical knife for total removal of the eyeball in cases of advanced eye tumors. Even the learned Wilhelm Fabricius had a copy made, based on Bartisch's description. But Fabricius improved it, in turn, when he found that Bartisch's instrument risked leaving parts of the eye tumor behind, which would start an even worse growth. Practical surgeons seemed to find Bartisch's book very useful. It was republished in the late sixteenth century and was to remain the major vernacular ophthalmologic textbook in Germany far into the eighteenth century.

Bibliography

Primary: 1583. *ΟΦΘΑΛΜΟΔΟΥΛΕΙΑ Das ist, Augendienst* (Dresden). [modern English trans. Oostende 1966, facsimile reprint Hannover 1983]; 1904. (Mankiewicz, Otto, ed.) *Kunstbuch darinnen ist der gantze gründliche, vollkomene, rechte, gewisse, bericht und erweisung vnnd Lehr des hartenn/ Reissenden, Schmertzhafftigenn, Peinlichenn Blasenn Steines . . .* (Berlin).

Secondary: Marré, Ernst, ed., 1985. *Georg Bartisch. Sein Leben, Werk und Vermächtnis* (Kamenz); Toellner, Richard, 1983. *Georg Bartisch (1535–1606). Bürger, Okulist, Schnitt- und Wundarzt zu Dresden und sein Werk 'Ophthalmodouleia das ist Augendienst'* [Supplement to the 1983 reprint] (Hannover); Holländer, Eugen, 1917. 'Marktschreizettel von Georg Bartisch. Reklame durch die Kanzel.' *Deutsche Medizinische Wochenschrift* 43: 1369–1370.

Michael Stolberg

BARTLETT, ELISHA (b. Smithfield, Rhode Island, USA, 6 October 1804; d. Smithfield, 19 July 1855) *medicine, philosophy.*

Bartlett's parents were Otis Bartlett and Waite Buffum Bartlett, leading members of Smithfield's Quaker community. After preparatory education he attended medical lectures in Boston and Providence and worked with practitioners in several smaller cities. He completed his MD degree at Brown University in 1826 and then spent a year in Paris. Upon his return, he settled in the growing industrial center of Lowell, Massachusetts. He was elected mayor of Lowell in 1836 and served two terms in the Massachusetts legislature beginning in 1840. Bartlett married Elizabeth Slater in 1829. They had no children.

In response to a critique of the Lowell factory system, Bartlett published an article noting the 'remarkable health' of the young women employed in the city's industry. Even Osler, however, in his laudatory sketch of Bartlett, acknowledged that there was another view, 'by no means a pleasant one, of the prolonged hours of the operatives and their wretched life in the boarding-houses' (Osler, 1900, p. 8).

Bartlett pursued the career of a peripatetic medical educator while maintaining his residence in Lowell. Over the course of twenty years he taught at eleven schools, for several years dividing his time between winter sessions in large cities and summer sessions in smaller country towns. In 1852, he accepted a chair at the College of Physicians and Surgeons in New York, his first permanent position.

In 1832 he founded the *Monthly Journal of Medical Literature and American Medical Students' Gazette,* intending it to go beyond case reports and to explore medical history and the medical literature. This journal survived for only three issues, but Bartlett quickly became involved in another new periodical that had some of the same features. In 1842 he published the first of several editions of a key text on typhoid and typhus fever. Osler points out that—in addition to providing an accurate clinical description of the diseases—Bartlett made clear that contemporary theories of fever were entirely speculative and suggested that the pathological basis of fever was yet to be understood.

Bartlett's *Philosophy of Medical Science* (1844) was the best American exposition of the methodology of the Paris school. Bartlett was adamant that doctors should generalize from observed facts and adopt theories only provisionally. He believed that absolute laws would not be found in medicine, but that 'approximative' principles would develop. In 1848 he published his *Inquiry into the Degree of Certainty in Medicine,* which was intended to demonstrate that some of the claims of medicine were justifiable and that, although disease usually runs its course regardless of the physician's action, there were some cases in which a doctor's intervention could effect or hasten a cure. Moreover, Bartlett insisted that the solace and hope that physicians provide was in itself an important contribution. Even so he was criticized for being too much of a therapeutic skeptic.

In 1854, while teaching in Kentucky, Bartlett began suffering from what Osler describes as 'some obscure nervous trouble' (Osler, 1900, p. 33). When this condition worsened during his second year in New York, he resigned his position and returned to Smithfield to die. He is remembered for a fluent writing style, which he utilized in an effort to raise the cultural level of the profession and to bring home to the USA the lessons of Paris.

Bibliography

Primary: 1842. *The History, Diagnosis, and Treatment of Typhoid and of Typhus Fever* (Philadelphia); 1844. *An Essay on the Philosophy of Medical Science* (Philadelphia); 1848. *An Inquiry into the Degree of Certainty in Medicine* (Philadelphia).

Secondary: Stempsey, William E., ed., 2005. *Elisha Bartlett's Philosophy of Medicine* (Dordrecht); Warner, John Harley, 1998. *Against the Spirit of System: The French Impulse in Nineteenth-Century American Medicine* (Princeton); Ackerknecht, Erwin, 1950. 'Elisha Bartlett and the Philosophy of the Paris Clinical School.' *Bulletin of the History of Medicine* 24: 34–60; Osler, William, 1900. *Elisha Bartlett: A Rhode Island Philosopher* (Providence); *DAMB.*

Edward T. Morman

BARTON, CLARA [CLARISSA] HARLOWE (b. North Oxford, Massachusetts, USA, 25 December 1821; d. Glen Echo, Maryland, USA, 12 April, 1912), *nursing, American Red Cross.*

Barton was the youngest of five children. Her father, a farmer and former soldier, was a socially aware, respected member of the community who was a believer in abolitionism and the importance of education. Her mother had a strong will, was outspoken on women's rights, and taught Barton the importance of thrift and cleanliness.

Barton's siblings assumed responsibility for her early education. From her sisters she learned spelling and geography. From her brothers she learned arithmetic and athletics. Her formal schooling began at age four, and she excelled in the classroom, but was exceptionally shy.

As an adolescent, her parents encouraged her to engage in charitable work, and she began to spend much of her free time actively assisting the ill and less fortunate. Day and night for two years, beginning when she was eleven, Barton nursed her brother, David, badly injured in an accident. At age seventeen, Barton embarked on an eighteen-year teaching career during which she taught in several schools and established several of her own.

Washington, D.C., became her home in 1854, where she worked as a clerk in the U.S. Patent Office. With the outbreak of the Civil War, Barton left the Patent Office to work as a volunteer. She collected supplies and provisions for the Union Army and delivered them to soldiers fighting on the front lines. Her work ministering to fallen soldiers earned her the title 'angel of the battlefield'.

In 1864 Barton was appointed superintendent of Union nurses. After the war ended, she began a campaign to search for missing soldiers and helped to reunite many soldiers with their loved ones. This project ultimately led to the identification and burial of thousands of Union prisoners of war.

In 1869 Barton went to Europe to rest and to regain her health. However, she soon found herself in the midst of the Franco-Prussian War. She began working with the International Red Cross, distributing supplies in France and Germany. She returned home in 1873 with the Iron Cross of Merit from the German emperor.

Barton saw the need for the Red Cross in the United States. Although the United States had not accepted the 1864 Treaty of Geneva, which made the Red Cross possible, Barton dedicated herself to bringing the Red Cross to the United States. She made speeches, distributed brochures, and called on cabinet heads and congressmen. Her efforts were successful, and in 1882 the Treaty of Geneva passed the U.S. Senate and was signed by President Chester A. Arthur.

Barton was the first president of the American Red Cross and directed its relief activities for the next twenty-three years. In the 1880s and 1890s the Red Cross assisted victims of fire, drought, earthquakes, tornadoes, and floods. In addition to disaster relief in the United States, the Red Cross also provided famine relief to Russia, Turkey, and Armenia.

In February 1898, Barton arrived in Havana, Cuba, to set up soup kitchens and supply hospitals, distribute clothing, and establish orphanages for the victims of the Spanish-American War. At age seventy-seven, she worked sixteen hours a day preparing food and nursing for victims of malaria, typhoid, dysentery, and yellow fever.

Barton believed in education and knew the importance of educating victims to look after themselves and rebuild their lives and homes after the Red Cross had left. Much of her efforts were directed toward teaching first aid and emergency preparedness. This initiative would prove correct. First aid practiced in the home would eventually help millions of people, and emergency preparedness would become a key element in disaster relief.

The last operation she personally directed was the relief effort for the victims of the 1900 Galveston, Texas, hurricane, at the time the largest natural disaster in American history.

In 1904, Barton was forced to resign as president of the American Red Cross. Her leadership style and financial management were under intense scrutiny and attack. She retired to her home in Glen Echo, Maryland, where she died of pneumonia.

A sometimes controversial figure, Clara Barton will always be remembered for her dedicated, compassionate relief of human suffering and her legacy of the American Red Cross.

Bibliography

Secondary: Oates, Stephen B., 1994. *A Woman of Valor: Clara Barton and the Civil War* (New York); Pryor, Elizabeth Brown, 1987. *Clara Barton, Professional Angel* (Philadelphia); *DAMB*.

C. Joan Richardson

BASAGLIA, FRANCO (b. Venice, Italy, 11 March 1924; d. Venice, 29 August 1980), *psychiatry*.

Basaglia was born in Venice into a wealthy family. The second of three children, he spent a happy childhood and adolescence in Venice, in the San Polo district. After completing grammar school he enrolled at Padua University, where he studied medicine and surgery, graduating in 1949.

During this period he was particularly interested in the works of Husserl, Heidegger, Merleau-Ponty, and Sartre. From Sartre he elaborated his idea of freedom, which led him toward asylum-based psychiatric work and the elaboration of patient rehabilitation practices tailored to individuals. In 1953 he specialized in mental and nervous diseases and qualified as a university professor in psychiatry in 1958.

Appointed director of the psychiatric hospital in Gorizia, Italy, in 1961, he approached phenomenological psychiatry through the works of Jaspers, Binswanger, and Minkowski. Starting from these sources, he worked on a further development of the best way to liaise with psychiatric patients, based on the conviction that they should be treated as people rather than clinical cases. To Basaglia phenomenology was important inasmuch as it placed emphasis on the antecedents of the patient, thus going beyond a merely positivist psychiatry.

The impact of the realities of asylum life on patients at the time was extremely hard; this motivated Basaglia strongly to strive for changes within psychiatric hospitals. He welcomed the ideas of the 'English' therapeutic community and, with regard to issues connected to psychiatric institutions, Basaglia largely referred to studies by Goffman and Foucault. While Basaglia worked at the asylum in Gorizia, physical restraint and the use of electric shock practices were abolished, and doors to and from the buildings were unlocked so that patients were free to move around, thus abolishing internal segregation.

In 1964 Basaglia went to London as part of the Italian delegation to the First International Congress on Social Psychiatry. There he presented a thesis based on 'The Destruction of the Psychiatric Hospital as a Place for Institutionalization', which was the basis of his subsequent work. In 1968 he edited a volume entitled *L'istituzione negata. Rapporto da un ospedale psichiatrico*, through which his work in Gorizia became known abroad, and thus also marks the birth of his anti-institutionalization movement.

After Gorizia, Basaglia was appointed director of the Colorno Hospital in Parma, and in 1971 he became director of the asylum in Trieste, where rehabilitation activities were set up for patients through painting and theater workshops. A social cooperative was also created to cater for working patients.

After striving to render asylum life more humane, Basaglia sought to establish the idea that it was possible to improve patients' future lives by closing the asylums and creating an external network of suitable alternative facilities. To Basaglia the closure of asylums entailed the destruction of the health service mechanism, which created the social divisions and sense of 'inferiority' that further invalidated the existence of the patient as an individual.

A political project thus became necessary to enable psychiatry to overcome the culture of asylum use. In 1973 he founded the movement for Democratic Psychiatry, and in 1977 he announced the closure of the psychiatric hospital in Trieste by the end of that year. In 1978 the Italian Parliament, almost unanimously, passed Law 180 on psychiatric reform, which, however, would prove to be extremely difficult to realize.

In 1979 Basaglia took part in various international congresses, especially in Europe and Brazil. Toward the end of that same year he left Trieste for Rome, where he became regional coordinator of the psychiatric services in Lazio. He died of cerebral cancer a few months later in Venice on 29 August 1980.

Bibliography

Primary: 1981. *Scritti, I: 1953–1968* (Turin); 1982. *Scritti, II: 1968–1980* (Turin); 1968. *L'istituzione negata. Rapporto da un ospedale psichiatrico* (Turin).

Secondary: Colucci, Mario, and Pierangelo Di Vittorio, 2001. *Franco Basaglia* (Milan).

Andrea Contini

BASEDOW, KARL ADOLPH VON (b. Dessau, Germany, 28 March 1799; d. Merseburg, Germany, 11 April 1854), *medicine.*

Basedow, son of the Regierungspräsident Ludwig von Basedow and Johanna Krüger, and grandson of the famous pedagogue Johann Bernhard Basedow, attended grammar school in Dessau and studied medicine at the university in Halle. Afterward, he spent two years of surgical service in Paris hospitals—the Charité and the Hôtel Dieu—graduating MD in 1821. In 1822 he settled in Merseburg as a physician. He was quickly respected as a brilliant and highly skilled helper in all branches of practical medicine, including obstetrics and pathology. He performed his own postmortem examinations and published findings on a number of difficult diseases. In 1830–31 he went to Magdeburg, in order to study the rampant cholera epidemic. In August 1834 he passed his physician's exam, the Physikatsprüfung, in Magdeburg. He was a sought-after physician and a well-respected medical officer of health, as well as a very prolific medical author. In 1844 he was appointed Sanitäts-Rath, the official consultant on medical affairs in Merseburg.

In German-speaking countries, Basedow's name is inexorably tied to exophthalmic cachexia, a disease accompanied by exophthalmos, thyroid gland enlargement (goiter), and an accelerated pulse (Merseburg Triad). Basedow is considered the first to describe this disease in German-speaking countries—the term 'Basedow's Disease' was coined by Georg Hirsch in *Clinische Fragmente* (Königsberg, 1858, vol. 2, p. 224). Basedow's famous contribution in the thyroid field appeared in1840, entitled 'Exophthalmos due to hypertrophy of the tissue in the orbit'. Exophthalmos, goiter, and palpitations of the heart have become known as the 'Merseburg Triad'. His claim to fame as the first to describe this affliction was contested by G. Flajani (1741–1808) in Italy and the Dublin clinician R. J. Graves (1797–1853). Basedow specifically called attention to the need to provide patients with iodine.

The articles he published attest to his capabilities as an active and competent physician who was acquainted with international medical publications and illustrated his theories with a diversity of cases, including pathological findings observed during his autopsies. That Basedow was a general practitioner who also took an active interest in his patients' living conditions can be concluded from his writing on the effects of wall paint emissions on general health. His interests were extremely varied, and during his lifetime he was involved in a great number of issues. Basedow's early death, presumably from a typhus fever infection, came three days after conducting an autopsy.

Bibliography

Primary: 1824. 'Über die Strictura ani spastica.' Graefe and Walther's *Journal der Chirurgie und Augenheilkunde* 7: 125–162; 1829. 'Einiges über das Zögern der Nachgeburt.' *Neues Journal für Geburtshülfe, Frauenzimmer- und Kinderkrankheiten* 9(1): 126–153; 1840. 'Exophthalmus durch Hypertrophie des Zellgewebes in der Augenhöhle.' *Wochenschrift für die gesammte Heilkunde* pp. 197–204, 220–228; 1848. 'Fernere Beobachtungen über die gesundheitsnachtheiligen Ausdünstungen der Zimmerfarben aus arseniksaurem Kupferoxyd.' *Wochenschrift für die gesammte Heilkunde* pp. 417–429, 436–448, 453–462.

Secondary: Meng, W., 1999. 'Carl Adolph von Basedow—zu seinem 200. Geburtstag.' *Zeitschrift für ärztliche Fortbildung und Qualitätssicherung* 93 (Supplement 1): 5–10; Medvei, V. C., 1982. *A History of Endocrinology* (Lancaster); Anon., 1935. *Medizinische Welt* 9: 34–36, 70–72; Anon., 1910. *Münchner Medizinische Wochenschrift* 57: 749.

Marion Hulverscheidt

BASSINI, EDOARDO (b. Pavia, Italy, 14 April 1844; d. Padua, Italy, 20 July 1924), *surgery.*

Bassini was son of Giovanni Battista Bassini and Luigia Rognoni. He studied medicine in Pavia, where he was trained by pathologist and histologist Giulio Bizzozero in the most recent microscopic techniques and by Luigi Porta in the newest surgical techniques. In 1866 he interrupted his studies to enroll in Garibaldi's volunteer troop fighting against the Austrian occupation of the Venetian region. In 1867 Bassini was seriously injured and saved by his master Luigi Porta. He then resumed his studies. Upon graduation he was trained in London by Joseph Lister and visited the clinical institutions of Thomas Spencer Wells at London, of Theodor Billroth at Vienna, and of Bernhard Langenbeck at Berlin. Back in Italy he became Porta's assistant (1874) and substitute professor of clinical surgery at the universities of Pavia (1876) and Parma (1879). After a short period as head surgeon at the hospital of La Spezia, he was called to the chair of surgical pathology (1882) and then of clinical surgery (1888) at the University of Padua. He retired in 1919 and died five years later at the age of eighty.

From Porta and his European masters, Bassini learned to treat surgery as an art, giving priority to high technology and to constant research and innovation. He introduced into Italian surgery the new techniques for nephropexy (surgical fixation of a floating kidney, 1882), for the operation of nasal polyps (1887), and for abdominal hysterectomy (1889), and also Lister's antiseptic sprinkling of the operative field and the hemostasis of the blood vessels with forceps. Moreover, Bassini was the first Italian to demonstrate the importance of normal and pathological histology for surgery, developing a series of new surgical techniques.

His most important innovation concerns the operation for inguinal hernia, one of the most frequent lesions of the human body. It was put into practice for the first time on 24 December 1884 at the Ospedale Maggiore of Padua and was made known at the congress of the Italian Surgical Society in 1887. Bassini was convinced that inguinal hernia was caused by a mechanical pathology and that hence an operative intervention had to reconstruct the abdominal side in order to restore a physical resistance to the mechanical factors. His new method consisted in a 'radical technique': the suture of the strata and the enforcement of the single anatomical plane on the abdominal side. The three anatomic layers of the posterior wall of the inguinal canal were sutured together in an overlapping fashion. Bassini's original technique found wide application until the 1980s. It was improved in the 1960s by Earl Shouldice and is as such still in general use today.

Bassini also distinguished himself as an excellent practical surgeon who, for the first time, followed up his postoperative patients. Thus he succeeded in reducing the cases of postoperative relapse from 20 percent down to 2.5 percent. His other important innovations concern procedures for femoral hernia (1883), the surgery of the thorax, the amputation of the uterus, and the resection of the segment between the small intestine and the appendix.

Like many of his Italian and European colleagues around the turn of the century, Bassini was socially engaged and donated, shortly before his death, his villa in Vigesia to the veterans of World War I affected by tuberculosis. He furthermore made a generous donation to an institution in Milan devoted to the assistance of humble people that had fallen ill with hernia, today known as the *Ospedale Bassini*.

Bibliography

Primary: 1889. *Nuovo metodo operativo per la cura dell'ernia inguinale* (Padua); 1893. *Nuovo metodo operativo per la cura radicale dell'ernia crurale* (Padua).

Secondary: Nyhus, L. M., 2001. 'Evolution of Hernia Repair.' *Hernia* 5: 196–199; Castellani, Carlo, 1989. *Medicina e sanità in Italia nel ventesimo secolo* (Rome); Vitali, E. D., 1965. 'Edoardo Bassini' in *Dizionario biografico degli italiani* vol. 7 (Rome) pp. 144–145.

Ariane Dröscher

BATEMAN, THOMAS (b. Whitby, Yorkshire, England, 29 April 1778; d. London, England, 9 April 1821), *dermatology*.

Bateman, the only son of a surgeon, was brought up in the Quaker faith. Little is known of his youth, but he did attend private school first at Whitby and then at Thornton. Before starting medical studies in London in 1797, possibly as a physician's pupil at Guy's Hospital, he had been apprenticed to an apothecary in Whitby. He then attended the Great Windmill Street School of Anatomy, listened to the lectures of Matthew Baillie (1761–1823), and participated in the activities of St George's Hospital. From 1798 to 1801, he matriculated at the University of Edinburgh, where his MD thesis (1801) was titled *Haemorrhoea petechialis*.

Instead of returning to Yorkshire, he made a permanent move to London. Obtaining a hospital appointment was difficult, and so he gravitated to the Public Dispensary on Carey Street, under the charge of Robert Willan (1757–1812), and in 1804 was appointed to the staff. There was now great concern about contagion, and Willan succeeded in having a fever hospital developed in Grays Inn Road, where Bateman served as his assistant.

Bateman would become not only Willan's best pupil but also his most devoted follower. Although Willan withdrew from most activities at the Carey Street Dispensary about 1805, Bateman remained very close to his mentor. He taught many pupils from the Continent, among them Laurent Biett (1781–1840), who created in Paris a rival school to the followers of Jean Louis Alibert (1768–1837). Like his teacher, Bateman was interested in the effect of climate and weather on disease, publishing his observations in the *Edinburgh Medical and Surgical Journal*, which he had helped to establish in 1805. Most of the papers were subsequently collected in the *Reports on the Diseases of London* (1819).

He became a licentiate of the RCP in 1805 and subsequently developed an important medical practice. Bateman was a keen observer and an even more commendable writer. His works reflect his knowledge of the ancients, and he was appointed Librarian of the Medical and Chirurgical Society of London, of which he was a founding member in 1805. (This was a breakaway group from the Medical Society of London and would later become the Royal Society of Medicine.) He was responsible for publishing a catalogue of the library in 1816. His honorary memberships included the Literary and Philosophical Society of London and New York. He was also a devotee of music and an accomplished organist. As a very religious man, Bateman wrote religious tracts, particularly after gravitating toward evangelical Christianity.

Bateman's major contributions are in the continuation and extension of Willan's classification of cutaneous disease, which had provided an orderly approach to the field. All was not so easy, for Willan's widow would not permit Bateman the possession of her late husband's work, instead fostering their potential publication by her son-in-law Ashby Smith. Eventually, Bateman was able to purchase the rights in 1817.

Bateman, along with his pupil Anthony Todd Thomson (1778–1849), published *A Practical Synopsis of Cutaneous Diseases According to the Arrangement of Dr. Willan, Exhibiting a Concise View of The Diagnostic Symptoms and the Method of Treatment* (1813); the title tells all. This was translated into French, German, Italian, and Swedish, with many American editions also produced. Five editions appeared in London, with the last being edited by Thomson (1849). So wide was the circulation of this volume that the Russian tsar ordered copies and rewarded Bateman with a diamond ring, valued at 100 guineas. A more extensive work appeared in 1817: *Delineations of Cutaneous Diseases*. Bateman introduced several skin diseases that came to be known as Bateman's disease: alopecia areata, ecthyma, molluscum contagiosum, and erythema multiforme (iris lesion). He seems also to have codified the term 'eczema'.

Bateman had what in contemporary parlance was called a delicate constitution, and his health began to fail. In 1816 he lost the sight in his right eye and the vision in the left was compromised, for which he sought a cure by the sulfur waters, possibly in Middleton, County Durham. When the problem, possibly mercury poisoning, seemed to have been resolved, he returned to London in 1817 to resume work at the Fever Institution. Unfortunately, this was only temporary and his health continued to deteriorate, and he left permanently for Yorkshire about 1819, dying two years later at the age of forty-two. There is no record of Bateman having married.

Bibliography

Primary: 1813. (with Thomson, Anthony Todd, and Robert Willan) *A Practical Synopsis of Cutaneous Diseases According to the Arrangement of Dr. Willan, Exhibiting a Concise View of the Diagnostic Symptoms and the Method of Treatment* (London); 1817.

(with Willan, Robert) *Delineations of Cutaneous Diseases; Exhibiting the Characteristic Appearances of the Principal Genera and Species Comprised in the Classification of the Late Dr. Willan and Completing the Series of Engravings Begun by That Author* (London); 1818. *A Succinct Account of the Contagious Fever of This Country, Exemplified in the Epidemic Now Prevailing in London with the Appropriate Method of Treatment as Practised in the House of Recovery: To Which Are Added Observations on the Nature and Properties of Contagion, Tending to Correct the Popular Notions on This Subject, and Pointing out the Means of Prevention* (London); 1819. *Reports on the Diseases of London, and the State of the Weather, from 1804 to 1816* (London).

Secondary: Holubar, K., 2004. 'The Compilation and Edition of the First Color Atlas of Dermatology by Robert Willan (1757–1812), Thomas Bateman (1778–1821), and Ashby Smith (–1831) from 1790 to 1817.' *Acta Dermatovenerol. Croat.* 12(1): 12–17; Levell, N. J., 2000. 'Thomas Bateman MD FLS 1778–1821.' *Br. J. Dermatol.* 143(1): 9–15; Leach, D., and J. Beckwith, 1999. 'The Founders of Dermatology: Robert Willan and Thomas Bateman.' *J. R. Coll. Physicians Lond.* 33(6): 580–582; Tilles, G., and D. Wallach, 1999. 'Robert Willan and the French Willanists.' *Br. J. Dermatol.* 140(6): 1120–1126; 1847. *Sketches of Eminent Medical Men* (Philadelphia); Rumsey, James, 1826. *Some Account of the Life and Character of the Late Thomas Bateman, M. D.* (London); Rumsey, James, 1822. *Brief Memoir of the Late Thomas Bateman* (Edinburgh); *Oxford DNB*.

Lawrence Charles Parish

BATTEY, ROBERT (b. Augusta, Georgia, USA, 26 November 1828; d. Rome, Georgia, USA, 8 November 1895), *medicine, gynecology.*

Battey, a younger son of Cephas Battey of New York state (whose Quaker ancestors were English) and Mary Agnes Magruder, was educated at Richmond Academy in Georgia and at Phillips Academy, Andover, in Massachusetts, before attending Booth's School of Analytical Chemistry, Philadelphia, and Jefferson Medical College, where he was taught by Charles D. Meigs. In the year commencing his medical studies, he married Martha Baldwin Smith (20 December 1849). Of their fourteen children, eight survived. After graduating from Philadelphia College of Pharmacy (1856) and from Jefferson (1857) and receiving the Obstetrical Institute of Philadelphia's diploma (1857), Battey concluded his medical studies by touring Britain, Ireland, and the Continent (1859–60). In Britain, he met Thomas Spencer Wells, then beginning his career as an ovariotomist.

During the American Civil War (1861–65), Battey served the Confederate Army as surgeon to the Nineteenth Georgia Volunteers and senior surgeon to Hampton's Brigade, both in the field and at hospitals in Atlanta, Rome, Macon, and Vineville, Georgia, and in Lauderdale, Mississippi. After returning to Rome, he established a Gynecological Infirmary, later enlarged to become the Martha Battey Hospital, named after his wife, who acted as surgical assistant and nurse. Battey performed his first ovariotomy (May 1869), successfully removing a thirty-pound dermoid cyst from a physician's wife. This procedure, pioneered in 1809 by Ephraim McDowell, was performed with increasing regularity following the introduction (1846) of anesthesia. It remained, nevertheless, a risky and controversial operation, breaching the peritoneal barrier and introducing 'foreign' suture material into the abdominal cavity. Battey, however, was considered one of the South's foremost surgeons.

On 17 August 1872 he performed a 'normal ovariotomy' on Julia Omberg, a thirty-year-old with amenorrhea and convulsions, pelvic cellulitis, and articular rheumatism, symptoms Battey associated with the effort to menstruate (menstrual molimen). Both 'functionally active' ovaries were removed as a *'dernier ressort'* to induce the menopause and relieve the patient's intense sufferings (she was, like a number of his patients, a morphine addict). The procedure became known as 'Battey's operation', although it was performed simultaneously in Germany by Alfred Hegar and in England by Robert Lawson Tait. In 1879 Spencer Wells reported a case of his own performed in 1865 for dysmenorrhea. At first, Battey used both an abdominal and a vaginal approach, devising a new self-retaining speculum for the purpose, but later advocated only the abdominal approach.

Battey was professor of obstetrics at Atlanta Medical College (1873–75) and editor of the *Atlanta Medical and Surgical Journal* (1873–76), but appears to have preferred private practice. Returning to Rome, he became president of the Georgia Medical Association (1876) and a founding member of the American Gynecological Society, serving as its president in 1889. He held fellowships of the British Gynaecological Society and the Obstetrical Society of Edinburgh. Between 1872 and 1890, he published over twenty articles on Battey's operation and, at the International Medical Congress in London (1881), reported 193 cases of bilateral oöphorectomy performed by forty-nine surgeons with an overall mortality of twenty per cent. Flagrant abuse of the procedure, which Battey claimed to have foreseen, and its performance particularly on institutionalized women for questionable indications, including insanity, epilepsy, nymphomania, and masturbation, caused Battey's operation to fall into disrepute. Its unquestionable contributions were to the development of pelvic surgery and to an understanding, prior to the discovery of the hormones secreted by the ovaries, of the role played by the ovary in menstruation and secondary sexual characteristics.

Throughout his career, Battey remained adamant that he operated with honorable intent 'to bring about a great physiological change in the system of the patient for the remedy of disease' (Battey, 1888, p. 837) and disliked the term 'oöphorectomy'. Nevertheless, as he later related, a group of townsmen, including physicians, waited during Julia Omberg's procedure to arrest him in the event of her death. As a surgeon, he was described as bold but prudent. A tall slender man, always plainly dressed and outwardly modest, he was considered to have much personal magnetism, which was combined with kindness and consideration for patients and acquaintances alike.

Bibliography

Primary: 1876. 'Extirpation of the functionally active ovaries for the remedy of otherwise incurable diseases.' *Transactions of the American Gynecological Society* 1: 101–120; 1880. 'Summary of the results of fifteen cases of Battey's operation.' *British Medical Journal* i: 510–512; 1881. 'Oöphorectomy—Battey's operation—spaying—castration of women.' *Transactions of the International Medical Congress* (London), 7th session, 4: 279–297; 1882. 'A new speculum.' *British Medical Journal* i: 194; 1888. (with Coe, Henry C.) 'Diseases of the ovaries' in Mann, Matthew D., ed., *A System of Gynecology by American Authors* vol. 2 (Edinburgh).

Secondary: Dally, Ann, 1991. *Women under the Knife: A History of Surgery* (London); Longo, Lawrence D., 1979. 'The Rise and Fall of Battey's Operation: A Fashion of Surgery.' *Bulletin of the History of Medicine* 53: 244–267; Reamy, Thaddeus A., 1896. 'In Memorium: Robert Battey, M.D., LL.D.' *Transactions of the American Gynecological Society* 21: 467–472; Watson, Irving A., 1896. *Physicians and Surgeons of America* (Concord); *DAMB*.

Carole Reeves

BATUT, MILAN JOVANOVIĆ (b. Sremska Mitrovica, Serbia, 22 October 1847; d. Belgrade, Yugoslavia (now Serbia), 11 September 1940), *social hygiene, bacteriology, public health, medical education.*

Batut (father Konstantin, mother Marija) studied in Vienna under professors Hyrtl, Rokitansky, Skoda, Bruecke, and Billroth, earning a PhD in 1878. As a student, he published several works on eugenics, as well as a book entitled *Zdravlje i napredak naše dece* [Health and Progress of our Children] in 1877. Following graduation, Batut began medical practice in Sombor (present-day northern Serbia and Montenegro). In 1882, with the support of Vladan Djordjevi, Batut was awarded a scholarship to study hygiene and bacteriology. He spent three years abroad, working in Munich with Max von Pettenkofer (a founder of scientific hygiene), in Berlin with Robert Koch, and in London with eugenist Francis Galton. Batut also spent several months with Pasteur in Paris, researching bacterial penetration of the placenta in collaboration with a Russian colleague, Bubnov.

In 1887 Batut was appointed professor of Public Hygiene and Forensic Medicine at the Great School (now Belgrade University) in Belgrade. Established in 1866, the Belgrade chair for public hygiene was among the first such professorships in Europe. Batut founded the first hygiene laboratory in Serbia, organizing the first bacteriological examinations of air, soil, and water in the country. During this period, he also began a long-term anthropometric study of the Serbian population. At the time, Serbia had one of the highest rates of neonatal mortality, and the infant mortality rate ran as high as 22 to 24 percent.

Understanding the importance of mobilizing the educated local populace in order to establish medical care and hygienic culture in a poor, agrarian country, Batut established a network of teachers, priests, and physicians. In 1880 he founded the periodical *Zdravlje* [Health], in Sombor (then part of Austria-Hungary), and later published the magazine in Belgrade in 1906. As president of the Society for the Protection of the People's Health, Batut traveled around the country, holding lectures and organizing hygienic exhibitions.

Batut published some 157 works in his lifetime, covering such topics as raising children, contagious diseases, and nutrition and pregnancy. They included nine monographs and three university textbooks, most notably *Pouke o cuvanju zdravla* [The Lessons about Health Protection] in 1884; and *Zdravlje I bolest* [Health and Disease] in 1922. His book on medical terminology (1886) contains more than 26,000 Serbian medical terms.

Batut's most significant contribution to medicine in Serbia, however, was the establishment of the Medical Faculty of Serbia in 1920, after two decades of determined effort. Batut served as the inaugural Dean of the Medical Faculty, as well as professor of hygiene. A member of all the relevant state bodies dealing with health care and disease prevention, Batut wrote the drafts of the Basic Sanitary Law (1929), the Prevention of Contagious Diseases Law, and the Chronic Diseases Containment Law.

Reflecting on his career, Batut wrote: 'I considered that the principal objective of my work was to bring more medical education into the family, as a foundation of survival and progress in every human community, and to direct physicians to get to know our people and its pathology, to live devoted to this people'. He was the recipient of numerous awards and distinctions, including the French Legion of Honor.

Bibliography

Primary: 1884. *Pouke o cuvanju zdravla* [The Lessons about Health Protection] (Belgrade); 1922. *Zdravlje I bolest* [Health and Disease] (Split).

Secondary: Jović, Pavle, 2002. 'Milan Jovanović Batut' in *Život i delo srpskih naunika*, 8 (Belgrade); 1972. *Spomenica Srpskog Lekarskog Društva* (Belgrade); 1961. *Medicinska enciklopedija*, 5 Hipos–Koma (Zagreb); Stanojevi, Vladimir, 1962. *Istorija medicine* (Belgrade).

Jelena Jovanovic Simic and Predrag J. Markovic

BAUDELOCQUE, JEAN-LOUIS (b. Heilly, Somme, France, 30 November 1745; d. Paris, France, 2 May 1810), *surgery, obstetrics.*

Baudelocque was the son of the physician and surgeon, Jean-Louis Baudelocque, and Anne-Marie Lavasseur. Two of his nephews, César-Auguste and Louis-Auguste, were also physicians. Baudelocque studied anatomy, surgery, and obstetrics at the Paris Faculty of Medicine. He became assistant to Solayrès de Renhac at the Charité hospital and took over the course when his teacher fell ill. As a professor at the Faculty of Medicine, he wrote a thesis in 1776 against the practice of symphyseotomy (surgical division of the pubic bones to enlarge the birth canal), which earned him admission to the College of Surgery.

During the Revolution, after the abolition of the Faculty of Medicine and the College of Surgery, Baudelocque became professor of obstetrics at the new *École de santé* and chief obstetrician at the Maternity of the Hôtel Dieu of Paris, which had just been transferred to Port-Royal, where it remains today. He was also responsible for the training of future midwives; his teaching clinic admitted some two thousand women in childbirth annually. He employed a lively question-and-answer method of instruction that demanded a lot of time, so he delegated a portion of his authority to a highly skilled midwife, Marie-Louise Lachapelle. With her expert help, he was able to train one hundred midwives per year and to create one of the most progressive schools of the period.

In 1806, Napoleon named Baudelocque to the chair of obstetrics, the first specialty professorship in France. He was obliged to give up private practice, but his reputation made him sought after by royalty. He became *accoucheur* to the queens of Spain, Holland, and Naples and to the court ladies of France. He died a short time before he was to deliver Empress Marie-Louise, who would give birth to Napoleon's son, the King of Rome.

Known as 'the new savior' of mothers and children, Baudelocque was the uncontested master of French obstetrics at the beginning of the nineteenth century, and his reputation extended over much of Europe. Imperious of temperament, he did not take criticism lightly, and he made many enemies, including Sigault and Leroy, the advocates of symphyseotomy, and Jean-François Sacombe, the leader of those who opposed cesarean sections for delivery. His followers drew support after Baudelocque's failure in a cesarean section resulted in the death of the mother and her baby. Baudelocque was against intervention to provoke labor in cases involving a narrow pelvic opening, a method favored by British obstetricians. Yet, unlike Levret, he cautioned against the use of the forceps, declaring 'There is nothing like the skillful use of the hands'. He placed complete confidence in podalic version (a maneuver in which the obstetrician turned the child in order to grasp a foot to make the delivery) followed by extraction, but he had recourse to the forceps in certain cases.

Baudelocque published two manuals—one in question-and-answer format for midwives, and the other for obstetricians. He was the first to describe with great precision the process of normal childbirth. But, obsessed by classification, he identified no fewer than ninety-four different positions in which the baby might present. Madame de Lachapelle reduced the total to twenty-two.

Baudelocque's contribution to obstetrics resided more in his scientific methodology than in any specific intervention. Along with contemporary British obstetricians, Baudelocque was responsible for introducing rigorous, precise, and clear guidelines for the practitioner.

Bibliography

Primary: 1775. *Principes sur l'art des accouchements*, 5 éditions (Paris); 1781. *l'Art des accouchements*, 6 éditions (Paris); 1787. *Principes sur l'art des accouchements en faveur des sages-femmes de la campagne* (Paris).

Secondary: Beauvalet-Boutouyrie, Scarlett, 1999. *Naître à l'hôpital au XIXe siècle* (Paris); Gélis, Jacques, 1988. *La sage-femme ou le médecin; une nouvelle conception de la vie* (Paris); Siebold, Eduard C. J. von, 1891. *Essai d'une histoire de l'obstétricie*, vol. 2 (Paris); Witkowski, G. J., 1891. *Accoucheurs et sages-femmes célèbres* (Paris).

Jacques Gélis

BAUER, KARL HEINRICH

(b. Schwärzdorf, Germany, 26 September 1890; d. Heidelberg, Germany, 7 July 1978), *surgery, oncology.*

Born as one of three children to a farmer and his wife in Upper Franconia, Bauer always wondered how his parents managed to grant two sons access to academic training. He attended Gymnasium in Bamberg, living in the house of a senior member of the student fraternity *Bubenruthia*. He joined that fraternity when he enrolled to study medicine at Erlangen in 1909. In a curriculum vitae written in 1946, Bauer claimed that he had always been skeptical about fraternity life, which was characterized by fencing competitions and heavy drinking, and often included chauvinistic sentiments. However, fraternities also provided their members with lifelong friendships and support networks. Bauer continued his studies in Heidelberg, Munich, and Würzburg, where he decided to specialize in surgery. After passing his state examination in 1914, he served in World War I, as did most graduates of his cohort. According to his own account, his experiences during battle and a serious injury in 1917 left a lasting impression.

In 1918 Bauer became an assistant to the eminent pathologist Ludwig Aschoff (1866–1942) at Freiburg, where he laid the foundations of his scholarly career. In 1919, after a brief stint as a countryside practitioner, he joined the surgical clinic at Göttingen, where in 1922 he received his Habilitation. In 1926 he was promoted to associate professor. Many of Bauer's publications during the Göttingen period were—unusually for a surgeon—dedicated to the then-fashionable issues of heredity and constitutional pathology. He published a much-discussed book, *Racial Hygiene: The Biological Foundations* (1926), which he regretted after the end of World War II, musing that 'Eugenics' might have been a better, less controversial title.

In 1933 Bauer accepted a call to the chair of surgery at Breslau. In his postwar CV, he emphasized that he received the call before Hitler assumed power, and he wrote that during the Nazi years he encountered difficulties because he spoke out for Jewish friends, and because of his wife's Jewish ancestry. Bauer styled himself as an enemy of the Third Reich, but he is probably better characterized as one of many German professors who initially sympathized with some aspects of the Nazi program but became increasingly disillusioned and eventually hostile to the regime. Most of these, however, chose 'inner emigration' over open resistance, and they adapted to the situation without much detriment to their careers. It probably helped Bauer that surgeons were needed during times of war. He continued to publish prolifically, including articles on the consequences of the Nazi sterilization law for surgeons (1934) and on the practice of sterilization (1935, 1936). In 1943 he accepted a call to Heidelberg.

Postwar Heidelberg saw Bauer excel as an administrator, starting with his election as first rector of the reopened university in 1945, and culminating in his championship of the large German Cancer Research Center (*Deutsches Krebsforschungszentrum*), which first opened its doors in 1964. Cancer had also become the main focus of Bauer's scholarly interest. He is hailed as one of the most influential German cancer specialists of the postwar era, not least because of his ability to communicate with nonspecialist audiences. Bauer never joined a political party, but he was an active participant in the public life of the Federal Republic, commenting, for example, on environmental cancer risks and the dangers of car traffic. He also served as a government expert on cancer. From 1945 to 1968 Bauer corresponded with the philosopher and physician Karl Jaspers (1883–1969) about academic, philosophical, and political issues.

Bibliography

Primary: 1949. *Das Krebsproblem* (Berlin).

Secondary: Herfarth, Christian, 1990. '100th Anniversary of the birthday of Karl-Heinrich Bauer.' *European Journal of Surgical Oncology* 16: 277–279; De Rosa, Renato, ed., 1983. *Karl Jaspers & K. H. Bauer, Briefwechsel, 1945–1968* (Berlin); Linder, Fritz and Wilhelm Doerr, eds., 1979. *Karl Heinrich Bauer: Konturen einer Persönlichkeit* (Berlin); Schwaiger, M., 1979. 'Karl Heinrich Bauer in Memoriam'. *Deutsche Medizinische Wochenschrift* 104: 441–443.

Carsten Timmermann

BAYLE, ANTOINE-LAURENT

(b. Vernet, Alpes-Maritimes, France, 13 January 1799; d. Paris, France, 29 March 1858), *mental pathology.*

Born into a landowning family that had been long established in the south of France, Bayle journeyed to Paris at sixteen. He hoped to embark on a career in medicine with the help of his uncle, Gaspard-Laurent Bayle, a leading figure among the first postrevolutionary generation of hospital clinicians. Unfortunately, Gaspard-Laurent lay dying of pulmonary tuberculosis at the age of forty-two. However, the elder Bayle's influential medical friends, notably his close colleague Laennec, were able to obtain a place for him at the Charité hospital. In 1817, again profiting from his late uncle's friendships, Bayle became an intern in the service of Royer-Collard at the mental asylum of Charenton, outside Paris.

Bayle defended his MD thesis, *Recherches sur les maladies mentales*, on 21 November 1822. It would become a landmark in the history of psychiatry and a striking application of the anatomo-clinical method advocated by his mentors. Here, Bayle demonstrated a correlation between chronic inflammation of the arachnoid membrane of the brain and progressive general paralysis of the insane (GPI). Bayle's description provided clear evidence of a long-supposed connection between insanity and organic disease of the brain. He identified stages of increasing neurological and mental impairment developing in tandem, beginning with impairment of speech, walking, and cognition, and terminating inevitably in an advanced state of paralysis, dementia, and death. Bayle based his description on six clinical case histories, four of whom displayed 'dominant or grandiose ideation'. He later made delusions of grandeur an important diagnostic feature of general paralysis of the insane.

In 1825, with the death of Royer-Collard, Bayle lost his position at Charenton. Not yet thirty years old, he found himself without a patron or a future in the emerging specialty of psychiatry to which he had made an epochal contribution. Bayle's career dead-end resulted in part from his not being a member of Esquirol's school of psychiatry, which held a virtual monopoly over the field. Moreover, his concept of an anatomical connection in mental illness ran counter to the reigning paradigm of Pinel, Esquirol, and their followers, who classified mental illness in terms of symptoms, signs, and functional impairment.

For the next two decades, Bayle devoted himself mostly to medical literary work. He served as assistant librarian to the medical faculty, but lost the competition for chief librarian. He edited his uncle's treatise on cancer and collaborated on various medical periodicals. He also was chief editor of the *Encyclopédie des sciences médicales*, within which he published a two-volume biographical dictionary of physicians from earliest times until his own day. By arranging the entries in chronological order of birth, Bayle sought to show the succession of medical errors, as well as advances.

In the 1850s Bayle defended his priority in the discovery of general paralysis. He discussed pathogenesis in greater detail, attributing manifestations of the ailment to compromised blood flow to and pressure on the brain. Not until late in the nineteenth century did physicians agree that syphilis was the cause of GPI. Bayle's unified conception of the disease, however, prevailed over rival theories that considered the progressive paralysis and the dementia to be either separate entities or late complications of mental illness. Bayle's long-term significance was to establish a specific precedent, indeed a model, for the doctrine equating mental illness with brain pathology.

Bibliography

Primary: 1822. Recherches sur les maladies mentales MD thesis, Paris; 1825. *Nouvelle doctrine des maladies mentales* (Paris); 1840–41. *Biographie médicale*, 2 vols., in *Encyclopédie des sciences médicales* (Paris).

Secondary: Brown, Edward M., 1994. 'French psychiatry's initial reception of Bayle's discovery of general paralysis of the insane.' *Bulletin of the History of Medicine* 68: 235–253; Semelaigne, René, 1930. *Les pionniers de la psychiatrie française*, vol.1 (Paris) pp. 244–249.

Toby Gelfand

IBN AL-BAYṬĀR, ḌIYĀ' AD-DĪN ABŪ MUḤAMMAD ʿABD ALLĀH IBN AḤMAD   (b. Malaga, Spain, *c.* 1197; d. Damascus, Syria, 1248), *medical botany.*

Ibn al-Bayṭār was born in Malaga and belonged to the family of the same name. His biography was preserved by Ibn Abī Usaibiʿa, his pupil from Damascus and a famous biographer of the Greek and Arabic doctors, with whom he collected plants. He studied in Seville under Abū 'l-ʿAbbās al-Nabāṭī, ʿAbd Allāh b. Ṣāliḥ, and Abū 'l-Ḥajjāj Yūsuf ibn Mūrāṭīr. In about 1220, he set out for the East, visiting North Africa, Asia Minor, and Syria. He lived in Egypt before settling in Damascus.

Useful sources for Ibn al-Bayṭār's biography are the names of places where he is known to have collected indigenous plants and herbs: Morocco, Algeria, Tunisia, and Tripoli (region, Libya). He also frequented many places in Syria, including Ghaza, Beirut, and Mt Lebanon. Some scholars believe he even went to Greece and India.

On his arrival in Egypt, the Ayyubid al-Mālik al-ʿĀdil appointed Ibn al-Bayṭār head of the Egyptian herbalists and later Doctor-in-Chief. His son, Mālik as-Ṣāliḥ Najm ad-Dīn, kept Ibn al-Bayṭār in his service, and Ibn al-Bayṭār started writing his major works while working for Mālik as-Ṣāliḥ Najm ad-Dīn. The books were dedicated to his patron. From Cairo, he undertook several scientific expeditions before moving to Damascus.

The two most important works by Ibn al-Bayṭār are the 'Collection of Simples' (*Jāmiʿ al-Mufradāt*) and the 'Sufficient' (*al-Mughnī*). The Collection of Simples comprises 2,330 paragraphs containing the names of 1,400 simples (herbs) arranged in alphabetical order, with their synonyms, descriptions, and properties. In this erudite volume he cited 150 authorities including al-Rāzī (400 times), Ibn Sīnā (300 times), and al-Ghafiqī (200 times). He also made use of Dioscorides' book of simples. The Collection of Simples became one of the standard books in the East and influenced many subsequent botanical works, including the Armenian Amin Dowlat's treatise on simples.

Apart from these two major works, Ibn al-Bayṭār authored 'The Druggist's Scales', a treatise about remedies, and 'A Chapter about Lemon'. Several other works, including a treatise on weights and measures and a book on veterinary medicine, are attributed to him.

Bibliography

Primary: 1987. *Traité des simples*/Ibn al-Bayṭār (traduction de Leclerc, Lucien) (Paris).

Secondary: Ullmann, Manfred, 1978. *Islamic Medicine.* trans. Jean Watt (Edinburgh); *DSB*; *Encyclopaedia of Islam*.

Nikolaj Serikoff

BEANEY, JAMES GEORGE (b. Canterbury, England, 15 January 1828; d. Melbourne, Australia, 30 June 1891), *surgery, sex education.*

Beaney, the son of George and Sarah 'Beney', completed his surgical indentures as an apprentice in Canterbury and later studied under James Syme in Edinburgh. As a young man he enlisted and served as a military surgeon with the 3rd Lancashire Regiment, based in Gibraltar, during the Crimean War. In 1857 he emigrated to Melbourne, working for eighteen months as assistant and partner to the pioneer Victorian obstetrician and pediatrician, John Maund (1823–58).

Beaney established a huge medical practice in Melbourne and became the richest doctor in Victoria, and probably in Australia. He practiced both heroic and conservative surgery and was one of the Australian pioneers of Listerian antisepsis. He was continually at the controversial forefront of innovations, not only in the technical aspects of medicine but in sociological developments that affected health. Beaney wrote the first Australian medical textbook, *Original Contributions to the Practice of Conservative Surgery* (1859).

Another of Beaney's significant contributions was his use, promotion, and teaching of anesthesia for surgery on children. In 1859 he wrote comprehensively about the various advantages and disadvantages of chloroform and ether. His cavalier surgical personality and willingness to embark on heroic surgery depended on relatively safe and prolonged anesthesia, a fact that he constantly acknowledged. He taught that the risks of anesthesia were age-dependent and that neonates could be safely anesthetized. He wrote the first two Australian textbooks on pediatrics. *Vaccination and its Dangers* (1870) decried arm-to-arm vaccination of children, and *Children: Their Treatment in Health and Disease* (1873) dealt with neonates, infants, and young children. Beaney also published the first textbook on family planning and contraception in Australia (1872) and the first Australian work on the history of medicine, *The History and Progress of Surgery* (1877).

Beaney's promotion of family planning and contraception was courageous, and it embroiled him in further controversy within the conservative *milieu* of Victorian Australia. In 1873 he published, in Melbourne, the first Australian text on sex education and family planning—*The Generative System and its Function in Health and Disease.* Childless himself, Beaney was an advocate for ameliorating the plight of poverty-stricken families, with the attendant degradation and misery of children. His promotion of family planning, contraception, and the public understanding of sexuality enmeshed him in fierce battles that resulted in ostracism by his peers in the medical establishment. *The Generative System* was reported in the *Australian Medical Journal* of 1879 as representative 'of that class of literature which honourable medical men shun'.

He was compassionate toward women who had suffered from 'back-yard' abortionists. Following his surgical intervention in an attempt to save one such victim, he was arrested following litigation brought by his bitter medical enemies. The resulting court case led *The Lancet* of 1866, which took his side, to note that 'nothing short of the highest legal ability could have saved an innocent man [Beaney] from the gallows'.

Beaney's personal appearance was ostentatious and flamboyant, and he affected a swept-up hairstyle—all of which were the subject of caricature in the hostile press of his day. He was a charismatic surgical teacher who endowed the first medical medals in Australia, fine gold and silver medals awarded to the top medical students who attended his surgical demonstrations at The Melbourne Hospital. He was a generous man, and he left bequests that have become his memorials. The Beaney Prizes for Surgery and Pathology bestowed annually by the University of Melbourne; a fine stained-glass window now at the Monash Medical Centre in Melbourne; the Beaney Institute and Free Library in Canterbury (UK); and a fine marble memorial in Canterbury Cathedral record his life and works.

Bibliography

Secondary: Pearn, J. H., 2004. 'Dr James George Beaney (1828–1891): A Pioneer Australian Paediatrician and Paediatric Surgeon'. *Journal of Paediatrics and Child Health* 40: 702–706.

John Pearn

BEARD, GEORGE MILLER (b. Montville, Connecticut, USA, 8 May 1839; d. New York, New York, USA, 23 January 1883), *neurology.*

Beard, son of the Congregational minister Spencer F. Beard, attended Andover College in Massachusetts and graduated from Yale College in 1862. After attending medical school in New Haven, he served for two years as assistant surgeon in the Navy during the Civil War, then completed his medical studies at New York's College of Physicians and Surgeons in 1866. He started to lecture on the nervous diseases at New York University only two years after he commenced practicing as a neurologist. During his short career, Beard contributed to the recently established specialty of neurology, was an advocate for the mentally ill, and published a tremendous number of articles and books. He was admired by some but criticized by many others for the superficial and repetitive nature of his writings and his often shameless self-promotion.

During the first part of his career, Beard was interested in electrotherapy or faradization, which used electricity to treat nervous disorders. Electricity was provided by a generator, while the patient's feet were placed on the cathode and the positive pole, in the form of the physician's hand or damp sponge, was moved over the patient's limbs. In 1874 Beard founded the *Archives of Electrology and Neurology* and participated in the establishment of the New York Society of Neurology and Electrology. In 1869 he coined the diagnosis of neurasthenia, or nervous exhaustion, for which he is most famous. Beard presented his views on this condition, which was defined as the depletion of nervous energy and characterized by a wide range of vague symptoms, including fatigue, insomnia, irritability, morbid anxiety, chronic indecision, dyspepsia, indigestion, headaches, impotence, and neuralgia. He mainly used electrical treatment to restore his patients to health.

According to Beard, neurasthenia was caused by a hereditary predisposition in combination with the social conditions inherent to modern civilization, which placed unprecedented demands on the nervous system. These conditions included 'steam power, the periodical press, the telegraph, the sciences, and the mental activity of women' (*American Nervousness*, p. vi) and mostly affected white, highly educated, urban, upper-middle class individuals who were engaged in brain-work. Their nervous exhaustion testified to the delicacy of their highly evolved nervous systems, and the high incidence of the condition in the United States demonstrated an extraordinary high level of social evolution in the country.

Beard exemplified the newly established profession of neurology, whose practitioners privately treated vague nervous complaints of well-to-do clients in the major urban centers. By providing a strictly somatic explanation for the symptoms of neurasthenia, he legitimized the complaints of sufferers and boosted the social standing of his discipline. The originality of his conception lies in the way he related social and cultural factors to the etiology of neurasthenia. His writings were thereby both medical theory and a form of social commentary or social critique of modernity. Despite the critique by Beard's contemporaries of his ideas and his personal style, his theories on the nature of neurasthenia have been pervasive and influential, and became part of the standard repertoire of physicians, psychiatrists, and neurologists.

Bibliography

Primary: 1869. 'Neurasthenia or Nervous Exhaustion.' *Boston Medical and Surgical Journal* 80: 217–221, 245–259; 1871. (with Rockwell, A. D.) *A Practical Treatise on the Medical and Surgical Use of Electricity* (New York); 1880. *A Practical Treatise on Nervous Exhaustion (Neurasthenia): Its Symptoms, Nature, Sequences, Treatment* (New York); 1881. *American Nervousness: Its Causes and Consequences* (New York).

Secondary: Rosenberg, Charles E., 1997. 'George M. Beard and American Nervousness' in Rosenberg, Charles, *No Other Gods: On Science and American Social Thought* (Baltimore); Sicherman, Barbara, 1977. 'The Uses of a Diagnosis: Doctors, Patients, and Neurasthenia.' *Journal of the History of Medicine and Allied Sciences* 32: 33–54; *DAMB*.

Hans Pols

BEAUMONT, WILLIAM (b. Lebanon, Connecticut, USA, 21 November 1785; d. St Louis, Missouri, USA, 25 April 1853), *military medicine, digestive physiology.*

In a series of 238 experiments, conducted intermittently over a period of eight years on a single human subject, the American army surgeon William Beaumont transformed the understanding of gastric physiology.

Beaumont was born on a farm in the small town of Lebanon, Connecticut, on 21 November 1785. Determined to better himself, he moved northward to Champlain, New York, in 1807 and taught school for three years, finally moving to St Albans, Vermont, where he served a two-year apprenticeship to a local physician, Benjamin Chandler. With the start of the War of 1812, an army unit was posted to Plattsburgh, New York, and Beaumont joined it as surgeon's mate shortly after becoming licensed by the Medical Society of Vermont. When the war ended in 1815, he went into practice in Plattsburgh, but after four years he reenlisted and was assigned as post surgeon to a fort on Mackinac Island on the upper Michigan peninsula, where he was the only physician within some 300 miles. He married Deborah Green Platt in 1821, and the couple would have four children.

On the morning of 6 June 1822, Beaumont was urgently called to see Alexis St Martin, a nineteen-year-old French-Canadian trapper employed by the American Fur Company, who had sustained an accidental shotgun wound to the left lower chest from a distance of about two feet. The resultant wound consisted of several smashed ribs and lacerations of the diaphragm, stomach, and lung, all of which could be seen through a hole some five inches in diameter. Despairing of his patient's life, Beaumont dressed the wound, and on returning to visit his patient the next day, was surprised to note that he was doing so well that he might be expected to recover. The wound took ten months to heal, leaving a physically exhausted patient with a gastric fistula about the size of a man's index finger.

Because the debilitated St Martin had no resources and was unable to earn a living, Beaumont took him into his home, cared for him, and continued to dress his wound. During this time and later, the young physician sought advice about the patient's treatment and observation from his friend, Joseph Lovell, Surgeon General to the United States Army. In May 1825 he began to use the fistula to conduct some experiments on gastric function, and in the following January published a report on the first four of them in the *Medical Recorder*. The following June, Beaumont was transferred to Fort Niagara and took St Martin with him, where he remained for a few months before leaving for Canada without notifying Beaumont of his intentions. It was not until 1829 that Beaumont was able to locate St Martin, who had since married and begun his family. The surgeon, who by then had been transferred to Fort Crawford at Prairie du Chien, Wisconsin, got him a job there with the American Fur Company and resumed his experiments for the next two years, until St Martin's wife insisted on the family's returning to Canada. St Martin came back about a year and a half later, and experiments continued until November 1833. By this time, Robley Dunglison of the University of Virginia and Benjamin Silliman of Yale had been sent samples of the gastric juice and determined that it contained free hydrochloric acid.

In April 1833 Beaumont published the book that would become a classic, *Experiments and Observations on the Gastric Juice and the Physiology of Digestion*. Though its value was appreciated even by the scientifically unsophisticated physicians of America, the book was absolutely hailed as an accomplishment of great significance by eminent European authorities within a few years of its appearance. Among Beaumont's discoveries were the fact that the gastric juice contains hydrochloric acid, the peristaltic action of the stomach, the way gastric mucosa responds to various stimuli, the manner in which the stomach contributes to digestion, and the difference between the mucosal and acid secretions of the gastric lining.

Beaumont was unable to convince his subject to allow further experiments. The surgeon's final posting, from 1834 to 1839, was at Jefferson Barracks near St Louis, after which he went into practice in that city. He died on 25 April 1853, from a head injury sustained by falling on the ice while leaving a patient's house.

Bibliography

Primary: 1833. *Experiments and Observations on the Gastric Juice and the Physiology of Digestion* (Plattsburgh, NY) (Facsimile of the original ed. with a biographical essay by Sir William Osler, 'A Pioneer American Physiologist', New York, 1959).

Secondary: Cummiskey, R. D., and J. P. O'Leary, 1996. 'William Beaumont.' *American Surgeon* 62: 690–693; Nelson, R. B., 1990. *Beaumont, America's First Physiologist* (Geneva, IL); Cohen, I. B., ed., 1980. *The Career of William Beaumont and the Reception of His Discovery* (New York); *ANB*; *DSB*; *DAMB*.

Sherwin Nuland

BEAUPERTHUY, LUIS DANIEL (b. Santa Rosa, Isle of Guadalupe, 26 August 1807; d. Bartica Point, Guyana, 3 September 1871), *yellow fever, leprosy.*

Beauperthuy was the son of the chemist and pharmacist Pierre Daniel Beauperthuy. He was sent to study in France, entering the Faculty of Medicine in Paris (1828). He carried out his clinical work at the Hôtel Dieu, taking complementary classes with the microscopist Donné, zoology with Flourens at the Musée d'Histoire Naturelle, physiology with Magendie at the Collège de France, and therapeutics and medicine with Alibert. He interrupted his studies in the early 1830s during General Lafayette's uprising against the Bourbon dynasty and the ensuing cholera epidemic, dedicating himself to the care of the wounded and ill.

Beauperthuy returned to Guadalupe in 1834, later moving with his brother Felipe to the town of Maturín in eastern Venezuela. He traveled up the Orinoco River and around the neighboring plains, finding frequent cases of yellow fever, dysentery, and hookworm that he studied clinically and included in his doctoral thesis. He also collected zoological, botanical, and mineral samples that were later donated to the Musée d'Histoire Naturelle. He returned to France and obtained his doctoral degree in medicine in 1837 from the Faculty of Medicine of Paris, with a thesis entitled *De la Climatologie*. During 1831–41 he worked as a traveling naturalist for the Musée d'Histoire Naturelle.

He established himself as general practitioner in Cumaná (Venezuela) in 1842, soon marrying a local young lady. He became professor of anatomy at the Colegio Nacional in Cumaná in 1850, chemical inspector of the mines in Carúpano (1852), and health officer during 1853–66, managing several epidemics of yellow fever and cholera. During a yellow fever epidemic in 1853, Beauperthuy experimented with mosquito nets, noticing that those who used them did not catch the disease. He pointed out in the *Official Gazette* of Cumaná (1854) that the fever was produced by an animal-vegetable virus originating in rotting matter and inoculating the human body through mosquitoes. In 1856 he sent an extensive review of this topic to the Académie des Sciences in Paris, but his pioneering proposal of insect vectoring remained unnoticed there. A summary of his work was published in *Comptes Rendus* under the name of Flourens, and was reproduced in the *L'Abeille Médicale*.

Between 1862 and 1871, as medical surgeon at the Lázaros de Cumaná Hospital (a leprosarium), he became interested in leprosy. His observations suggested that the illness was curable and not hereditary, and that it could be addressed with a two-step therapy. To dissolve the albuminous secretions of the leprosy lesions he recommended Van Swieten liquor, a mercury bichloride solution that could be substituted with potassium bicarbonate and small amounts of quinine and potassium hydrate if the wounds did not dry up, or if the patient experienced intestinal upset. For tubercle cauterization he used cashew-nut oil (*Anacardium occidentales*), reinforced with a silver nitrate application, in order to destroy parasites and other germs. The second-stage therapy was a diet of meat (excluding pork and salted fish) and fresh vegetables; moderate exercises; the use of mosquito nets to avoid insect stings; baths twice a week with soap and water; and skin rubbing with oily substances.

At the beginning he had encouraging results that drew the attention of the French and English governments (1868–69). The latter supported his founding of an experimental hospital for the treatment of leprosy in Kao Island, Guyana (1871), and he moved to Bartica Point, which was near the facility. His last days were tense, a consequence of his arduous hospital work and the expectations aroused by his therapy, possibly leading to the stroke that finally caused his death.

Bibliography

Primary: 1891. *Travaux Scientifiques* (Bordeaux).

Secondary: Lemoine, Waleska and María Matilde Suárez, 1984. *Beauperthuy. De Cumaná a la Academia de Ciencias de Paris* (Caracas); Sanabría, Antonio and Rosario Benedetti de Beauperthuy, 1981. *Beauperthuy: un ensayo biográfico* (Cumaná); Llopis, José María, 1965. *Luis Daniel Beauperthuy: crónicas de una vida* (Caracas).

Yajaira Freites (translation by Claudio Mendoza)

BECK, CLAUDE SCHAEFFER (b. Shomokin, Pennsylvania, USA, 8 November 1894; d. Euclid, Ohio, USA, 14 October 1971), *surgery.*

Beck graduated MD from Johns Hopkins in 1921. His formative years were spent in Boston, Massachusetts. He was later Professor of Cardiovascular Surgery at Western Reserve University, Cleveland, Ohio, and was President of the prestigious and elite American Association for Thoracic Surgery. The theme running throughout his contributions is that of finding practical surgical solutions to prevalent diseases or clinical problems.

Between 1923 and 1929 in Boston, Massachusetts, at the Peter Bent Brigham Hospital, he was involved in a series of operations to relieve mitral stenosis, a narrowed heart valve occurring as a sequel to rheumatic fever, which was very common at the time. Since the beginning of the century there had been interest in surgical relief of this disease. The London physician Thomas Lauder Brunton (1844–1916) had observed that the cusps of the valve, adherent edge to edge, could easily be freed after death and speculated that this could be done in life. The first case report was from the more senior surgeon, Elliot Cutler (1888–1947) who cut the valve blindly with a knife inserted through the apex of the heart. Encouraged by an initial success, Cutler and Beck did several more similar operations, which all resulted in deaths within a few days. In 1929 they wrote up the series as a 'last report', and from then until the late 1940s there was effectively a moratorium on surgery within the heart, with successive editions of medical textbooks becoming ever more strongly opposed to it. Then the sequence of operations in 1948 by Charles P. Bailey (1910–93), Dwight Harken (1910–93), and Russell C. Brock (1903–80) was followed by wide dissemination of surgical relief of mitral stenosis by valvotomy, which was soon performed in large numbers throughout the world.

During the 1920s Beck also studied the problem of constrictive pericarditis, another prevalent disease, occurring as a sequel to tuberculosis. Together with R. Arnold Griswold, he mimicked the condition in dogs. A common theme of his time was to attempt to recreate the constellation of symptoms and signs of a human disease in an animal as a 'model', so that experiments could then be performed in an attempt to relieve the problem. He emphasized the features of pericardial constriction, namely increased venous pressure, abdominal fluid accumulation due to ascites, hydrothorax, edematous swelling of the legs, and a small quiet heart due to the thickening around it.

Through the 1930s Beck, along with others of that era, most notably Laurence O'Shaughnessy (1900–40), experimented in the laboratory and in patients with ways of bringing new blood flow to the heart, in order to relieve angina. He tried a combination of the methods that were being explored at the time, which included abrading the pericardium to cause adhesion, introduction of irritants (he used coarsely ground asbestos), partially obstructing the exit of blood by narrowing the coronary sinus with a ligature, and attaching pedicles of muscle, pericardium, or abdominal fat. All were intended to cause the body to generate collateral flow. He reported some relief of symptoms, but with a high (up to 50 percent) perioperative mortality. His methods were all abandoned for want of demonstrable efficacy. Arthur M. Vineberg's (1903–88) method of tunneling the internal mammary artery into the heart muscle had had more success, but was never widely taken up. Another alternative to increasing the blood supply to the heart was to reduce the demand placed upon it by irradiating the thyroid gland. The patients were thereby made myxoedematous, which was not an acceptable outcome. Following the development of cardiopulmonary bypass in the 1950s and then of coronary artery bypass grafting in the 1960s, all other surgical methods were discontinued.

Amazingly, throughout the years during which these hazardous operations on the heart were being performed, there was no means of reversing the situation if the heart lost its pumping action due to fibrillation. It appears that at the time the surgeons stood by helplessly. Beck took a serious interest in resuscitation techniques, including opening the chest to perform internal massage of the heart. He is credited with ushering in an era in which doctors were encouraged to cut open the chest, with a penknife if necessary, to perform internal massage. His first success with electrical defibrillation was in 1947.

Bibliography

Primary: 1941. 'Resuscitation for Cardiac Standstill and Ventricular Fibrillation Occurring during Operation.' *Am. J. Surg.* 54: 273.

Secondary: Shumacker, H. B., 1992. *The Evolution of Cardiac Surgery* (Bloomington and Indianapolis); *DAMB.*

Tom Treasure

BEDDOES, THOMAS (b. Shifnal, Shropshire, England, 13 April 1760; d. Clifton, Bristol, England, 23 December 1808), *chemistry, medicine.*

Beddoes, the son of Richard Beddoes, a tanner, and Ann Whitehall, was educated at Bridgnorth grammar school, where he received a solid grounding in classics. He attended Pembroke College, Oxford, starting in 1776, added French, Italian, and German to the earlier Latin and Greek, and graduated BA in 1779. He then moved to London to work at the Great Windmill Street school of anatomy and the chemical laboratory of Bryan Higgins in Greek Street. In 1784 he both translated the work of Lazzaro Spallanzani (1729–99) and went up to Edinburgh University to study medicine.

Already persuaded that medicine needed a new chemical foundation and that the work of Joseph Black was more important than the respectable albeit dated approach of William Cullen (1710–90) and his school, Beddoes returned to Oxford in 1786 to take his MB and MD and continued to translate European chemical works. In the summer of 1787 he visited France; while there he sought out the work of Louis Bernard Guyton de Morveau (1737–1816) on the purification of air (conducted at the academy in Dijon) and met Antoine Lavoisier (1743–94) in Paris. He also became acutely aware of the political developments of the day and of the growth and organization of antimonarchical and democratic political forces. His sympathy with these pre-Revolutionary movements was very strong. After his return to Oxford he was appointed reader in chemistry in 1788. Archival evidence for his lectures in the next few years in Oxford is slim but he lectured on both chemistry and geology. In the latter subject he expressed firm support for those who identified the primary agent of geological power as heat (as opposed to water and events such as the Noachian deluge); some of this commitment was based on fieldwork done in Cornwall. Beddoes's years in Oxford were vexed; he was angry that the books purchased by Bodley's librarian were consistently antiprogressive and thus obstructed new curricula in chemistry and medicine. He was also dismayed at the political events in France with the collapse of the reformist democratic hopes of the Revolution's early years into bloodshed, terror, and eventually war.

In 1793 Beddoes left Oxford, with a reputation of being a short (and short-tempered) radical with some grand but elusive ideas for a new medicine. He took up residence in the spa of Clifton, near Bristol. There, drawing on financial support from members of the Wedgwood pottery dynasty as well as on moral backing from members of the Lunar Society of Birmingham, he planned a Pneumatic Institute in Dowry Square, Hotwells. Beddoes's alliance with the Lunar Society was further cemented by his marriage in April 1794 to Anna (1773–1824), daughter of Richard Lovell Edgeworth (an active member of the Society); the Institute opened in 1799.

Beddoes had by now developed a combined program for a new kind of medicine. Chemistry—the new chemistry—had led to new understandings of human physiology, respiration, and health. In collaboration with men such as the inventor James Watt (1736–1819), Beddoes had even developed the apparatus to carry out a variety of chemical experiments. Alongside this medicine—pneumatic medicine—was a fuller understanding of the social nature of illness. Illness was of course rooted in poverty and exploitation, but it was also generated by the very consumer society that seemed to be the height of modernity and fashion at the time. Snobbery, empty fashion crazes, the exhaustions of grand living, all combined with older but also apparently endemic disorders—the drunkenness of agricultural workers, for example—to produce a wholesale social pathology. Only a new kind of doctor could see this, free of the prejudices of politics and the blindness of the consumer. However, it was to be a moot point—Beddoes's fate—whether enough people would share these insights and promote social progress as a result.

At the heart of the Pneumatic Institute and the icons of its age and moment were a young man and a new discovery: Humphry Davy (1778–1829) and nitrous oxide. Gases were to be the royal road to medical relief, for both people of high society and the deserving poor. But Beddoes's dream was not to be. Davy left for London in 1801. Beddoes became more despairing of the idiocies of both the poor and the rich. His marriage was never happy. His writings from the early 1800s onward were full of despair and anger. He and his circle were easily satirized by political opponents as a crowd of gas-filled radicals whose delusions had led them into bad medicine and even worse politics. Their time had come and gone. Most of Beddoes's private papers were destroyed and some of the gloom of the father's life seemed to have passed on to his son—the medical man, poet, and eventual suicide, Thomas Lovell Beddoes (1803–49).

Bibliography

Primary: 1802–03. *Hygëia: or essays moral and medical, on the causes affecting the personal state of our middling and affluent classes* 3 vols. (Bristol).

Secondary: Porter, Roy, 1991. *Doctor of Society: Thomas Beddoes and the Sick Trade in Late Enlightenment England* (New York and London); Stansfield, Dorothy, 1984. *Thomas Beddoes, MD 1760–1808: Chemist, Physician, Democrat* (Dordrecht and Boston); Stock, J. E., 1811. *Memoirs of Thomas Beddoes MD* (Bristol) (reprinted 2003); *DSB; Oxford DNB.*

Michael Neve

BEECHAM, THOMAS (b. Curbridge, Oxfordshire, England, 3 December 1820; d. Southport, Lancashire, England, 6 April 1907), *patent medicines.*

Beecham was the eldest of seven children of Joseph Beecham, a laborer and then a shepherd, and his wife Sarah Hunt. From his early years Beecham was exposed to cottage cures, village fairs, and country markets. He was sent to a country school at age seven, where he started learning to read and write, but at eight he was pulled from school and set to work in the fields tending sheep. At the age of twelve he went to work on a farm in Cropredy, near Banbury.

It was while looking after animals that he learned about herbs and their medicinal properties. He experimented with other ingredients, including aloes and ginger, and also learned the art of pill-making. He collected herbs from the meadows, rolled his pills, and took them to the market to sell. He continued working as a shepherd until the age of twenty.

Beecham continued making and peddling his pills, and by the end of 1846 had made sufficient money to go north. Wages there were higher than in the south because of the competition provided by mines and factories. By the spring of 1847 he was living in Liverpool. There he met his first wife, Jane Evans, and in the summer of 1847 they moved to Wigan in Lancashire. A year later their son Joseph was born.

He began touring the surrounding towns, selling his products at markets, particularly that at St Helens, Lancashire, where he sold his main product, *Beecham's Pills*, for 6d (2½p) per box. The basic ingredients of the pills—aloes, ginger, and soap—remained the same until the product was withdrawn in 1998. The pills were sold wholesale and retail. Business flourished, and Beecham acquired permanent premises.

Beecham made full use of the power of advertising. The first advertisement appeared in the *St Helens' Intelligencer* in 1859. The pills were advertised as 'one box sent post free for eight stamps to any address'. He had already adopted the slogan 'Worth a Guinea a Box', said to have been the unsolicited testimonial of a woman in St Helens market.

Testimonials were an important component of his advertisements: that in the *St Helens' Intelligencer* carried one from a Mr Mason, boot and shoemaker. But they never referred to its discovery, nor used patrons or celebrities.

Beecham spent massive sums on advertising. Expenditure went from £22,000 in 1880 to over £120,000 in 1891. Fourteen thousand newspapers around the world carried his advertisements. His other promotional activities included a reference for students called 'Help to Scholars'. Between 1889 and 1959 over 47 million copies were distributed. In promoting *Beecham's Pills* as a family remedy he published over twenty songbooks, featuring such songs as 'Men of Harlech', 'St Helen's Waltz' and the 'Guinea-a-Box Polka'.

The business continued to expand. By 1875 he was exporting to Africa and Australia. His staff included his son, Joseph, as business manager. Beecham was known as a benevolent and generous employer. His employees were given a medical examination on employment; and for one penny per week, if ill, they were treated in their homes, and guaranteed their jobs. A new factory was built in 1887 in the Queen Anne style at a cost of £30,000. This enclosed a floor space of some 1,600 square yards and had three imposing frontages. Beecham designed much of the machinery used.

Beecham retired from the business in 1895. In 1893 he moved to Southport on the Lancashire coast, but continued to visit the factory on a regular basis until his death in 1907. He left two sons; Joseph, who followed him into the family business, and William, who qualified as a medical practitioner.

When Sir Joseph Beecham died the business was carried on by his executors. In 1924 Beecham Estates and Pills Limited was formed. The Beecham family were bought out and ceased to have any connection with the business. In 1928 it became Beecham Pills Limited, and in 1955 Beecham Pharmaceuticals Limited. It later changed its name to Beecham Proprietary Medicines, becoming part of GlaxoSmithKline.

Bibliography

Secondary: Lazell, H. G., 1975. *From Pills to Penicillin: The Beecham Story* (London); Francis, Anne, 1968. *A Guinea a Box: A Biography.* (London); 1961. *Beecham Group Journal* 1(3): 1–6; 1960. *Beecham Proprietary Medicines* (Lancashire) p. 2; 1907. Obituary. *The British and Colonial Druggist* 12 April: 308; *Oxford DNB.*

Stuart Anderson

BEECHER, HENRY KNOWLES (b. Peck, Kansas, USA, 4 February 1904; d. Cambridge, Massachusetts, USA, 25 July 1976), *anesthesia, ethics.*

Of German stock, Beecher was born with the name Harry Unangst, which he changed at the age of twenty. He trained in chemistry at Kansas University, entering Harvard in 1928 and graduating MD in 1932. In 1936, after a surgical residency at Massachusetts General Hospital, he was selected to develop the new specialty of anesthesiology. Save for a traveling fellowship and wartime service (including at the Anzio bridgehead) Beecher spent the rest of his life at Harvard, becoming Dorr Professor of Anesthesia Research in 1941 and training many later chairmen of anesthesiology departments; in retirement he wrote the medical school's history.

Active in research even as a student, by 1960 Beecher had written over 200 papers and several books, notably on the physiology of anesthesia, battlefield trauma, and the placebo response. His interest in human research ethics arose out of his own experience and the reports of the Nazi atrocities. His concerns were documented in a 1959 report to the American Medical Association Council on Drugs and in *Experimentation in Man* (1960). Little attention was aroused, however, until he presented anonymized examples of ethical lapses in research at a conference on drug research in March 1965. So concerned were some colleagues at the public furor that they convened a press conference to refute Beecher's views. Not given the opportunity to respond, he determined to expose the reports to professional scrutiny. He incorporated twenty published studies out of fifty ethically questionable examples he had collected 'easily' into an article and submitted it to the *Journal of the American Medical Association.* After external peer review, the latter rejected it for its excessive length and muddled presentation. Beecher then turned to the *New England Journal of Medicine*, providing the editor with the articles for assessment. The compromise was to publish fewer details from the case histories.

The *NEJM* then had a lesser public impact than it would later have, so Beecher informed influential publications such as the *New York Times* about his article. He had been advised that documenting his cases might lay the research workers open to litigation, so his article contained no references. Nevertheless, it was clear that the studies were conducted in major research and academic centers, mostly in the USA (though two were in Britain), and characteristically would not have benefited the subjects, who had been unable to make an informed choice during their participation in the research. Given a similar exposé in the UK by Maurice Pappworth, the response was immediate and far-reaching, resulting in the concept of truly informed consent and scrutiny of projects by institutional review boards (research ethics committees). And, equally importantly, in 1968 Beecher was chosen to chair the Harvard committee into the definition of brain death, which had assumed great importance with the developments in organ transplantation.

A man of contradictions, Beecher was dour ('never convicted of a sense of humor', to quote an obituarist) and uninterested in teaching or clinical anesthesia, yet had many admirers. He fell out over several issues with the American Society of Anesthetists, becoming a member only in 1938 given his lack of formal training. Colleagues have recorded that he found informed consent an obstacle in his own research. His occasional claim to kinship with distinguished Beechers probably went along with his vision of Harvard man, along with the Brooks Brothers tweeds and the buttonhole Legion d'Honneur ribbon. But without his proselytizing, the worldwide protection of patients against unethical research practices would have been longer delayed.

Bibliography

Primary: 1938. *The Physiology of Anesthesia* (New York and London); 1960. *Experimentation in Man* (Springfield, IL); 1966. 'Ethics and Clinical Research.' *New England Journal of Medicine* 274: 1354–1360; 1968. 'A Definition of Irreversible Coma.' *Journal of the American Medical Association* 205: 337–340; 1977. (with Altschule, Mark D.) *Medicine at Harvard: The First Three Hundred Years* (Hanover, NH).

Secondary: Kopp, V. J., 1999. 'Henry K. Beecher, M.D. Contrarian (1904–1976).' *American Society of Anesthesiologists Newsletter* 63(9): 9–11; Rothman, D. J., 1991. *Strangers at the Bedside* (New York); *DAMB*.

Stephen Lock

BEERS, CLIFFORD WHITTINGHAM (b. New Haven, Connecticut, USA, 30 March 1876; d. Providence, Rhode Island, USA, 9 July 1943), *mental health advocacy.*

Beers was instrumental in organizing the National Committee for Mental Hygiene, which promoted the development of psychiatry and the extension of mental health care services. He was the son of Robert A. Beers, a wholesale merchant, and Ida Cooke. He graduated from the Sheffield Scientific School at Yale University in 1897. After working at the New Haven Tax Commission Office, he moved to New York City, where he worked for an interior decorating firm. In the summer of 1900 he returned to his parents' home after suffering from depression, agitation, and delusions. After a failed suicide attempt, he was institutionalized in a proprietary mental hospital. During the following three years, he was committed to a private and a public mental hospital as well. Initially, Beers suffered from severe depression; later, this turned into mania. He witnessed the deplorable conditions in mental hospitals at the time and several instances of abuse. Beers related his experiences and observations in his autobiography, which was published in 1908 under the title *A Mind that Found Itself.* At the same time, he organized a reform movement aimed at improving the conditions in mental hospitals. Beers was able to establish contact with several leading psychiatrists, academics, and philanthropists. The influential psychiatrist Adolf Meyer, the psychologist William James, the Johns Hopkins physician William H. Welch, and the former Harvard University president Charles W. Eliot were among his supporters.

In 1909 the National Committee for Mental Hygiene was founded in New York City. Beers was appointed secretary, a position he held until 1939. During his tenure at the National Committee, Beers was engaged in fund-raising and the international expansion of the mental hygiene movement. During the four decades of its existence, the National Committee focused on public health education and the development of preventive measures within psychiatry, and was instrumental in the professionalization and the expansion of the discipline of psychiatry. It received generous funding from several philanthropic organizations, in particular the Rockefeller Foundation. During the first decade of its existence, the National Committee surveyed mental health care facilities in a large number of states and advocated their improvement and the establishment of outpatient clinics. During the 1920s, when American psychiatry was influenced by psychoanalysis, the National Committee was instrumental in establishing Child Guidance Clinics in many cities. It also undertook a number of initiatives within the educational system. During the 1930s, the Committee arranged funding for research into schizophrenia and developed ideas on community mental hygiene programs. The National Committee was successful in raising the public image of psychiatry, increasing the discipline's standing within medicine, and advocating the treatment of mental disorder in outpatient settings. The community mental health movement, which became prominent in the United States in the 1960s, was based on ideas developed by members of the National Committee.

Beers had many conflicts during his tenure as secretary of the National Committee for Mental Hygiene, which were mostly due to his desire to maintain tight personal control over its affairs. During the summer of 1939, Beers suffered a mental breakdown and a relapse of his mental illness. He was institutionalized at Butler Hospital in Providence, Rhode Island, where he died four years later.

Bibliography

Primary: 1908. *A Mind That Found Itself: An Autobiography* (New York); 1931. 'An Intimate Account of the Origin and Growth of the Mental Hygiene Movement.' *Mental Hygiene* 25(4): 673–684.

Secondary: Dain, Norman, 1980. *Clifford W. Beers: Advocate for the Insane* (Pittsburgh); Cross, Wilbur L., ed., 1934. *Twenty-five Years and After: Sidelights on the Mental Hygiene Movement and Its Founder* (New York); Farrar, Clarence B., 1933. 'Twenty-five Years of Mental Hygiene: A Tribute to Clifford W. Beers, Author of "A Mind That Found Itself", and Founder of the Mental Hygiene Movement.' *American Journal of Psychiatry* 13(3): 695–698; *DAMB*.

Hans Pols

BEHRING, EMIL VON (b. Hansdorf, East Prussia (now Germany), 15 March 1854; d. Marburg, Hessen-Kassel, Germany, 31 March 1917), *bacteriology, hygiene.*

The eldest son of a village schoolmaster, Behring received medical training thanks to a scholarship to the Military Medical Academy in Berlin. In return, he was required to spend a number of years in the army after obtaining his MD in 1878. Receiving his license to practice medicine in 1880, Behring was posted to serve as a military doctor in a number of different garrisons. He continued his military career, passing the examination to become a military officer in 1885 and completing a course in bacteriology in 1886. In 1889, Behring was assigned to the Hygiene Institute, headed by Robert Koch, at Berlin University, and in 1891 he followed Koch to the newly founded Institute for Infectious Diseases.

From the early 1880s, Behring took an interest in the problems of hygiene and sepsis in the context of his military medical activity. In particular, his studies focused on the ability of different iodine compounds to render harmless the germs responsible for infection. This work led to the idea of using disinfectants of that sort to neutralize poisons acting within the body, a concept known as *inner disinfection.* His transfer to Carl Binz's laboratory of pharmacology at the University of Bonn in 1887 gave Behring the chance to improve his knowledge of chemistry and to hone his laboratory skills, which were further enhanced by his move to Berlin to work with Robert Koch. Starting in 1891, he also worked with Georg Gaffky and Friedrich Loeffler in the new Institute.

In 1890 Behring published important new discoveries made in collaboration with the Japanese bacteriologist Shibasaburo Kitasato, who was a member of Koch's research group in Berlin. They observed that treatment of experimental animals with increasing doses of sterilized diphtheria cultures rendered them resistant to the toxin generated by the cultures. They also demonstrated that the serum of a resistant animal could be used to cure another animal infected with the disease.

The use of this diphtheria antitoxin serum marked the discovery of a new, specific curative principle. In order to apply the discovery to the treatment of human disease, however, the antitoxic efficacy had to be improved, and a means for large-scale production had to be developed. With the assistance of Erich Wernicke, Behring entered into a race with a group working with Emile Roux at the Institut Pasteur in Paris to develop the treatment for humans. Most of the animal experiments in Berlin were carried out by Behring and Wernicke at their own expense, under an archway of Berlin's S-Bahn. Paul Ehrlich also contributed to the development of a system for producing the serum, using horses made resistant to the diphtheria toxin.

Behring resisted moves to establish a state monopoly of serum production, and he signed a contract with the dyestuffs company Hoechst that would allow him to finance further research. The first successful human trials of the serum took place in 1893, and large-scale manufacture began the following year.

Behring was now able to advance rapidly in his academic career, under the patronage of the powerful Prussian undersecretary Friedrich Althoff (1839–1908). In 1894 he was appointed associate professor in Halle, and in 1895 he became full professor at Marburg and was discharged from the army.

Behring's relationship with Hoechst proved profitable, allowing him to become the leading partner in a serum research and production center in Marburg. After winning the Nobel Prize in 1901, Behring took over the serum production facility in Marburg.

Although the serum for the treatment of tuberculosis that Behring announced in his Nobel lecture was a failure, that venture had already succeeded in poisoning his relationship with Koch. Questions of priority and property rights also led to a certain bitterness on the part of Ehrlich and Wernicke. Furthermore, biographical studies written during the Nazi period sought to minimize the significant contributions made by Ehrlich (and others), a bias that has begun to be redressed in more recent work.

Bibliography

Primary: 1892. *Blutserumtherapie* (Leipzig); 1893; 1915. *Gesammelte Abhandlungen* (Leipzig).

Secondary: Zeiss, H., and R. Bieling, 1940. *Behring, Gestalt und Werk* (Berlin); *DSB*.

Volker Hess

BEKHTEREV, VLADIMIR MIKHAILOVICH (b. Sorali, Russia, 20 January [1 February] 1857; d. Moscow, Russia, 24 December 1927), *neuropsychology.*

Bekhterev, one of four children, grew up in the Russian province of Viatka and was raised by his mother after his father's death in 1866. In 1873 he entered the Military-Medical Academy in St Petersburg, where he specialized in nervous and mental illnesses under I. P. Merzheevskii (1838–1908). After earning the title of university lecturer in 1884, Bekhterev toured Europe, visiting the laboratories of Wundt, Fleschsig, and Charcot (among others). While visiting Meynert's laboratory in Vienna, Bekhterev learned that he had been offered a professorship in the Russian city of Kazan. Forced to decide between remaining in Europe (where he had received several job offers) and going to Kazan, the 28-year-old Bekhterev responded that he would accept the position only if the Russian government supplied him with a fully equipped laboratory for the study of nervous illness. To his lasting surprise the government agreed, and Bekhterev spent the next nine years building a thriving research center at Kazan University.

Bekhterev's most lasting contributions came from his studies of the physiology and morphology of the nervous system, a subject that drew his attention while still a student in St Petersburg. Using newly developed methods of staining brain tissue and nerve cells, Bekhterev discovered a number of previously unknown structures, most notably the superior vestibular nucleus (Bekhterev's nucleus). The results of his research were published in 1896 in his two-volume *Provodiashchie puti spinnogo i golovnogo mozga: Rukovodstvo k izucheniiu vnutrennikh sviazei mozga* [Passages of the Spinal Cord and the Brain].

Bekhterev's fame, however, is in large part due to his extraordinary capacity for creating and managing scientific enterprises. In his nine years at Kazan University he founded a research laboratory for the study of nervous illnesses, introduced new methods of treatment at the psychiatric clinic, established several scientific journals, and founded a society for neuropathologists and psychiatrists that is still in existence—all the while earning a reputation as a researcher and lecturer. When his mentor Merzheevskii retired in 1893, Bekhterev was offered chair of mental and nervous illnesses at the Military-Medical Academy. There he developed a thriving community of researchers and became a leading figure in the Russian medical profession, as well as a sometimes outspoken (and controversial) critic of the tsarist government. (In an influential 1905 speech he famously suggested that capitalism and the tsarist regime were damaging the mental health of Russian citizens.)

As a professor in St Petersburg, Bekhterev applied his skills as an organizer to his long-held dream of placing clinical psychiatry and neurology on a scientific foundation. Using the concept of the conditioned reflex, he developed what he first referred to as 'Objective Psychology' (the title of his 1907 book). It was an eclectic combination of physiology, experimental psychology, anthropology, and even philosophy that Bekhterev hoped to turn into a new discipline called 'reflexol-ogy', which he hoped would supersede psychology as the science of human mind and behavior. To develop his vision, Bekhterev founded his own private institute—the Psycho-Neurological Institute (later referred to simply as The Bekhterev Institute)—which opened for classes in 1906. At first the institute struggled to survive under the suspicious eyes of the tsarist authorities, but in the 1920s it blossomed into a thriving (if eclectic) center of research where, with the support of the Bolshevik regime, he and his colleagues attempted to develop a Marxist approach to the study of the mind.

Bekhterev's sudden death in 1927 has long been rumored to have come at Stalin's orders (Bekhterev supposedly diagnosed the dictator as suffering from pathological paranoia), but these claims have never been substantiated.

Bibliography

Primary: 1903–1907. *Osnovy uchenia o funktsiakh mozga* [Bases for Study about the Functions of the Brain] 7 vols. (St Petersburg); 1926. *Obschie osnovy refleksology cheloveka: Rukovodstvo k obektivnomu izucheniyu lichnosti* [The General Bases of the Reflexology of Man: A Guide to the Objective Study of the Personality] 3rd ed. (Petrograd); 1928. *Avtobiografiia* [Autobiography] (Moscow).

Secondary: Joravsky, David, 1989. *Russian Psychology: A Critical History* (Oxford); Iudin, Tikhon I., 1951. *Ocherki istorii otechestvennoi psikhiatrii* [Studies in the History of the Homeland's Psychiatry] (Moscow); Kannabikh, Iurii V., 1928. *Istoriia psikhiatrii* [History of Psychiatry] (Moscow).

Benjamin Zajicek

BELIOS, GEORGE DEMETRIOU (b. Athens, Greece, 27 March 1909; d. Athens, Greece, 15 December 1995), *public health, malariology.*

The Belios family originated from the Aegean island of Sifnos, but George was born and grew up in Athens. As a child he enjoyed spending long hours at the printing business where his father, Demetrios, worked. Reading books that had just come off the press triggered in young George a lifelong interest in learning.

Belios benefited from a French Government scholarship by studying medicine at the Sorbonne (University of Paris), graduating with an MD in 1933. He undertook his postgraduate studies at the Athens School of Hygiene (DPH, 1939) and at the London School of Hygiene and Tropical Medicine (DTM&H, 1952).

Belios first joined Greece's antimalaria efforts in 1936. When Mussolini's Italy invaded Greece in 1940, he joined the army's medical service and participated in the effort to resist the invasion. As a communist, he was arrested by the Germans when the Axis powers occupied Greece and spent part of the occupation period in prison.

After liberation in 1944, he returned to antimalaria work, taking part in Greece's successful nationwide antimalaria campaign by serving as a regional malariologist in the Peloponnese. The campaign coincided with the Greek Civil

War (1946–49), and during this period Belios never hid his distaste for the monarchy. Because of his political views, he was sent into exile.

Following a year's service with the WHO, which took him to the Middle East and to India, Belios returned to Greece in 1950 to become deputy director of the Malaria Division at the Ministry of Social Welfare. Two years later, he became director of the division and, in 1959, professor of malariology at the Athens School of Hygiene. He served as dean of the School during 1966–68.

While he was at the Ministry, and subsequently as an Athens School academic, Belios worked energetically to guide Greece's antimalaria efforts. During a period when the Greeks considered the control of malaria a fait accompli, Belios sought to persuade them that organized antimalaria work was still needed to secure what had already been achieved. In order to reach even higher levels of malaria control, he maintained the need to marshal the limited resources available for antimalaria work so as to obtain maximum benefit.

In 1951–52 Belios voiced concern over the decision to terminate Greece's house-spraying program. The program had to restart in 1954, but its temporary interruption had already contributed to the shaping of the WHO's malaria eradication policy.

Not the least important problem troubling Greek antimalaria work in the 1950s and 1960s was the development of DDT resistance by the *Anopheles* mosquito, which soon extended to other insecticides. That resistance phenomenon was identified, for the first time anywhere, in Greece in 1951. Belios and colleagues studied it extensively and modified spraying protocols accordingly.

Following the launch of the WHO's malaria eradication campaign in 1955, Belios guided the reorientation of Greece's program from malaria control to malaria eradication. Financial shortcomings continued to hamper the program after its reorientation, but Belios stressed the continuous need for an adequate number of malariologists and entomologists to be part of the effort. He organized courses to provide basic knowledge of malariology to the majority of physicians serving in rural Greece and emphasized the need for Greece to cooperate with the WHO.

Belios downplayed the importance of all honors and distinctions he received during his career, including Greece's King George I medal (1962). He remained a scholar to the end, passionate about the latest scientific and medical advances and most interested in the implications those advances could have for public health.

George Belios and his wife Astero, a medical technician, had no children.

Bibliography

Primary: 1978. 'From Malaria Control to Malaria Eradication: Problems, Solutions' *Archeia Hygienes* 27: 54–59 (in Greek).

Secondary: Vassiliou, Maria, 2005. 'Politics, Public Health, and Development: Malaria in Twentieth-Century Greece', DPhil thesis, University of Oxford.

Maria Vassiliou

BELL, CHARLES (b. Fountainbridge, Edinburgh, Scotland, 8 November 1774; d. Hallow Park, Worcester, England, 28 April 1842), *anatomy, physiology, surgery.*

Early Life

Bell was the youngest of the six children who survived infancy, five sons and one daughter, of the Reverend William Bell (1704–79), who for many years was the Episcopalian minister at Doune, Perthshire. They were the grandchildren of the Reverend John Bell, minister of the parish of Gladsmuir, East Lothian. Bell received much of his early general and artistic education from his mother, Margaret Morice (aka Morrice), his father's second wife, and she from her grandfather, Bishop White, Primus of Scotland. The rest of his education was from the example set by his brothers, although he spent some years at the High School in Edinburgh.

Bell was left fatherless from the age of five. Two of his brothers entered the legal profession: Robert (1757–1816), his oldest brother, became an advocate and later was elected Professor of Conveyancing to the Society of Writers to the Signet, while George Joseph (1770–1843) became Professor of the Law of Scotland at the University of Edinburgh. Bell's brother John (1763–1820) became a distinguished anatomist and surgeon, and for twenty years was said to have been the leading operating surgeon in Britain and throughout the world. Information is lacking about the fifth son, James (1767–1830), and Bell's sister, Margaret (1765–1832). Throughout his life, Bell suffered bouts of depression and lacked self-confidence. He often sought the advice of his older brother George, even in matters relating to medicine. Almost thirty years after Bell's death, his wife published a selection of the correspondence between Charles and George.

Bell went to Edinburgh University to study medicine, but did not graduate with the MD degree. He was at the same time apprenticed to his brother John, who trained him in anatomy and surgery at his Anatomy School in Edinburgh. Bell's indenture to John was dated 26 September 1792. While still a student, Bell prepared *A System of Dissections* illustrated with his own drawings, and published it in 1798–99. He addressed this book to the students of practical anatomy. He was already a talented artist, having studied under the Edinburgh artist, David Allan (1774–96). Bell was admitted a Freeman Surgeon Apothecary of the Royal College of Surgeons of Edinburgh on 1 August 1799, without having previously taken their LRCSEd diploma. For about a year afterward, as FCSEd, he was allowed access to the surgical wards of the Royal Infirmary of Edinburgh.

John withdrew from teaching anatomy in 1799 and confined himself to private surgical practice. There was much jealousy and political opposition to John Bell, principally led by James Gregory (1753–1821), professor of the practice of physic (medicine) at the university, and a manager of the Infirmary, largely due to John's surgical success. As neither John nor Bell was elected to surgeoncies in the Infirmary in 1800, and because Bell was unable to establish himself as a teacher of anatomy in Edinburgh, on the advice of brother George he traveled to London, arriving on 28 November 1804. Before he left Edinburgh, in 1803 and 1804, Bell collaborated with John on the third and fourth volumes in John's series, *The Anatomy of the Human Body.* John had previously published his *Engravings of the Arteries, of the Nerves, and of the Brain* (1801–02).

The Great Windmill Street School and London Surgical Career

Despite written introductions to well known anatomists and surgeons in London, and despite having published a series of anatomical texts, Bell could find no employment, and had to be supported financially by George during this period. He first lived at 22 Fluyder Street; then, in 1805, he established a school at his house in Leicester Street, formerly occupied by Speaker Onslow (1691–1768), where he taught anatomy and surgery to medical men and anatomy to painters. He also expanded the anatomical museum that had been packaged and sent down to him from Edinburgh by George. This museum collection had largely been prepared and used by John for his teaching, and contained many pathological preparations of the skeleton. Bell also had the assistance of a number of house pupils who undertook the dissections needed for his classes. He purchased bodies from grave robbers as and when required, this being many years before the 1832 Anatomy Act. During this period, Bell completed the plates for the first edition of what became his extremely popular *Anatomy of Expression in Painting.* This was published in 1806 with the support of Benjamin West (1738–1820), then President of the Royal Academy. His book was widely read at the time by artists and others, including the Queen.

Although short of money, Bell nevertheless enjoyed the London theatrical and intellectual scene. In 1807, he was able to spend much of his spare time researching the anatomy of the nervous system. Early in 1812, he purchased from James Wilson (1762–1821) a part share in the Hunterian, or Great Windmill Street, School of Anatomy, and from that time until 1826 he was both its co-owner and lecturer on anatomy. From the first, Bell had the assistance of Benjamin Brodie (1783–1862), who was at that time assistant surgeon at St George's Hospital. The addition of Bell's museum to Wilson's greatly enhanced its usefulness and value. In 1826, Bell sold his share in the Hunterian School to Herbert Mayo (1796–1852) and Caesar Hawkins (1798–

1884), and withdrew from teaching. He also sold many of the anatomical and pathological preparations in his museum collection to the RCSEd for the then large sum of £3,000.

Bell volunteered to attend the sick and wounded following their retreat from Corunna, Spain in January 1809, some thousands of whom had been disembarked at Portsmouth and Plymouth. The Medical Board gratefully accepted his offer. He had very much regretted not attending the wounded from the battle of Trafalgar in 1805. He made an impressive series of preliminary oil sketches from his observations of these casualties while they were housed at Haslar Hospital, and these sketches are now displayed in the Playfair Hall of the RCSEd. His *Dissertation on Gunshot Wounds* was largely based on his experiences during this period.

After Waterloo in 1815, Bell traveled with his brother-in-law, John Shaw (1792–1827), to Brussels, 'their only passports being their surgical instruments'. They arrived eleven days after the battle, and found that many of the French wounded were still unattended on the battlefield. Bell was said to have attended 300 of them. As the situation of many of these men was extremely poor, not surprisingly, a high proportion of those whom Bell operated on died shortly after surgery. He operated in the Gens D'Armerie Hospital, and was assisted on some occasions by Robert Knox (1791–1862), who stated afterwards that 'only one of C. Bell's lived'. Bell never claimed to be other than an enthusiastic amateur, rather than a military surgeon such as George Guthrie (1785–1856), John Pringle (1707–82), or John Hennen (1779–1828).

After John Shaw's sudden death in 1827, his brother Alexander (1804–90) took his place and assumed his teaching responsibilities, lecturing for some years at the Great Windmill Street School. John Shaw, in addition to being one of Bell's house pupils, had also acted as his research assistant and prepared many of the specimens in his anatomical museum. Alexander also acted as Bell's research assistant, and was later appointed a surgeon at the Middlesex Hospital. He was the author of a number of works that publicized Bell's research and discoveries on the nervous system.

London Scientific Career

Bell moved to 34 Soho Square in May 1811, and in June married Marion Shaw, of Ayr. Her sister had earlier married his brother George, and her brother John was then one of Bell's house pupils. Soho was at that time the home of a number of important anatomical schools. Principally between 1811 and 1821, Bell was engaged in scientific enquiry into the anatomy and physiology of the nervous system. In 1811 he published his *Idea of a New Anatomy of the Brain*, in which he indicated his views on the structure and functions of the nervous system. He particularly emphasized that different parts of the brain, such as the cerebrum and cerebellum, had different functions. He always avoided vivisection where possible, as he was wary of the findings obtained in this way. Consequently, most of his information came from anatomical findings alone. One of his important neurological observations was on the different functions of the anterior and posterior spinal roots. Additonal work in this area was conducted by the French physiologist, François Magendie (1783–1855), who finally established that the anterior roots were motor in function, while the posterior roots had a sensory function (subsequently termed the Bell-Magendie Law).

Bell was also appointed to the surgical staff of the Middlesex Hospital in 1814, succeeding the recently deceased Henry Witham, and maintained a considerable consulting practice. Many of his students at Great Windmill Street completed their medical studies at the Middlesex Hospital. On 17 November 1826, Bell was elected FRS, and three years later was awarded their Gold Medal for his research into the nervous system. In 1827 he was appointed professor of anatomy, surgery, and physiology at the University of London, and gave the inaugural address at the opening of its Medical School. He resigned from his chair of surgery and clinical surgery in September 1830, and later that year he was relieved of his physiology teaching.

From about 1827, he was involved with the Society for the Diffusion of Useful Knowledge, and produced a number of works of a religious character. These included his Bridgewater Treatise on *The Hand* (1833), illustrated with his own drawings, and in 1836, his and Lord Brougham's annotations on William Paley's (1743–1805) treatise on *Natural Theology*.

In 1831, on the accession to the throne of William IV, Bell was knighted in the Guelphic Order of Hanover. In 1835 he saw the establishment of the Middlesex Hospital Medical School, and taught surgery and anatomy there. In 1836, at age sixty-two, he returned to Edinburgh, to the chair of surgery. This was not a successful move, and he additionally suffered from ill health with repeated episodes of angina. He died while visiting friends at Hallow Park in 1842, and was buried in the local churchyard. His wife was awarded a pension of £1,000 by Robert Peel's government.

Bibliography

Primary: 1798–99. *A System of Dissections* (Edinburgh, Glasgow, and London); 1803. *The Anatomy of the Human Body* vol. 3 (London); 1804. *The Anatomy of the Human Body* vol. 4 (London); 1806. *Anatomy of Expression in Painting* (London); 1814. *A Dissertation on Gunshot Wounds* (London); 1833. *The Hand, Its Mechanism and Vital Endowments, as Evincing Design* (London).

Secondary: Gordon-Taylor, G., and E. W. Walls, 1958. *Sir Charles Bell: His Life and Times* (Edinburgh and London); Bell, C., 1870. *Letters of Sir Charles Bell, K.H., F.R.S.L. & E. Selected from his Correspondence with his Brother, George Joseph Bell* (London); Shaw, A.,

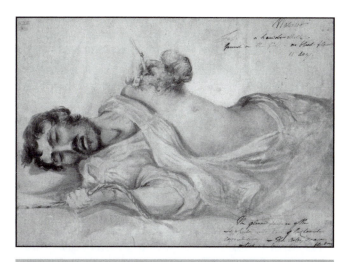

Soldier severely wounded at the Battle of Waterloo whose left arm has been shot off at the shoulder, gripping a rope for pain relief with his right hand. Watercolor by Sir Charles Bell, dated 11 August 1815. Archives and Manuscripts, Wellcome Library, London.

1844. *An Account of Sir Charles Bell's Classification of the Nervous System* (London); Pettigrew, T. J., 1839. 'Sir Charles Bell' in *Medical Portrait Gallery* 4 vols. (London) vol. 3(2): 1–22; Shaw, A., 1839. *Narrative of the Discoveries of Sir Charles Bell in the Nervous System* (London); *DSB*; *Oxford DNB*.

Matthew Howard Kaufman

BELL, MURIEL EMMA (b. Murchison, New Zealand, 4 January 1898; d. Dunedin, New Zealand, 2 May 1974), *nutrition, dietetics.*

Modestly born, Muriel Bell graduated MB ChB from the University of New Zealand's medical school at Otago University in 1922. Four years later, she became the first woman to graduate with an MD from that school, presenting a thesis on basal metabolism in goiter. Soon appointed to a lectureship in physiology, Bell was later described as 'Professor (John) Malcolm's right-hand man.' In 1930 a scholarship took her to University College, London, to research vitamins under Jack Drummond. There she published with the New Zealand biochemist Elizabeth Gregory, who was completing her doctorate with Drummond.

Bell returned to Otago University's physiology department in 1935 and soon found herself appointed to the New Zealand government's Board of Health. When that agency became the funding channel for a new Medical Research Council (MRCNZ) in 1936, Bell became a council member. She held that position until 1965.

Politically, MRCNZ was the new Labour government's response to the League of Nations' call for an integrated research and action agency to tackle nutritional problems arising from the 1930s depression. Thus, the first MRCNZ committee to start work focused on nutrition research. Bell soon replaced John Malcolm, the committee's first chair. Directing this committee's research work at Otago, she channeled her research results to wide social audiences through her parallel appointment as government nutritionist. She was helped in that effort by Elizabeth Gregory, now Dean of Home Science in Otago's School of Home Science.

Muriel Bell's nutritional science stood at the frontier of current knowledge. Building on her earlier work, she undertook and oversaw investigation into a string of locally significant issues, including dietary problems caused by mineral deficiencies in New Zealand soils, and the vitamin contents of fruit, vegetables, and fish. But simply producing research results was never enough—they had to be transmitted to public audiences, and Bell used a huge range of means to that end. In 1940 she edited the first edition of *Good Nutrition*, a handbook outlining the best current nutritional practice, combined with recipes. Cowritten by Elizabeth Gregory and her staff and published in large numbers by the Health Department, three new editions appeared over the next sixteen years. Throughout World War II, Bell spread nutritional advice through her regular column in the Broadcasting Department's influential magazine, *The New Zealand Listener*.

Bell campaigned successfully on many issues rooted in nutritional science. She was an advocate for iodized salt to ease endemic soil-based goiter problems; for a government requirement that millers increase flour extraction rates to increase dietary roughage; for safe and cheap milk supplies; and for water fluoridation to reduce dental caries. At the same time, her Nutrition Research Unit also bridged the life and social sciences. Inheriting an earlier Home Science School-based survey program on dietary inadequacy among low-income groups in New Zealand, Bell's unit undertook parallel investigations of diet among the Maori people, and on certain Pacific islands.

But the political climate inside MRCNZ grew steadily colder toward public health research. As medical researchers gained greater autonomy from state surveillance, so priorities shifted toward 'blue skies' biomedical investigation. The announcement that Bell's Nutrition Research Unit would close when she retired in 1963 caused a political furor. Implementing that decision threw Bell into a depression from which she never recovered. Debating the abolition of MRNCZ in 1989, health minister Helen Clark called it 'a biomedical old boys club'. Bell was long dead, but that description would have pleased her. She was always warm, caring, and determined to give women sound scientific advice about nutrition, but she felt that her life had been wasted. It had not.

Bibliography

Primary: 1940. Bell, Muriel, ed., *Good Nutrition* (Wellington); (anon.) 1963. 'The Work of the Nutrition Research Unit'. MRCNZ Annual Report 1962, *Appendix to the House of Representatives* H31-B: 6–11.

Secondary: Carter, Ian, 2004. 'The Missing Link.' *New Zealand Sociology* 19(2): 197–219; *DNZB*.

Ian Carter

BELLINI, LORENZO (b. Florence, Italy, 3 September 1643; d. Florence, 8 January 1704), *anatomy, physiology, medical theory.*

Born into a modest merchant family, Bellini graduated in philosophy and medicine from the University of Pisa on 14 September 1663. A disciple of Giovanni Alfonso Borelli (1608–79), to whose iatromechanic conceptions he fully adhered, he was also influenced by the Galilean and Gassendist Antonio Oliva, and by the mathematician Alessandro Marchetti, translator of Lucretius. While still an undergraduate at Pisa he was made extraordinary lecturer, a position given only to the most gifted students, and in 1663 he became lecturer of logic. He held that post until 1668, when he was given the chair of anatomy that he occupied until 1703. During this period he still continued to practice medicine with great success, holding the position of chief physician to the Grand Duke Cosimo III.

Bellini was a pioneer in applying mechanical philosophy to provide explanations for the functions of the human body. His first essay, *Exercitatio anatomica . . . de structura et usu renum* (1662), published when he was only nineteen years of age, was an important study of the structure and function of the kidneys and was accompanied by an excellent collection of illustrations.

In the kidney Bellini discovered a canalicular system terminating in tubules that open into the apex of the papillae by means of capillary pores, through which the urine flows into the renal pelvis. These tubules (later called 'Bellini's tubules') run through the kidney from the external surface to the edge of the papillary body, where they open their meatuses. By injecting colored liquids, Bellini demonstrated that the vascular ramifications reached the external surface of the kidney. There they formed a system of varicosities (*sinuli vermiculares et tortuosi*) that established the junction between arterioles, venules, and uriniferous tubules, in which the arterial blood is separated into urinous and sanguineous portions. The urinous portion is drawn into the tubule by capillarity, whereas the purified venous blood is returned to the circulatory system through the venules. The separation of urine, therefore, was found not to be the work of the hypothetical 'faculties' postulated by Galen; it could be explained mechanically as a consequence of the differences in width and configuration between the openings of the two ducts (tubule and vein).

These anatomical discoveries and the application of mechanical principles to physiology won Bellini widespread fame in Italy and abroad. In 1665 he published the work *Gustus organum*, containing his researches on the lingual gustatory papillae, which had recently been discovered by Marcello Malpighi (1628–94) and Fracassati. Regarding the function of taste, he followed the atomistic Democritean conception.

Thereafter, Bellini accomplished no further important anatomical research, preferring to devote himself mostly to studies of medical theory and physiology. In his *De urinis et pulsibus* (1683), he considered blood as a fluid exhibiting several elementary physical properties—such as density, viscosity, and impulse—that could be expressed in mathematical terms. He postulated that health depended on a well-ordered circulation, and that disease implied an increased or diminished velocity of the blood.

Bellini developed his iatromechanic themes in his *Opuscula aliquot* (1695), dedicated to the Scottish physician Archibald Pitcairne (1652–1713). In this work, organized into postulates, theorems, and corollaries, he applied the laws of mechanics systematically to all of the most important physiological phenomena. *Opuscula aliquot* was to have a profound influence on medicine in the first part of the eighteenth century, in particular upon Giorgio Baglivi (1668–1707), and on Herman Boerhaave (1668–1738), who studied with Pitcairne at Leiden.

Bibliography

Primary: 1708. *Opera omnia* 2 vols. (Venice); 1662. *Exercitatio anatomica . . . de structura et usu renum* (Florence); 1665. *Gustus organum . . . novissime deprehensum* (Bologna); 1683. *De urinis et pulsibus* (Bologna); 1695. *Opuscula aliquot* (Pistoia).

Secondary: Grondona, Felice, 1963. 'L'esercitazione anatomica di Lorenzo Bellini sulla struttura e funzione dei reni.' *Physis* 5: 423–463; Nardi, Giuseppe Michele, 1937. 'L'organo del gusto nelle ricerche ed osservazioni di Lorenzo Bellini.' *Omnia medica* 15: 141–175; *DSB*.

Giuseppe Ongaro

BENE, FERENC VON (b. Mindszent, Hungary, 12 October 1775; d. Pest, Hungary, 2 July 1858), *medicine, medical education, medical scholarship.*

The son of a village notary (a minor official, but from an ennobled family) in a town with few educational resources, Bene was first schooled in nearby Szeged and then sent to board in Pest (German: Ofen). Inadequately challenged after a year at the university in Pest, he continued his medical studies in Vienna. Diminished funds dictated a return to Pest, where he earned his MD in 1798. He worked in Johann Peter Frank's clinic during another brief sojourn in Vienna and was encouraged to stay. He soon settled in Pest, however, where he spent the remainder of his long career.

Bene climbed the professional ladder rapidly (he began teaching in 1799, only a year after qualifying in medicine) and taught a stunningly wide array of subjects. In short order he replaced the professor of anatomy, took over the chair in the theory and practice of medicine, and was made professor of forensic medicine. He taught the theory of medicine to surgeons and stepped in for the professor of physiology. After three years of teaching special pathology and therapy on a temporary basis, he was appointed permanently to that chair. Over a period of nearly three decades (1813–41), Bene taught thousands of students.

Yet this massive contribution to the teaching of medicine in Hungary is not all that accounts for Bene's importance. His scholarship was remarkably broad and deep (he read both Greek and Latin), and his output as an author was unmatched among his contemporaries. Through journals and books he stayed abreast of developments across Europe. He traveled for both pleasure and professional purposes, staying weeks at a time in different European capitals. He wrote and published in Latin, German, and Hungarian, and many of his works were translated into other languages (including Serbian, Romanian, Slovakian, and Croatian), further promoting Hungarian medicine. His *Elementa medicinae practicae* [The Elements of the Practice of Medicine]—a five-volume work edited by his son, Ferenc Bene, Jr.—was widely used within Hungary and elsewhere, perhaps most notably in Russia. Together with two other major Latin-language texts (on forensic medicine and on public health), this monumental work made Bene widely known and helped educate generations of physicians, not only in Hungary but throughout central and eastern Europe.

Arguably his greatest contribution to medicine in Hungary was introducing smallpox vaccination to his colleagues and his countrymen. In 1800, he wrote a booklet entitled *A himlő veszedelme ellen való oltás* [Vaccination, Effective Protection Against the Danger of Smallpox], and the medical faculty had a thousand copies distributed to physicians and surgeons, and to schools. On 27 August 1801, Bene performed the first smallpox vaccination in Hungary, inoculating the nine-month-old daughter of a colleague.

In 1841 Bene was responsible for the first joint gathering of natural scientists and physicians in Pest, thus creating another forum for medical education. His leadership role at that meeting was no surprise; at various stages of his career he had served as (among other things) director of the city hospital, dean of the medical faculty, *Rector Magnificus* (president) of the university, and director of medical and surgical studies. He was made an 'honored member' of the Hungarian Academy of Sciences in 1831, he was a member of the royal council, and the King-Emperor conferred on him the Order of Leopold. Of his ten children, two sons became physicians.

Bibliography

Primary: 1800. *A himlő veszedelme ellen való oltás* [Vaccination, Effective Protection Against the Danger of Smallpox] (Buda); 1807. *Elementa politiæ medicæ* (Buda); 1811. *Elementa medicinæ forensis* (Buda); 1833–34. Ferenc Bene, Jr., ed., *Elementa medicinæ practicæ e prælectionibus illius publicis* (Pest).

Secondary: Albert, E. et al., eds., 1929–34. *Biographisches Lexikon der hervorragenden Ärzte aller Zeiten und Völker*, vol. 1: 452–453 (Berlin); 1858. 'Nekrolog' [Obituary] *Wiener med. Wochenschr.* 8: 547–549.

Constance Putnam

BENIVIENI, ANTONIO (b. Florence, Italy, 3 November 1443; d. Florence, 2 November 1502), *pathological anatomy.*

Antonio Benivieni, the eldest son of Paolo Benivieni—a notary—and Nastagia de' Bruni, was born into an ancient and noble Florentine family. At first he was drawn to a literary career, and in this period he wrote the *'Εγκώμιον Cosmi.* It was dedicated to the young Lorenzo de' Medici on the death of his grandfather (1464), but not published until 1949. Benivieni then turned to medicine, studying at the University of Pisa but also attending lessons at the University of Siena. Around 1470 he started to practice medicine in Florence and soon became very famous, counting such men as Angelo Poliziano (1454–94), Marsilio Ficino (1433–99), Lorenzo the Magnificent (De'Medici, 1449–92) and Girolamo Savonarola (1452–98) as his friends, and sometimes his patients.

The work which made Benivieni famous was his *De abditis nonnullis ac mirandis morborum et sanationum causis,* published posthumously in 1507. The title would appear to have been suggested by Celsus's 'abditae morborum causae' (cf. Celsus, *De medicina,* Bk. I, *Proemium*). Conceived by the author as a collection of 300 observations made during his medical practice, the *De abditis* was published by his brother Girolamo—with the help of the physician Giovanni Rosati—in an incomplete form with only 111 observations. The work was translated into Italian by Carlo Burci (1843), and in 1855 Francesco Puccinotti published the original dedication to the physician Lorenzo Lorenzi (known as *Laurentianus,* d. 1502), along with forty-seven unpublished observations. A partial nineteenth-century copy of the original manuscript of the *De abditis* survives in the Biblioteca Nazionale of Florence. In 1963 that copy was studied by A. Costa and G. Weber, who clearly documented the Celsian humanism of the *De abditis.*

For the most part, Benivieni's observations have a clinical character and reveal his ability in medicine, as well as in surgery and obstetrics. Among other things, he performed the ligation of vessels in the stump of amputation instead of following the usual practice of cauterization, and he performed bony resections and lithotripsy in women. The fundamental element of the work, however, which makes Benivieni a forerunner of pathological anatomy, is the fact that in various observations the clinical findings are accompanied by necroscopic ones that, apart from their conciseness, show just how he examined the cadavers for the cause of death and attempted to establish a parallel between the clinical symptomatology and the anatomical lesions.

Benivieni's work, therefore, besides providing precious documentation of the importance already attributed to autopsy at that time, constitutes the first appearance of the anatomical-clinical method, which would evolve slowly over the following centuries to definitively establish itself with Giovanni Battista Morgagni's *De sedibus* (1761). Benivieni performed at least twenty autopsies and observed gallstones, urinary calculi, scirrhous cancer of the stomach, cardiac lesions, peritonitis arising from intestinal perforation, chronic intestinal ulcers, mesenteric abscesses, osseous lesions, and the transmission of syphilis from the mother to the fetus. Some of his observations concerned malformations.

Benivieni left other works in manuscript, and among these are the two hygienic-prophylactic treatises *De regimine sanitatis ad Laurentium Medicem,* published by L. Belloni (1951), and *De peste* (1938).

Bibliography

Primary: 1507. *De abditis nonnullis ac mirandis morborum et sanationum causis* (Florence) [Italian trans. Burci, Carlo (Florence, 1843); English trans. Singer, Charles, and Esmond R. Long, *The Hidden Causes of Diseases* (Springfield, IL, 1954)]; 1855. *Observationum medicarum centuria secunda inedita* in Puccinotti, Francesco, ed., *Storia della medicina,* vol. II/I (Leghorn) pp. 233–255.

Secondary: Siraisi, Nancy G., 2001. *Medicine and the Italian Universities, 1250–1600* (Leiden) pp. 226–252; Stefanutti, Ugo, 1966. 'Benivieni, Antonio' *Dizionario biografico degli Italiani,* vol. 8 (Rome) pp. 543–545; Costa, Antonio and Giorgio Weber, 1963. 'L'inizio dell'anatomia patologica nel Quattrocento fiorentino, sui testi di Antonio Benivieni, Bernardo Torni, Leonardo da Vinci'. *Archivio De Vecchi per l'anatomia patologica e la medicina clinica* 39: 429–878; Major, Ralph H., 1935. 'Antonio di Pagolo Benivieni'. *Bulletin of the History of Medicine* 3: 739–755; DSB.

Giuseppe Ongaro

BENNETT, JOHN HUGHES (b. Exeter, Devon, England, 31 August 1812; d. Norwich, England, 25 September 1875), *physiology, medicine.*

Bennett was the son of John Stokes Bennett, an actor and musician, and his wife Julia Hughes, an actress from an established theatrical family. His grandfather was what would now be called a theater impresario, owning a number of theaters in London, including Sadler's Wells. Although the performing arts were still not considered a respectable occupation in conservative circles, the Bennetts were successful enough to establish a middle-class lifestyle, and John, their only son, received a solid classical education at Exeter grammar school and at Mount Radford School in Exeter. His lifelong interest in the fine arts has been attributed to his mother's influence.

In 1829 Bennett was apprenticed to the surgeon William Sedgwick in Maidstone, Kent. The five-year apprenticeship required by law was often supplemented by 'walking the wards' in the London hospitals, and Bennett worked as an assistant in medical dispensaries in north London. He seems to have quarreled with Sedgwick, allegedly over carrying out an unauthorized postmortem, but Sedgwick later wrote him a good recommendation, as did William Kingdon, a consulting surgeon with whom he worked in London. In 1833 Bennett began attending classes at the

University of Edinburgh, studying with James Syme (1799–1870), Charles Bell (1774–1842), and Robert Christison (1797–1882). He appears to have looked for ways to distinguish himself, seeking out like-minded, scientifically inclined medical students, several of whom, like John Goodsir (1814–67) and John Reid (1809–49), later became medical professors. Bennett was very active in student societies, including the Royal Medical, the Royal Physical, and the Anatomical and Physiological societies. In 1836 he published his first paper, 'On the Anatomy and Physiology of the Otic Ganglion' (*London Medical Gazette*, July 30 1836). He graduated MD in 1837, receiving a gold medal for the best clinical report of surgical cases.

After Edinburgh, Bennett spent two years studying at the Paris hospitals, at that time the center of scientific-based medical education. He founded the Paris-based English medical society, modeled on the student societies at Edinburgh. He then spent two years in Germany, studying at both Heidelberg University and at the Charité hospital in Berlin. In 1841 he returned to Paris. Fascinated with the new discoveries in microscopy, such as those on the structure of the cell by Mathias Schleiden (1804–81) and Theodor Schwann (1810–82), Bennett studied with Alfred Donné (1801–78) and others to master the new field of microscopy and its use in both physiology and pathology.

Bennett returned to Edinburgh in 1841, determined to introduce both histology, defined as 'the minute structure of organized tissues', and the use of the microscope into the medical curriculum. François Xavier Bichat (1771–1802), whose classification of human anatomy into distinct tissues had initiated the study of histology, had regarded the microscope as little more than a toy, but by the 1840s the microscope was widely used in both physiology and pathology in urban medical centers in France and Germany. Bennett did not have a position with Edinburgh University, but like many other ambitious medical men, he began by offering private lectures, in the hope that this would one day lead to a professorial chair. Bennett offered a set of lectures in Edinburgh on 'Histology with reference to Anatomy, Physiology, Pathology, and the Diagnosis of Disease', the first set of its kind in Edinburgh.

As a complement to the lectures, he offered a practical course on the use of the microscope. To Bennett, hands-on experience with the microscope, including 'the optical and mechanical arrangements of microscopes, illumination, mensuration, optical illusions, mode of displaying objects, and every information necessary for the medical inquirer', was as important a part of medical education as hands-on experience with chemical techniques. Each student was provided with a microscope and a set of prepared slides, illustrating 'inflammation, tubercle, and the ultimate structure of all the morbid products'. Bennett's object was to make microscopy so familiar to students that it became, in effect, a sixth medical sense for interpreting pathological anatomy, so that every student knew his microscope, 'as a trained soldier knows his rifle', and could describe what he saw with it carefully and accurately 'so as to give a correct picture of the cell, tissue, or organ seen' (Jacyna, 1997, pp. 14–15). He was certain that microscopy held the key to advancements in pathology, a view that was vindicated by 1858 with the publication of Rudolf Virchow's *Cellular Pathology*.

Bennett's private lectures did not attract many students, who already had enough required courses to more than occupy their waking hours. He was disappointed that the medical faculty did not provide more encouragement for them, and even more disappointed when he was passed over for the position of pathologist and superintendent of the Royal Infirmary of Edinburgh. In 1844 those two positions were separated, and Bennett was appointed pathologist. In 1845 he was appointed lecturer in medicine at the University and, in 1848, professor of the institutes of medicine. In these more established positions, he attracted many devoted students. Unlike many of his more conservative colleagues at Edinburgh, he supported medical education for women.

In 1845, Bennett published the paper that assured his posthumous reputation, 'Case of Hypertrophy of the Spleen and Liver in which death took place from suppuration of the Blood'. It was the first unambiguous description of leukemia in the medical literature. In the early nineteenth century, pathological alterations in the blood were generally attributed to either inflammation or pus, with the latter predominating in cases which we would now diagnose as leukemia. In 1844, an alert consulting physician to the Royal Infirmary noted the similarities between the case of John Menteith, aged twenty-eight, who was admitted with an enlarged spleen, fever, and joint pain, and that of a previously admitted patient who had died within a few months. When Menteith died, Bennett performed the postmortem examination, paying close attention to the state of the blood cells. His work indicated that neither pus nor inflammation were responsible for the changes that had taken place in the blood. Using the microscope, he clearly described the white blood cells. The modern diagnosis would probably be chronic granulocytic leukemia. In 1852, Bennett published a systematic review of the subject, entitled *Leucocythemia or White Cell Blood*, which included a list of thirty-seven case studies. His drawings of the white blood cells, taken from Menteith's case, were the first illustrations of the cells in a patient with leukemia. The following year, Virchow in Berlin independently described his postmortem analysis of the blood in a similar case, probably chronic lymphocytic leukemia. Although some contemporary physicians assumed a priority dispute between the two men, both Bennett and Virchow agreed on the sequence of publications, and spoke highly of each other's abilities.

Bennett was a fluent and able writer, publishing 105 articles and editing the *London and Edinburgh Monthly Journal of Medical Science* for many years. His *Clinical Lectures on the Principles and Practice of Medicine* (1850) went through five

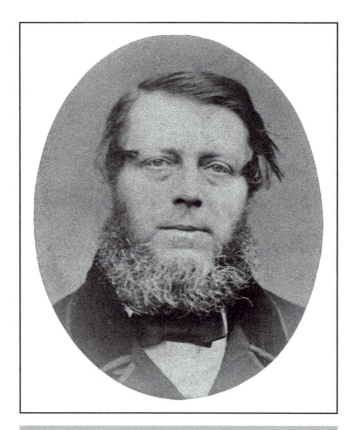

John Hughes Bennett. Photograph, Iconographic Collection, Wellcome Library, London.

British and six American editions. It was translated into French, Russian, and Hindi. His *Textbook of Physiology* (1871, 1872) was translated into French. Bennett's book, *Introduction to Clinical Medicine: six lectures on the method of examining patients, and the means necessary for arriving at an exact diagnosis* (1853), exemplifies the mid-nineteenth-century shift to greater reliance on diagnostic tools.

Bennett also exemplifies the shift among mid-nineteenth-century medical professors from part-time practitioner to full-time scientist, since he had little private practice. It is nonetheless striking that he became well known for two assertions regarding therapeutics. The first involved bloodletting, which he denounced to his classes from 1855. Although venesection had been declining as a therapy since the 1820s, many physicians felt that it was because changes in diseases, and in human constitutions, made it less useful in practice. Bennett declared vehemently that bloodletting had never been therapeutic, but instead always had resulted in unnecessary death. Although defended by older physicians, venesection continued to decline, although leeches as a therapy for fever continued to be practiced in rural areas until World War II.

Bennett's second therapeutic dictum called for what he called the 'restorative treatment' of pulmonary disorders such as pneumonia and tuberculosis. This was related to his opposition to bloodletting, since the standard treatment involved leeches as well as other harsh remedies. Instead, he argued, the goal of the medical practitioner should be to support the body's own natural healing powers, and the way to do that was to promote healthy nutrition. He therefore recommended cod-liver oil for its restorative powers, and his example was widely followed by patients and practitioners looking for alternatives to existing remedies. Twentieth-century research later showed cod-liver oil to be rich in vitamin D, suggesting a physiological reason for its therapeutic properties.

Bennett was a member of the Royal Society of Edinburgh and the Académie de Médecine in Paris. In 1874 the University of Edinburgh awarded Bennett the honorary degree of LLD. In September of the same year, continued illness required Bennett to submit to a lateral lithotomy to remove a stone. He died nine days later on 25 September. In 1901 one of his daughters, Harriet Cox, donated money to the University of Edinburgh to establish the John Hughes Bennett Laboratory.

Bibliography

Primary: 1841–44. (editor) *London and Edinburgh Monthly Journal of Medical Science* (London); 1850. *Clinical Lectures on the Principles and Practice of Medicine* (Edinburgh); 1852. *Leucocythemia or White Cell Blood* (Edinburgh); 1853. *Introduction to Clinical Medicine: six lectures on the method of examining patients, and the means necessary for arriving at an exact diagnosis* (Edinburgh).

Secondary: Jacyna, L. S., 2001. 'A Host of Experienced Microscopists: The Establishment of Histology in Nineteenth-Century Edinburgh.' *Bulletin of the History of Medicine* 75(2): 225–253; Jacyna, L. S., 1997. 'John Hughes Bennett and the Origins of Medical Microscopy in Edinburgh: Lilliputian Wonders' in Piller, G. J., ed., *John Hughes Bennett and the Discovery of Leukemia* (Edinburgh) pp. 12–21; Piller, G. J., 1997. *John Hughes Bennett and the Discovery of Leukemia* (Edinburgh); *Oxford DNB*.

Lisa Rosner

BENTLEY, CHARLES ALBERT   (b. Chipping Norton, Oxfordshire, England, 25 April 1873; d. Carshalton, England, 23 November 1949), *parasitology, tropical medicine*.

Charles Bentley pursued his early education at University College, Liverpool, completed his MB CM from Edinburgh (1898), and the DPH and the DTMH both from Cambridge (1905). He began his career as a junior surgeon in the Royal Southern Dispensary, Liverpool (1898). He moved to India in 1900, where he served for seven years as the chief medical officer for the Empire of India and Ceylon Tea Company in Assam.

It was in the Assamese tea plantations that Bentley began his research. He found that 'ground itch' was caused by larvae of *Ancylostoma duodenale* nematodes present in contaminated soil passing through the skin of the workers' feet and lower limbs (1902). He discovered the first known leucocytozoan (a blood parasite of birds) in 1903 and determined that the newly discovered Leishman-Donovan parasites were present in patients suffering from fever and enlarged spleens, helping to complete the etiology of the infectious disease kala azar (1904). He was a member of the Dooars (or Duars) Blackwater Fever and Malaria Commission (1907–9) and worked with Samuel Rickard Christophers, trying to determine what role quinine played in the etiology of blackwater fever. His detailed knowledge of the tea-growing district proved especially valuable.

Bentley was appointed to the Bombay Malaria Enquiry Commission (1909–11). Based on systematic investigations of Bombay city, he recommended covering the numerous wells and breeding fish to control mosquito larvae as antimalaria measures. He urged that quinine should be sold at a loss, if necessary, to bring it within reach of the poor. From 1911 to 1915, he served Bengal as deputy sanitary commissioner, and as director-general of public health for Bengal he organized the inoculation of more than two million people against cholera in 1928. From 1915, he prepared the annual public health reports. He married Gwendoline Mary Harper in 1916, and they had two sons and two daughters.

While in Bengal, Bentley prepared a scheme for the control of malaria in that region. Apart from the application of specific measures against the malaria parasite, he held that there was immense potential in carrying out antimalarial projects based on the principles underlying Italian *bonificazione,* which embodied measures with a dual purpose—to improve agriculture and health simultaneously. He pointed out that since the country had gone dry, it was essential to restore a healthy flow of water, which could be achieved by improving irrigation. Thus, he contended that malaria could be controlled by the improvement of agriculture.

Bentley was awarded the Kaiser-I-Hind medal in 1916 and the CIE in 1929. In 1931 he retired from India and went to Cairo as professor of hygiene at the Egyptian University, becoming professor emeritus in 1937. That same year he was honored as Commandant of the Order of Nile.

Bibliography

Primary: 1902. 'On the Causal Relationship Between "Ground Itch", or "pani-ghao", and the presence of the larvae of *Ankylostoma Duodenale* in the soil.' *British Medical Journal* i: 190–193; 1904. (with Leishman et al.) 'Discussion on the Leishman-Donovan body.' *British Medical Journal* ii: 642–658; 1909. (with S. R. Christophers) 'The Human Factor in Malaria.' *Transactions of the Bombay Medical Congress* (Bombay); 1911. *Report of an Investigation into the Causes of Malaria in Bombay and the Measures Necessary for Its Control* (Bombay); 1913. *Report on Malaria at Dinajpur* (Calcutta); 1916. *Report on Malaria in Bengal* (Calcutta); 1925. *Malaria and Agriculture in Bengal* (Calcutta); 1925. *The English Sanitary Reformation: A Study in the Dynamics of Public Health* (Calcutta); 1928. *Quinine Policy* (Calcutta).

Mridula Ramanna

BERENGARIO DA CARPI, GIACOMO   (b. Carpi, Italy, *c.* 1460; d. Ferrara, Italy, 24 November 1530), *surgery, anatomy.*

Berengario (or Barigazzi) was one of the five children of Faustino Barigazzi and Orsolina Forghieri. His father, a barber and surgeon, taught him the rudiments of surgery at a very early age, and he received a sound education in the humanities from Aldo Manuzio (1449–1515), who was in Carpi between 1469 and 1477 as tutor to Alberto Pio, son of the Prince of Carpi. On 4 August 1489 he received a degree in philosophy and medicine from the University of Bologna, and in 1502 he was appointed lecturer in surgery and (later) in anatomy at the same university. He continued to teach there with great success and popularity until 1527, notwithstanding his quarrelsome and violent character. He also became surgeon at the ducal court of Ferrara, a post that he held until his death.

An extremely competent surgeon and anatomist, Berengario's first work (1514) was an edition of Mondino dei Liuzzi's (*c.* 1270–1326) *Anothomia* (*c.* 1316), accompanied by his critical observations. In 1517 he was summoned to Ancona to attend Lorenzo dei Medici, the Duke of Urbino, who had received a gunshot wound and an occipital skull fracture at the siege of Mondolfo. This experience resulted in Berengario's writing his *Tractatus de fractura calvae sive cranei* (1518), which met with great success and was continually reprinted until almost the middle of the eighteenth century. In that work, Berengario examined the various types of skull fractures and their relevant symptomatology, diagnosis, prognosis, and treatment, as well as the indications and the technique of craniotomy. His *Tractatus* also presented the first organic and systematic illustrations of the instruments to be employed.

Berengario was certainly the greatest of the pre-Vesalian anatomists, believing that the study of anatomy should be acquired above all by performing dissections. In 1521 he published a thorough and detailed commentary to Mondino's *Anothomia*, with numerous references to his own professional experience, and a year later he published a handy and clear anatomic compendium for his students entitled *Isagogae breves*. Both of those works were illustrated by a score of anatomical woodcuts that were substantially identical from book to book, except for some variations and additions. In effect, they were the very first illustrations in a book of anatomy.

Berengario pointed out many anatomical particularities, such as the first mention of the vermiform appendix and the first description of the two arytenoid cartilages. He also provided the first good account of the thymus, denied the medieval belief in the seven-celled uterus, and demonstrated that nerves originated from the brain and spinal cord. He described two of the ossicles of the ear—the malleus and the incus—studied the action of the cardiac valves, and was the first to describe the sphenoidal sinus. It is particularly significant that he claimed he had never been able to demonstrate the *rete mirabile* in the human brain, which constituted a fundamental point of Galen's anatomical-physiological system.

Berengario preferred to treat syphilis with mercury, but he also encouraged the use of a new antiluetic (anti-syphilitic) remedy—guaiac wood (the so-called 'holy wood/tree', or guaiacum). He proposed this remedy in a new edition (1521) of Huldrich von Hutten's (1488–1523) small treatise *De guaiaci medicina et morbo gallico* (1519). Berengario also published an edition of Galen's *De crisi* (1522) and a collection of Latin translations of some Galen's anatomical works (1529).

Bibliography

Primary: 1514. *Anothomia Mundini noviter impressa ac per Carpum castigata* (Bologna); 1518. *Tractatus de fractura calvae sive cranei* (Bologna); 1521. *Commentaria cum amplissimis additionibus super anatomia Mundini* (Bologna); 1522. *Isagoge breves perlucide ac uberrime in anatomiam humani corporis* (Bologna) [English trans. Lind, L. R., 1959. *A Short Introduction to Anatomy* (Chicago)].

Secondary: Lind, L. R., 1975. *Studies in Pre-Vesalian Anatomy* (Philadelphia) pp. 157–165; Putti, Vittorio, 1937. *Berengario da Carpi. Saggio biografico e bibliografico seguito dalla traduzione del 'De fractura calvae sive cranei'* (Bologna); *DSB*.

Giuseppe Ongaro

BERGER, HANS [JOHANNES] (b. Neuses bei Coburg, Germany, 21 May 1873; d. Jena, Germany, 1 June 1941), *neuropsychiatry, electroencephalography.*

Berger was the son of the physician Paul Friedrich Berger and Anna Rückert, youngest daughter of the poet and orientalist Friedrich Rückert. He studied medicine at the universities of Würzburg, Jena, and Kiel and graduated with an MD from Jena in 1897. In the same year, he joined the Jena psychiatric clinic as assistant physician under director Otto Binswanger and was finally named successor to Binswanger in 1919. He spent his entire academic career at the psychiatric clinic of Jena, where he also served as rector of the university during the academic year 1927–28. In 1929 Berger published the first of fourteen reports on the human electroencephalogram (EEG), his most significant achievement. He retired in 1938 and committed suicide in a state of depression on 1 June 1941.

Berger found the lasting theme of his scientific work in the graphic registration of the physiological signs of psychic states. He started by investigating intracerebral blood circulation, which he recorded noninvasively in patients with skull defects caused by previous illnesses or accidents (as introduced by the Italian physiologist Angelo Mosso). His monumental *The Bodily Concomitants of Psychic States* (1904–07) employed the graphic recording of pulsations for psychophysiological investigations. In his next project, Berger aimed at identifying a quantum of psychic energy as part of the brain's metabolism by recording minute temperature changes within the brain (Berger, 1910). Again he observed distinctive changes in relation to psychic processes, but he failed to demonstrate the independent physiology of psychic processes as he had hoped to do.

By that time, Berger had already engaged in a series of experiments to record the electric activity of the human brain. Electric brain activity had been observed by Richard Caton in animal experiments in 1875 and recorded by Vladimir Pravdich-Neminsky in 1913, but similar studies had not been pursued in humans. According to his own account (Berger, 1929), Berger had started as early as 1902 with such experiments, which proved exceedingly difficult because of the minute nature of the currents, their unknown characteristics, and Berger's expectations regarding those potentials. In a long series of attempts he gradually adapted the experimental system and his conceptualization of electric brain activity to produce a new physiological trace—the human EEG—which he first published in 1929. With confirmation of the EEG by Edgar Douglas Adrian in 1934, and with the observation of pathognomonic wave patterns for brain tumors and epilepsy in 1936, EEG soon became a major research method in the neurosciences and a diagnostic routine in neuropsychiatric practice. EEG radically transformed the understanding of the epilepsies and changed, for example, the approach to behavior disorders.

Between 1929 and his retirement in 1938, Berger published on a vast variety of EEG phenomena in his fourteen reports *On the Electroencephalogram of Man* (summarized in Berger, 1938), but he hesitated to implement the new method in clinical practice. Furthermore, his hope of finding a proof of his psychic energy concept in the electrical activity of the brain was not to be fulfilled. Berger was elected to the German Academy of Scientists and Physicians Leopoldina in 1937 and was nominated for the Nobel Prize in 1940. The prize was not awarded that year because of World War II.

Bibliography

Primary: 1904–07. *Über die körperlichen Äußerungen psychischer Zustände* 2 vols. [plus 2 atlases] (Jena); 1929. 'Über das Elektrenkephalogramm des Menschen'. *Archiv für Psychiatrie* 87: 527–570; 1938. *Über das Elektrenkephalogramm des Menschen* [Nova Acta Leopoldina NF 6, Nr. 38] (Halle/Saale); 1940. *Psyche* (Jena).

Secondary: Gloor, Pierre, 1969. 'Hans Berger and the Discovery of the Electroencephalogram' in Gloor, Pierre, ed., *Hans Berger on the Electroencephalogram of Man* [*Electroencephalography and Clinical Neurophysiology* Suppl. 28] pp. 1–35; Jung, Richard, 1963. 'Hans Berger und die Entdeckung des EEG nach seinen Tagebüchern und Protokollen' in Werner, Roland, ed., *Jenenser EEG-Symposion. 30 Jahre Elektroenzephalographie* (Berlin) pp. 20–53.

Cornelius Borck

BERGMANN, ERNST VON (b. Riga, Russia (now Latvia), 16 December 1836; d. Wiesbaden, Germany, 25 March 1907), *surgery.*

Bergmann was the eldest of eight children of a German family of clerics settled in Latvia for centuries. He broke with tradition by reading medicine at the German University of Tartu/Dorpat (Estonia), where he graduated in 1860. After an internship in surgery, he became a Privatdozent with his dissertation on fat embolism (1863). He then received a grant for a fourteen-month study trip to the West (1865).

Although Viennese surgery seemed old-fashioned to him, Bergmann was impressed by the pathological anatomy and dermatology practiced in Vienna. In Berlin he was attracted by Rudolf Virchow, the pathologist, Albrecht von Graefe, the ophthalmologist, and Bernhard von Langenbeck, the surgeon, but he was somewhat disappointed by Langenbeck's lectures. Although he demonstrated brilliant operative skills, Langenbeck failed to discuss diagnostic issues and postoperative problems, let alone the fate of postoperative patients. Nevertheless, Bergmann dropped his plans to visit Paris and stayed in Germany. In 1866 he acquired practical experience during the Austro-Prussian War. In the Franco-Prussian War of 1870–71, he worked under Theodor Billroth and Richard Volkmann. It was Volkmann who was instrumental in introducing Joseph Lister's antiseptic treatment with carbolic acid to Germany.

After the war, Bergmann was prepared to follow his teacher and father-in-law, Georg Adelmann, in the surgical chair of Tartu. He reformed the hospital according to modern hygienic principles and introduced a program of research that included chemical laboratory methods. In 1877 he served in another war, this time with the Russian army against Turkey. A year later he moved to Würzburg, where again he was a successful reformer. Bergmann finally succeeded Langenbeck in the prestigious Berlin chair (1882), Theodor Billroth having declined the offer.

Bergmann's standing in surgery initially stemmed from studies of military surgery and wound disease and on the generation and propagation of cancer, as well as his experiments with blood transfusions and intravenous saline (1883). Later, his assistant, Kurt Schimmelbusch, introduced bacteriological research at the Berlin Clinic, thus transforming Lister's chemical antisepsis into asepsis by the physical method of steam sterilization. Whereas his predecessor, Langenbeck, had been an idiosyncratic genius who invented and performed operations himself, Bergmann systematized procedures in order to render them teachable. He introduced a military-style discipline that seemed indispensable in running an a(nti)septic surgical service. A fourth achievement was his work on brain surgery, accompanied by laboratory experiments on intracranial pressure. His 1888 treatise on the surgical treatment of brain *diseases*, rather than brain injuries only, was the first textbook in this nascent field, and it brought Bergmann international repute. Working as a relict from preanesthetic and preantiseptic times, he operated quickly and radically. He left the delicate gastrointestinal interventions developed in the 1880s by Billroth's Viennese school to younger collaborators.

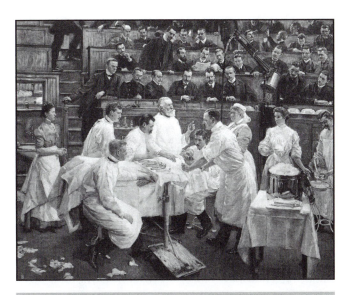

Ernst von Bergmann demonstrating to students in Berlin. Oil painting by Franz Skarbina, 1906. Iconographic Collection, Wellcome Library, London.

In 1887–88 the prominent professor from the capital became involved in the nationalist medico-political tug-of-war about the treatment of the German Crown Prince (later Emperor) Frederick III. Bergmann clinically confirmed the prince's ultimately fatal disease as a laryngeal carcinoma and recommended radical surgery, in contrast to the advice of the British laryngologist, Morell Mackenzie. Understandably, the prince and the princess, who was a daughter of the British Queen Victoria, preferred Mackenzie's conservative treatment, which was supported by his biopsies that did not exhibit signs of cancer, in Virchow's view.

Bergmann had extensive literary influence as coeditor of two surgical periodicals and a four-volume handbook, but he lacked scientific instinct when publicly disapproving of Themistocles Gluck's bone transplants and metal implants or Carl Schleich's local anesthesia. Nevertheless, as an international authority at a time when German surgery enjoyed prestige at home and abroad, he became a life member of the Prussian *Herrenhaus* (upper chamber of parliament) in 1906 and was a much sought-after consultant from Turkey to Russia to Spain.

Bibliography

Primary: 1883. *Die Schicksale der Transfusion im letzten Decennium* (Berlin); 1888. *Die chirurgische Behandlung der Hirnkrankheiten* [3rd ed. 1899] (Berlin); 1899 (ed. with von Bruns and Mikulicz-Radecki). *Handbuch der speziellen Chirurgie* 4 vols. [English ed. 1904] (Stuttgart).

Secondary: Buchholtz, Arend, 1912. *Ernst von Bergmann* (Leipzig).

Ulrich Tröhler

BERNARD, CLAUDE (b. Saint Julien de Villefranche, Beaujolais, France, 12 July 1813; d. Paris, France, 10 February 1878), *physiology.*

Bernard holds a well-deserved place in the history of science because he made concrete discoveries and systematized revolutionary concepts that led to a better understanding of the human body. Born into a winemaking family in a small town near Lyon, this man of science later described the beautiful Beaujolais countryside with admiration and fondness from his family home, where he spent his infrequent vacations and prolonged convalescences from illness. He received his early education from the parish priest and, later, in a Jesuit school. At the age of eighteen, the family's economic circumstances obliged him to abandon his studies, so he found work as a pharmacist's apprentice in Lyon. In reality, Bernard aspired to be a writer, and after a vaudeville piece he composed, *La Rose du Rhône,* was well received, he left for Paris (1832). There he presented a play entitled *Arthur de Bretagne* to a theater critic named Saint-Marc Girardin, whose advice was that Bernard should learn a trade that would allow him to earn a living.

In 1834 he enrolled in the Faculty of Medicine in Paris, where he soon came into contact with François Magendie, a professor involved in animal research at the margins of the academic programs, who encouraged his students to undertake experimentation. Bernard won Magendie's confidence, serving as his intern at the *Hôtel Dieu* (1840) and his preparer at the *Collège de France* (1841). Medicine was not yet considered a science because it had not acquired the necessary experimental character, but French clinical medicine was at its apogee thanks to the work of many physicians, such as Jean-Nicholas Corvisart (on percussion) and Théophile Laennec, the inventor of the stethoscope. Bernard, opted not to join the ranks of these distinguished clinicians, however, but chose instead to concentrate on research.

By the time he concluded his studies (1843), Bernard had already published three articles. Nevertheless, gaining entry into the world of science was no easy matter. He was passed over for a post as adjunct professor in the Faculty of Medicine, and failed to gain admission as a member of the Academy of Medicine. After this series of setbacks, he resigned himself to returning to his hometown to work as a rural doctor. But his friend Théodore Jules Pelouze convinced him to stay on in Paris and persist in his quest to do science. In 1845 he married Marie Françoise Martin, with whom he had three children—one son and two daughters, though the boy died in infancy. We know that Bernard was unhappy with his family life, that he eventually left his wife, and that his daughters were active in antivivisectionist movements.

Vivisection and Philosophy

Bernard believed it was necessary to study the phenomena of life in the context in which they develop, a conviction that included experimentation with live animals. Through *in vivo* experimentation it was possible to reproduce such phenomena in conditions that approximated natural states, yielding results that were similar, if not identical. That type of experimentation also allowed researchers to manipulate physiological processes in order to discover responses to different circumstances. Bernard's great manual dexterity allowed him to operate efficaciously at a time when modern anesthetics were unavailable.

The language he used to inquire into nature was that of experimental physiology. In many of his discoveries, he inferred physiological or normal states from observations of pathological states that he created experimentally. For him, experimentation was a dialogue with nature through which ideas were adjusted to the evidence of fact.

Bernard understood the link between *primary observation* (what he called 'intuition' or 'a feeling') and *prior knowledge and reasoning*, which leads to an abstract concept of a phenomenon and then to the elaboration of an hypothesis ('experimental' or *a priori* ideas). After that, the true test comes with deduction, for which scientific curiosity was all important. One must not discard preconceived concepts nor eliminate premature ideas, he argued—new doubts and questions were to be addressed through experimental work. That orientation evolved from his work in the laboratory—for him a kind of sanctuary—and was articulated in his magnum opus: *Introduction à l'étude de la medicine expérimentale* (*Introduction to the Study of Experimental Medicine*) (1865).

In 1859 an intense abdominal pain forced Bernard to abandon his laboratory and return to Saint Julian to rest. That time of forced inactivity gave him an opportunity to think about writing a treatise on experimental medicine. Bernard considered that the process of physiological inquiry should not be very different from that of other experimental sciences, but that its argumentation should be structured on a methodology that included research on living animals. Thus, his principal contribution consisted of systematizing, synthesizing, and enunciating with philosophical clarity the meaning of his scientific experience, and also creating a model for laboratory conduct. He also contributed certain elements of the mental processes that guide scientists to their findings and pushed experimental rigor in medicine to its ultimate consequences.

For Bernard, the experimental method had three fundamental, interdependent elements: feeling, reason, and experiment. His writings reveal a rejection of all research bereft of feelings, because he believed that the human capacity to be amazed was necessary, and that the imagination stimulates intuition and propitiates a sensitive attitude toward our surroundings. Reason, in turn, allows us to approximate the proportions of natural phenomena and the (almost) mathematical mechanisms that control them, whereas experiment makes it possible to probe nature's secrets through directed observation in certain conditions, for the purpose of proving a hypothesis.

In this process of exploration, it is indispensable to maintain a free spirit and be able to doubt, but not to the point of skepticism. Philosophical doubt believes in the determinism of things, in their 'order', and in the absolute relations that prevail among them, but doubt also suggests that scientists must question themselves and be suspicious of their interpretations. Determinism is the absolute relation that exists between the effect of a phenomenon and its cause. Effects can be perceived, but understanding the immediate or ultimate causes of events, not to mention the underlying laws that govern them, requires experimental analysis. Bernard defined determinism as the operating principle of phenomena that are always the same while conditions remain unchanged, that emerge when identical conditions are reproduced, and that fail to occur if these tenets are not met. For him, the latter operation was a 'counter-proof'.

These deterministic principles allowed experimenters to generate new conditions. Determinism exists in both physical and biological phenomena, but its laws vary because these two classes of phenomena deal with different realities, and because spontaneity is a factor in the case of living beings. In Bernard's view, determinism made the use of statistics unnecessary in physiological research.

Digestion

Bernard was interested in the process to which food is subjected from the moment of ingestion, through assimilation, to expulsion. He called this process 'nutrition', equivalent to the modern term 'intermediate metabolism'. Basic to this research was his ability to suggest physiological interpretations for the chemical phenomena he observed in the laboratory.

Bernard's first grand discovery (1848) was that the pancreas is capable of breaking down neutral fats in the diet. That was also one of his most beautiful discoveries because it was fortuitous, and because he recognized right away that he had isolated a function of the organ that up to then had been shrouded in mystery. By demonstrating that the pancreas produces enzymes that break down sugars, fats, and proteins, Bernard discovered its exocrine function. He defined glucogenesis (1850) by observing that glucemia is normal and does not depend on alimentation—the liver produces glycogen that, when broken down, liberates glucose into the bloodstream. This discovery was fundamental to his later elaboration of the principle of internal secretion, and it earned him his doctoral degree in natural sciences. He also discovered extrahepatic glucogenesis, gluconeogenesis, and the formation of lactic acid in the muscles, in addition to observing that a lesion in a certain area of the floor of the fourth ventricle causes glycosuria, which he called *picûre diabétique*.

Toxicology

Bernard was also an important pioneer in the study of toxic and pharmacological substances, such as opium, strychnine, and anesthetics. For example, he studied the action of curare, a poison used by some hunters in South

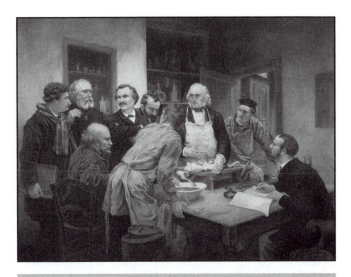

Claude Bernard, watched by his pupils, experiments on a rabbit. Oil painting after Léon-Augustin L'Hermitte, 1889. Iconographic Collection, Wellcome Library, London.

America, which immobilizes animals so that they die without ever reacting. He discovered that curare acts on the muscles of frogs, an observation that led him to discover the neuromuscular plate (1864). He also found that carbon monoxide displaces oxygen from erythrocytes by observing the red-colored blood in the veins of dogs that had died from carbon monoxide poisoning (1856). That discovery allowed him to confirm his theory of organic combustion.

The Nervous System

One of Bernard's most important discoveries was the existence of the vasomotor nerves (1852–53). While studying the pink ears of rabbits, he cut the cervical sympathetic nerve in an attempt to observe its participation in regulating tissue temperature. He found that the temperature rose throughout the area innervated by the severed nerve and inferred that the sympathetic nervous system thus caused chemical changes, and not vasoconstriction. In 1853 he won the Academy of Sciences Award for his research on the influence of the greater sympathetic nervous system on animal heat. Later, he discovered the vasodilator nerves, established the notion of physiological equilibrium between two antagonistic innervations, discovered active-reflexive vasodilatation, described the ocular syndrome now known as Claude Bernard-Horner syndrome, elaborated the notion of local circulation, and formulated the hypothesis of dual reciprocal innervation that acts through excitation and inhibition.

In 1855 he was accepted into the Academy of Sciences, and following Magendie's death he was named professor of the experimental physiology program at the *Collège de France*.

Bernard also studied animal thermogenesis, the mechanism of death caused by temperature elevation, the decrease in vital processes at low temperatures, the mechanism of fever, rigor mortis, alcoholic fermentation, and the metabolism of muscles.

The Interior Milieu

The apogee of Claude Bernard's thinking came with his notion of the 'internal medium (or milieu)' (1857), which he considered to be the condition of free life, of equilibrium, of the regulating mechanism. According to Bernard, cells have a highly complex organization because they are covered with liquids that characterize their internal medium. This obliges them to maintain an internal equilibrium and to utilize certain compensatory mechanisms that make them independent of the external medium (within certain limits). This autonomy is not unrelated to events that occur in the rest of the body, however. There is a relationship between the organs and their cells through which they become integrated into a functional whole that Bernard called 'organic unity'. This idea toppled the belief that an organism was made up of a series of independent organs, unrelated to each other. According to Bernard, modern scientific medicine was based on the concept that life was dependent on its internal medium.

Bernard received many honors during his life and after his death. He died of a kidney ailment at his home on *Rue des écoles*, across the street from his laboratory at the Collège de France. He was a human being with qualities and defects, but also with a certain *je ne sais quoi* that made him truly exceptional.

Bibliography

Primary: 1865. *Introduction à l'étude de la médecine expérimentale* (Paris) (English trans. Greene, Henry Copley, 1927 (New York)); Grmek, Mirko, 1967. *Catalogue des Manuscrits de Claude Bernard* (Paris).

Secondary: Grmek, D. Mirko, 1997. *Le legs de Claude Bernard* (Paris); Holmes, Frederic Lawrence, 1974. *Claude Bernard and Animal Chemistry: the Emergence of a Scientist* (Cambridge, MA); Olmsted, James M. D., and E. Harris Olmsted, 1952. *Claude Bernard and the Experimental Method in Medicine* (New York); *DSB*.

Ana Cecilia Rodríguez de Romo

BERNARD OF GORDON (aka BERNARDUS DE GORDONIO, BERNARDUS GORDONIUS) (b. Gourdon de Quercy?, France, c. 1258; d. Montpellier?, France, before 1330), *medicine*.

Bernard was a French physician, one of the most famous masters in the medical faculty of Montpellier, France, in the golden age (1250–1350) of this important center of medical teaching during the Middle Ages. It was a time of high scholastic medicine, as developed in Western Europe. A sign of the early acknowledgment and fame of Bernard is the quotation from the *Canterbury Tales'* Prologue, where Bernard of Gordon was named among the most distinguished physicians known at the time of Chaucer, the English poet. He developed a prominent career as a practitioner and professor of medicine and wrote many medical treatises, of which the preeminent text is the *Practice Called Lily of Medicine* or, simply, *Lily of Medicine*.

Life

Despite his contemporary fame, Bernard of Gordon's biographical data are limited and stem from his own writings, which are practically the only source of information about him. As he tells us in the preface to his *Lily of Medicine* (started in 1303), he began that work after twenty years as professor of medicine. That bit of information leads us to conclude that he started his teaching activity in 1283. From that date, his birth has been set at about 1258, considering that a master at that time could begin teaching in the University at the age of twenty-five. The year of his death is also uncertain; we can locate it between the conclusion of his last dated work, the *Book on the Preservation of Human Life*, which he finished in 1308, and the year 1330. The latter date comes from a notarial document, where, speaking of a certain Gulielmus Gordonius, our subject was already mentioned in the past tense.

Scholars have speculated that the surname 'Gordon' suggests a possible Scottish origin, but it seems more likely that he came from a village in southern France called Gourdon (Latin *Gordonium*) in Quercy (*départment* of Lot), about two hundred kilometers from Montpellier. This hypothesis is supported not only by the Latin form of his surname (*de Gordonio*), but also by the analysis and consideration of different data extracted from his writings that point to a French origin—specifically, to Provençal.

Regarding his education, it is likely that Bernard began his studies with the Cistercian monks, who in 1261 founded an abbey in Gourdon de Quercy. He then received his medical training at Montpellier. We can say little more about his life than that he seems to have dedicated himself to the exercise of medicine and educational activities, and that he seems not to have married or to have served any contemporary powerful person, as did his colleague, Arnald of Vilanova (d. 1311). One of the reasons proposed to explain the silence that surrounds Bernard's life is the critical attitude he maintained toward some of his colleagues and certain medical practices of his time. For example, he criticized the scorn that some doctors showed for the examination of urine, and he decried the preference that others had for becoming rich treating diseases, rather than preventing them with a suitable regime.

Works

Bernard's dedication to teaching is reflected in the format of his works, all written in Latin, in which he tended to tackle the main subjects of the curriculum at the faculty of medicine. In his writings, there is a combination of theoretical knowledge and practical application. He carefully selected and interpreted the sources available in his time, with the heritage of Greek authors (Hippocrates and, mainly, Galen) occupying a preeminent place. Other sources included the Judeo-Arabic texts, especially Avicenna (Ibn Sīnā), and Salernitan authors. To this traditional knowledge, he usually added his own contributions, the fruit of his personal experience.

Bernard's writings that have been recognized and accepted as authentic are worthy of comment. As was usual with famous authors of that time, several manuscripts circulated with texts attributed to him.

His first work was the *Treatise on Regimen of Acute Diseases*, dated 1294. Divided into three parts, its objective was to offer general principles of treatment for acute diseases. His source was the Hippocratic work on the same subject, but Bernard's contribution lies in organizing the matter in a more logical arrangement and in documenting it with references to the later medical tradition.

The *Compendium on Regimen of Acute Diseases* (also from 1294) was derived from the same source but covered the subject more briefly, as its title suggests. Bernard dedicated it to his colleague, Johannes de Confluente.

The *Treatise on Crisis and Critical Days*, also known as the *Book on Prognostics*, was finished 25 January 1295 and dealt with medical prognosis, in which the doctrine of crisis and critical days played a decisive role. This work, articulated in five books, served as a manual describing how to perform accurate prognostication of disease. It included all of the factors a physician must consider in making a prognosis, always from the viewpoint of a medieval doctor.

On 22 December 1295, Bernard completed his *Treatise on Reduction of Geomancy to the Orb*, the only nonmedical work he wrote. Specifically, it was a Latin translation of an Arabic treatise about divination that was attributed to the Greek Ptolemy. Bernard's translation was likely made from Provençal, the language of the Montpellier region, because he does not seem to have had familiarity with other languages. In spite of its title, the system of divination described in the treatise was not really typical of geomancy, but of a different *astrologic* geomancy. The basic idea was to know the fate of past, present, or future events. Accordingly, the work included a list of several questions regarding, for example, the outcome of a trip, or the whereabouts of stolen property. It also included some questions related to medicine, such as whether a patient was likely to die, or if it was wise for the physician to take care of a particular patient, or not.

In *On the Ten Methods to Cure Diseases* (finished in July 1299)—a brief treatise that the author also entitled *Table of Methods*—Bernard of Gordon set forth ten methods of treating and curing illnesses, based on works by Hippocrates, Galen, Haly Abbas (Al-Mājūsī), and Avicenna. But this was no mere compendium; rather, it added many of Bernard's own ideas and adapted transmitted textual knowledge to the circumstances of the time and region where he worked.

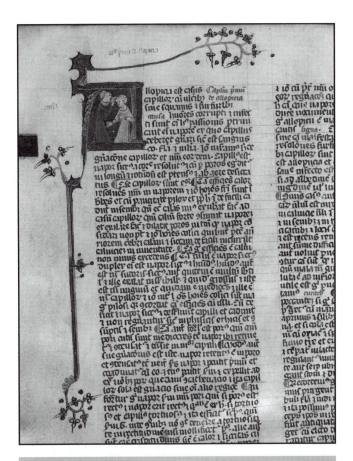

Bernard examines head of a patient with alopecia (baldness). Illuminated MS 1189, *Lilium medicinae*, folio 21 verso, 14th century. Universität Leipzig, Universitätsbibliothek.

The *Treatise on Degrees* (composed in the first half of 1303) was a work devoted to pharmacology. It dealt with the qualities and properties of medicaments in order to determine their effect on the patient, following the then-current therapeutic principle that 'contraries cure'. The title was derived from the classification of medicines into different degrees, according to their qualities.

Bernard's magnum opus, the *Lily of Medicine* (started in July 1303 and finished on 5 February 1305), was a compendium of practical medicine. In principle, it was for the young and inexperienced physician, but because of its clarity, concision, and order the *Lily* also enjoyed great popularity among experienced practitioners, and it had an important influence on subsequent medicine. It was his most extensive and complete work and was divided into seven books—the number of petals in a lily's flower. Bernard dealt with different human diseases in the traditional 'head to foot' arrangement, that is, by following the location of illnesses in the human body from the head to the feet. Each book was divided into chapters that, for the most part, were organized in a systematic schema according to six aspects of the illness—its description, causes, diagnosis, prognosis, treatment, and clarifications.

Evidence of the *Lily*'s wide distribution included the great number of surviving manuscripts; the numerous editions printed from 1480 until the seventeenth century; and the diverse languages (French, Provençal, Hebrew, Spanish, English, Irish, and German) into which it was translated very early on. Nevertheless, a critical and modern edition is still not available.

Between 1305 and 1306, Bernard composed the *Treatise on Theriac*, a monograph of a predominantly theoretical nature, about the popular medicinal compound used as an antidote to all poisons and toxic substances.

The *Book on the Preservation of Human Life*, started on 22 February 1308 and finished on 9 November 1308, was a treatise in four parts that commonly appeared separately in the manuscript tradition and the Renaissance editions, because each piece deals with a clearly differentiated subject: *On Phlebotomy, On Urines, and On Pulses*, and *Regimen of Health*—the latter giving the reason for its general title.

Finally, we cite a brief work of a speculative and theoretical nature, the *Treatise on Marasmus*, known to have been written after 1308. It dealt with illness related to the consumption of bodily moisture by desiccation.

All of Bernard's work is characterized, in general, by its concision, clarity, and logical organization, but there is also an observable evolution whose intermediate point is marked by the *Lily of Medicine*. His first treatises are distinguished by brevity, an essentially practical nature, and a rigorous arrangement of the material. By contrast, the writings of his later period are more extensive, more speculative, and more poorly organized. On the other hand, he rarely referred to his sources in the first treatises, but later he named his sources more frequently. Finally, his works showed an adherence to the University of Montpellier curriculum at the beginning, but that characteristic was attenuated with the passage of time.

In summary, Bernard of Gordon was a physician and professor of medicine who produced a broad and important body of literature that has had enduring influence. Consequently, his work is a fundamental source for understanding how late medieval medicine developed in Western Europe.

Bibliography

Primary: 1574. *Opus, Lilium medicinae inscriptum, de morborum prope omnium curatione, septem particulis distributum, una cum aliquot aliis eius libellis, quibus de novo accesserunt libri, de phlebotomia, de conservatione vitae humanae, de floribus diaetarum, omnia quam unquam antehac emendatiora et in novum ordinem distributa, ut sequens pagina indicabit, cum indice amplissimo* (Lyon); 1895. *Tractatus de gradibus* in Pagel, Julius L., ed., 'Über die Graden der Arzneien nach einer bisher ungedruckten Schrift des Bernhard von Gordon aus dem Jahre 1303.' *Pharmaceutische Post* 28: 65–67, 131–133, 142–144, 180–182, 221–225, 257–262; 1992. *Tractatus de marasmode* in Demaitre, Luke E., ed., 'The Medical Notion of "Withering" from Galen to the Fourteenth Century: the Treatise on Marasmus by Bernard of Gordon.' *Traditio* 47: 288–307; 2003. *Tractatus de crisi et de diebus creticis* in Alonso Guardo, Alberto, ed., *Los pronósticos médicos en la medicina medieval: El 'Tractatus de crisi et de diebus creticis' de Bernardo de Gordonio* (Valladolid) pp. 116–449.

Secondary: Cull, John, and Brian Dutton, eds., 1991. *Un manual básico de medicina medieval. Bernardo Gordonio. Lilio de medicina* [edición crítica de la versión española, Sevilla 1495] (Madison, WI); Demaitre, Luke E., 1980. *Doctor Bernard de Gordon: Professor and Practitioner* (Toronto); Wickersheimer, Ernest, 1979. *Dictionnaire biographique des médecins en France au Moyen Âge. Nouvelle édition sous la direction de Guy Beaujouan* [Supplément by Danielle Jacquart] (Geneva); Dulie, Louis, 1975. *La médecine à Montpellier*, vol. 1: *Le Moyen Âge* (Avignon).

Alberto Alonso Guardo

BERNHEIM, HIPPOLYTE (b. Mulhouse, France, 27 April 1840; d. Paris, France, 22 February 1919), *psychotherapy.*

Bernheim was the second of four children born to Corneille Bernheim, a successful merchant, and Sarah Lévy. He came from a thriving industrial town in Alsace where many Jewish families, including his own, enjoyed rapid upward social mobility. After studies in Mulhouse, Bernheim earned his MD from Strasburg in 1867. He studied for two years in Paris and six months in Berlin, then returned to Strasburg with the rank of *agrégé* (assistant professor). A French patriot, Bernheim served on the battlefield during the disastrous war with Prussia. Rather than remaining in Alsace after the annexation of the region by the victorious Germans, he moved, along with most of his colleagues, to the new university established in Nancy in 1871. By the end of that decade, Bernheim had obtained the rank of professor and had published in various fields of clinical medicine and pathology, including infectious diseases, cardiac and respiratory ailments, and reforms in medical education.

In 1882 Bernheim's career took a decisive turn when he encountered Ambroise Liébault, a country doctor who had remarkable success with hypnotic therapy, then a discredited procedure in academic medicine. Embracing Liébault's methods, Bernheim devoted the rest of his career to the promulgation and wide application of verbal therapy. In 1884 he published *De la suggestion*, a collection of his earlier articles. Bernheim believed that 'suggestion in the waking state', could be as effective as hypnosis in relieving the symptoms of hysteria and other nervous system ailments in which there was no organic pathology. In 1886, he published a vastly expanded second edition that included one hundred case histories. In 1891, he added the word 'psychotherapy' to the book's title, the first such use of the term.

For Bernheim, psychotherapy was synonymous with therapeutic suggestion. Suggestion itself, he asserted, was the fundamental psychological and cerebral mechanism responsible for individual and group behavior. Bernheim cited the extraordinary cures at the Catholic shrine at Lourdes as an example. He concluded that hypnotic therapy was merely a special case of suggestion in a sleep-like state.

During the 1880s Bernheim established the so-called Nancy school of hypnotism. That group challenged the prevailing doctrines of the Paris school, led by the neurologist Jean-Martin Charcot. According to Charcot, hypnotism was an induced neurological disease akin to hysteria. Indeed, he believed that only hysterics were hypnotizable, and he used the technique on his hospital patients in public lessons to display the presumed cerebral mechanisms of hysteria. Charcot cautioned against the danger of hypnotic therapy, but Bernheim, in contrast, asserted that most people could be hypnotized and that hypnosis and psychotherapy offered powerful therapeutic techniques. The Nancy school rejected Charcot's typology of hypnotic states and ultimately reduced his somatic interpretation of hysteria itself to a cultural artifact. The Nancy school warned that crimes, including murder, might be instigated via posthypnotic suggestion, whereas the Parisians largely dismissed that possibility.

Bernheim's psychological therapy won wide acceptance, but his publications after the turn of the century tended to be repetitions of earlier work. He defended a didactic and rather authoritarian form of suggestion and persuasion, while showing little appreciation for the new psychodynamics of the unconscious that were advocated by Sigmund Freud and Pierre Janet. Bernheim retired to Paris in 1910. His marriage with Maxime Schiama of Bordeaux, fifteen years his junior and said to be nearly twice her husband's diminutive height, was childless.

Bibliography

Primary: 1884. *De la suggestion dans l'état hypnotique et dans l'état de veille* (Paris); 1886. *De la suggestion et ses applications à la thérapeutique* (Paris); 1889 [trans. Christian A. Herter]. *Suggestive Therapeutics* (New York and London); 1891. *Hypnotisme, suggestion et psychothérapie* (Paris); www.medecine.uhp-nancy.fr/professeurs/Bernheim_H.htm

Secondary: Harris, Ruth, 1989. *Murders and Madness. Medicine, Law, and Society in the Fin de Siècle* (Oxford); Ellenberger, Henri R., 1970. *The Discovery of the Unconscious: the History and Evolution of Dynamic Psychiatry* (New York).

Toby Gelfand

BERT, PAUL   (b. Auxerre, France, 19 October 1833; d. Hanoi, Tonkin (now Vietnam), 11 November 1886), *physiology, politics.*

The son of Auxerre attorney Joseph Bert and Jeanne Henriette née Massy, Bert attended elementary school and Collège Auyot in Auxerre. In 1853 he went to Paris, where he entered the Collège Sainte Barbe with the intention of entering the École Polytechnique. At his father's urging, he studied jurisprudence instead, obtaining a law degree in 1857. He was dissatisfied with the law and began to study medicine while working as a law clerk. Bert obtained his MD degree in 1863 with a thesis that examined the transplantation of tissues between individuals of the same species and of different species. His experiments included skin grafts joining two rats and the regrafting of a rat's tail onto its own back, noting the reestablishment of circulation and the regrowth of bone. He then began to study physiology with Claude Bernard, serving as his laboratory assistant and opting, as did Bernard, for a purely research career. Bert received a doctorate in natural sciences in 1866 with a thesis in which he exposed animal tissue to different environments, thereby demonstrating the survival of individual cells after the death of the animal itself. That study was awarded the physiology prize from the Académie des Sciences.

Bert married Josephine Clayton in 1865. Soon after that, with Claude Bernard's support, he went to teach physiology in the Faculty of Sciences at Bordeaux, where he published prolifically on physiological topics. In 1868 he returned to Paris to take over the comparative physiology course of Pierre Flourens at the Museum of Natural History, and the following year he succeeded Claude Bernard in the chair of physiology at the Sorbonne.

Over the next six years, Bert began a series of studies on the role of oxygen in respiration and the effects of changing barometric pressure on animals and humans. He developed various pieces of apparatus to study those effects, including an anesthetic chamber in which a patient could be placed under increased pressure. His studies were awarded the biannual prize by the Institut de France in 1875, and a more comprehensive version of the work appeared two years later as *La Pression Barométrique*, considered by many to be his masterpiece. Bert was elected to the Académie des Sciences in 1881.

Claude Bernard had hoped that his favorite student would devote his entire life to science, but with the onset of the Third Republic, Bert became more and more involved in political life. An admirer and friend of the politician Léon Gambetta, he edited the scientific section of Gambetta's journal *La Republique Française*, including articles on Darwinism. He was elected deputy to the National Assembly from Auxerre, a position that he maintained until his death. In 1881 Gambetta named him minister of education, and although he held that position for only nine weeks, he worked hard to expand scientific education. During this period, however, he continued to teach, to publish, and to serve as head of the Société de Biologie.

An advocate of a 'scientific' and progressive colonialism, Bert was named the first governor general of Indochina in early 1886. He declared that he would use the 'scientific method' to improve economic and social life in the colonies by educating the population in secular schools. Shortly before his death (from dysentery) in Tonkin, he restated his long-held belief that the social sciences were fundamental to politics in the same way that physiology was fundamental to medicine.

Bibliography

Primary: 1863. *De la greffe animale.* Doctor of medicine thesis (Paris); 1866. *Recherches expérimentales pour servir an l'histoire de la vitalité propres des tissus animaux* (Paris); 1877. *Recherches expérimentales sur l'influence que les modifications dans la pression barométrique, recherches de physiologie expérimentales* (Paris); 1881. *Leçons de zoologie professées à la Sorbonne. Anatomie physiologie* (Paris).

Secondary: Kotovtchikine, Stéphane, 2000. *Paul Bert et l'Instruction publique* (Dijon); Dejours, Pierre, Maurice Fontaine, Jean-Pierre Rocher, Jean-Pierre Soisson, and G. Decuyper, 1983. *Paul Bert. Savant, homme politique, administrateur* (Auxerre); *DSB.*

Joy Harvey

BERTILLON, (LOUIS-) ADOLPHE (b. Paris, France, 1 April 1821; d. Paris, 28 February 1883), *medical statistics, demography, anthropology.*

Bertillon was the son of a chemical distiller, Jean-Baptiste Bertillon, and his wife, Pierette Garinot. Against his father's wishes, he entered the Paris École de Médecine and took whatever laboratory courses he could find, both at the medical school and at the Collège de France. He became the laboratory assistant of Amédée Deville, through whom he met Paul Broca. The 1848 revolution intervened, and Bertillon became active in one of the republican clubs. There he met the botanist and statistician, Achille Guillard, joined him in organizing welfare for the poor, and soon married Guillard's daughter, Zoe. Considered a threat to the new Empire, Bertillon and Guillard were imprisoned for a number of months, during which time the two studied statistics together. When he was released, Bertillon finished his medical studies with a thesis completed in 1852 on the topic he continued to pursue throughout his life—medical statistics on longevity.

From 1854 to 1860, Bertillon was a hospital doctor in Montmorency and also had a large private practice. He was twice a laureate of the Académie des Sciences (1856 and 1858), the second time for a statistical proof of the usefulness of vaccination. By 1860 Bertillon had left Montmorency for Paris, where he devoted himself to the study of medical statistics. He was one of the first members of the Société de Statistique, publishing extensively in that organization's journal, in the *Annales de démographie*, and in the medical press. During the siege of Paris by the Prussian army in 1870, he served as mayor of the 5th arrondissement.

Bertillon collaborated on a number of medical projects, as well on two major medical dictionaries: Dechambre's *Dictionnaire encyclopédique des sciences médicales* and Littré and Robin's *Dictionnaire de médecine.* As Broca's close friend and associate he was active in Broca's Société d'Anthropologie as a member of the council and vice-president of the society, and he took part in the evolutionary debates of 1870. Later, he was an editor of the *Dictionnaire Encyclopédie des Sciences Anthropologique*, which was published after his death. Bertillon established the field of medical demography at Broca's new École d'Anthropologie in 1876 and held the chair in that subject until his death. He also established the Société de Démographie and was a member of the short-lived Société de Sociologie established by Émile Littré. He performed statistical studies for the Paris Municipal Council and helped to establish the Bureau of Statistics under the Préfecture de la Seine in 1880. A strong anticleric, he insisted on a civil burial for his wife and bequeathed both his skeleton and his brain to Broca's Museum of Anthropology.

His son, Jacques Bertillon, continued his father's statistical studies after receiving a medical degree in 1883. He took over the statistical work for the City of Paris and eventually became head statistician. Both Louis-Adolphe and Jacques Bertillon wrote about causes of the decline in the French population. In 1891, Jacques pointed out that a decline in mortality would not necessarily increase the population growth, because high mortality was often found in regions that also had the highest birth rate. He argued that the best way to reverse population decline was to provide a payment from the state to both parents for each birth. His later pronatalist writings (in 1896 and 1911) have caused some historians in recent years to criticize both father and son for failing to consider the important role of women in controlling the birth rate.

In 1893 Jacques Bertillon presented suggestions for a uniform statistical system to classify causes of death, later adopted as the Bertillon System of Classification. As chair of the International Statistical Institute, he oversaw the adoption of that classification system and its subsequent revisions throughout the Americas and much of Europe. After his death, the World Health Organization supervised later revisions that became the basis of the current International Classification of Disease (ICD), which from 1948 began to include nonfatal diseases.

Bibliography

Primary: [Adolphe Bertillon] 1857. *Conclusions statistiques contre les détracteurs de la vaccine; précédées d'un Essai sur la méthode statistique appliquée à l'étude de l'homme* (Paris); 1866. 'Des diverses manières de mesurer la durée de la vie humaine.' *Journal de la Société de Statistiques de Paris* 7: 45–64; 1874. *La démographie figurée de la France: ou Étude statistique de la population française avec tableaux graphiques traduisant les principales conclusions. Mortalité selon l'âge, le sexe, l'état-civil, etc. etc.* (Paris); [Jacques Bertillon] 1891. 'Discussion sur la natalité.' *Bulletins Société d'Anthropologie de Paris* 2(4): 366–385; 1896. *La dépopulation de France et les remèdes à apporter* (Paris); 1900. *Nomenclatures des maladies (statistique de morbidité, statistique des causes de décès) arrètées par la Commission internationale chargée de reviser les nomenclatures nosologiques (Paris, 18–21 août 1900) pour être en usage à partir du 1 janvier 1901* (Paris); 1910. *International classification of causes of sickness and death/Rev. by the International commission at the session of Paris, July 1 to 3, 1909, for use beginning January 1, 1910, and until December 31, 1919* (Washington).

Secondary: Hecht, Jennifer Michael, 2003. *The End of the Soul: Scientific Modernity, Atheism and Anthropology in France* (New York) pp. 147–167; Dupaquier, Michel, 1983. 'La famille Bertillon et la naissance d'une nouvelle science sociale: la démographie.' *Annales de démographie historique*, pp. 293–311; Bertillon, Suzanne, 1941. *Vie d' Alphonse Bertillon, inventeur de l'anthropométrie* (Paris); [Anon.], 1883. *La Vie et les Oeuvres du Docteur L.-A. Bertillon* (Paris).

Joy Harvey

BETHUNE, HENRY NORMAN

BETHUNE, HENRY NORMAN (b. Gravenhurst, Ontario, Canada, 3 March 1890; d. Hijuang Shiko, Shansi Province, China, 12 November 1939), *surgery.*

Born to the Reverend Malcolm Nicholson Bethune and his wife Elizabeth Ann, Bethune learned to enjoy the outdoors in the frontier communities where the family lived as they moved from parish to parish. He early showed his independence, rebelliousness, and athleticism; he wrote, 'My father was an evangelist and I come of a race of men violent, unstable, of passionate conviction and wrongheadedness, intolerant yet with it all a vision of truth and a drive to carry them on to it even though it leads, as it has done in my family, to their destruction' (MacLeod et al., 1978, p. 25).

Bethune insisted he be called by his middle name, the name of his physician grandfather. After graduating with honors from Owen Sound Collegiate in 1907, he went to work as a lumberjack and for six months taught in a one room schoolhouse. He began a science course at the University of Toronto, but after two years quit in boredom and taught at the northern Frontier College, where he worked as an ax-man and lived with immigrant workers while teaching them English and Canadian history. Following a trip through the American Midwest, he enrolled at the University of Toronto as a medical student; but before graduating, he enlisted in the Royal Canadian Army Medical Corps and went overseas as a stretcher bearer. He was wounded at the second Battle of Ypres, and upon discharge returned to his medical studies in Toronto, graduating in 1916. He then enlisted as a Surgeon-Lieutenant in the Royal Navy. Following the war he briefly began pediatric studies at the Hospital for Children at Great Ormond Street in London, but his restlessness brought him back to a general practice in Canada. He then joined the Canadian Air Force, but after six months returned to studies at London and Edinburgh hospitals. Back in London he met and married the wealthy Frances Campbell Penney. After spending most of her inheritance on a long honeymoon, they settled in Detroit where he established a busy practice. Their relationship was strained by his busy schedule and their argumentativeness.

In 1926 Bethune was diagnosed with tuberculosis, and became a patient at the Trudeau Sanatorium in the Adirondack Mountains of northern New York. During this time his wife filed for divorce, and as he worsened he became depressed, convinced he was dying, and contemplated suicide. A talented artist, he had been painting murals and other art works, many of them allegories of his life and experiences, and in one he painted a tombstone marked 'Norman Bethune. Died 1932'.

After he convinced the medical staff to give him the new procedure of artificial pneumothorax, he recovered well enough to become a surgical assistant to Edward Archibald at the Royal Victoria Hospital in Montreal. During his five years there he invented about a dozen surgical instruments, including a compact pneumothorax machine. Although liked by his patients, his relationship with Archibald soured and his outspokenness, casual dress, and surgical flair that many considered reckless resulted in his being asked to leave. He was lonely for Frances and convinced her to marry him again, but this marriage also ended in divorce. Although his life seemed a series of disappointments, Bethune was given the opportunity to become the chief of thoracic surgery at Sacred Heart Hospital, where he did not have to answer to others. Again he offended his colleagues and local supporters, but continued to approach surgery with inventiveness and a skill that increased his reputation outside the institution. His outspoken and blunt comments at national and international meetings were seen by some as refreshing.

Meanwhile, Bethune was writing short stories and poems and gaining some success with his painting. He started an art school for poor children. Aware of the effects of the Great Depression on the poor, he held meetings in his apartment where discussions centered on the inadequacy of political systems. Now interested in politics, he began writing and speaking to physicians about the necessity of a government-supported medical system for all, with elimination of the fee-for-service system, and with physicians and health care workers paid by the state. He was distressed that not only physicians but political and religious leaders criticized his views.

Bethune joined the Communist Party in 1935, and as he learned more about the Spanish Civil War, determined to organize a medical service for the Republican side. He wanted something that would be more creative and challenging than just acting as a military surgeon, something that would capture the public's attention. He organized a mobile transfusion service that provided acute care at the front. His tireless work and travels in dangerous territory gained him wide attention. Returning to Canada on a speaking and fundraising tour, he continued his pattern of irritating his audiences and even his supporters. When he wished to make public that he was a Communist, even the Communist Party wanted him to remain silent, which he didn't accept.

His restlessness continued and he determined not to return to Spain, so when he learned more about Japan's invasion of China and Mao Zedong's Great March, he decided to join Mao's 8th Route Army. He was put in charge of the medical services and organized mobile medical units, further demonstrating the value of providing immediate care at the front. He organized teaching of health workers, and planned a Model Hospital and a medical school. When Pai-ch'iu-en, as Bethune was known to the Chinese, died of septicemia as a result of a cut during surgery, he became a legendary Chinese hero, memorialized in statues, school teachings of his life, and writings about his dedication, heroism, and service to others. The eulogy written by Mao is familiar to all Chinese schoolchildren. He is buried in the Mausoleum of Martyrs, Shih Cha Chuang, southeast of Peking, near the Bethune International Peace Hospital and Bethune Medical School. Recognition came later in Canada, and a life-sized statue now stands in Montreal, donated by the Chinese people.

Bibliography

Primary: 1975. *We Are the Heirs to Norman Bethune* (Toronto) [a collection of Bethune's writings].

Secondary: Stewart, Roderick, 2002. *The Mind of Norman Bethune* (Ontario); Wilson, John, 2001. *Norman Bethune, Homme de caractère et de conviction* (Montreal); Hannant, L., 1998. *The Politics of Passion: Norman Bethune's Writings and Art* (Toronto); Shepard, David A. E., 1982. *Norman Bethune: His Times and His Legacy* (Ottawa); MacLeod, W., L. Park, and S. Ryerson, 1978. *Bethune: The Montreal Years: An Informal Portrait* (Toronto); Stewart, Roderick, 1974. *Norman Bethune* (Ontario); Allen, T., 1974. *The Scalpel and the Sword: The Story of Dr. Norman Bethune* (Toronto).

Jock Murray

BEVAN, ANEURIN (b. Tredegar, Monmouthshire, Wales, 15 November 1897; d. Asheridge, Buckinghamshire, England 6 July 1960), *politics, health reform.*

Born into a Welsh mining family, Nye (as he was known), was the sixth of ten children, four of whom died before reaching adulthood. Although he displayed strong intellectual ability at school, he left at fourteen to work in the local colliery. From an early age he was politically active, taking classes with the social scientist Sydney Jones in a mix of official Labour Party and Marxist philosophies. He was elected as a delegate to the South Wales Miners' Federation and took an active antiwar stance during World War I. His reputation as a public speaker grew when he was sent to the national conference of the Miners' Federation of Great Britain during the 1926 dispute.

In 1922 Bevan had won a seat as a Labour councilor on Tredegar urban district council. He built up a core of loyal support, and in 1929 was returned as Labour MP for Ebbw Vale at the age of thirty-two. His sharp intellect and witty debate found their home at Westminster, and senior parliamentarians such as Lord Beaverbrook noticed him. His love of high living and wide social life occasionally drew barbed comments from both his opponents and colleagues, but he appeared at ease with his background, politics and place in London life. He married fellow Labour MP Jennie Lee in 1934.

Bevan did not always accept the party line, and in 1939 he was briefly expelled from the Labour Party's National Executive Committee for sharing a platform with Communists. His outspoken views on World War II did not, however, prevent his appointment as Minister of Health and Housing in the new Labour government of 1945. This was a significant cabinet post, which he used to push through the construction of over one million new homes by 1950.

However, it is for his determination to implement Sir William Beveridge's report *Social Insurance and Allied Services* (1942) that Bevan is best remembered. The prewar health services in Britain were fragmented between various systems. Bevan took forward the vague outline drafted by his predecessor, the Conservative Henry Willink, for a national, state-run health service. In less than a year, Bevan had fleshed out a National Health Service Bill, which was passed in November 1946. Without his intellect and persuasive abilities, it is unlikely that the medical profession would have been convinced to participate. The British Medical Association held out until February 1948 before agreeing to work within a modified NHS, which finally came to life on 5 July 1948.

Bevan's basic principles were enshrined within the NHS: a comprehensive, free at the point of delivery service, funded through central taxation rather than insurance. It provided a massive morale-boost at the end of World War II and attracted international admiration. However, within two years the costs had escalated to such an extent, that charges were introduced for glasses, dentures, and prescriptions although this was partly to fund the deployment of British troops in Korea. Bevan opposed the war and wanted to control NHS spending by different means. He resigned in protest from the government in April 1951. Although he continued to be active within the Labour Party, his views on trade unions and defense were out of line with opponents such as Gaitskell, and he failed to revive his authority. Despite support from Jennie Lee and other colleagues, he eventually succumbed to stomach cancer in 1960.

The National Health Service is undoubtedly the greatest socialist achievement in twentieth-century Britain, and it is inextricably linked with Bevan. Despite repeated restructuring, no political party has yet had the temerity to openly suggest that it could be replaced by a better system.

Bibliography

Primary: 1952. *In Place of Fear* (London); Webster, Charles, ed., 1991. *Aneurin Bevan on the National Health Service* (Oxford).

Secondary: Webster, C., 2002. *A Political History of the NHS* (Oxford); Campbell, J., 1987. *Nye Bevan and the Mirage of British Socialism* (London); Foot, M., 1962 (2nd edn., 1973). *Aneurin Bevan: A Biography* (London); *Oxford DNB*.

Sally Sheard

BEVERIDGE, WILLIAM HENRY   (b. Rangpur, Bengal, India, 5 March 1879; d. Oxford, England, 16 March 1963), *medical reform, social reform.*

Beveridge was born in Bengal, where his father was a district sessions judge in the Indian Civil Service, and his mother a pioneer of education for Hindu women. He was sent to a Unitarian boarding school in Worcestershire at the age of five, and saw little of his parents during his childhood. At the age of eleven he won a scholarship to Charterhouse school, where he excelled at mathematics and classics, although his real passion was for natural science and astronomy.

He went as an exhibitioner in 1897 to Balliol College, Oxford. After a year working with a commercial barrister in London, he went to University College Oxford on a prize fellowship and took a bachelor of law degree in 1903. However, he switched careers to investigate social problems from a position as sub-warden at Toynbee Hall—a settlement in the East End of London, staffed by Oxford University personnel. This move had been inspired by Beveridge's reading of T. H. Huxley (1825–1895), who claimed that social problems required the rigorous application of social science techniques, in much the same way as the natural sciences used their techniques.

At Toynbee Hall Beveridge formed close alliances with a number of key reformers, especially Sidney (1859-1947) and Beatrice Webb (1858-1943), the Fabian socialists. Beveridge took a particular interest in the campaigns for a national minimum wage and old age pensions. Between 1904 and 1909, he researched and subsequently published a pioneering study: *Unemployment: A Problem of Industry.* In 1905 he began to write for the *Morning Post*, producing nearly 1,000 leading articles on socio-economic issues.

In 1907 Beveridge was introduced by the Webbs to Winston Churchill (1874–1965), the new Liberal President of the Board of Trade, and the following year he became a civil servant, working on the Labour Exchanges Act of 1909 and the National Insurance Act of 1911. During World War I he was seconded to the Ministry of Munitions, but his poor relations with the unions meant that he was not transferred as he hoped to the new Ministry of Labour. Instead he went to the Ministry of Food, where he became one of the youngest Permanent Secretaries in 1919. He resigned from the civil service in 1919 to take up the directorship of the London School of Economics (LSE).

Beveridge attracted a number of social sciences experts to the LSE, including H. J. Laski. In 1937 he moved as Master to University College Oxford. With the threat of war, he was keen to return to a policymaking role, but it was not until December 1940 that he achieved this. He then exploited a broad brief to conduct a social services inquiry in June 1941 to accomplish one of the most significant surveys of the twentieth century. Published to unexpected widespread public acclaim in 1942, Beveridge's report, *Social Insurance and Allied Services*, exposed Britain's problems with the 'five giants' of idleness, ignorance, disease, squalor, and want.

Beveridge reinforced the work of earlier social scientists such as Edwin Chadwick (1800–1890), Charles Booth (1840–1916), and Joseph Rowntree (1801–1859) in showing that there were clear links between low income, poor housing, and poor health. He interviewed hundreds of working class families, who along with leading economists, testified to the impact of the inter-war economic depression and fragmented health care system on the nation's health. Furthermore, the wartime Emergency Medical Service had demonstrated that it was possible to provide an integrated, state-run service. The 1942 report provided a blueprint for universal social insurance, including a comprehensive national health service, free at the point of delivery, along with family, unemployment, and old age benefits. More than 70,000 copies were sold in the first few days after publication, putting considerable pressure on the government.

Beveridge actively promoted his plans and entered parliament as a Liberal MP for Berwick upon Tweed. He lost his seat after only a year, and went to the House of Lords in 1946. Aneurin Bevan, new Minister of Health and Housing in the 1945 Labour government, adopted his plan for a national health service. After a period of bitter negotiations with the medical profession, Bevan succeeded in passing the NHS Act in 1946, and the service came into operation on 5 July 1948.

Bibliography

Primary: 1942. *Social Insurance and Allied Services* (London); 1953. *Power and Influence* (Oxford).

Secondary: Harris, José, 1997. *William Beveridge: A Biography* (Oxford); Beveridge, Janet, 1954. *Beveridge and His Plan* (London); *Oxford DNB*.

Sally Sheard

BEVERWIJCK, JOHAN VAN   (b. Dordrecht, the Netherlands, 17 November 1594; d. Dordrecht, 19 January 1647), *medicine, anatomy, surgery.*

Born into a distinguished family in Dordrecht, van Beverwijck was a typical self-confident burgher of the Protestant Dutch Republic. His father was a cloth merchant, and his mother, Maria Boot van Wezel, was a distant relative of the sixteenth-century anatomist Andreas Vesalius. At the Dordrecht Latin school, the famous scholar Gerardus Vossius taught van Beverwijck the principles of classical rhetoric, which can be traced throughout his writings. He started his medical studies at Leiden (1611–15) and completed his training at several European universities, including Paris, Lyon, Montpellier, Bologna, Padua (graduation, probably 1617), Basel, Heidelberg, and Leuven.

In 1618 he started to practice as a family doctor and chemist in Dordrecht, where he joined the local elite and held many official medical and nonmedical positions. In 1625 he became the official town physician, and from 1634 until 1643 he lectured anatomy to surgeons and laymen. He also trained and examined midwives. In his extensive social network we find politicians (he was the private doctor of the De Witt family), lawyers, clergymen, writers, and medical colleagues.

Van Beverwijck was well-read in the history of medicine and he eagerly conducted experiments, especially in the field of anatomy. He was the first Dutch physician to acknowledge William Harvey's ideas on the circulation of the blood; he expanded on them in a treatise on bladder and renal stones (*De calculo renum & vesicae liber singularis*, 1638; translated into Dutch as *Steen-stuck*).

He wrote widely on medical subjects, but also on topics such as history or the qualities of the female sex. Between 1636 and 1645 he published the famous trilogy *Schat der Gesontheyt, Schat der Ongesontheyt,* and *Heel-konste* [*Treasury of Health, Treasury of Illness,* and *Surgery*]. This first complete and often reprinted medical encyclopedia in Dutch offered doctors and laymen a systematic survey of conditions of health, as well as the causes and treatments of all known diseases. It was based on the classical Galenic doctrine of the four humors and supplemented with the ideas of Harvey.

Van Beverwijck's trilogy was written in a clear, matter-of-fact style, with many humorous observations, and his explanations followed a steady pattern. First of all, he was confident that God has enabled mankind to guard its health. Next, he observed each disease critically, comparing historical and contemporary medical reports with his own experience. He also took into account whatever useful information he could get from other sources, including the Bible, books on mythology and world history, travel stories, novels, and poetry. With regard to the latter, he received help from a friend, the popular poet Jacob Cats, who enriched the text with verse summaries. Accordingly, this medical encyclopedia offered useful insights and practical advice, but was also a book of miscellaneous content, full of fascinating stories that perfectly demonstrated the well-known Renaissance combination of *utilis* [useful] and *dulcis* [attractive].

Bibliography

Primary: 1651–52. *Alle de wercken, soo in de medicyne als chirurgye: Schat der gesontheyt; Schat der ongesontheyt; heel-konste* (Utrecht and Amsterdam); 1638. *De calculo renum & vesicae liber singularis* (Leiden); 1992. (Gemert, Lia van, ed.) *De schat der gezondheid. Met gedichten van Jacob Cats* (Amsterdam).

Secondary: Gemert, Lia van, 1998. 'Johan van Beverwijck' in Frijhoff, Willem, Hubert Nusteling, and Marijke Spies, eds., *Geschiedenis van Dordrecht van 1572 tot 1813* (Hilversum) pp. 260–261; Gemert, Lia van, 1994. 'The Power of the Weaker Vessels. Simon Schama and Johan van Beverwijck on Women' in Kloek, Els, Nicole Teeuwen, and Marijke Huisman, eds., *Women of the Golden Age. An International Debate on Women in Seventeenth-century Holland, England and Italy* (Hilversum) pp. 39–50; Gemert, Lia van, 1992. 'Johan van Beverwijck als "instituut".* De zeventiende eeuw* 8: 99–106.

Lia van Gemert

BIAN QUE 扁鹊 (aka QIN YUEREN 秦越人) (b. Mo 鄚, Bo Hai 渤海 [now Renqiu 任邱] Hebei, China; fl. *c.* sixth to fifth century BCE), *Chinese medicine.*

Bian Que was a physician whose deeds and achievements are documented in many Chinese sources. The most detailed description is in Sima Qian's 司馬遷 (*c.* 145 or 135 BCE) 'Biography of Bian Que' recorded in *Shiji* 史记 [Records of History], the first general history of China presented in a series of biographies. Sima Qian recorded only one other biography—that of the Han physician Chunyu Yi 淳于意, who lived some three centuries later than Bian Que's putative dates. Before these two biographies, there were just two brief accounts of physicians, Yi He 醫和 and Yi Huan 醫缓. They were recorded in *Zuo Zhuan* 左传 a commentary on the chronicle of the reigns of the twelve dukes of the state of Lu 魯 (722 BCE).

Despite Bian Que's reputation for being an outstanding physician with wide-ranging experience, scholars differ in their interpretations of Sima Qian's account, and there is no consensus about the details of Bian Que's name, place of birth, and lifespan. The main themes that emerge in that account are summarized here, with evidence from my own research, including an introduction to the life and achievements of Bian Que.

Sima Qian's account is the source for Bian Que's name and place of birth, which lay at the borders of the states of Qi 齊, Zhao 趙, and Yan 燕 during the Spring and Autumn and Warring States periods (770–221 BCE). When Bian Que was young, he was the manager of a hotel in Mo 鄚 (now in Ren Qiu county, Hebei Province). Over a ten-year period, one customer, Chang Sang Jun 長桑君, would often stay at the hotel when traveling to and from the town. Bian Que believed his customer to be an extraordinary man, and Chang Sang Jun also had respect for Bian Que.

One day, Chang Sang Jun invited Bian Que for a private interview. He told Bian Que that since he was very old, he would like to pass on some secret prescriptions that had been handed down in his family for generations. Bian Que accepted the offer with due gratitude and propriety. Later, he changed his occupation, becoming a physician who traveled through the states of Qi, Zhao, and Yan to offer his services. He was skilled in remedies and techniques for the treatment of a variety of illnesses, providing not only internal medicine—herbs and drugs—but also whatever surgical, gynecological, and pediatric care the local people needed. His therapies were of such excellence that he was held in high repute.

Bian Que's original name was Qin Yueren, which he used when practicing, and he was called Bian Que when he was practicing in the state of Zhao. At that time, Bian was an unusual surname and Que was rarely used as a given name. So why was Qin Yueren nicknamed Bian Que by the people of Zhao? First, the ancient Chinese character for Bian 扁 was interchangeable with 遍, in that these graphic variants shared a common pronunciation and application.

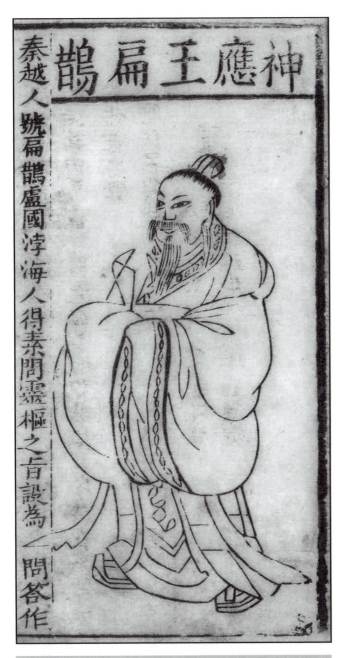

Portrait of Bian Que from *Tai yiyuan zengbu xhenzhu nang yaoxing quan fu zhijie tai yi yuan.* **Revised by Luo Biwei. Late Qing period.**

Bian 遍 means 'widespread', and according to *Xunzi* 荀子 (*c.* fourth to third century BCE), the term *bian* also suggested that wherever one went there would be a good result. According to *Mengzi* 孟子 (*c.* third century BCE), the term *bian* could also signify a joyful and happy appearance. Que is a kind of magpie—the so-called 喜鵲 [Happy Magpie] that flies around, cheering and bringing happiness and good news, and is taken to be a symbol of happiness. Thus we have the traditional Chinese saying, 'The Happy Magpie will certainly bring you good news.' Second, according to

Zhao's ancestral lineages, the local people took the bird as their totem, and the ancestors had human faces and bird beaks. In short, there is copious evidence of their high regard for birds. Just like the Happy Magpie that brings good news, Sima Qian's story about Qin Yueren suggests the popularity of this physician who traveled widely, offering his medical services to relieve suffering and illness. The nickname given to him by the people of Zhao was actually an expression of their warmth and respect for the excellence of his medical practice. This nickname, which he deserved, was spread together with his popularity, and as a result, people were happy to call him Bian Que rather than Qin Yueren.

There is also archaeological evidence of Bian Que's (Qin Yueren's) popularity. In 1971 a stone relief dating from the later Han Dynasty was recovered in Shandong Province, in the former state of Qi. Central to that carving is a human-headed bird with arms holding a needle above a human figure, in a gesture suggesting that he is about to administer acupuncture.

According to Sima Qian's account, when Bian Que was passing through the state of Jin 晉 while pursuing his medical practice (*c.* sixth century BCE), he was told of a high official named Zhao Jianzi 趙簡子 who had fallen ill and had been in a coma for five days. His subordinates were terrified and thought that Zhao Jianzi was already dead. Using the man's pulse as his main diagnostic method, Bian Que ascertained that the patient was still alive and predicted that he would revive in three days. Afterward, when Zhao Jianzi recovered, he granted Bian Que 40,000 *mu* 亩 (*c.* 6,590 acres) of land to express his gratitude.

Bian Que continued to practice medicine as he passed through the state of Guo (*c.* fifth century BCE). Anxious local people told him that the Prince of Guo had been dead for half a day. After Bian Que asked about everything that had happened and examined the Prince by feeling his pulse, he concluded that the Prince was not in fact dead but had fallen into *shijue* 尸厥, a syndrome that induced coma. He explained the mechanism of the disease according to the complex theories of Yin, Yang, and the channels. Bian Que then ordered one of his disciples, Ziyang 子阳, to 'sharpen needles and needling stone to stimulate the *outer three Yang and five meetings*', which were points on the top of the head. He ordered another disciple called Baozi to use medicated ironing therapy (a kind of treatment using a metal instrument with boiled herbs) to heat the patient's flanks. After a short time, the Prince was able to sit upright. Bian Que then gave his patient a decoction to regulate Yin and Yang, and the Prince recovered completely within twenty days.

Bian Que excelled at all four of the diagnostic methods promoted in Chinese traditional medicine: inspection, auscultation and olfaction, interrogation, and feeling pulses. He was especially good at pulse diagnosis, and according to Sima Qian's account, he was the first to master pulse diagnosis in ancient China. Later books that discuss pulse diagnosis cited

Bian Que, generally acknowledging him as the founder of pulse teaching in ancient China. He was also famous for his skills in internal medicine, surgery, gynecology, pediatrics, etc. Bian Que was an expert and pioneer in combination therapy, using many techniques including acupuncture, drugs, massage, and medicated ironing.

Bian Que is credited with development of the theory of the channels and their collaterals. Before his time, the theories of Yin, Yang, and the channels were embryonic. Yi He had used Yin, Yang, and the six *qi* in order to explain the causes of disease in the sixth century BCE, but his theories were simplistic. The second-century BCE silk books from Mawangdui 馬王堆 set out theories of the channels, but the channels were not at that time associated with the inner organs. When Bian Que treated the Prince of Guo, he explained the cause of his disease with reference to the theory of Yin and Yang in their association with the internal organs. That was the foundation upon which theories of the channels in Chinese traditional medicine were constructed.

As a renowned physician, Bian Que was thought to be able to revive the dead. It seems that he rejected hollow praise, however, maintaining that his patients had originally been alive and only *seemed* to be dead. The story suggests that he was above using his medical skills in the pursuit of fame and gain. In later ages we can see the influence of the figure of Bian Que, when grateful patients would send their doctor a horizontal board inscribed with the words 'The Ways of Bian Que'.

In ancient China, a group of healers known as *wu* 巫 played important roles in healing. They were diviners, spirit mediums, or ritual specialists whose work might involve dealing with those ancestors, deities, demons, and spirits that could influence a person's health. Before Bian Que, some physicians such as Yi He and Yi Huan had already rejected the work of the *wu*, and although there are magical elements in Sima Qian's account of Bian Que, he also was resolutely set against the work of the *wu*. Among the 'six hard to cure'—six kinds of illnesses that were difficult to treat—Bian Que included one that involved 'believing in *wu* rather than medicine'.

Various sources recorded or cited texts in the name of Bian Que, among them *Bian Que nei jing* 扁鵲內經 [Bian Que's Inner Classic] and *Bian Que wai jing* 扁鵲外經 [Bian Que's Outer Classic] in *Han Shu yiwen zhi* 漢書藝文志 (first century), and the bibliographic treatise of *Han Shu*, the standard 'History of the Han Dynasty'. Similar records and citations can be found in the bibliographic treatises of the later standard histories of the Sui Dynasty and the Tang Dynasty: *Sui Shu jing ji zhi* 隋書經籍志 (636) and *Jiu Tang Shu jing ji zhi* 舊唐書·經籍志 (940–45).

The two books thought to have been written by Bian Que were lost long ago, but many classics of Chinese traditional medicine such as *Nei jing* 內經 [Inner Canon] and *Mai jing* 脈經 [The Pulse Classic] (third century) contain quotations from his writings on pulse diagnosis. Another important text, *Nan jing* 難經 [Classic of Medical Catechisms], is traditionally ascribed to Qin Yueren (Bian Que), but my research shows that it was composed later by an unknown author using Qin Yueren as a pseudonym.

Bian Que was an outstanding representative of Chinese medical expertise. Unfortunately, he was murdered by a palace doctor inferior to him, Li Xi 李醯,who envied his prodigious medical skill. In later ages, many temples and stelae were erected to commemorate Bian Que and make his achievements known.

Bibliography

Primary: Sima Qian 司馬遷, *c.* 145 or 135 BCE. Biographies of Bian Que and Chuang Gong 扁鵲倉公列傳 in Records of History 史記, vol. 105. [Modern edn., 1972, Shanghai].

Secondary: Kang Wenhai 亢文海, ed., 1999. *Huaxia yizu Bian Que* 華夏醫祖扁鵲 [Bian Que, the Medical Ancestor of China] (Beijing); Cao Dongyi 曹東義, ed., 1996. *Shenyi Bian Que zhi mi* 神醫扁鵲之迷 [Mystery of the Wonderful Doctor Bian Que] (Beijing); Ma Kanwen 馬堪溫 1955. 内媚县神头村扁鹊庙调查记 ['An Investigation into the Temple of Bian Que at Shen Tou Village of Nei Qiu County']. 中华医史杂志 *Journal of Chinese Medical History* 2: 100–103; Yang Shixing 楊世興, ed., 1991. *Dongzhou weida yixue kexuejia—Qing Yueren-Bian Que* 東周偉大醫學科學家—秦越人扁鵲 [The Great Medical Scientist of the Eastern Zhou Dynasty, Qing Yueren-Bian Que] (Xi'an).

Kan-Wen Ma

BICHAT, MARIE-FRANÇOIS-XAVIER (b. Thoirette, Jura, France, 14 November 1771; d. Paris, France, 22 July 1802), *anatomy, physiology, pathology.*

Bichat was born in a small village near Lyons, the first child of the physician Jean-Baptiste Bichat and his wife (and cousin), Jeanne-Rose (sometimes identified as Marie-Rose). The couple had three other children, a son and two daughters. Jean-Baptiste Bichat was a medical graduate of the University of Montpellier in southern France, where the philosophy of vitalism was strongly advocated throughout the latter half of the eighteenth century. Vitalism held that the phenomena of living bodies are caused by specific properties inherent in living matter, and that these properties are radically different from those of nonliving matter. That view was reflected in all of Xavier Bichat's writing, and it is likely that he was first introduced to it by his father.

Bichat received his early education at a college operated by the Josephist order in Nantua, which he began attending in 1781. He was a diligent student and won many prizes, but with the outbreak of the French Revolution in 1789 his education was disrupted. His devout parents removed him from the college in 1790 when its director accepted the civil constitution of the clergy—a measure introduced by the Revolutionary government to bring the church under state control. Bichat was then sent to Lyons to complete his final year of study, which was devoted to philosophy, at the Saint-Irénée seminary of the Sulpician order. A Father Bichat, one of his uncles, was the superior there. During that year he excelled particularly in the study of mathematics and natural history.

In 1791 Bichat began his medical education at the Hôtel Dieu hospital in Lyons. He studied anatomy and surgery with the chief surgeon, Marc-Antoine Petit (1766–1811), but the events of the Revolution soon overtook him. With the commencement of war in 1792 the Saint-Irénée seminary was converted to a military hospital, and Bichat was conscripted to serve there as a surgical assistant. Shortly afterward, in early 1793, the southeastern regions of France—including Lyons—rebelled against the government in Paris. That uprising developed into a civil war lasting several months, during which Bichat served with the antigovernment party in both a combatant and a medical capacity. He left the city at the beginning of August 1793, before it came under siege from the central government's Army of the Alps, and went to the nearby town of Poncin, where his father's medical practice was located.

Arriving in Poncin, Bichat was pressed into the Army of the Alps as a junior surgeon. After several months' service at Grenoble and Bourg, he was discharged and made his way back to join his family at Poncin. Although his father had been a deputy of the Third Estate in the early days of the Revolution, the family was now under suspicion for lack of patriotism, leading Bichat to volunteer for military ambulance service as a demonstration of loyalty. In the summer of 1794, however, he left for Paris. There he joined his aunt, uncle, and cousin Buisson, who had moved there from Lyons the previous August to escape the siege.

Paris and the New Medical School

The ancient faculties of medicine throughout France, the royal academies, and many other institutions associated with the old regime had been closed by the Revolutionary government in 1793, so there was no system of formal medical instruction operating in Paris when Bichat arrived there. In order to continue his education, he apprenticed himself to the eminent surgeon, Pierre-Joseph Desault (1738–95), with whom his former surgical teacher in Lyons, Petit, had once studied. Bichat impressed his new master and was taken into the Desault household.

At the beginning of 1795 a new medical school was established in Paris, with Desault as Professor of Clinical Surgery. But in the summer of that year Desault died of fever, leaving behind a number of manuscripts that Bichat edited for publication with the encouragement of Desault's friend, Jean-Nicolas Corvisart des Marets (1755–1821), the Professor of Clinical Medicine. These articles appeared in the final volume (1795) of the *Journal of Surgery*, which Desault had founded. Some time later (1798–99), Bichat also brought out a multivolume collection of Desault's surgical works and prefaced it

with a eulogy for his deceased teacher. For the remainder of his life, Bichat continued to live in the Desault household, where Desault's widow treated him as an adopted son.

After the fall of the radical Jacobin government late in 1794, the political climate became more moderate in Paris, and professional groups were less likely to be denounced as elitist. In that climate, a number of new medical and scientific societies were formed as voluntary organizations to replace the previously suppressed royal academies. Bichat was a member of several of these groups, and he was particularly active in one that he cofounded in 1796—the *Société médicale d'émulation* [Society for Medical Improvement is an approximate English translation]. Originally conceived as a scientific society for younger medical men, it soon attracted more senior figures as well. Among them were Philippe Pinel (1745–1826), Antoine-François Fourcroy (1755–1809), Pierre-Jean-Georges Cabanis (1757–1808), and Desault's friend Corvisart—all men who were leaders in the new approach to medicine and medical education then being developed in France.

Both the Society and the new medical school were guided by the prevailing French philosophy of the time, known as 'ideology'—so named for its commitment to the analysis of ideas. Building on the work of the most influential philosopher of eighteenth-century France, Étienne Bonnot de Condillac (1715–80), ideology was based on the premise that all ideas are derived from simple sensations, which are in turn variously combined in the human mind to form complex thoughts. The 'method of analysis', or the process of tracing back all ideas to their constituent primitive sensations, was regarded as a way not only of revealing the empirical content of each idea, but also of correctly understanding the relationships between ideas. These relationships were then 'fixed' or stabilized in the mind by the use of a precise nomenclature that would give an accurate linguistic reflection of the order of ideas.

Both Cabanis and Pinel in their medical doctrines, and Fourcroy more particularly in his collaboration as a chemist with Antoine-Laurent Lavoisier (1743–94), took Condillac's method of analysis as a model for the development of scientific knowledge. Indeed, after the success of Lavoisier's *Elementary Treatise of Chemistry* (1789) and the reformed chemical nomenclature that Lavoisier had devised in collaboration with Fourcroy and others, the 'new chemistry' was taken as a practical demonstration of the validity of Condillac's approach. That same model served to guide the pedagogy of the new medical school in Paris, which unified surgery with medicine and emphasized clinical instruction over textbook learning.

Bichat was never enrolled as a student at the Paris medical school, nor did he ever formally teach there. But he seems to have fully assimilated its ethos through his brief association with Desault and his ongoing interaction with senior figures from the school in the *Société médicale d'émulation*. These connections enabled him to teach private courses in anatomy and physiology from 1797 and, in 1801, to secure an appointment to the Hôtel Dieu hospital in Paris, which had been renamed the Grand Hospice d'Humanité by the Revolutionary government. His reputation for extraordinary productivity was established in 1798–99, when he completed the editing of Desault's collected works and published six articles of his own in the *Mémoires* of the *Société médicale d'émulation*. Three of these memoirs were on surgical topics, which had been Bichat's primary area of interest up to 1797, but the other three signaled the new direction his thought was taking, with a focus on anatomy and physiology.

First Major Publications

The last years of Bichat's life (1800–02) saw the publication of three major works from his pen and part of a fourth one. Together they were a grand synthesis of all his accomplishments to that point, and they were completed after his death by two of his students: his cousin Mathieu-François-Regis Buisson (1776–1804) and Philibert-Joseph Roux (1780–1854). These works fall naturally into two groups. The first two books, published in 1800, were single volumes elaborating on memoirs he had previously presented to the *Société médicale d'émulation*. The last two, published in the period 1801–03, were multivolume, systematic treatments of anatomy and physiology.

Bichat's first book, the *Treatise on Membranes in General, and on Various Membranes in Particular*, appeared early in 1800. In it he developed ideas outlined in two articles he had published in the *Mémoires* of the *Société médicale d'émulation* in 1798–99: his 'Memoir on the Synovial Membrane of the Joints' and his 'Dissertation on the Membranes and on the General Relations of Their Organization.' In the second of these articles he noted that there existed no systematic account of membranes as an anatomical category. Individual membranes had been studied along with their associated organs—the pericardium with the heart, the peritoneum with the abdominal viscera, and so forth—but the characteristics of membranes as a group had not been investigated. Citing the 'philosophical manner' in which Pinel had classified the inflammations, but arguing that it needed to be taken further, Bichat undertook to distinguish and characterize the types of membranes on the basis of their anatomical structure and their physiological functions (Bichat, 1798–99b, p. 372).

Pinel, in his *Philosophical Nosography, or the Method of Analysis Applied to Medicine* (1798), had grouped inflammations according to the nature of the organs that they affected (membranes, muscles, glands, etc.), rather than according to the broad region of the body in which they occurred (head, thorax, abdomen, etc.). That approach had been a feature of Pinel's teaching since the early 1790s, probably as a result of his familiarity with work published at the beginning of that decade by the British physician James Carmichael Smyth

(1742–1821). Pinel did not directly cite Smyth, however, and Bichat seems not to have known of him.

Bichat commended the approach taken by Pinel, but he regarded Pinel's grouping of anatomical organs as insufficiently precise. Both Bichat and Pinel worked at the level of gross anatomy, without attempting a microscopic examination of anatomical specimens, but Bichat based his classification of membranes on a much wider range of observational criteria than did Pinel. He outlined that classification in his 'Dissertation on the Membranes' of 1798–99, and in his *Treatise on Membranes* of 1800 he elaborated it in greater detail, again giving credit to Pinel's work for suggesting the overall approach employed (Bichat, 1800a, p. 4).

Bichat's second book, also published in 1800, was entitled *Physiological Researches on Life and Death*. Here again, Bichat developed material first published in 1798–99—in this case his 'Memoir on the relations that exist between organs of symmetrical form and those of irregular form'. He had argued that the organs pertaining to what he called the exterior life of an animal, or its relations with the surrounding world (functions such as sensation, locomotion, and vocalization), are always symmetrically paired about the median line of the animal's body (Bichat, 1798–99c, pp. 478, 482). But organs pertaining to an animal's interior life, or the life that animals share with plants (functions such as nutrition, circulation, and respiration), are always asymmetrical with respect to the median line, according to Bichat (*Ibid.*, pp. 478, 484). The reproductive organs pertain to neither the exterior life nor the interior life, in a strict sense, but in his view they are symmetrical. That symmetry is consistent with the process of sexual reproduction, which requires interaction with another animal from the external world (*Ibid.*, p. 487).

This doctrine of the two lives, and the anatomical generalizations that went with it, served as the starting point for Bichat's *Physiological Researches*. In the first half of that book, following a methodology based almost entirely on observation, Bichat sought to give a comprehensive account of the phenomena of the two lives, now referred to as the animal life and the organic life. He outlined not only the differences of symmetry and asymmetry in the organs associated with the two lives, but also the mode and duration of the actions of these organs. In addition, for each of the two lives he discussed their relationship to habits, intellect, and emotions; their vital properties (i.e., forms of sensibility and contractility found only in living bodies); their tissue properties (i.e., the extensibility and contractility that the tissues retain after death, before decomposition sets in); their origin and development; and their natural death. Then in the second half of the book, employing a predominantly experimental methodology, Bichat investigated the phenomena of violent death. In particular, he wished to elucidate the sequence of events leading to death when the functioning of one of the three primary organs—the brain, heart, or lungs—is suddenly interrupted.

The *Treatise on Membranes* and the *Physiological Researches* were immediate successes when published, exciting both acclaim and envy. Those who admired Bichat's work called for him to write an elementary textbook on physiology, a course of action that apparently did not interest him at the time. Those who were critical of his work questioned its originality or accuracy. But controversy of that kind was again something that seemed to hold no interest for Bichat, and in the preface to his *Physiological Researches* he dismissed both forms of criticism. On the matter of originality, he stated that the works of his predecessors were so well-known that it was unnecessary for him to show how they had been misquoted by his critics. As for the charge of inaccuracy, he asked anyone who had been swayed by such criticism to inspect some cadavers and verify for themselves the accuracy of his findings. But he was more scathing toward the critics themselves, saying that he did not expect them to benefit from further inspection of the evidence because they had all been present at his dissections and had already seen him demonstrate his discoveries.

Physiology, Philosophy, and Religion

In the preface to his *Physiological Researches*, Bichat advised that his goal was 'the art of allying the experimental method of Haller and Spallanzani with the broad and philosophical views of Bordeu' (Bichat, 1800b, p. ii). Given Bichat's later fame, it is easy to overlook the audacity of that statement at the time it was made. Here was a young man of twenty-eight from the provinces, a private lecturer in anatomy and physiology with no formal qualifications and no formal hospital or teaching appointments, seeking to place himself alongside such internationally celebrated luminaries of physiology as Albrecht von Haller (1708–77), Lazzaro Spallanzani (1729–99), and Théophile de Bordeu (1722–76). Haller and Spallanzani, as Bichat suggested, were known for their careful use of experimentation, whereas Bordeu was one of the founding figures of Montpellier vitalism, which opposed experimentation in medicine. Reconciling these two discrepant approaches was indeed a challenge, but one that Bichat successfully met.

Bichat's interest in the 'broad and philosophical views' of the Montpellier vitalists was genuine. So was his interest in philosophy, in the sense intended when he praised Pinel's 'philosophical manner' of classifying inflammations—that is, in the sense of Condillac's method of analysis. Accordingly, he presented his *Physiological Researches* as a self-consciously 'philosophical' treatise. That work did in fact succeed in establishing his philosophical standing—not just among philosophers with a commitment to 'ideology', such as Cabanis (who also shared Bichat's medical orientation) and Antoine-Louis-Claude Destutt de Tracy (1754–1836), but also among many other nineteenth-century philosophers with widely differing outlooks, such as Arthur Schopenhauer (1788–1860) and Auguste Comte (1798–1857).

One unexpected result of Bichat's venture into philosophy, however, was a threatened breach with his parents back

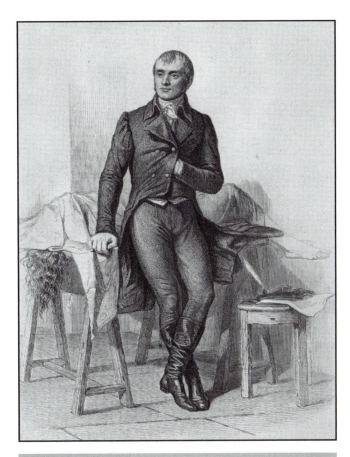

Marie-François-Xavier Bichat in the dissecting room. Line engraving by Wacqua after E. Béranger. Iconographic Collection, Wellcome Library, London.

in Poncin. Even before seeing a copy of the *Physiological Researches*, they wrote to accuse him of abandoning his religion and adopting instead 'all the principles of the day' from fashionable Parisian society—'principles', as Bichat wrote to his father, 'which you believe are leading me to perdition' (quoted in Kervella, 1931, pp. 50–51).

It is likely that the information that upset Bichat's family came from Buisson, Bichat's cousin and collaborator, whose religious outlook was firmly orthodox and who disapproved of the views of Cabanis and Pinel. Buisson presented his thesis to the Paris medical school only a few months after Bichat's death in 1802, and in that document he criticized his cousin's *Physiological Researches* for failing to distinguish appropriately between humans and animals. And Roux, Bichat's other collaborator, reported that Buisson once tore up the proofs of a section of Bichat's work that offended his religious sensibilities. Given this evidence and the complaints of Bichat's parents that he had failed to write to them for some time, it is plausible that the family would have sought and obtained information from Buisson, either directly or through Buisson's family in Paris.

There is no suggestion in the *Physiological Researches* that Bichat had adopted a position of irreligious materialism, although the vital properties that he identified in that work were treated as properties of living matter, rather than as properties of an immaterial soul or spirit. In any case, Bichat reassured his parents that his principles were not opposed to theirs, but in fact always had been and always would be the same as theirs (quoted in Kervella, 1931, p. 52).

Final Works and Uncompleted Projects

The approach Bichat took in his *Treatise on Membranes* formed the basis of his last completed work, *General Anatomy Applied to Physiology and Medicine*, which appeared in 1801. Analyzing the living body as a whole, not just the membranes, Bichat identified twenty-one simple tissues that, in different combinations, make up the various organs. He distinguished those tissues from one another not just by simple observation of their appearance and texture, but also by subjecting them to a wide range of relatively standardized tests—exposure to acids and alkalis, boiling, desiccation, and so forth. In four substantial volumes, Bichat characterized those tissues and their locations within the body, and then described their vital properties in accordance with the scheme he had developed in his *Physiological Researches*.

Bichat proposed that the twenty-one tissues were the fundamental components of living organisms in the same way that chemical elements were the fundamental components of nonliving matter. Just as the structure of each organ arose from the combination of tissues that composed it, so too did the function of each organ derive from the vital properties of its constituent tissues. Moreover, diseases were predominantly seated in tissues rather than in whole organs, and they were caused by alterations of the vital properties that could—in principle—be specified for each pathological condition. Effective therapeutic intervention, therefore, would involve returning those vital properties to their natural state. In sum, Bichat's conception made the tissues and their properties the key to physiology and medicine.

Whereas the *General Anatomy* undertook the analysis of the body, concentrating on individual tissues and their properties, the *Treatise on Descriptive Anatomy* that followed provided the complementary synthesis. The *Treatise* was organized according to the classification of functions in the *Physiological Researches*, with functions of the external life being treated first, followed by those of the internal life, and finally those relating to generation. The group of organs contributing to each of the functions was described, with each organ being characterized structurally in terms of the tissues that composed it and functionally in terms of the vital properties of those tissues.

Originally planned as a four-volume work like the *General Anatomy*, the *Descriptive Anatomy* ultimately ran to five volumes, only two of which were published before Bichat's death. Bichat was directly responsible for volume one (1801), volume two (1802), and for a large part of volume three (1802), which was finished by Buisson. The remaining two volumes (1803) were completed in conformity with Bichat's original plan—the fourth by Buisson and the fifth by Roux.

The sequence of events leading to Bichat's premature death at age thirty was initiated on 8 July 1802. After working with anatomical specimens in the midsummer heat, he fell while descending a staircase in the Hôtel Dieu and was unconscious for several minutes. Bichat's health while in Paris had never been robust; he suffered from chronic gastric problems and was once bedridden for an extended period after an episode of spitting blood. His condition deteriorated rapidly after his fall, and he experienced extreme fatigue, gastric symptoms, and severe headaches. Corvisart attended him, but treatment with emetics and leeches was ineffectual. Bichat died on 22 July 1802, a fortnight after the accident. His death was felt as a great loss by the entire Parisian medical community, and more than 500 people attended his funeral. A few days later, Napoleon (then First Consul) ordered that a monument jointly honoring Desault and Bichat be placed in the medical school. Accordingly, a marble plaque was installed in the amphitheatre.

At the time of his death, Bichat was seeking to develop pathological anatomy and therapeutics on the basis of his tissue theory. He had presented lecture series on both of those subjects, and a set of student notes from his lectures on pathological anatomy was eventually published in 1825. He had also been conducting extensive clinical and postmortem studies in both areas. Bichat's appointment to the Hôtel Dieu in 1801 gave him the official access to hospital patients that he needed for such research programs, and at that time he seemed to have had no interest in private practice.

In addition to those projects, he was said to be planning a substantial revision of his *Physiological Researches*. A new 'experimental' first half was to be written, devoted to the study of pathological conditions. The contents of the original 'philosophical' first half were to be integrated into a separate treatise on physiology that he had begun to draft. That new treatise, presumably, was where Bichat intended to locate new material linking physiology with philosophy, such as a chapter on esthetics that he had foreshadowed.

In the decades after his death, Bichat's understanding of physiology as the science of vital properties was rendered obsolete by the criticisms of François Magendie (1783–1855) and others, who carried forward his experimental methodology while abandoning his explanatory concepts. His most lasting contribution was his tissue theory, which was widely accepted. The doctrine that the tissues are the loci of physiological and pathological phenomena was not entirely original with Bichat, but it was highly influential in the form he gave it, serving historically as the foundation of histology and histopathology.

Bibliography

Primary: 1798–99a. 'Mémoire sur la membrane synoviale des articulations.' *Mémoires de la Société médicale d'émulation* 2: 350–370; 1798–99b. 'Dissertation sur les membranes, et sur leur rapports généraux d'organisation.' *Mémoires de la Société médicale d'émulation* 2: 371–385; 1798–99c. 'Mémoire sur les rapports qui existent entre les organes à forme symétrique, et ceux à forme *irrégulière.' Mémoires de la Société médicale d'émulation* 2: 477–487; 1800a. *Traité des membranes en général et de diverses membranes en particulier* (Paris); 1800b. *Recherches physiologiques sur la vie et la mort* (Paris); 1801. *Anatomie générale, appliquée à la physiologie et à la médecine* 4 vols. (Paris); 1801–03. *Traité d'anatomie descriptive* 5 vols. (Paris); 1825. *Anatomie pathologique. Dernier cours de Bichat d'après un manuscrit autographe de P.- A. Béclard* (Paris).

Secondary: Haigh, E., 1984. *Xavier Bichat and the Medical Theory of the Eighteenth Century* [*Medical History*, Supplement No. 4] (London); Albury, William Randall, 1977. 'Experiment and Explanation in the Physiology of Bichat and Magendie.' *Studies in History of Biology* 1: 47–131; Kervella, Emile-Jean, 1931. *La vie et l'oeuvre de Bichat* (Paris); Levacher de la Feutrie, A. F. T., 1803. 'Éloge de Marie-François-Xavier Bichat.' *Mémoires de la Société médicale d'émulation* 5: xxvii–lxiv; Buisson, M. F. R., 1802. 'Précis historique sur Marie-François-Xavier Bichat' in Bichat, M.-F.-X., 1801–03. *Traité d'anatomie descriptive* 5 vols. (Paris) vol. 3, pp. vii–xxviii; *DSB.*

W. R. Albury

BIDLOO, GOVARD

(b. Amsterdam, the Netherlands, 12 March 1649; d. Leiden, the Netherlands, 30 March 1713), *anatomy, military medicine, poetry.*

Govard Bidloo was the second son of Mennonite parents, Govert Bidloo and Maria Lamberts Feliers. He is best known for the anatomical work that he began in 1670, when he became a surgical apprentice and attended lectures by Frederik Ruysch. Even before his graduation as a medical doctor at the University of Franeker (1682), Bidloo started working on an anatomical atlas that became famous for its 'realistic' depictions. The plates, made by the painter Gerard de Lairesse, included ropes, books, blocks, pins supporting body parts, and even a fly creeping across a dissection of the abdomen. They were intended to be lifelike imitations of what became visible during a dissection. The Latin atlas appeared in 1685, and a Dutch translation followed in 1689. Bidloo's other project was a refutation of the thesis that *spiritus animales* exist and circulate through the nerves. In 1688 he was appointed professor of anatomy in the Hague, followed in 1694 by an appointment to the anatomy chair in Leiden.

The anatomical atlas infuriated Ruysch, who accused Bidloo of inaccuracies in depicting the glands, valves and tubes in the skin, the coronary system, spleen, gall bladder, and the brain. The conflict with his former anatomy teacher ended in bitter accusations involving each other's morals and character. Another enemy of Bidloo was the English anatomist William Cowper, who in 1698 published the plates of Bidloo's anatomical atlas (*The Anatomy of Humane Bodies*) under his own name and supplemented with his own commentary. Bidloo was furious that Cowper never acknowledged him as author of the original atlas, even though his name was mentioned sixty-nine times in Cowper's version.

After the death of Paulus Hermannus in 1695, Bidloo assumed responsibility for clinical teaching at Leiden University, in addition to his anatomical work there. In 1702, he

also became *professor chirurgiae.* Bidloo regularly complained to the curators of the university about the shortage of cadavers for dissection. The curators, in turn, reprimanded Bidloo for his frequent absences and the subsequent decline in medical teaching, particularly during his travels to England in 1695, 1699, and 1701–02.

Politically, Bidloo trimmed his sails according to the wind. He started his career as a republican, but he changed his tune when he became a favorite of William III. In 1690 William III entrusted him with supervision of the military hospitals in the Netherlands; two years later, Bidloo was awarded the same post in England. In 1701 he became physician to William III in England, and he served the king in London until the latter 'died in Bidloo's arms' in 1702. In his often polemic literary writings Bidloo stepped on many toes, and William III regularly intervened to keep him out of trouble—and even out of prison.

Bidloo's Mennonite descent and his adherence to the 'Lammist' group within the Mennonite Church are visible in his literary works. Most notably, his *Brieven der gemartelde apostelen* [Letters of the Tortured Apostles] of 1675, 1698, and 1712 reflect the Mennonite fascination with martyrdom.

Govard Bidloo died at the age of sixty-four, leaving his wife, Hendrina Kiskens, and a son, Gerrit Bidloo. At the widow's request, there was no funeral oration.

Bibliography

Primary: 1715. *Opera omnia anatomico-chirurgica, edita et inedita* (Leiden);1685. *Anatomia humani corporis* (Amsterdam); 1697. *Vindiciae quarundam delineationum anatomicarum* (Leiden); 1708. *Exercitationum anatomico-chirurgicarum decades duae* (Leiden).

Secondary: Knoeff, Rina, 2003. 'Over "het kunstige, toch verderfelijke gestel". Een cultuurhistorische interpretatie van Bidloo's anatomische atlas'. *Gewina* 26: 189–202; Dumaître, P., 1982. *La curieuse destinée des planches anatomiques de Gérard de Lairesse* (Amsterdam); Vasbinder, Willem, 1948. *Govard Bidloo en William Cowper* (Utrecht).

Rina Knoeff

BIDLOO, NIKOLAI

(b. Amsterdam, the Netherlands, 1670; d. Moscow, Russia, 23 March [3 April] 1735), *anatomy, surgery.*

Bidloo was born into a Dutch medical and academic family. In 1697 he defended his dissertation on the delay of menstruation (*Disputatio medica inauguralis de menstuorum suppressione…*) at Leiden University. He had a medical practice in Amsterdam until 1702.

In 1702 he moved to Russia, under contract to 1708, in the capacity of physician in ordinary (personal doctor) to Tsar Peter I. In May 1706 he complied with the tsarist decree to plan and supervise construction of the Moscow hospital, the first state clinical institution in Russia. The hospital was opened in 1707 and was initially expected to treat 300 patients, but Bidloo's letters to the tsar reveal that 1,996 were admitted from

1708 to 1712. The hospital treated skin and psychiatric illnesses, as well as diseases and injuries requiring surgery.

The hospital school was the first institution in Russia for medical education, and it prepared physicians for the army and navy. As head doctor of the hospital and head of the hospital school, Bidloo himself taught anatomy, internal illnesses, and surgery with dressings. He is considered to have been the first in Russia to practice and teach obstetrics. An anatomical theater, where Peter I often attended postmortem examinations, was also built at the hospital school, and there was a pharmaceutical garden where medicinal herbs were grown. The required examination and preparation of unidentified bodies was performed at the theater by special state decree. Bidloo also put together a collection of pathological-anatomical preparations, part of which was transferred to the St Petersburg *Kunstkamera*.

For students, clinical experience included their presence on doctors' rounds, their participation in the execution of medical assignments and the preparation of medications, and shift work in hospital wards. During the life of Bidloo the Moscow hospital school produced ten graduates, giving Russia 102 credentialed physicians. He cared about the professional growth of his students. When a question arose in 1715 regarding the oppression of Moscow hospital school graduates at the St Petersburg hospital, Bidloo sent a petition to the tsar, and the affair was resolved in the Senate in his favor.

Because there were no textbooks, the initial integrated sources of knowledge for students were the lectures that Bidloo dictated. In 1710 he created a textbook for surgery. Its 1,306-page manuscript is preserved in the archive of the Military Medical Academy and was published in 1979. A significant part of the book was devoted to the surgical care of the injured, and it can be considered the first textbook in Russia on surgery. Bidloo also wrote about the surgical particularities of the structure of the womb and placenta, the technique of cutting the umbilical cord, and operation by cesarean section.

Bidloo was not only an expert doctor, but also a connoisseur of art, music, theater, and architecture. Thanks to him, the first Russian play dedicated to Peter I was performed by students of the Moscow hospital school. Bidloo designed several arches that were raised in Moscow and St Petersburg, and he designed and built his own country estate. That eighteen-page design, capably executed by Bidloo himself on sheets approximately twenty-five by fifty centimeters, is preserved in the archive of Leiden University. It was published in 1975.

Bibliography

Primary: 1702. Rossiskaia gosudarstvennaia biblioteka [Russian state library], Nauchno-issledovatel'skii otdel rukopisei [Scientific research department of manuscripts]. 'File about the admission of Doctor Bidloo . . .' f. 334, op. 440, d. 1, ll: 6–8 (Moscow); 1712. Rossiskii gosudarstvennyi arkhiv drevnykh aktov [Russian state archive of ancient documents]. '. . . of Doctor Bidloo to Tsar Peter I about the opening of the hospital and a report on 5 years of work.' f. 9, Cabinet of Peter I, department II, d. 15, ll: 144–146 (Moscow); 1713. [Russian state archive of ancient documents]

'The file about the dispatch by Doctor Bidloo of exhibits for the Kunstkamera.' f. 248, d. 27, l: 626 (Moscow).

Secondary: Bidloo, N., 1979. *Nastavlenie dlia izuchaiushchikh khirurgiiu v anatomicheskom teatre* [*Instructions for Studying Surgeons in the Anatomical Theater*] (Moscow); Willimse, D., 1975. *The Unknown Drawings of Nicholas Bidloo, Director of the First Hospital in Russia* (Voorburg); Alelekov, A., 1907. *Istoriia Moskovskogo voennogo gospitalia v sviazi s istorieiu meditsiny v Rossii k 200-letnemu ego iubileiu 1707–1907 gg.* [*History of the Moscow Military Hospital in Connection with the History of Medicine in Russia on Its 200th Jubilee 1707–1907*] (Moscow); Chistovich, Ia., 1883. *Istoriia pervykh medistinskikh shkol v Rossii* [History of the First Medical Schools in Russia] (St Petersburg).

Mikhail Poddubnyi

BIEGANSKI, WLADYSLAW (b. Grabow on Prosna, Poland, 28 April 1857; d. Czestochowa, Poland, 29 January 1917), *occupational medicine, philosophy of medicine.*

Born into a working class family, Bieganski studied medicine and philosophy at the University of Warsaw. After his graduation in 1880, he worked for two years as a physician in central Russia, and in 1883 he traveled to Berlin and Prague to study medicine.

At that time Bieganski was interested in scientific research. He specialized in the study of neurological disorders and aspired to an academic career, but academic jobs were very rare in occupied Poland. Unable to obtain a university position, he settled in Czestochowa, a rapidly growing industrial center. At first he elected to take only waged jobs (he worked for the municipality of Czestochowa and for several local factories) in order to keep regular work hours and to have free time for scientific research. But Bieganski became increasingly interested in occupational medicine. He published several studies on occupational diseases and on links between occupation, ethnic origins, social class, and health. He also promoted hygiene and health education in Czestochowa. An indefatigable worker and writer, Bieganski was the author of a well-known textbook of internal medicine (1891) and a monograph on the treatment of acute infectious diseases (1901).

In parallel, Bieganski produced a body of critical thinking on medical knowledge and medical practice. His best-known work in this area, *The Logic of Medicine* (1908), was translated into German and Russian. In it he argued that 'clinical logic' is different from—but not inferior to—scientific logic. Consequently, clinicians should strive to develop specific forms of medical understanding that are grounded in observations made at the bedside. Clinical science, he added, should not be confused with experimental biology. Medicine incorporates elements of the biological sciences, but only a small fraction of the factors that determine human health and illness can be studied in the laboratory. Accordingly, Bieganski was opposed to the reductionist tendencies of late nineteenth-century medicine. He proposed that medical science should focus on the sick person, not on isolated organs or tissues, and that a physician should never lose sight of medicine's ultimate goal—the reduction of pain and suffering.

Bieganski placed parallel emphasis on the moral dimension of medicine. He published studies on medical ethics, among them the highly popular (and still quoted in Poland) *Thought and Aphorisms on Medical Ethics* (1899). In the late nineteenth and early twentieth century the term 'medical ethics' was often synonymous with deontology, and writings on the subject focused on rules that regulated competition among doctors. Bieganski strongly criticized such corporatist attitudes. He affirmed, for example, that a patient who is dissatisfied with her doctor is entitled to a second or third opinion. Doctors who refuse to provide such opinions, in the name of solidarity with their colleagues disguised as 'professional ethics', are actually behaving in a deeply unethical way. Bieganski wrote that 'ethics requires that the consideration of good intraprofessional relations should be subordinated to the highest goal: the well-being of the patient'.

Bibliography

Primary: 1897. *General Problems of the Theory of Medical Sciences* [Polish] (Warsaw); 1899. *Thought and Aphorisms on Medical Ethics* [Polish] (Warsaw); 1908. *The Logic of Medicine or The Critique of Medical Knowledge* [Polish] (Warsaw).

Secondary: Löwy, Ilana, 2000. *Medical Acts and Medical Facts: The Polish Tradition of Practice-Grounded Reflection on Medicine and Science* (Cracow) pp. 45–67; Ziemski, Grzegorz and Marian Stanski, 1971. *Wladyslaw Bieganski, Physician and Philosopher* [Polish] (Poznan); Bieganska, Mieczyslawa, 1930. *Wladyslaw Bieganski, Life and Work* [Polish] (Warsaw).

Ilana Löwy

BIERNACKI, EDMUND FAUSTYN (b. Opoczno, Poland, 19 December 1866; d. Lwow, Ukraine, 29 December 1911), *internal medicine, hematology.*

Born into a family of impoverished Polish nobility, Biernacki developed a strong interest in scientific research during his medical studies. At first he became interested in physiology. He won the Gold Medal of Warsaw University for his studies of intravenous hydration with a saline solution, a method he proposed to apply to the treatment of diseases that induce a rapid loss of fluids. After his graduation in 1889, Biernacki received a scholarship to complete his medical training in Germany and in France. He studied physiology and hematology with Kühne in Heidelberg, Reigel in Giessen, and Hayem in Paris.

Back in Warsaw, however, Biernacki was unable to obtain an academic position. He worked as a clinician at the Wolski Hospital, opened a small private practice, and pursued in parallel investigations in physiology and hematology. He was probably the first to describe modifications in the sedimentation rate of red blood cells in numerous disorders and to propose (in 1897) the diagnostic use of the sedimentation test—a phenomenon later described independently by other hematologists. In 1902 Biernacki was named docent of pathology at the

University of Lwow (a city under Austrian occupation at that time). He also held a summer job at the health resort of Carlsbad, and in 1908 he was appointed to the chair of general pathology at Lwow University. He died three years later.

Between 1896 and 1905, Biernacki wrote articles and books that analyzed recent changes in medicine—especially the 'scientific turn' of medicine under the impulsion of physiology, and then bacteriology. The originality of those works was rooted in Biernacki's sharp awareness of the gap between the rapid progress of medical science and slow changes in the art of healing. The important advances in the understanding of pathological states had but limited effect on physicians' capacity to alleviate the sufferings of their patients.

In his best-known theoretical work, *The Essence and the Limits of Medical Knowledge* (1899), Biernacki argued that patients systematically confuse 'knowledge about disease' with the ability to cure it. They look for a physician who will make an accurate diagnosis, mistakenly believing that putting the right name on their suffering will automatically open the way to efficient elimination of its source. Alas, Biernacki explained, although doctors now know much better how to recognize a disease, they may not know how to cure it. They possess only a handful of truly efficient drugs and therapies, and in the great majority of cases they can only provide symptomatic treatment (such as painkillers) and psychological support. For that reason, the most successful physicians are often not those who are familiar with the latest developments in medicine, but those who know how to provide hope and consolation.

Biernacki concluded that there are three reasons why medicine, i.e., the art of curing diseases, cannot be transformed into a true science. One is the intrinsic complexity of human pathologies. The second is the impossibility of dissociating physiological and psychological determinants of disease—in his words, 'suggestion can influence in a positive way even the most material perturbations of vegetative functions of the organism'. The third reason is the close link between health and socioeconomic variables, or, as Biernacki put it, 'the best treatment for tuberculosis is money'.

Bibliography

Primary: 1899. *The Essence and the Limits of Medical Knowledge* [Polish] (Warsaw); 1900. *The Principles of Medical Understanding* [Polish] (Lodz); 1905. *What Is a Disease?* (Lwow).

Secondary: Löwy, Ilana, 1990. *The Polish School of Philosophy of Medicine: From Tytus Chalubinski (1820–1889) to Ludwik Fleck (1896–1961)* (Dordrecht) pp. 37–67; Zwozniak, Wladyslaw, 1964. 'The History of the Medical Department of Lwow University.' [Polish]. *Archiwium Historii Medycyny* 27: 193–226; Wrzosek, Adam, 1912. *Edmund Biernacki, 1866–1911* [Polish] (Krakow).

Ilana Löwy

BIGELOW, HENRY JACOB (b. Boston, Massachusetts, USA, 11 March 1818; d. Newton, Massachusetts, USA, 30 October 1890), *surgery.*

Bigelow's parents were Jacob Bigelow, a leading Boston physician, and Mary Scollay Bigelow. After completing his BA at Harvard in 1837, he attended medical lectures while serving an apprenticeship with his father. In 1840 he went to Cuba to recuperate from a respiratory problem, and subsequently traveled to Paris. He earned his MD at Harvard in 1841, and set out again to the French capital. Among the young English-speaking doctors there, he became particularly adept in the use of the stethoscope. Atypically, he was skeptical of Pierre Louis's numerical method.

In 1844 Bigelow returned to Boston and opened the 'Charitable Surgical Institution'. Work in this dispensary helped Bigelow develop a reputation as a skilled surgeon. He began teaching at the Tremont Street Medical School, and quickly became known as a talented teacher as well. Soon he was appointed visiting surgeon at Massachusetts General Hospital (MGH).

After witnessing the first use of inhalation ether in October 1846, Bigelow became a supporter of its application as an anesthetic and, as controversy developed about the relative merits of ether and other anesthetics, Bigelow experimented until he satisfied himself that ether was the safest. Interestingly, he remained a conservative operator, and expressed fear that the availability of anesthetics might encourage unnecessary surgery. He believed in avoiding pain whenever possible, especially as a patient was dying.

Bigelow married Susan Sturgis in 1847. She died in 1853, and Bigelow never remarried. Their one child, William Sturgis Bigelow, became a physician.

Within a year of his 1849 appointment as Professor of Surgery at Harvard, Bigelow was confronted with the case of Phineas Gage, a railroad worker who survived a crowbar pushed through his head. Bigelow's paper on Gage's case contributed to his renown. In 1852 he performed an excision of the hip, and he was associated with hip surgery for the rest of his career.

Bigelow was conservative in his thinking about medical education. He resisted Harvard President Charles Eliot's effort to introduce laboratory work to the curriculum, maintaining that vivisection would desensitize students to suffering. Believing in medicine as a beneficent calling, Bigelow opposed allowing attending staff at MGH to charge their private patients for care given in the hospital.

In surgery and surgical instrument design, he remained an innovator through the end of his career. In 1878, after three years of experimentation satisfied him that the urethra could be dilated sufficiently, he published a paper describing an improved instrument for crushing stones within the bladder and promptly washing them out. This device won him international acclaim. Bigelow resigned from Harvard in 1882, and from MGH in 1889.

Known as a brilliant operator with a dramatic style, Bigelow was the dominant surgeon in New England for several decades. His experiences in France as a young man left their mark on him in more ways than one, and he was perceived throughout his life as having a 'French manner'. He was a pioneer of surgical pathology, and one of the earliest Americans to make regular use of a microscope.

A patron of the arts, Bigelow was one of the first trustees of the Boston Museum of Art. He was a charismatic character, a great teacher, and played an important role on the Boston scene.

Bibliography

Primary: 1846. 'Insensibility during surgical operations produced by inhalation.' *Boston Medical and Surgical Journal* 25: 311–317; 1869. *Mechanism of Dislocation and Fracture of the Hip, with the Reduction of the Dislocations by the Flexion Method* (Philadelphia); 1871. *Medical Education in America: Being the Annual Address Read before the Massachusetts Medical Society, 7 June 1871* (Cambridge, MA).

Secondary: Macmillan, Malcolm, 2000. *An Odd Kind of Fame: Stories of Phineas Gage.* (Cambridge, MA); Mayo, William J., 1921. 'In the Time of Henry Jacob Bigelow.' *JAMA* 77: 597–603; Bigelow, William Sturgis, 1900. *A Memoir of Henry Jacob Bigelow, AM, MD, LLD* (Boston); *DAMB*.

Edward T. Morman

BIGELOW, JACOB (b. Sudbury, Massachusetts, USA, 27 February 1787; d. Boston, Massachusetts, USA, 10 January 1879), *botany, technology, medicine.*

Bigelow's parents were Jacob Bigelow, a clergyman and farmer, and Elizabeth Flagg Bigelow. As a child, Bigelow taught himself about the local flora, built devices such as animal traps and, against his father's advice, studied Latin. After graduating from Harvard College in 1806, he attended medical lectures at Harvard. In 1809, Bigelow went to the University of Pennsylvania to study medicine and take classes with botany professor Benjamin Smith Barton. He returned to Boston after earning his MD degree, joining the medical practice of James Jackson in 1811. In 1814, he published *Florula Bostoniensis*, based on his own botanical collections. In 1815 he was appointed lecturer in material medica at Harvard, and between 1817 and 1855 he served as professor in that subject. Bigelow's groundbreaking *American Medical Botany* appeared in 1817—the first American book to feature illustrations printed in color, using an aquatint technique developed by Bigelow himself.

In that same year Bigelow married Mary Scollay, with whom he had three children. One, Henry Jacob Bigelow (1818–90), became a leading surgeon.

Bigelow was a leader in the effort to produce the first edition of the *United States Pharmacopoeia*. Two years later he published 'Bigelow's Sequel', in which he urged a conservative approach to the remedies described in the pharmacopoeia. Over time, he became one of America's leading exponents of therapeutic skepticism. His gentle approach to treatment helped him develop an enormous consulting practice.

In the course of the first cholera pandemic to reach North America (1832), Boston's death toll was only one hundred, compared to the 8,000 in New York City. Despite the risk involved, Bigelow joined a three-man medical committee sent to New York to learn what they could from the devastation.

In 1825 Bigelow took the lead in establishing the earliest planned cemetery in the United States, at Mount Auburn. In doing this he was motivated by the common fear that crowded graveyards in densely populated areas endangered the public health—but also by an interest in providing a park-like space in Boston's outskirts. Bigelow himself landscaped this innovative facility.

In 1816 Bigelow became Professor of the Application of Science to the Useful Arts at Harvard College, a chair endowed by and named for Baron Rumford. This was the first effort to introduce engineering education at Harvard, and Bigelow created his own models and drawings to illustrate his lectures. In 1829 he published his Rumford lectures as *Elements of Technology*, the work that introduced the word 'technology' into common English discourse. He was later among the strongest supporters of the establishment of the Massachusetts Institute of Technology. He brought attacks on himself when, in 1865, he advocated abandoning the classics in higher education in favor of technical subjects.

Bigelow enjoyed a long and active retirement and retained his mental acuity until his final illness.

In medicine, Bigelow was most important for rejecting heroic remedies and articulating the notion of self-limited diseases. Thus, ironically, Bigelow's chief accomplishment in his main field of endeavor—based on his own clinical experience and his familiarity with contemporary French developments in pathology—led him to deny the efficacy of much of what he was supposed to teach.

Bibliography

Primary: 1817. *American Medical Botany, Being a Collection of the Native Medicinal Plants of the United States* . . . (Boston); 1829. *Elements of Technology* . . . (Boston); 1835. *A Discourse on Self-Limited Diseases* . . . (Boston).

Secondary: Wolfe, Richard J., 1979. *Jacob Bigelow's American Medical Botany, 1817-1821: An Examination of the Origin, Printing, Binding, and Distribution of America's First Color Plate Book* (North Hills, PA); Jarcho, Saul, 1969. 'Jacob Bigelow on Physical Diagnosis.' *American Journal of Cardiology* 23: 446-452; Ellis, George E., 1880. *Memoir of Jacob Bigelow, M.D., LL.D* (Cambridge, MA); *DAMB*.

Edward T. Morman

BIGGS, HERMANN MICHAEL (b. Trumansburg, New York, USA, 29 September 1859; d. New York, New York, USA, 28 June 1923), *bacteriology, public health.*

Descended from late seventeenth-century English immigrants to New England, Biggs attended Cornell University (1879–82), where he wrote a baccalaureate thesis on regulatory sanitation and the role of government in promoting public health—themes that would shape his entire later career. In 1883, Biggs earned his MD degree from Bellevue Hospital Medical College in New York City and, after a one-year internship at Bellevue, spent two years studying in Germany. For part of this time he worked in the laboratory of Robert Koch, the researcher who first isolated the tubercle bacillus.

Upon returning to the United States, Biggs was put in charge of the Carnegie Laboratory of the Bellevue Hospital Medical College. At the College, Biggs became lecturer on pathology (1886), professor of pathology (1889), professor of material medica and therapeutics (1892), professor of therapeutics (1898), and professor of the practice of medicine (1898).

In 1889 Biggs achieved notoriety as one of the coauthors of a report on steps to be taken to protect the people of New York City from tuberculosis. Three years later, he was appointed Director of Bacteriological Laboratories of the Department of Health of New York City. From this position, Biggs launched what would become a lifelong campaign to prevent the spread of tuberculosis through the regulatory means of city sanitation and surveillance of disease, coupled with the new laboratory-based bacteriological techniques that he had learned in Germany. Toward these ends, Biggs implemented a policy of compulsory notification of all cases of tuberculosis to the city's health department. At the New York City Health Department, he instituted school nursing, tuberculosis nursing, a tuberculosis clinic service, and a tuberculosis sanitorium. In 1894, he introduced the use of the diphtheria antitoxin and, in 1910, began a campaign to pasteurize New York City's milk supply. In 1911, Biggs launched a program of mandatory reporting of cases of venereal disease.

In 1913 Biggs resigned from the New York City Health Department to become Commissioner of Health for the State of New York. As commissioner, he developed a division of infant and maternity welfare. During World War I, Biggs served as a consultant to a number of institutions. He consulted with the Rockefeller Foundation in its effort to establish the first professional school for public health at Johns Hopkins University, and headed a Rockefeller Foundation commission that investigated tuberculosis in France. He also advised the Army Surgeon General's office on tuberculosis.

Biggs is widely regarded as one of the pioneers who implemented a new scientifically based public health system that was made possible because of advances in bacteriology in the latter half of the nineteenth century. The municipal bacteriological laboratory that Biggs created in New York City has been characterized as one of the first such laboratories in the world, and his methods of dealing with public health problems have been widely emulated.

Bibliography

Primary: 1904. 'Preventive medicine; its achievements, scope, and possibilities.' *Journal of the American Medical Association* 42 (June 11, 1904): 1550; 1907. 'Compulsory Notification and registration of tuberculosis. A discussion before the Advisory Council of the National Association for the Study and Prevention of Tuberculosis.' *Transactions of the National Association for the Study and Prevention of Tuberculosis* 3: 39; 1910. *The Administrative Control of Tuberculosis* (New York).

Secondary: Miller, Everett B., 1990. 'Bibliographic Briefs on Hermann M. Biggs, M.D., and Three Other Physicians—All Honorary Members of the American Veterinary Medical Association.' *Veterinary Heritage: Bulletin of the American Veterinary History Society* 13(2): 35–57; Winslow, C. E. A., 1929. *The Life of Herman M. Biggs, M.D., D.Sc., LL.D, Physician and Statesman of the Public Health* (Philadelphia); *DAMB*.

J. Rosser Matthews

BILLINGS, JOHN SHAW (b. near Allensville, Indiana, USA, 12 April 1838; d. New York, New York, USA, 11 March 1913), *military medicine, military surgery, public health, hygiene, medical bibliography, medical history.*

Billings's parents, James Billings and Abby Shaw Billings, were easterners who moved to rural Indiana a few years before his birth. Not meeting financial success in what was still a pioneering community, the family relocated to New York state, and then Rhode Island when Billings was a toddler. Both as a child in Rhode Island and after the family returned to Indiana when he was ten years old, Billings participated in his father's economic endeavors. He engaged in farm work, helped in storekeeping, and learned shoemaking, leaving him little opportunity for formal primary schooling. He read widely on his own, however, and studied Latin with a young clergyman. In order to pass the entrance examination for Miami University (Oxford, Ohio), he taught himself geometry and Greek. With a minimal level of financial support from his father, he earned his BA in 1857, at a time when very few American physicians took a liberal arts degree before entering medical school.

After graduation from Miami, he spent a year earning money for medical school by traveling and giving lectures illustrated by lantern slides. He entered the Medical College of Ohio (now the University of Cincinnati College of Medicine) in 1858, and completed his medical degree in 1860. Billings found the lectures less than useful, and spent his time on independent reading and seeking opportunities for dissection and clinical work. Upon completing the course, he was offered the position of demonstrator of anatomy.

Billings left Cincinnati for Washington, D.C., in September 1861, to join the Union Army as a contract surgeon. In 1862 he was commissioned as a lieutenant, and he also married Katharine Mary Stevens. The couple had four daughters and one son, who himself became a physician.

Billings's early postings were to supervise hospitals in Washington and Philadelphia, but in March 1863 he was reassigned to the Army of the Potomac. At the particularly bloody battles of Chancellorsville and Gettysburg, he distinguished himself by his surgical skill. After a few months, feeling the stress of battle, he was reassigned to various hospitals in or near New York. Following a secret mission to accompany back to the United States a group of blacks who had been taken from Virginia and abandoned in Haiti, he

rejoined the Army of the Potomac in March 1864, and served under Grant during the siege of Richmond. In August he began work on sections of the *Medical and Surgical History of the War of the Rebellion.*

In December 1864, a few months before the end of the Civil War, Billings was assigned to the office of the Surgeon-General, where his first assignment involved demobilizing the Army's medical department: organizing the Army's medical records, phasing out the system of army hospitals, and paying off the contract surgeons. In his free time he taught himself German. Assignment to Washington was a crucial development in Billings's career, enabling his administrative skills and interest in documentation to flourish. His most notable achievements there were connected with his leadership of the Library of the Surgeon-General's Office, based on his explicit intention to transform the collection of 2,000–3,000 poorly catalogued books into a national medical library.

Billings became skilled in Washington politics and, in a relatively short time, found the money that would allow him to purchase large numbers of monographs, periodicals, and pamphlets for the library. By the end of the nineteenth century, thanks to Billings's efforts, the Surgeon-General's library was the largest medical library in the United States; today, as the National Library of Medicine, it is the largest in the world.

Two projects that stand out as uniquely American contributions to both medicine and librarianship resulted from Billings's efforts in Washington. In 1879, as a private venture but based on the collection of the library, he began publishing the *Index Medicus*, a monthly classified index to the world medical literature. It survived until 2004, and is effectively continued by the MEDLINE database (from which it was compiled for several decades). Billings's other masterpiece of bibliography was the *Index-Catalogue of the Library of the Surgeon-General's Office*, an official publication funded by Congress, of which the first volume appeared in 1880. The *Index-Cat* was an author-subject catalog of the books and pamphlets in the collection, supplemented by interfiled subject entries for journal articles thought to be of lasting significance. The first series was published over the course of sixteen years, alphabetically listing acquisitions indexed up to the date of publication of each volume. A second series was begun in 1896, and a third in 1918. Arguably the single most valuable reference source for historians of medicine, the *Index-Cat* gained new life when, in April 2004, the National Library of Medicine announced a web-based digitized version.

Billings was also responsible for the expansion of the Army Medical Museum (which later evolved into the Armed Forces Institute of Pathology), and remained in charge of the museum and the library until his retirement from the Army in 1895. In addition to specimens, Billings accumulated an important collection of instruments, most notably microscopes. Again using his lobbying skills, he convinced

Congress to fund a new building to house both the museum and the library.

In no way were Billings's accomplishments during his thirty years in the Surgeon-General's Office limited to what he achieved in the library and museum, or even more broadly as a military medical officer. In 1869 and 1870, he surveyed the marine hospital system that had been established in 1798 to care for merchant seamen, and was operated by the Treasury Department. Based on his experience in the Civil War, Billings undertook two sanitary surveys of army camps. In 1872, Billings was among the founders of the American Public Health Association, and served as president of the organization in 1880. With others, he proposed a general sanitary survey of the United States in 1875, but funding was not forthcoming and the project was abandoned.

Billings was appointed Vice-President of the newly established National Board of Health (NBH) in 1879. Congress had authorized the NBH specifically for the purpose of coordinating port quarantine administration, which up to that time was fragmented among the states. Billings's vision of the NBH was much more expansive: he organized a sanitary survey of Memphis, Tennessee, where yellow fever had recently raged; he hoped to have the Board intervene more in matters of communicable disease, and to take on responsibility for both vital statistics and medical research. As it turned out, Billings resigned after a short time because of conflict between the NBH and the director of the Marine Hospital Service. The NBH was disbanded after only a few years and, ironically, the U.S. Public Health Service, successor to the Marine Hospital Service, ultimately took on many of the functions Billings had proposed for the NBH.

Billings's work in military hospital design and administration earned him a reputation in the civilian hospital world, and in 1875 he was one of five people invited to submit plans for the newly endowed Johns Hopkins Hospital. His proposal covered not only building design, but also plans for staffing and organization. Although the hospital did not open for another fourteen years, Billings was engaged as advisor to the trustees. He worked closely with Daniel Coit Gilman, the first President of Johns Hopkins University (which opened in 1875 as an entity distinct from the Hopkins Hospital), planning how to integrate training at the university's medical school with care in the hospital. An advocate of preclinical education in the basic sciences, he helped Gilman recruit William Osler and William Henry Welch to the hospital staff and as faculty members at the Johns Hopkins School of Medicine.

Billings's work with the Hopkins medical institutions certified him as an expert on design of building with sanitation and healthfulness in mind. In 1884 he published *Principles of Ventilation and Heating*, and was commissioned to design a new ventilation system for the United States Capitol building.

In 1870, with Joseph Janvier Woodward (a colleague in the Surgeon-General's Office and principal compiler of the *Medical and Surgical History of the War of the Rebellion*), Billings began addressing the problem of imperfect mortality statistics in the United States. He aggressively took on the problem of birth and death registration, and was responsible for vital statistics supplements to the 1880 and 1890 federal censuses. In the course of this work, Billings suggested the development of punched cards to Herman Hollerith, a statistician in the Census Bureau, and subsequently was responsible for the introduction of Hollerith cards for use in the 1890 census. While collection of vital statistics remained a state or local concern, Billings proposed the notion of a 'registration area' for the entire country, which local jurisdictions would be encouraged to join by improving their work in this field. It was not until 1933 that all states were included in the registration area. Current estimates are that more than 99 percent of births and deaths in the United States are recorded.

Billings did not apply himself greatly to laboratory research, although his interest in microscopy and photomicrography did lead to some interesting publications. On the other hand, he was among the most active proponents of scientific medicine in the United States. He made himself familiar with all advances in pathology and bacteriology, wrote and lectured extensively, and saw it as his responsibility to pass on to the larger medical and public health communities what he had learned from his own reading. In 1892 he planned the bacteriology laboratory at the University of Pennsylvania, and briefly served as Professor of Hygiene after leaving the Army in 1895. As a personal advisor to Andrew Carnegie, he helped develop the Carnegie Institute of Washington.

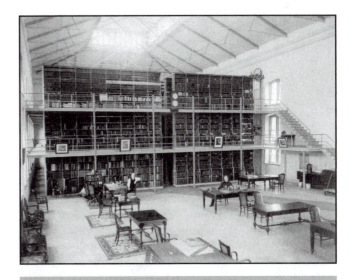

Library of the Surgeon General's Office. John Shaw Billings is seated at a table (center) with Thomas W. Wise to the left. Photograph, *c.* 1887–94, courtesy of the National Library of Medicine.

In 1878 Billings was among the founding members of the Cosmos Club, which fashioned itself as the gathering place for Washington's scientific and intellectual elite. He was elected to the National Academy of Sciences in 1883, and served as a member of its council from 1896 to 1907.

Billings left Washington in 1895 and, following his brief sojourn in Philadelphia, took on his final major project: consolidating three major private collections into the research libraries of the New York Public Library, and serving as its first director. As in so many of his endeavors, this project involved planning buildings as well as organizational structure. In his role as library director, he took advantage of his relations with Andrew Carnegie to convince him to provide the $5 million to build circulating branch libraries. Billings remained with the New York Public Library until his death.

The breadth of Billings's interests, the range of his accomplishments, and the depth of his vision make it impossible to assign him to any one field of endeavor. Perhaps what most unified his career was his post-Civil War view of the United States as a single unit, best served by national institutions of the highest quality and scientific integrity.

Bibliography

Primary: 1870. *A Report on Barracks and Hospitals; with descriptions of military posts* (Washington); 1883. 'Medical Bibliography.' *Transactions of the Medical and Chirurgical Faculty of Maryland* 85: 53–80; 1890. *Description of the Johns Hopkins Hospital* (Baltimore); 1891. 'The Conditions and Prospects of the Library of the Surgeon-General's Office and of its Index-Catalog.' *Transactions of the American Association of Physicians* 6: 251–257; 1965. (Rogers, Frank Bradway, ed.) *Selected Papers of John Shaw Billings* (Chicago).

Secondary: Chapman, Carleton B., 1994. *Order Out of Chaos: John Shaw Billings and America's Coming of Age* (Boston); Lydenberg, Harry Miller, 1924. *John Shaw Billings: Creator of the National Medical Library and Its Catalogue; First Director of the New York Public Library* (Chicago); Garrison, Fielding H., 1915. *John Shaw Billings: A Memoir* (New York).

Edward T. Morman

BILLROTH, CHRISTIAN ALBERT THEODOR (b. Bergen/Island of Rügen, Germany, 26 April 1826; d. Abbazia, Austria [now Opatija, Croatia], 6 February 1894), *surgery, musicology*.

Theodor was the eldest of five sons of a Lutheran pastor. After his father's death, when Theodor was only five, the mother moved to Greifswald, where her father, the mayor of the city, provided for his grandsons' education. Musically inclined, Billroth was only a below-average pupil at the *Gymnasium* because the piano was of greater interest to him. But his mother and Wilhelm Baum, the local surgery professor and friend of the family, insisted that Billroth attend a university. When, after one term at Greifswald, his mentor

took over the surgical chair at the University of Göttingen, Billroth followed him (1844).

Baum introduced the young man to the professorial circles of Göttingen. Georg Meissner, the future anatomist, was a stimulating senior medical student and a good violinist who became Billroth's lifelong friend. Together they accompanied the professor of physiology and anatomy, Rudolf Wagner, on a trip to the Adriatic to study the nervous system of certain fish. Thus, Billroth quickly acquired scientific interests, especially in histology. Nevertheless, he was an accomplished pianist, and he unforgettably accompanied the famous soprano, Jenny Lind, in a private concert.

Following his mother's death, Billroth moved to Berlin, where he obtained his MD (1852). In order to complete his education, he visited Vienna and Paris, the leading continental medical centers of the time. In Paris, and a few years later in London, the brutality with which hospital patients were treated shocked him. Unsuccessful as a general practitioner in Berlin, he became an assistant at the university surgical clinic headed by Bernhard Langenbeck. Billroth developed pathological histology with the aim of classifying tumors, thereby becoming Privatdozent for surgery and pathological anatomy (1856). Subsequently, he declined the chair of pathological anatomy in Greifswald and failed to obtain the Berlin one, which went to Rudolf Virchow. Accordingly, when offered the professorship of surgery in Zurich, Billroth chose a clinical rather than a research career (1860).

In Zurich he found a congenial environment and the possibility of developing his manifold talents as a reformer and teacher. Like Langenbeck, Billroth was preoccupied with improving wound healing at a time when suppuration and even sepsis were so frequent that mortality in major operations reached 80 percent in some Parisian hospitals. He introduced routine measurement of the body temperature in order to catch the beginning of a complication. Aware of the school of 'cleanliness and cold water' propagated by Thomas Spencer Wells in London, Billroth demanded 'cleanliness' for his sphere of activity. In 1865 Spencer Wells performed Switzerland's first ovarectomy as a guest in Billroth's clinic, where they discussed Wells's impressive results. In fact, precisely in that year, Wells published the results of his first 114 ovarectomies. He courageously faced criticism, for many still considered the abdominal cavity a *noli me tangere*, and he had had many failures in the beginning. But Wells 'rightly [made an] enormous impression' with his statistical honesty, and Billroth concluded, 'We ought to work more methodically' (Billroth, 1869, pp. 9, 12).

Billroth indeed followed Wells's example. His regular and complete reports of *all* the treatments in his clinic, grouped according to diagnosis, were a major accomplishment in surgical accountancy and publication practice, at least in German-speaking countries (from 1869). Although they were not the first statistical hospital reports, Billroth's were remarkable for their self-criticism in analyzing both successes and failures. Their author later regretted not having pursued the insight that to properly evaluate an intervention, one ought to compare its long-term outcome with the natural course of the disease. Billroth's frankness was also manifest in his concert reviews for a local newspaper.

Although the Zurich facilities seemed modest, Billroth rapidly gained international recognition. His textbook (1863) was re-edited and eventually translated into ten languages. He received offers from German universities, but since the local government was generous in regard to his requirements for working conditions and salary, he stayed in Zurich. However, he could not refuse the call in 1867 from the 'cosmopolitan city' of Vienna. His wife, Christel, the daughter of a Berlin court physician, was not demanding, but she was happy to leave the narrowness of Zurich, which she associated also with the death of their only son from scarlet fever.

In Vienna, Billroth continued to study ever-threatening wound disease. He knew Lister's papers on antiseptic surgery from the late 1860s, but considered Lister's methods an empirical fashion with insufficient scientific rationale. During the 1870 summer break, he gained practical experience in wartime wounds while volunteering in the Franco-Prussian War. His own theoretical work seemed to show that microscopic living beings (*Coccobacteria septica*) played only an incidental role in 'wound-fever', which he believed to be caused by the chemical processes of putrefaction (1874). Billroth's practical success with 'open-air treatment' and the known toxicity of carbolic acid caused him to belittle 'Listerism' for years. Convinced by Richard von Volkmann in Halle to at least give antiseptic surgery a try, he sent his assistants, Johannes von Mikulicz-Radecki and Anton Wölfler in 1877 and 1879, respectively, to visit Lister in London. When Mikulicz returned to Vienna enthusiastic, his mentor systematically introduced 'improved' antiseptics. Billroth was a scientific rationalist rather than an empiricist, and he was definitely convinced when Robert Koch's studies (admittedly influenced by Billroth's own research) established the causal connection between specific microorganisms and wound suppuration (1878). Koch's results came just in time for Billroth's next exploits in abdominal surgery.

Billroth also pursued statistical reporting. In 1879 his final report on the Vienna clinic, including the Zurich years, summarized sixteen years of experience. His book on *Krankheiten der Brustdrüse* [Diseases of the Mammary Gland] (1880) contained rates of recurrence, mortality, and cure of mammary disease. Cancer became his great challenge, and he focused even more decidedly on expanding the domain of operative surgery. The rationale behind an aggressive surgical approach to cancer lay in the prevalent medical theory of the time—cellular pathology. The extirpation of pathological tissues as extensively as possible seemed logical.

Besides holding a professorial chair, Billroth was the director of the *Operationsbildungsinstitut,* an institution that enabled licensed doctors to train in surgery at government expense for three years. He recruited collaborators from that elite group to work on his team. Laryngoscopy, for example, was well advanced in terms of diagnosis and conservative therapy, particularly in Vienna, so Billroth's group attempted excisions of the esophagus and the larynx in large canines. In that they followed Spencer Wells's practice. With an instrument-maker they studied gadgets that could make speech possible. Despite criticism, Billroth felt justified in extirpating the esophagus for the first time in 1872. It had been considered a hopeless case, but was successful in that the patient survived for some time. In 1873 Billroth had Carl Gussenbauer report on the first excision of the larynx and the use of an artificial larynx. Such generosity toward one's collaborators was quite unusual for the medical world at the time, but Billroth was proud of his 'family school'.

He initiated proven experimental procedures to attack gastrointestinal cancer, work that addressed several critical issues: What about the physiological consequences of partial resection of the stomach? How could the residual stump be united with the duodenum's much smaller lumen? Would the sutures withstand the acidity of gastric acid? Such questions were answered satisfactorily in the laboratory and published jointly (1876) by Billroth's assistants, Gussenbauer and Alexander Winiwarter.

Around the same time, Mikulicz was experimenting with electrically operated esophago-gastroscopes to improve diagnostics. Yet Billroth cautiously and responsibly waited until January 1881, when he had a patient whose advanced pyloric cancer seemed to warrant a daring resection of the stomach. The patient, a mother of eight living children, agreed. In contrast to earlier attempts by colleagues, Billroth's operation was a success: the patient survived for eighty-four days. That sensational outcome, still known as 'Billroth I', opened the way to gastrointestinal surgery. Wölfler followed in the same year with direct gastro-enterostomy, an operation circumventing an inoperable, obstructive stomach carcinoma. In 1885 Billroth used the same method after resection of the stomach ('Billroth II'). In 1890, he presented a report to one of those huge medical congresses (that he disliked attending) about the 124 resections on the gastrointestinal canal that had been performed in his clinic—eighty-three of them by himself. Those achievements in visceral surgery required, among other things, delicate suture technique, and they added enormously to his reputation. His Vienna clinic drew students and visitors from all over the world, particularly from the United States, and his pupils obtained key positions in many countries.

Initially enthusiastic about his and others' new possibilities for surgical cancer treatment, he gradually became skeptical—even depressed—when considering the long-term results of radical intervention. After becoming severely ill with pneumonia and 'heart disease' (1887), Billroth spent several weeks at a time in his country home in the Austrian lake district. In his later publications, he devoted himself to general issues of medicine, health care, philanthropy—and music. In his view, the scientific approach to medicine was not an end in itself, but a means to achieve patient welfare. In that spirit, he wrote a monograph (1876, followed by *Aphorisms*, 1886) on nuisances and abuses in the teaching and learning of medicine in German lands. It was translated into English in the context of Abraham Flexner's efforts to reform American medical education around 1910. The work generated a ministerial reprimand and public debate, in part because of some nationalistic comments that were interpreted as anti-Semitic in the atmosphere of contemporary Vienna. But Billroth certainly had no prejudices in that respect—one of his sons-in-law and his highly esteemed collaborators, Robert Gersuny and Anton Wölfler, were Jewish, as were many of his good friends.

The reform of the Austrian health system was of great concern to Billroth, and for that reason he was committed to the construction of the *Krankenanstalt Rudolfinerhaus*. It was to be a model hospital, with its own school for secular nurses who were to assume new roles in operative surgery. To promote the project he wrote a manual on nursing (1881) that saw its seventh edition as late as 1905. The hospital project faced fierce opposition, despite being supported by Crown Prince Rudolf (d. 1889), but it finally succeeded. Both the hospital and the nursing school are still in operation.

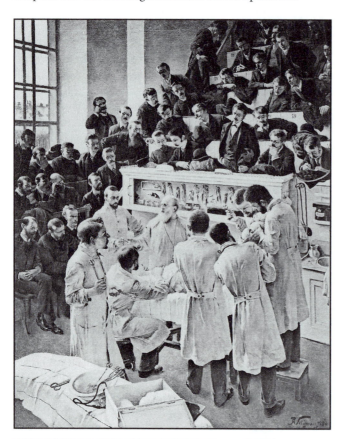

Theodor Billroth operating before students in Vienna, 1890. Painting by R. Seligman. Wellcome Library, London

Billroth continued to be an ardent musician. In his Zurich days, he had befriended Joseph Joachim and Johannes Brahms (who now lived in Vienna). Many of Brahms's new compositions were first heard in Billroth's home, a center of social activity that brought together leading artists and intellectuals of the culturally flourishing imperial capital. Billroth's psychophysiological treatise, *Wer ist musikalisch?*, was edited posthumously by his close friend Eduard Hanslick, the best-known Viennese music critic and theorist of the time. Such a colorful life reflected Billroth's generous, intuitive, sometimes exuberant, sometimes melancholy nature, and it was one of the reasons why he twice refused calls to prestigious chairs in Berlin (1869, 1882).

In 1887 he was appointed a member of the Austrian *Herrenhaus* [Upper Chamber]. He wrote that he was 'the first surgeon of the German nation, perhaps the world's most celebrated surgeon', yet he made only a tenth of the income of less-famous colleagues in Paris, London, St Petersburg, and Moscow (Kern, 1994, pp. 268–269). In fact, in 1889 he had to sell his house in Vienna, bought fourteen years earlier.

Billroth died during one of his much-desired stays on the Adriatic, survived by his wife and three of their four daughters. His cautious approach to great achievements in medicine; his self-critical attitude toward medical issues; his ability to foster teamwork; and his multifaceted, artistic personality are still considered exemplary and exceptional. Street names in Zurich and Vienna remind us of him.

Bibliography

Primary: 1863. *Die allgemeine chirurgische Pathologie und Chirurgie in fünfzig Vorlesungen* [16th edn., 1906; English edns., 1871, 1883] (Berlin); 1869–79. *Chirurgische Klinik* 4 vols [English edn., 1881] (Berlin); 1876. *Über das Lehren und Lernen der medicinischen Wissenschaften an den Universitäten der deutschen Nation* [English edn., 1924] (Vienna); 1881. *Über die Krankenpflege im Hause und im Hospitale* [English edn., 1890] (Vienna); 1881. 'Offenes Schreiben . . .' (on his first stomach resection) in *Wiener Medizinische Wochenschrift* 31: cols. 161–165.

Secondary: Kern, Ernst, 1994. *Theodor Billroth . . . Biographie anhand von Selbstzeugnissen* (Munich); Absolon, Karel B., 1979–87. *The Surgeon's Surgeon: Theodor Billroth*, vols. 1–3 (Lawrence, KS); vol. 4 (Rockville, MD); *DSB*.

Ulrich Tröhler

AL-BĪRŪNĪ (BERUNI) ABŪ RAYHĀN MUḤAMMAD B. AḤMAD (b. Beruni, Kath, Khwarazm, Uzbekistan, 15 September 973; d. Ghazna [now Ghazni], Afghanistan, 13 December 1048/1050), *medical botany.*

A universal scholar, Bīrūnī spent the first twenty-five years of his life in his native Kath, a suburb (*berun*) of Hwarizm. He was taught by Abū Naṣr Mansūr b. 'Alī b. Iraq Gilānī, the mathematician and Prince of the Banu Iraq family. Bīrūnī spoke the Iranian dialect of Khwarizm but deliberately chose to use the Arabic language in his scientific writings, though some later works may have been written in

Persian, or in both Arabic and Persian. Bīrūnī's biography can be traced from his records of astronomical events and the occasional dedications of his works to his patrons. Because of his command of various languages and an ingenious mind, he was entrusted with delicate political duties.

The period of the late tenth and early eleventh centuries was one of unrest in the region of Khwarazm. In 995 Bīrūnī fled Kath with the outbreak of civil war. Between 995 and 997, he probably spent some time in the cities of Rayy and Gilan. Later, from 1000 to 1003 (according to his works), he was at Gurgan, southeast of the Caspian Sea, and supported by Qābūs, the ruler of the Ziyarid state. The Prince 'Alī ibn Ma'mūn and his brother 'Abū'l 'Abbās Ma'mūn had ruled over Khwarazm. Through their marriages they were related to the great Maḥmūd, ruler of state at Ghazna (971?–1030), which would eventually take control of Khwarazm. Both 'Alī ibn Ma'mūn and 'Abū'l 'Abbās Ma'mūn were patrons of the sciences and provided generous support for Bīrūnī's scientific work. Next came a strange period during which there is evidence, in Bīrūnī's own writings, that he suffered great hardships, even though supported by Maḥmūd of Ghazna for his scientific work from 1018 until 1030, when Maḥmūd died. The relationship between Maḥmūd and Bīrūnī is unclear. It is likely that he was essentially Maḥmūd's prisoner and not free to leave. He may also have been a court astrologer. However, Maḥmūd's military excursions into India in 1022 meant that Bīrūnī was taken to the northern parts of that country. He may have wished for better treatment from Maḥmūd, but Bīrūnī's scientific work certainly benefited. His work *India* was written as a direct result of the studies he made while in that country.

Maḥmūd's son and successor, Mas'ūd, proved to be a ruler who treated Bīrūnī more kindly than his father had done. Bīrūnī dedicated his so-called *Mas'ūdic canon*—which contained a table with the coordinates of 600 places, almost all of which he had direct knowledge—to Mas'ūd. Mas'ūd was murdered in 1040 and succeeded by his son Mawdūd, who ruled for eight years. By this time Bīrūnī was an old man, but he continued his enormous output of scientific work right up to the time of his death.

Bīrūnī was an extremely accurate observer and an ingenious logician, making him an original thinker. Many of his discoveries were made through careful calculations. His ideas frequently originated in discussions and arguments with other eminent scholars (e.g., his teacher Abū Naṣr Manṣūr, Avicenna, and as-Sijzī). Some forty of Bīrūnī's works survived; however, during his lifetime he produced around 180 works on different subjects: mathematics, cartography, spherical trigonometry, geometry, astronomy, astrology, calendars, weights and measures, chronology, history, literature, and medicine. He was amazingly well read, having knowledge of Greek and Sanskrit literature, and his sharp observations of the use of Arabic script for scientific purposes are remarkable. His medical writings comprise various remarks on medical or related subjects in numerous works, as well as

his famous *Ṣaydala fī 't-Ṭibb*. This is the work of a mature master who had an exhaustive personal knowledge of materia medica as well as an appreciation of the world's scholarship on this subject. *Ṣaydala fī 't-Ṭibb* includes an alphabetical list of drugs along with descriptions of their properties.

Bibliography

Primary: 1914. (ed. Sachau, E. C.) *Alberuni's India: an account of the religion, philosophy, literature, geography, chronology, astronomy, customs, law and astrology of India about A.D. 1030* (London); 1973. *Al-Bīrūnī's book on pharmacy and materia medica* (Sa'id, Hakim Muhammed, Sami Khalaf Hamarneh, and Rana Ihsan Ilahi, eds., and English translation) (Karachi); 1991. *In den Gärten der Wissenschaft: ausgewählte Texte aus den Werken des muslimischen Universalgelehrten* (al-Bīrūnī, übersetzt und erläutert von Gotthard Strohmeier) (Leipzig).

Secondary: Rosenfeld, B. A., and E. Ihsanoglu, 2003. *Mathematicians, Astronomers and Other Scholars of Islamic Civilisation and Their Works (7th–19th c.)* no. 348 (Istanbul); *DSB*.

Nikolaj Serikoff

BIZZOZERO, GIULIO CESARE

BIZZOZERO, GIULIO CESARE (b. Varese, Italy, 20 March 1846; d. Turin, Italy, 8 April 1901), *pathology, histology, hematology.*

Bizzozero, son of Felice Bizzozero, a small manufacturer, and Carolina Veratti, attended the humanities Lyceum at Milan. Then he studied medicine at Pavia under Eusebio Oehl, Arnaldo Cantani, and Salvatore Tommasi, all strongly connected to the emerging German medicine. After graduating with honors in 1866, he enrolled as a volunteer in Garibaldi's army. Bizzozero's academic career was characterized by strong obstacles, but also by strong support. After the unification of the Italian Kingdom (1860), the Ministry of Education was in search of young, promising physicians and scientists to carry out the necessary institutional and didactical reforms. It was people like Bizzozero in whom the Ministry invested. In 1868, he obtained an Italian government scholarship to improve his skills in the laboratories of microscopist Heinrich Frey (Zurich) and cellular pathologist Rudolf Virchow (Berlin). In 1869, at the age of twenty-three, he replaced his master, Paolo Mantegazza, in lecturing on general pathology and histology. In 1872 he became ordinary professor of general pathology in Turin, where he remained for the rest of his life, offering also practical courses in histology and microscopy.

During the first years at Turin, Bizzozero had to overcome great institutional obstacles. For the first three years he was obliged to install a laboratory in his private house. Through his perseverance and political talent, in 1876 he obtained a small laboratory and, in 1881, a 'gabinetto'. Bizzozero was an exhilarating teacher, attracting numerous students from all over Italy, among them Camillo Golgi, Pio Foà, Guido Tizzoni, Edoardo Bassini, and Carlo Forlanini. He supplied them with thorough theoretical instruction, and excellent

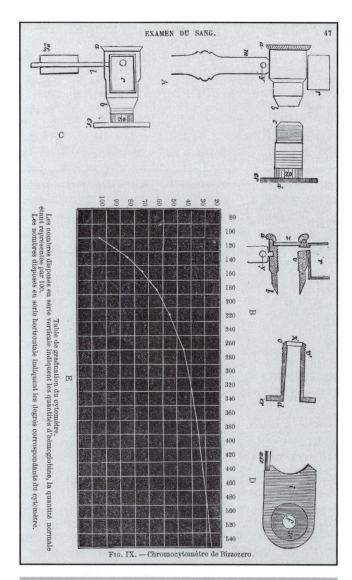

EXAMEN DU SANG.   47

Fig. IX. — Chromocytomètre de Bizzozero.

Bizzozero's chromocytometer and haemoglobin graduation graph. Lithograph from *Manuel de microscopie clinique . . .*, 2nd edition, Paris, 1885. Wellcome Library, London.

training in normal histology and cytology, and in clinical microscopy, transforming Turin in the 1880s into the center of Italian pathology and cytology. Bizzo- zero's importance for the introduction of microscopy and cytology into Italian medicine earned him the title of 'Italian Virchow'.

Bizzozero's research was basically morphological, and covered a wide range of histological topics. Combined with his mastery of microscopical techniques, he made several extraordinary discoveries (many of them rediscovered and appreciated only decades later). In 1876 he founded the journal, *Archivio per le scienze mediche*, to propagate the results of the new positivistic medical research. In 1897 he became editor of *Rivista d'igiene e sanità pubblica*, a journal that gave voice to physicians engaged in diffusing social medicine and public health. Bizzozero made use of his political influence to call phy-

sicians like Cesare Lombroso, Pio Foà, and Camillo Bozzolo to Turin, and to promote many of his students to academic chairs. In 1885 he was elected rector of the University of Turin. In this period he was also appointed member of many governmental committees, member of the Akademie der Wissenschaften of Berlin (1888), and senator of the Italian Kingdom (1890).

Connective Tissue, Epithelia, and Epithelioma

In 1862, at the age of sixteen, Bizzozero published his first scientific paper while working in the laboratory of experimental pathology of Paolo Mantegazza at Pavia. In the 1860s, Pavia was one of the main centers of microscopical studies in Italy, but also one of the strongholds of the advocates of spontaneous generation. With the intention of disproving Rudolf Virchow's aphorism, *Omnis cellula e cellula* [all cells from cells], Mantegazza charged his assistant Bizzozero to furnish him with the illustrations for his work on inflamed connective tissue. Bizzozero, however, confirmed Virchow's maxim, and made his first important discoveries (1865–66): the structure of loose connective tissue and the role of the mobile cells, discovered three years earlier by Friedrich Daniel von Recklinghausen. Bizzozero called them 'wandering polyplastic cells', and described their capacity to regain, under certain conditions, the functions of embryonic (stem) cells. In 1866, he demonstrated that granulation tissue originated as a consequence of the proliferative activity of these mobile cells, accompanied by a neoformation of blood capillaries.

His work on epithelial tissues was likewise important. In 1864, 1870, and 1886, he published studies on the cells of the Malpighian layer and of the stratified squamous epithelium. He also investigated the epithelium of the gastric and intestinal glands of mammals (1888–93). In 1872, Bizzozero showed that epitheliomas originate in the epithelial tissue. Thus he proved their homologous origin. Likewise he confuted the exclusive role of connective tissues that Virchow had assigned them for the origin of tumors. In the same year, Bizzozero published a paper that related all known types of neoplasm to their respective tissues of origin. In the 1880s, directing or collaborating with many of his students, he continued to study the role of connective tissue for normal and pathological histology, demonstrating the presence of karyokinetic figures around inflamed foci (1885), and developing a new technique for the quantification of the mitotic activity of various tissues (1886).

Hematology

Since his time as a student of Mantegazza, Bizzozero had made observations on the histology of the bone marrow. During this period he noticed colorless cells showing amoeboid movements. Focusing his attention on these cells, he furnished evidential proof for the hypotheses about their function that had been made of late by other researchers. In 1868, Bizzozero published *Sulla funzione ematopoietica del midollo delle ossa*, a paper that made him prominent contemporaneously but independently from Ernst Neumann, the discoverer of the hemato-poietic function of the bone marrow. A decade later, in 1879, Bizzozero developed a new apparatus, the chromocytometer, to quantify the hemoglobin in the blood.

In 1881 Bizzozero made his most famous discovery, the blood platelets, and published articles in various Italian, German, and British journals. The platelets had already been described by Max Schultze (1865), Louis Ranvier (1873), and Georges Hayem (1878), but these researchers had given a distorted image and completely ignored the function of the observed 'granular masses'. Bizzozero developed a new technique that enabled him to investigate the histology of the blood in living guinea pigs. He noticed very small, oval or round, colorless bodies circulating in addition to the elements already known. Thus, Bizzozero demonstrated that platelets represented a normal and constitutive element of mammalian blood. In a subsequent series of experiments, he proved the temporal concomitance between the beginning of coagulation and the morphologic alteration of the platelets, concluding that they carried out an important function in the phenomenon of thrombosis.

Phagocytosis

Between 1870 and 1872, Bizzozero treated the much-discussed question of the origin of pus granules in a series of papers. Many influential physicians, such as Julius Cohnheim (1867), had expressed themselves in favor of an endogenetic origin of the purulent corpuscles in infected tissues. Even Rudolf Virchow, the most famous opponent of the spontaneous generation of cells, admitted an exception in this special case. Bizzozero's *Saggio di studio sulla cosidetta endogenesi del pus* appeared in 1872. Experimentally inducing a hypopyon— an inflammation causing the accumulation of pus in the anterior chamber of the eye—in a rabbit, Bizzozero observed that the pus did not originate spontaneously inside the 'bigger cells' generally observed to appear in inflamed tissues. Rather, he showed that the big, mobile, and contractile cells, originating from the connective tissue and moving into the inflamed tissues, actively incorporated the purulent corpuscles. Thus, Bizzozero was the first to have exactly described the process of phagocytosis. He had already observed a similar phenomenon occurring in bone marrow with pigment granules and erythrocytes. He even intuited that the phenomenon constituted a mechanism to absorb and eliminate extraneous elements. About ten years later, Elie Mechnikov, quoting and praising the work of Bizzozero, redescribed the phenomenon, interpreted it correctly, and transformed it into his well-known theory of phagocytosis (1882).

Classification of Tissues

After 1890, Bizzozero's eyesight was impaired by a serious form of choroiditis, preventing him from proceeding with his microscopical investigations. He then published many contributions on public health and vaccination, and devoted himself to a program to combat infectious diseases

that he had been developing since 1883. He likewise overcame his profound reticence to the formulation of theories, which he considered nonscientific speculations, and turned his attention toward more general aspects of his many years of research. On the occasion of the Eleventh International Medical Congress held in 1894 in Rome, Bizzozero proposed a new classification of cells based on their capacity to reproduce and regenerate. He distinguished three groups of cells: the 'labile cells', that continue to multiply throughout their life with a succession of apoptosi and regeneration; the 'stable cells', that multiply until they have reached a certain degree of specificity; and the 'perennial cells', that have lost their capacity to reproduce. It was his last scientific contribution. In April 1901 Bizzozero fell ill with acute pulmonary pleura, and died a few days later at the premature age of fifty-five.

Bibliography

Primary: 1905. *Le opere scientifiche di Giulio Bizzozero. Introduzione del prof. Camillo Golgi* 2 vols. (Milan); 1880. *Manuale di microscopia clinica. Con aggiunte riguardanti l'uso del microscopio nella medicina legale* (Milan) (2nd edn., 1882; 5th edn., 1901; translated into German, French, Russian, Danish, Spanish, and Japanese).

Secondary: Accademia di Medicina di Torino, 2001. *Convegno per il centenario della morte di Giulio Bizzozero* (Turin); Dröscher, Ariane, 1998. 'La Cellularpathologie (1858) di Rudolf Virchow e il rinnovamento della medicina italiana nella seconda metà dell'Ottocento.' *Annali dell'Istituto storico italo-germanico in Trento* 24: 87–112; Dianzani, Mario Umberto, 1994. 'Bizzozero and the Discovery of Platelets.' *American Journal of Nephrology* 14: 330–336; Gravela, Enrico, 1989. *Giulio Bizzozero* (Turin); *DSB*.

Ariane Dröscher

BLACKLEY, CHARLES HARRISON   (b. Bolton, Lancashire, England, 5 April 1820; d. Southport, England, 4 September 1900), *allergy, homeopathy, medicine.*

Blackley was born in Bolton but was raised and educated in Manchester after his father died when Charles was only three years old. He worked initially as an apprentice printer and engraver to the firm of Bradshaw and Blacklock, but he also attended evening classes in chemistry, botany, and Greek, and developed a particular interest in homeopathy. In 1855, he left the printing business and enrolled at the Pine Street Medical School in Manchester. After qualifying in 1858, Blackley practiced as a general practitioner in Hulme, Manchester, but became increasingly committed to the study and practice of homeopathy. He was a member of the British Homoeopathic Society, and an honorary member of the Manchester and Salford Homoeopathic Dispensary. In addition, he edited the *Manchester Homoeopathic Observer*, and published articles on homeopathy in professional journals. In 1874, Blackley completed a doctorate of medicine at the University of Brussels.

In 1859, Blackley had begun a series of detailed experiments on the etiology and pathogenesis of hay fever, from which he had himself suffered for many years. Like contemporaries in North America, such as Morrill Wyman (1812–1903) and George Beard (1839–83), Blackley was particularly concerned to determine the precise cause of hay fever. Although most writers acknowledged that predisposing constitutional factors played a crucial role, there were disputes about the relative contributions of a range of precipitating or exciting causes of individual attacks of the disease. Using both himself and his patients as subjects, Blackley effectively dismissed previous accounts of hay fever which had emphasized the role of benzoic acid, coumarin, various odors, animal danders, ozone, dust, and the influence of heat and light. In an expansive monograph first published in 1873, Blackley emphatically concluded that hay fever was the direct product of exposure to pollen. Accordingly, he advised patients to alleviate their symptoms by traveling to coastal or mountainous regions (or in some cases to the center of a large town) in order to avoid pollen clouds during the summer months.

Blackley's investigations were notable for the assiduity with which he assessed and eliminated competing causes of hay fever; for his elaboration of novel apparatuses for collecting, measuring, and charting the seasonal distribution of pollen in the atmosphere; and for his careful description of skin testing for pollen sensitivity. Although Blackley's publication was favorably reviewed in medical journals, his belief that pollen was the sole proximate cause of hay fever was not universally accepted by his contemporaries. Drawing on the explanatory power of germ theories of disease in this period, some authors stressed the role of organisms in the nasal secretions of hay fever sufferers, or emphasized the impact of modern lifestyles. In 1903, however, Blackley's preoccupation with pollen found influential support from the research of William P. Dunbar (1863–1922), an American physician who was Director of the State Hygienic Institute in Hamburg.

Believing that hay fever was largely 'an aristocratic disease' which was particularly prevalent among members of the learned professions such as theology and medicine, Blackley suggested that rising trends in hay fever could be traced in part to the shifting agricultural practices and demographic transformations wrought by the processes of industrialization. In addition, however, he presaged modern debates about allergies by linking trends in hay fever to the growth of civilization, warning that 'as population increases and as civilisation and education advance, the disorder will become more common than it is at the present time' (Blackley, 1873, p. 162).

Bibliography

Primary: 1873. *Experimental Researches on the Causes and Nature of Catarrhus Aestivus (Hay-Fever or Hay-Asthma)* (London); 1880. *Hay Fever: Its Causes, Treatment, and Effective Prevention: Experimental Researches* (London); 1882. 'On the influence of infinitesimal quantities in inducing physiological action.' *Homoeopathic Review* 26: 604.

Secondary: Jackson, Mark, 2006. *Allergy: The History of a Modern Malady* (London); Waite, Kathryn, 1995. 'Blackley and the Development of Hay Fever as a Disease of Civilization in the Nineteenth Century.' *Medical History* 39: 186–196; Emanuel, M. B., 1988. 'Hay Fever, a Post Industrial Revolution Epidemic: A History of Its Growth during the Nineteenth Century.' *Clinical Allergy* 18: 295–304; Taylor, G., and J. Walker, 1973. 'Charles Harrison Blackley, 1820–1900.' *Clinical Allergy* 3: 103–108.

Mark Jackson

BLACKWELL, ELIZABETH (b. Bristol, England, 3 February 1821; d. Hastings, Sussex, England, 31 May 1910), *medical education, medicine.*

Blackwell was the third of nine children of Samuel Blackwell (sugar refiner, Congregationalist, and anti-slavery campaigner) and Hannah Lane. At her father's insistence, she and her four sisters received an education from private tutors comparable to that of their brothers; all absorbed their father's interest in moral reform.

Because of business difficulties, Samuel Blackwell moved the family to the United States in 1832; he died in 1838 leaving little. Blackwell and her two older sisters set up a school to support the family, and she continued to teach, although she disliked it. Her decision about 1844 to enter the medical profession stemmed from several considerations: the suggestion of a friend dying of uterine cancer, who would have consulted a doctor sooner had there been a woman doctor; Blackwell's search for an engrossing, worthwhile activity; her desire to dissociate the term 'female physician' from abortionists; and her desire to avoid dependence on a man through marriage.

Fulfilling her ambition was difficult. Alongside teaching, she studied medicine privately with doctors, and made sixteen unsuccessful applications to medical schools. Finally, a small medical school in Geneva, New York, accepted her; she graduated MD in 1849. Later that year she traveled to Paris for further training, enrolling at La Maternité, the leading school for midwives. She contracted purulent ophthalmia from a patient and lost one eye and part of the sight in the other, ending her ambition to be a surgeon, but leaving her determined to practice as a physician. In 1850 she visited London, worked under Sir James Paget at St Bartholomew's hospital, and was welcomed in social circles surrounding the emerging women's movement.

Blackwell set up practice in New York City in 1851. She had few patients, but opened a dispensary for poor women, extending it in 1857 with her sister Emily (1826–1910) and Marie Zakrzewska (1829–1902), to establish the New York Infirmary for Women and Children, run by women where many early, formally qualified women doctors in the United States gained clinical experience.

In 1858 Blackwell visited Britain. A clause in the new Medical Act recognized doctors with foreign degrees practicing in Britain before 1858; thus she became the only woman on the medical register when it was initiated in 1859. During the visit she lectured extensively, influencing Elizabeth Garrett Anderson (1836–1917) who, in 1865, became the second woman on the medical register.

Blackwell returned to New York in 1859, where she developed the Infirmary both as a hospital and a place of education. During the Civil War (1861–65), she organized nursing services for the Union Army. In 1868 the Infirmary's medical school (Woman's Medical College of the New York Infirmary) formally opened, but relations with her sister Emily became strained. In 1869 Blackwell returned to Britain, where she lived on income from investments, first in London and from 1879 in Hastings, with summers in Scotland, where she is buried.

Although largely retired from medical practice after 1869, Blackwell was a member of the council and lecturer at the London School of Medicine for Women when it formally opened in 1875. Wider social reform absorbed her energies. She helped found the National Health Society, promoting sanitary and hygiene instruction with the slogan, 'prevention is better than cure;' she campaigned against the Contagious Diseases Acts in the 1870s, and in favor of social and sexual purity in the 1880s; and she opposed animal experimentation and germ theories. Two basic views underlay her writing and career: disease was due to failure to adhere to the moral laws of healthy living, in contrast to materialist medicine where ill health resulted from a chance encounter with germs or physiological malfunctions; and women were guardians of social purity and hence health, with women doctors uniquely contributing to society by safeguarding the links between medicine and morality, and emphasizing prevention through hygiene. Such views brought her into conflict with medical women who followed her, such as Elizabeth Garrett Anderson and Mary Putnam Jacobi (1842–1906), who did not oppose germ theory, animal experimentation, or major abdominal surgery. These differences represent distinct approaches to medicine and women in medicine that have been passed on to succeeding generations.

Bibliography

Primary: 1895. *Pioneer Work in Opening the Medical Profession to Women: Autobiographical Sketches* (London); 1898. *Scientific Method in Biology* (London).

Secondary: Morantz-Sanchez, R. M., 1985. *Sympathy and Science: Women Physicians in American Medicine* (New York); Forster, M., 1984. *Significant Sisters: The Grassroots of Active Feminism, 1839–1939* (London); Morantz-Sanchez, R. M., 1982. 'Feminism, Professionalism and Germs: the Thought of Mary Putnam Jacobi and Elizabeth Blackwell.' *American Quarterly* 34: 459–478; *DAMB; Oxford DNB.*

Marguerite Dupree

BLALOCK, ALFRED (b. Culloden, Georgia, USA, 5 April 1899; d. Baltimore, Maryland, USA, 15 September 1964), *surgery.*

Blalock graduated MD from Johns Hopkins (Baltimore) in 1922. He was professor of surgery at Vanderbilt University 1938–41 but returned to Johns Hopkins, where he

remained for the rest of his career. He was President of the American Association for Thoracic Surgery (1951). He died three months after his retirement from a professional career characterized by energy and zest. He was evidently a popular and likeable man, appearing in photographs with an engaging smile and sporting a cigarette in a holder.

His early career was already distinguished by surgical achievements such as performing the dissection of a pneumonectomy in a three-year-old, and relieving myasthenia by removing a tumor of the thymus gland. The relationship between myasthenia, thymic tumors, and the removal of the thymus gland remains incomprehensible. He was interested in research in shock, and placed great emphasis on an understanding of physiology. He cautioned against rushing to open the chest after a stabbing or other penetrating injury, advocating the practice of drawing blood out of the pericardium with a needle and returning it to the circulation, hoping that the bleeding would be contained and cease. This was in line with instructions to army medical officers (1942) in the management of heart injuries. Blalock's theory presented a difficulty to Dwight Harken (1910–93), the young Boston surgeon who was working in the military hospital in Cirencester, England, removing bullets from the hearts and great vessels of soldiers.

While at Vanderbilt, Blalock had been experimenting with surgical diversion of arterial blood flow to create pulmonary hypertension. This led to experiments in the relief of coarctation by diverting the subclavian artery to bypass a narrowing created in a dog. His pediatrician colleague, Helen Taussig (1898–1986), was concerned with treating blue babies. In particular, these were children with Fallot's tetralogy, where the combination of a hole in the heart (a ventricular septal defect) and obstruction of the pulmonary blood flow allows deoxygenated blood to bypass the lungs. Taussig is credited with the idea of surgically diverting blood back toward the lungs. Blalock worked on this with his black technician, Vivien T. Thomas (1910–1985). When it came to surgery on children, Thomas was close in behind Blalock, and there is no doubt that his advice on how and where to place sutures was gladly taken by Blalock. This relationship was eventually recognized in Thomas's obituaries.

At the time, a close relationship existed between Guy's Hospital (London, England) and Johns Hopkins, and surgical traveling by the leading surgeons was usual. Blalock performed a series of these operations in London, and Russell C. Brock (1903–80) did the first mitral valvotomy operations in Baltimore. The first child operated on in London was taken to a public meeting in a nurse's arms, an event reported in all of the accounts. These surgical 'firsts' were widely publicized, and the surgeons lionized.

An additional eponymous operation was the Blalock-Hanlon shunt (1950). In another form of congenital heart disease causing 'blue babies', transposition of the great arteries, life is sustainable only if the right and left sides can mix. This operation allowed the blood to mix in the atria, as opposed to the arterial mixing created by the Blalock-Taussig operations.

Perhaps Blalock's preference for conservatism in the management of penetrating wounds of the heart is in keeping with the fact that his surgical career was dominated by the palliation of cyanotic heart disease (blue babies), and noted for the two operations that bear his name. He preferred these to the more direct approach to correcting the heart itself, as favored by his British contemporary, Brock. At the time, operations were being performed on the great vessels around the heart, but surgery within the heart itself was not being attempted.

Bibliography

Primary: 1945. (with Taussig, Helen) 'The surgical treatment of malformations of the heart in which there is pulmonary stenosis or pulmonary atresia.' *JAMA* 128: 189–202; c. 1966. (Ravitch, Mark M., ed.) *The Papers of Alfred Blalock* 2 vols. (Baltimore, MD).

Secondary: Shumaker, H. B., 1992. *The Evolution of Cardiac Surgery* (Bloomington, IN); *DAMB*.

Tom Treasure

BLAND, WILLIAM   (b. London, England, 5 November 1789; d. Sydney, Australia, 21 July 1868), *surgery, invention, politics.*

The second son of Robert Bland, a gynecologist, William Bland attended Merchant Taylors' School before being apprenticed to his father. In 1809 he qualified as a surgeon's mate in the Royal Navy and was promoted to surgeon three years later. While serving in India, he was involved in a duel with a fellow officer resulting in that man's death. Convicted of murder, Bland was sentenced to seven years in a penal colony. He arrived in Australia as a convict early in 1814. There were no private medical practitioners in Sydney, so Bland was pardoned in 1815 to begin the first full-time medical practice in the colony. He was soon in court again, however, after an officer eloped with his wife; he was never able to collect the damages awarded.

Always an impetuous, argumentative man, within three years Bland was convicted for publishing defamatory pamphlets about Governor Macquarie and was sentenced to twelve months' imprisonment. After completing that sentence, Bland resumed medical practice, beginning a long association with the Benevolent Society (1821–63). He was also on the staff of the Sydney Dispensary (1826–45) and dispensed medicines to the poor from his home. In 1859 he became the first president of the original Australian Medical Association.

Bland was a resourceful surgeon, improvising his own instruments for complex procedures such as repairing aneurysm of the subclavian artery (1832). He was also noted for his ability in removing cataracts from eyes and stones from the bladder.

His inventive mind devised solutions for other problems that beset the English antipodes. In 1843 he published proposals for suppressing spontaneous fires in ships carrying wool from Australia by circulating carbon dioxide gas through the holds of the ships. That procedure would eventually become standard fire-fighting practice. In 1855 he published designs for an even more ambitious project, an 'Atmotic Ship' that he imagined would reduce the journey from Australia to England to less than a week. That invention was a prototype Zeppelin, consisting of a large, gas-filled balloon powered by steam engines and sails: models of those devices attracted much interest when they were exhibited in London.

Bland's restless energy was channeled into politics as well. Given his background, it is not surprising that he advocated trial by jury, and an elected government in place of autocratic rule by the colonial governor. He was elected to Australia's first representative body in 1843, serving on the Legislative Council on three occasions until 1861. Although he was nominated for the Senate of the University of Sydney, that appointment did not proceed because there was vehement resistance to the notion of a former convict being connected with university administration.

Bland was able to help in the educational development of the colony in other ways, notably through his involvement in the establishment of Sydney College and the School of Arts. He amassed considerable wealth that enabled him to be a generous supporter of those institutions and the Church. Bland's elegant carriage, painted a dazzling yellow, was a familiar sight as he conducted his medical rounds in mid-nineteenth-century Sydney. His philanthropy and his extravagant lifestyle resulted in bankruptcy in 1861. Nevertheless, he continued active medical practice until his death from pneumonia in 1868, when he was accorded a state funeral.

A daguerreotype image of William Bland in the Mitchell Library, Sydney, is the earliest known photograph taken in Australia (c. 1845).

Bibliography

Primary: 1832. 'Operation of tying the arteria innominata'. *Lancet* ii: 97–101; 1848. 'Report of a case of snake-bite'. *Lancet* i: 71–72.

Secondary: McIntosh, A. M., 1954. 'The Life and Times of William Bland.' *Bulletin of the Post-Graduate Committee in Medicine* (Sydney), 10(6): 109–152; Dunlop, N. J., 1926. 'Dr William Bland.' *Journal of the Royal Australian Historical Society* 11: 321–351; *AuDB*.

Peter J. Tyler

BLANKAART, STEVEN   (b. Middelburg, the Netherlands, 24 October 1650; d. Amsterdam, the Netherlands, 23 February 1704), *anatomy, botany, pharmacology, lexicography.*

Blankaart was the eldest son of Maria Eversdijck (1628–74) and Nicolaas Blankaart (1624–1703). He began his career as an assistant apothecary in Amsterdam. In 1671 he went to study medicine in Franeker, where he graduated in philosophy and medicine on 18 December 1674. He set up a medical practice in Amsterdam, where he worked on a long list of publications. His works included Dutch editions of Hippocrates, Lucianus, Santorio, Digby, Descartes, and others; a French edition of Bontekoe; and many works of his own on geographical names, insect anatomy, botany, chemistry, pathology, pharmacology, human anatomy, surgery, and other subjects. On 3 March 1682, Blankaart married Isabella de Carpentier (1644–1730). The couple had two sons, Nicolaas (1682–88) and Willem (1683–1748). Blankaart died in Amsterdam in 1704 and was buried in the Westerkerk on 28 February.

Blankaart explained the workings of the human body in iatromechanical and partly iatrochemical terms. Health depended on the flow and agitation of the liquid and airy substances contained in the body's organs, vessels, and nerves. However, as the preface to his *Kartesiaanse academie* (*Cartesian Academy*) of 1683 indicates, the term 'Cartesian' merely suggested an approach to medicine that was based on natural philosophy, not an allegiance to any particular school. As such, the connotation of the term 'Cartesian' was similar to the contemporary qualification 'scientific'.

Significantly, Blankaart published his account of syphilis together with alternative accounts by Sylvius, Sydenham, and others. Though his suggestions for treating the disease were based on his own experience, his mechanistic views had no bearing on the type of medication prescribed. The substances he tried on his patients were all the usual drugs. They had either proved more or less successful in practice or were in some way still linked to Galenic theory—for instance, in regard to the supposed benefits of diuretics and diaphoretics. Because they relied on processes taking place at microscopic levels, both the iatromechanical and the iatrochemical models were doomed to remain highly speculative, and neither resulted in any successful new treatments.

On the other hand, there was plenty of room for innovation in other fields. The indefatigable Blankaart contributed to the biological and medical sciences by gathering precise data on plants and insects, which he published in popular works with fine illustrations. His *Collectanea medico-physica* was the beginning of a scientific journal that conveyed all sorts of observed and reported medical cases, as well as astronomical observations, reports on earthquakes, etc. Blankaart confidently presented his journal as a Dutch equivalent to the transactions of philosophical societies abroad.

His most noteworthy contribution to medicine was the Greek-Latin lexicon of medical terms that he finished on his twenty-ninth birthday. It combined ancient and modern terminology with the latest findings in anatomy, surgery, botany, and pharmacology, and it was intended to be used by medical practitioners. The book was first published with equivalent phrases in Dutch, and Blankaart himself added German, French, and English equivalents for a 1690 edition. By that time, the lexicon had already appeared in a German edition (1683), with German phrases instead of Dutch, and in a complete English translation (*A Physical Dictionary*, 1684). A final edition was issued by Karl Gottlob Kühn as late as 1832.

Bibliography

Primary: 1701. *Opera medica, theoretica, practica et chirurchica* 2 vols. (Leiden); 1679. *Lexicon medicum Graeco-Latinum, in quo termini totius artis medicae, secundum Neotericorum placita, definiuntur vel circumscribuntur* (Amsterdam); 1680–88. *Collectanea medico-physica oft Hollands jaarregister der genees- en natuur-kundige aanmerkingen van gantsch Europa* 4 vols. (Amsterdam).

Secondary: Ruler, Han van, 2003. 'Blankaart, Steven (1650–1704)' in Bunge, Wiep van, et al., eds., *The Dictionary of Seventeenth and Eighteenth-Century Dutch Philosophers* 2 vols. (Bristol) 1: 106–110; Huisman, Frank, 1999. 'Medicine and Health Care in the Netherlands, 1500–1800' in Berkel, Klaas van, et al., eds., *A History of Science in the Netherlands: Survey, Themes, and Reference* (Leiden) pp. 239–278; Jarcho, Saul, 1982. 'Blankaart's Dictionary. An Index to Seventeenth-Century Medicine.' *Bulletin of the New York Academy of Medicine* 58: 568–577.

Han van Ruler

BLASCHKO, ALFRED (b. Freienwalde an der Oder, Germany, 4 March 1858; d. Berlin, Germany, 26 March 1922), *dermatology, venereology*.

Blaschko was the second child of the assimilated Jewish physician Hermann Blaschko and Babette Mannheimer. In 1871, after the foundation of the German Reich, the Blaschkos moved to Berlin, which was more liberal and tolerant toward Jews. Blaschko studied medicine at the University of Berlin (1876–81), wrote his doctoral thesis on the visual center of frogs in 1880, and qualified in 1881. In the following two years he worked as assistant to a surgeon in Stettin and subsequently set up his own practice as a physician in Berlin, but he also continued to be an active researcher. Besides physiology and anatomy, Blaschko became increasingly interested in dermatology and venereology, in which he specialized. He was ideally located in Berlin, where he was able to become acquainted with leading researchers in dermato-venereology such as Paul Ehrlich and August Paul von Wassermann. In 1888 Blaschko worked with Moritz Kaposi in Vienna and published papers on occupational skin diseases. In the 1890s, he also published on leprosy in Prussia. At the 1901 Congress of the German Dermatological Society, Blaschko presented his observations on various linear dermatoses that became known as the *Lines of Blaschko*. He saw no anatomical basis for those lines, but they were consistent between different patients and diseases. Blaschko therefore proposed an embryonic origin for them.

In 1896 Blaschko married Johanna Litthauer, the daughter of the physician Marcus Mosse. They had three children: Charlotte (1898–1933), who also became a physician; Hermann

[Hugh] (1900–93), FRS, who also studied medicine and had a distinguished British academic career in physiology and pharmacology; and Margarete Felicia.

In addition to his private practice, Blaschko established a large and well-equipped clinic [*Poliklink*] for dermatology and venereology in 1893, where he treated poorer patients and workers insured through the compulsory health insurance system. His very successful clinic had fourteen beds and extensive laboratory facilities by 1900, and it expanded even further over the years. It not only provided Blaschko with the facilities he needed for his research, but also put him in the position to offer specialist training to other doctors.

Politically, Blaschko established close links with the revisionist wing of the German socialist party (SPD)—without becoming a formal party member—and with the radical wing of the German women's movement. He was also on good terms with Friedrich Althoff, one of the most important civil servants in the Prussian Department for Science and Education. Blaschko's socialist convictions and his Jewish origin kept him from an academic career and other high-ranking positions. However, in 1904 the Prussian state made him *Sanitätsrat* (*Geheimer Sanitätsrat* in 1918), and in 1908 he was given the title of professor.

By the end of the nineteenth century, Blaschko had become increasingly interested in the social problems connected to the spread of venereal diseases (VD). He published on social and public health issues related to VD, such as prostitution, VD control, and the treatment of VD patients in hospitals and in the health insurance system. Together with other leading German dermato-venereologists, he founded the German Society for Combating VD [*Deutsche Gesellschaft zur Bekämpfung der Geschlechtskrankheiten,* DGBG] in 1902 and became its general secretary and president in 1916. Blaschko was the driving force in the DGBG and became an influential advisor to the government in the long-lasting debates about the Imperial Act for Combating VD. That measure was finally passed by the German parliament in 1927, five years after Blaschko's death. In 1914 Blaschko was also invited to give evidence to the British Royal Commission on VD in London.

Bibliography

Primary: 1890. *Die Behandlung der Geschlechtskrankheiten in Krankenkassen und Heilanstalten* (Berlin); 1893. *Syphilis und Prostitution vom Standpunkte der öffentlichen Gesundheitspflege* (Berlin); 1897. *Die Lepra im Kreise Memel* (Berlin); 1900. *Die Geschlechtskrankheiten—ihre Gefahren, Verhütung und Bekämpfung. Volkstümlich dargestellt* [eighth edn., 1919] (Berlin).

Secondary: Sauerteig, Lutz, 1999. *Krankheit, Sexualität, Gesellschaft: Geschlechtskrankheiten und Gesundheitspolitik in Deutschland im 19. und frühen 20. Jahrhundert* (Stuttgart); Weindling, Paul, 1992. *Alfred Blaschko (1858–1922) and the Problem of Sexually Transmitted Diseases in Imperial and Weimar Germany: A Bibliography* (Oxford); Tennstedt, Florian, 1979. 'Alfred Blaschko: das wissenschaftliche und sozialpolitische Wirken eines menschenfreundlichen Sozialhygienikers im Deutschen Reich.' *Zeitschrift für Sozialreform* 25: pp. 513–523, 600–613, 646–667.

Lutz D. H. Sauerteig

BLEULER, EUGEN (b. Zollikon-Zurich, Switzerland, 30 April 1857; d. Zollikon, Switzerland, 15 July 1939), *psychiatry*.

Bleuler was the son of the farmer and businessman Johann Rudolf Bleuler and his wife, Pauline. He attended medical school at the University of Zurich, graduating in 1881. For his training in psychiatry, he worked at the psychiatric university clinics and hospitals in Bern, Munich, and Zurich; he also spent a longer period studying psychiatric institutions and practicing in London and in Paris (with Charcot). At the age of twenty-nine, in 1886, he was appointed director of the psychiatric hospital Rheinau (near Zurich). In 1898 he succeeded his teacher Auguste Forel as professor, and as director of the Burghölzli hospital at the University of Zurich, a position he held until his retirement in 1927.

Under Forel, the Burghölzli had already been established as one of the earliest—and very successful—models of a university department of psychiatry, with research focusing on hypnotic psychotherapy and the social dimensions of psychiatric practice, such as alcoholism and forensic issues. Bleuler continued and extended these activities, and he was the first prominent academic psychiatrist who systematically integrated psychoanalytical concepts into both his research and his therapeutic practices. In 1901 he asked his assistant (and later deputy) Carl Gustav Jung to report on Freud's *Interpretation of Dreams* to the staff of the Burghölzli. Later, Bleuler formulated important contributions to psychodynamic approaches in the psychotherapy of psychoses. From 1909 until 1913, he coedited (with Freud) the *Jahrbuch für psychoanalytische und psychopathologische Forschung.*

In 1908 Bleuler coined the term and concept of schizophrenia ('split mind' disorder), modifying Emil Kraepelin's notion of dementia praecox as one of the basic categories of psychiatric classification. Whereas Kraepelin had abstained from any psychological considerations regarding the etiology and symptoms of dementia praecox, Bleuler postulated a basic psychological dysfunction—a disorder of associations (*Assoziationsstörung*) that in turn caused secondary psychopathological processes. Those processes included autism and ambivalence, in particular, as well as the symptoms of the disorder, such as delusions or hallucinations. Although he did not deny a somatic correlate of the basic psychological dysfunction (indeed, he took it for granted), Bleuler focused his further research and therapeutic approaches on the psychological dimension of the disorder.

During the twelve years of his work at the Rheinau mental hospital, Bleuler had lived as a bachelor in the same building as his patients. Accordingly, he had developed an intimate knowledge of both the living conditions in contemporary psychiatric institutions, and the concerns of the patients. Next to his contributions to psychiatric conceptualizations, his main interest and efforts were devoted to the social ramifications of psychiatric prevention and care. Those ramifications included occupational therapy and employment for the patients, housing conditions, and forensic issues. Because efficient preventive and therapeutic measures were lacking, the later stages of Bleuler's career found him increasingly convinced of the necessity of eugenic measures. Regarding forensic issues, Bleuler propagated the idea that punishment should not be based on moral guilt, but rather on the prospect of curing the perpetrator.

In 1919 Bleuler published *Das autistisch-undisziplinierte Denken in der Medizin*, a description and detailed analysis of both insufficient methodologies and self-reflection in medical practice and research, combined with a polemic against the widespread self-righteousness among the medical profession. The book had almost no resonance within psychiatry, but it had some impact on later discussions and developments in medical theory, and on the methodology of clinical research.

Bibliography

Primary: 1908. 'Die Prognose der Dementia praecox (Schizophreniengruppe).' *Allgemeine Zeitschrift für Psychiatrie* 65: 436–463; 1911. *Dementia praecox oder Gruppe der Schizophrenien* [English edn., 1950] (Leipzig and Vienna); 1919. *Das autistisch-undisziplinierte Denken in der Medizin und seine Ueberwindung* (Berlin).

Secondary: Bernet, Brigitta, 2005. 'Assoziationsstörung: Zum Wechselverhältnis von Krankheits—und Gesellschaftsdeutung im Frühwerk Eugen Bleulers' in Nolte, Karin, and Heiner Fangerau, eds., 'Moderne' Anstaltspsychiatrie im 19. und 20. Jahrhundert—Legitimation und Kritik* (Göttingen) pp. 167–192; Hell, Daniel, Christian Scharfetter, and Arnulf Möller, eds., 2001. *Eugen Bleuler. Leben und Werk* (Bern).

Volker Roelcke

BLOODGOOD, JOSEPH COLT (b. Milwaukee, Wisconsin, USA, 1 November 1867; d. Baltimore, Maryland, USA, 22 October 1935), *surgery.*

Although Bloodgood is primarily remembered as having been one of William Stewart Halsted's chief residents, he did in fact make several significant clinical contributions during his lifetime. His interests in the microscopic pathology of tumors, surgical training, radiotherapy, and the education of the public in the prevention and treatment of cancer and other diseases made his name well known among his medical colleagues and the laity.

Bloodgood was born in Milwaukee to prosperous parents. His father had a successful law practice, later joined by two of his sons. Having received his Bachelor of Science degree from the University of Wisconsin, Bloodgood went on to medical school at the University of Pennsylvania, from which he graduated in 1891. Influenced by William Osler's move from Philadelphia to the new Johns Hopkins Hospital, and recommended to the chief of surgery by Osler, he became Halsted's fourth assistant resident, serving from June to November 1892. At the conclusion of that six-month period, he was encouraged by Halsted to spend a year at the great surgical centers of Europe. He visited the clinics of Kocher, von Recklinghausen, and Bassini, among others, but seems to have been most impressed by Theodor Billroth, perhaps the world's leading surgeon and surgical teacher at the time. It seems to have been Billroth's avid interest in microscopic pathology that most intrigued Bloodgood and influenced his subsequent career. He brought home a microtome designed for making frozen sections during operative procedures or immediately afterwards, in order to avoid the long wait for the results of permanent sections.

Returning to Baltimore, Bloodgood served as chief resident in surgery at Johns Hopkins from 1893 to 1897, during which time he was asked by his chief to organize a section of surgical pathology, the first of several subspecialties that Halsted would create. Succeeded as chief resident by Harvey Cushing (who would later organize the subspecialty of neurosurgery), Bloodgood was appointed associate in surgery. Among his duties in his capacity as the chief's primary assistant was the study and correlation of the statistics of Halsted's new operations for hernia and breast cancer.

The Johns Hopkins program frowned on starting a family during the early, productive years of a medical career, and thus Bloodgood did not marry until he was forty-one years old. His wife, Edith, was a social worker and the daughter of New York publisher Henry Holt, and although she and Joseph later had two children, she remained very active in numerous medical contexts, most notably the welfare of the blind. Bloodgood went on to become adjunct professor of surgery at the Johns Hopkins Medical School, and assistant visiting surgeon at its hospital. He created the second surgical residency program in the nation—after Halsted's—at St Agnes Hospital in Baltimore, having become chief of staff there in 1906, a position he held until his death of heart failure at the age of sixty-seven.

During his busy career, Bloodgood became known for his assiduous follow-up studies of tumor treatment, keeping accurate records of long-term results, and describing them in the surgical literature. In time, his laboratory had between 25,000 and 30,000 case reports classified by organ and diagnosis, setting a precedent for the tumor registries of a later era. His primary interest in this regard was in malignancies of bone and breast. He published some sixty articles on the former, and approximately eighty on the latter. It was his contention that cancer begins in a focus of tissue that has become abnormal, meaning that the disease is curable in its earliest stage if the abnormality can be recognized and treated. The dysplasias and colonic polyps so diligently pursued today are examples of his thesis.

In the final five years of his life, Bloodgood was subjected to severe criticism by medical colleagues for carrying his message about cancer prevention and treatment to the public through articles in the lay press, radio broadcasts, and similar means. Although he was in the vanguard of a movement now recognized to have enormous benefits, the importance of such efforts by outstanding members of the medical profession was not appreciated at the time. Another unappreciated means of combating cancer was the use of radiation therapy, advocated by Bloodgood and Howard Kelly, Chief of Gynecology at Johns Hopkins, for which the two surgical leaders were severely castigated. In each case, Bloodgood's position eventually came to be accepted as the correct one.

Bibliography

Primary: Bloodgood, E. H., and V. H. Long, 1936. *Index to the Writings of Joseph Colt Bloodgood* (Baltimore).

Secondary: Marmon, L. M., A. K. Mandal, D. Goodman, and G. R. Hoy, 1993. 'The Life of Joseph Colt Bloodgood, M.D., Public Surgeon.' *Surg. Gyn. and Obst.* 177: 193–200; Geschickter, C. F., 1956. 'Joseph Colt Bloodgood, Biographical Sketch.' *Clin. Ortho. Rel. Res.* 38: 3–8; *DAMB*.

Sherwin Nuland

BLUMENBACH, JOHANN FRIEDRICH (b. Gotha, Germany, 11 May 1752; d. Göttingen, Germany, 22 January 1840), *anthropology, comparative anatomy, natural history.*

Blumenbach was the son of Heinrich Blumenbach, professor and pro-rector at the Gymnasium Ernestinum in Gotha, and his wife, Charlotte Eleonore Hedwig Buddeus, daughter of a senior government employee and the granddaughter of a Jena theologian. Thus Blumenbach grew into a cultured, wealthy Protestant family and was exposed to both literature and natural science. After completing his schooling (1769), he first studied medicine at the University of Jena. There he attended the lectures of the mineralogist Johann Ernst Immanuel Walch (1725–78), the author of *Naturgeschichte der Versteinerungen* [Natural history of petrifactions], which motivated Blumenbach to study fossils. He also received an excellent education in philosophy and the classics.

University Career

Blumenbach soon transferred to the university in Göttingen, however, where he came into contact with Christian Wilhelm Büttner (1716–1801), a learned scientist renowned for his linguistic skills. Büttner's brilliant travel writing and his descriptions of foreign people had a strong influence on Blumenbach's doctoral dissertation, giving him the impetus to start his widely admired anthropological-ethnographic collec-

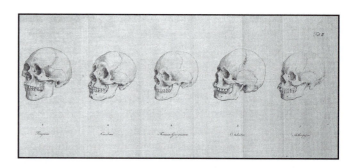

Blumenbach's five racial varieties as defined by cranial differences. Left to right: Mongolian, American, Caucasian, Malaysian, and Ethiopian. From *De Generis Humani Varietate Nativa*, 1795. Rare Books, Wellcome Library, London.

tion. Even today, that collection contains the key specimens on which he based his classifications. He received his MD in 1775, and only one month later he presented his first lecture. Blumenbach started his university career that same year, and in 1776 he became extraordinary professor at Göttingen and curator of the natural history collection. At the age of twenty-six he became full professor of medicine (1778), a post he held for sixty-two years until his death. The subjects he taught included mineralogy, botany, and, especially, zoology.

Through marriage (1778), Blumenbach became the son-in-law of Georg Brandes, who held an influential position in the university administration, and a brother-in-law to Christian Gottlieb Heyne (1729–1812), the classics scholar. Those connections helped strengthen Blumenbach's influence at the university. In 1816 he was appointed 'professor primaries' of the faculty of medicine. In 1784 he became a member of the *Königliche Societät der Wissenschaften zu Göttingen*, and permanent secretary to the academy of science (1812). Blumenbach was either a regular or a corresponding member of more than seventy other academies and scientific organizations, including the *Institute de France*, the Royal Society of London and the Linnean Society of London, the *Königliche Akademie zu Berlin*, the Imperial Academy of St Petersburg, and the American Philosophical Society. He celebrated his fiftieth doctoral anniversary in 1825.

Blumenbach carried out extensive correspondence with scientists, including Albrecht von Haller (1708–77) and the Swiss zoologist Charles Bonnet (1720–93). Although he traveled relatively little, he made journeys through Switzerland (1783), to the Netherlands (1791), and to England. After the occupation of Göttingen by the French army (1806), he visited Paris in order to influence Napoleon favorably. Blumenbach was a personal friend of the great poet Johann Wolfgang von Goethe (1749–1832). Even though he had discovered the Os intermaxillare himself in 1786, Blumenbach nonetheless avoided a priority controversy with Goethe.

He was unusually successful as a teacher, and many of his students claimed that Blumenbach had given them the decisive impetus for the formation of their ideas. He certainly realized the value of empirical knowledge in the natural sciences, and he gave his students many opportunities to participate in scientific expeditions. Students influenced by Blumenbach included Alexander von Humboldt (1769–1859) and Karl Ernst von Baer (1792–1876).

Besides Buffon and Linné, Blumenbach was one of the greatest natural scientists of his time. His view of nature was a philosophical one; he searched for the underlying causes of things, not satisfied with the mere counting and description of phenomena. Blumenbach was the first university lecturer to teach comparative anatomy. He was a highly original character whose vivid spirit captured the attention of his audience.

Anthropology

Johann Friedrich Blumenbach is generally regarded as the founder of physical and scientific anthropology. His dissertation (1775) *De generis humani varietate nativa liber* [On the Natural Varieties of Mankind] became world famous as one of the basic works in anthropology. In it Blumenbach classified mankind into four races, as Carl von Linné (1707–78) had done, based on selected combinations of different facial configuration. He was the first to use the word 'race' to classify humans. Blumenbach also coined the term 'Caucasian', because he believed that the Caucasus region of Asia Minor produced 'the most beautiful race of men'. Blumenbach defined the Caucasian race as the basic race of all human races (*Stammrasse*). Both he and Linné stated that human beings are one species, and Blumenbach commented on the arbitrary nature of his proposed categories. In his classification of the subdivisions of the human race, Blumenbach was the first to utilize facial configuration as well as skin color, and his system has survived to the present with little modification. His most important anthropological work was a collection of sixty human skulls described in his *Collectionis suae craniorum diversarum gentium illustrate decades* (1790–1828).

Blumenbach approached anthropology with the mind of the natural scientist. He recognized that just as domestic animals come in varieties, all known groups of mankind originated from one common, basic race. But for the second edition of his dissertation (1781), Blumenbach found it necessary to expand his discussion to allow for *five* races, even though his famous terms for the different races were not used until the third edition (1795). His classification into Caucasian (key object: female skull of a Georgian), Mongolian (male skull of a Tungusen), Ethiopian (female skull from Guinea), Malayan (male skull from Tahiti), and American (male skull of a Caribbean) established the modern theory of human races.

Blumenbach was one of the first scientists to view man as an object of natural history, and he saw in man the most perfect of all domesticated animals. He wrote, 'the causes and ways of degeneration, and the analogous phenomena of degeneration in the other domestic animals, brings us to

that conclusion. . . . That no doubt can any longer remain but that we are with great probability right in referring all and singular as many varieties of man as are at present known to one and the same species' (Blumenbach, 1865, p. 276). On the other hand, he gave special emphasis to the gap between man and animal and attacked all political or social abuses of anthropological ideas, in particular that black people were on a lower level of humanity than white people. In his dissertation one can find the first reliable survey of the characteristics and distribution of the human races; its most significant points were included in almost all later anthropological classifications.

Natural History and the Nisus Formativus

Blumenbach's *Handbuch der Naturgeschichte* (*Elements of natural history*, 1779), is the first book grounded on an anatomical-physiological basis. It went through many editions and was translated into many languages. Although Blumenbach tended to follow the Linnean system, this Handbuch opened a new era in natural history. It contains many new morphological and ecological details and hitherto insufficiently evaluated findings, from which Blumenbach drew conclusions that led to a more modern concept of the plant and animal kingdoms. Influenced by Kant's rational philosophy, he began by defining the specific, basic biological terms such as *genera, species, races,* etc. He concluded from the spread of certain parasites found only in the domestic pig that such parasites did not exist unless pigs were domesticated, and therefore that they could not possibly have existed since the creation of the world. Such ideas, revolutionary in their day, were carefully presented in various places in the *Handbuch*, and were demonstrated by concrete examples.

In connection with the morphological analysis and geological dating of fossil plants and animals, Blumenbach developed ideas that were still unknown to most of the scientists of his day and were touched upon by only a few others, among them Jean-Louis Soulavie-Giraud (1752–1813), the French abbot and author of the *Histoire naturelle de la France* (1781). Blumenbach came to the conclusion that there had been groups of plants and animals, now extinct, that could not be classified in the system of recent forms of life, and he even attempted to draw up a geological-paleontological time scale. His book *Beyträge zur Naturgeschichte* [Contribution to natural history] contained several essays on the 'variability' of nature, a concept that was not understood very well in his day. It also showed that the earth, with all its flora and fauna, had a very long history. Blumenbach was one of the earliest thinkers to recognize the historicity of nature, and therefore he occupies an important place in the history of evolution theory, development, and embryology. He was also one of the founders of comparative anatomy and the first to lecture on the topic. Blumenbach's noteworthy book on human osteology (1807) contains his original description of the base of the skull (*clivus Blumenbachi*).

In connection with the problems of embryonic development, regeneration, and self-healing, scientists widely discussed the controversial problem of a mechanistic explanation of organic life. Many of them favored a vitalistic approach in analyzing these phenomena. They introduced a specific organic force called *Lebenskraft* [vital force] that was analogous to Newtonian gravitation. Blumenbach himself interpreted the living organism in terms of the body's three-fold constitution. He saw it as comprising *materials* (represented by fluids), *structure* (represented by solids), and *vital powers*, which enabled motor interactions between fluids and solids. Those three constituents seemed to him to be ontologically independent, but causally interdependent. Blumenbach substituted the term *Bildungstrieb* (*Nisus formativus*) for *Lebenskraft*. In his 1781 work *Über den Bildungstrieb und das Zeugungsgeschäft* [On Nisus formativus and the procreation], Blumenbach rejected the 'preformation' theory of Albrecht von Haller. Instead, he advocated Caspar Friedrich Wolff's (1734–94) theory of epigenesis as the true explanation of the phenomenon of embryological development.

Blumenbach's ideas on *Bildungstrieb* (*Nisus formativus*) made a great impression on his contemporaries, as well as on later scientists. Those ideas are historically significant, because in the controversy surrounding epigenesis versus preformation they introduced some new arguments in favor of the epigenetic theory. Even the great philosopher Immanuel Kant (1724–1804) discussed Blumenbach's arguments in connection with Kant's philosophical debate about the concept of vital force. However, those arguments were very short-lived, and did not exert a lasting influence.

Bibliography

Primary: 1775. *De generis humani varietate nativa liber* (Göttingen); 1779. *Handbuch der Naturgeschichte* (Göttingen); 1781. *Über den Bildungstrieb und das Zeugungsgeschäft* (Göttingen);1806–11. *Beyträge zur Naturgeschichte* 2 vols. (Göttingen); 1865. (Bendyshe, Thomas, trans. and ed.) *The Anthropological Treatises* (London).

Secondary: Dougherty, Frank William Peter, 1996. *Gesammelte Aufsätze zu Themen der klassischen Periode der Naturgeschichte* [Collected Essays on Themes from the Classical Period of Natural History] (Göttingen); McLaughlin, P., 1982. 'Blumenbach und der Bildungstrieb. Zum Verhältnis epigenetischer Embryologie und typologischen Artbegriff.' *Medizinhistorisches Journal* 17: 357–372; Lenoir, Timothy, 1982. *The Strategy of Life. Teleology and Mechanics in Nineteenth-Century German Biology* (Dordrecht); Marx, K. F. H., 1843. 'Zum Andenken an Johann Friedrich Blumenbach' trans. Bendyshe, Thomas, 1865 (listed in primary bibliography).

Brigitte Lohff

BOERHAAVE, HERMAN (b. Voorhout, the Netherlands, 31 December 1668; d. Leiden, the Netherlands, 23 September 1738), *medicine, chemistry, botany*.

Boerhaave was the eldest son of Hagar Daalders and the Reformed pastor Jacobus Boerhaave. His mother died in 1673; one year later, his father married Eva du Bois, with whom Herman had a good relationship. While Boerhaave was still very young, his father started teaching him Latin and Greek, using the grammar of Vossius, the dialogues of Erasmus and the comedies of Terence, the New Testament, and universal history as expounded in the 'Theatre' of Christian Matthias. When he was eleven years old, Boerhaave was fluent in Latin, and he was particularly interested in etymology.

In 1682 his father sent the fourteen-year-old Boerhaave to the Latin grammar school in Leiden. The Latin school was considered necessary preparatory training for a university education; moreover, Leiden offered the boy better medical treatment for a malignant ulcer on his left thigh, which had developed a few years earlier. Boerhaave proved to be a bright pupil; within one year he won two prizes and was ready to start his university education. But that beginning was delayed by the untimely death of his father in 1683 and the troublesome ulcer on his leg (which ultimately he cured himself, using a mixture of salt and his own urine).

In 1685, the States of Holland awarded Boerhaave a free scholarship to study at the Leiden faculties of theology and philosophy. On the recommendation of Jacobus Trigland Jr. and Daniel van Alphen Simonszoon, Boerhaave became a pupil of Wolferd Senguerd, who taught him logic, the use of globes, natural philosophy, metaphysics, and ethics. Boerhaave also continued to study Latin and Greek, and he followed classes in rhetoric, history, geography, Hebrew, and Chaldaic. Under the supervision of Senguerd, Boerhaave held four public 'disputations', one on cohesion and three on the human mind—*De cohaesione corporum* (1687) and *De mente humana prima* (1687), *secunda* (1688), *et tertia* (1688). In 1687 Boerhaave added mathematics (geometry and trigonometry) to his studies, and it is likely that he also attended demonstrations in the physics laboratory of Burchard de Volder. He was given the opportunity to hold a public 'oration' in 1689, which was a much higher distinction than a disputation. His oration on Cicero's right interpretation of Epicurus's maxim of the highest human good (*De bene intellecta Ciceroni sententia Epicuri de summo hominis bono*) was awarded a gold medal. With a thesis on the distinction between the mind and the body (*De distinctione mentis a corpore*), Boerhaave finished his philosophy education in 1690.

When his scholarship expired, Boerhaave obtained a supervisory post in the university library, in order to be able to continue his studies in theology. Meanwhile, he started studying medicine. He read the medical authors in chronological order, starting with Hippocrates through to Sydenham, and he vivisected animals. He attended only a few lectures by Drélincourt and anatomical dissections by Anton Nuck. In 1693 Boerhaave took his medical degree in Harderwijk, where–according to a contemporary rhyme—it was as easy to buy a degree from the university as a fish in the market. Not long after his return to Leiden, Boerhaave was accused of being a Spinozist. That was a serious accusation, and it severely damaged Boerhaave's chances to obtain a position in the Church. Accordingly, he decided to pursue a full-time career in medicine.

Lecturer in Medicine

In the years between 1693 and 1701, Boerhaave's medical practice was not very busy, which meant that he had plenty of time to continue his studies in mathematics, physics, anatomy, botany, and chemistry. In 1701, while the curators of the University of Leiden were still looking for a professor in (theoretical) medicine (they appointed Bernhard Albinus to the chair in 1702), Boerhaave—considered too young and too inexperienced to be given the chair— was appointed lecturer (*lector*) in medicine. He took up his office with an oration on the study of Hippocrates (*De commendando studio Hippocratico*). He considered the example provided by the 'Father of Medicine' to be of prime importance in medical education and practice. What Boerhaave admired most in Hippocrates were his detailed and meticulous clinical observations and his devotion and concern for his patients. In Boerhaave's view, medicine since Hippocrates had deteriorated into a speculative and theoretical discipline. Although he appreciated the value of theory, Boerhaave intended to reintroduce clinical experience into the medical curriculum, and he urged his students to study the Hippocratic Corpus before starting the practice of medicine. Hippocrates remained important to Boerhaave until the end of his career.

In 1731, upon stepping down from his position as Chancellor (*rector magnificus*) of the University for the second time, Boerhaave once more spoke about Hippocrates as a prime example for the medical practitioner. Hippocrates, in his view, best followed and served Nature as his own guide. 'Nature', in Boerhaave's medical system, referred to the sum total of phenomena in the world. It included the movements of those phenomena and the laws regulating them, and the vital force innate in all living beings. Along that line, Boerhaave argued that the body is like a circle, in which all organs function in mutual dependence. His assertion that no part of the body was worth more than another denied contemporary opinion that the heart was the most important organ. Boerhaave's emphasis on Nature as an organic, living system had direct consequences for his clinical practice. He started from the premise that Nature has a tendency to always move to a position that is best for her, which in the case of illness means that the body always seeks relief, and so tries to cure itself. The physician cannot do more than assist Nature in her task. Thus, a doctor should never forbid a patient to eat and drink what he likes, for that is how the body clarifies what it needs to get better. Boerhaave considered Nature to be the most important medical teacher, which meant that medicine should be based upon meticulous (Hippocratic) observation of Nature.

Boerhaave began his public and private lectures on the 'Institutes of Medicine' with a short history of the discipline. The majority of both his lecture series and the *Institutiones medicae* (published in 1708) is about physiology, which he considered a neglected subject. In the textbook, Boerhaave began the section on the animal economy with the process of digestion, followed by a discussion of circulation. He proceeded with the lungs and respiration before going on to the organs of the lower abdomen and the sense organs. The process of generation he dealt with last.

His teaching was directed not only at the theoretical foundations of medicine, however; it also included 'practical' subjects such as pathology, symptomatology (semiotics), and therapy. In his *Aphorismi de cognoscendis et curandis morbis* [Aphorisms on the Diagnosis and Treatment of Diseases], published in 1709, Boerhaave stressed the importance of clinical medicine. Furthermore, the curators gave him permission to teach anatomy and chemistry privately. They were happy to do so because Govard Bidloo was neglecting his duties as professor of anatomy, and the number of students attending the chemical instructions of Jacob le Mort was declining. Although Boerhaave was to continue his chemistry teaching in later years, his interest in anatomy came to the fore with his editing of the work of Eustachius (1707), Vesalius (1725), and Swammerdam (1737).

Boerhaave's medical teaching did not go unnoticed. In 1703 he was offered a professorship in Groningen. He declined, but the Leiden curators were so anxious to keep him that they doubled his salary and promised to give him the first chair that became vacant in the medical faculty. To mark the occasion, Boerhaave delivered an oration on the use of mechanistic reason in medicine (*De usu ratiocinii mechanici in medicina*). He argued that medicine paid too little attention to (Newtonian) mechanics, even though—in his view—the healthy life and motion of the body depend on the mechanical motion of the humors through the tubes and vessels. The tone of Boerhaave's oration was optimistic. He compared the body to a clock—once the inner mechanisms are known, the physician can correct its structure and repair defects.

The Boerhaavian body was built of fibers (long threads of earthlike particles) woven together into membranes. These membranes, when rolled up, form small vessels (*vasa minora*), which in turn are woven together into bigger vessels (*vasa maiora*). Ultimately, the vessels build up the organs and other parts of the body, and it follows that the whole body is built of vessels. The smallest vessels cannot be seen; their existence can only be deduced. All the vessels are directly or indirectly connected to the left ventricle of the heart, so that all bodily fluids except excretions ultimately return to the heart. As long as the fluids move regularly through the channels, the body is alive and healthy. However, when the movements of fluids are obstructed or cease altogether, the body falls ill and dies.

Eleven years later, on the occasion of his resignation from a one-year office as Chancellor (*rector magnificus*) of the

University (1715), Boerhaave was far less optimistic about the possibilities of knowing the nature of the body. In his oration on the achievement of certainty in physics (*De comparando certo in physicis*), he paradoxically argued that 'the first principles of nature [such as atoms, the Cartesian principle of extension, the void, Newtonian gravity, motion, the working of seeds, and even the emergence and growth of a single hair] are wholly hidden from us' and 'only from the observation of our senses can knowledge of their properties be gained'. All claims to understand these hidden principles of nature are blasphemous, because they equate the fallible knowledge of man with the omnipotent wisdom of God. Thus, instead of emphasizing the mechanical laws of bodies, Boerhaave devoted more attention to the essentially incomprehensible vital powers of bodies. For instance, he pointed to what was originally the Stoic concept of 'seminal principles' as the prime subject for natural philosophical research. As a consequence, mechanics was pushed into the background and chemistry became increasingly more important in Boerhaave's natural philosophy. He considered chemistry to be best suited to reveal the latent powers of bodies.

Professor of Botany

In 1703 Boerhaave had been promised the first available professorship in the medical faculty, but he had to wait another six years before Peter Hotton died and the chair of botany became vacant. The curators preferred Boerhaave to Johannes Jacobus Scheuchzer, appointing him *ordinaris professor medicinae et botanices*. His salary was set at 1,000 guilders, plus 300 guilders for maintaining his botanical correspondence.

In accordance with his lifelong motto *simplex veri sigillum* (Simplicity is the Hallmark of Truth), Boerhaave began his professorship with a nonbotanical oration on the simplicity of true medicine (*Oratio qua repurgatae medicinae facilis asseritur simplicitas*) that was particularly devoted to practical medicine, diagnosis, treatments, and remedies. Its main assumption was that everything has a single, essentially simple nature, and that medical knowledge should be based on these simple, natural phenomena as the only way to attain perfection and truth. He argued that medical practice should be based on the simplicity of nature. For example, an extensive and complicated pharmacopoeia that describes infinitely many remedies is unnecessary, because when the physician knows the essential (simple and true) nature of the body, he will know what to do in case of illness.

Although Boerhaave had little knowledge of botany at first, he quickly familiarized himself with the Botanical Garden in Leiden and its medicinal plants. Immediately after his appointment, he started corresponding with botanists all over Europe (e.g., Sébastian Vaillant, William Sherard, and in later years, Linnaeus), and he was soon able to enlarge the Garden with seeds and plants given to him by his new botanical friends. In the year 1725, for example, Boerhaave received 1,416 parcels of seeds for the Garden. Moreover, he installed a new heating system that he had invented and was able to grow tropical plants in the hothouses. The Botanical Garden soon proved to be too small, and in 1710 the curators gave Boerhaave permission to plant trees at the Maliebaan, a now nonexistent street along a canal. In a period of ten years, Boerhaave increased the number of plant varieties cultivated in the Botanical Garden to 5,846.

During the summer, Boerhaave inspected the plants and seedlings early in the morning, followed by a botanical lecture in the Garden (or, in case of bad weather, in the Gallery) at 7 A.M. For the purpose of his teaching and correspondence, Boerhaave published a catalog of the trees, plants, and herbs cultivated in the Botanical Garden (1710). Since that work was written in haste, and because of the subsequent enlargement of the Garden, Boerhaave composed a second—enlarged—catalog ten years later. In the index of 1710, Boerhaave followed the Carpological System of Hermann, describing only a few new plants. In the later *Index alter* (1720), he described twenty-eight new species, noting the characteristics of genera more accurately. Yet, as Boerhaave wrote in his preface to the *Index alter*, he was 'not yet able to build a complete general system'—nor would he ever have been able to, even if he had grown very old and devoted himself entirely to it. Boerhaave's descriptions, therefore, were eclectic, as were his works on medicine and chemistry. According to Linnaeus, he combined the taxonomic systems of Hermann, Ray, and Tournefort.

Professor of Practical Medicine

In 1714 Boerhaave also took on clinical teaching responsibilities (*collegium medico-practicum*). Unlike the medical professors, the curators were keenly aware of the need for bedside instruction. Boerhaave and Frederik Dekkers were appointed to reinvigorate practical education, which had declined after the death of Bidloo in 1713. The hospital wards were on the first floor of St Caecilia Hospital. The twelve-bed teaching ward (six beds for male and six for female patients) had viewing galleries along the walls. Twice a week Boerhaave, accompanied by the city doctor and students, walked along the beds questioning and examining each patient. The patients had been carefully selected beforehand from the other six wards in the hospital. Usually, Boerhaave would select a patient for a special examination and demonstration. He discussed the signs and symptoms, the prognosis, and the treatment of the disease. Often he invited a student from the gallery to come down, and while discussing the case, he would test the student's medical knowledge. Afterward, he discussed the patient's diet and medication with the matron of the ward. After the death of a patient, Boerhaave also carried out the postmortem examination in the presence of students.

Although Boerhaave has been praised for his clinical teaching at St Caecilia Hospital, not many clinical lessons actually took place. The number of patients declined from

1721 onward, and no patients were admitted at all during the period 1732–36. Boerhaave's famous pupils Albrecht von Haller and Gerard van Swieten scarcely referred to clinical instruction in Leiden, and Boerhaave himself wrote to his friends J. B. Bassand and Jourdain that he became less active in medical practice after 1723, and that he had little time to visit patients.

However, one area of clinical instruction remained important throughout Boerhaave's life. Up until his death, he gave clinical advice in his extensive correspondence. Among his 'paper patients' were princes and princesses, but also ordinary people with complicated ailments that their doctors could not easily solve. It is likely that Boerhaave's fame as a clinician is based on his medical correspondence, rather than on the clinical instruction at St Caecilia Hospital.

Professor of Chemistry

In 1718 a third professorship was added to Boerhaave's duties. After the death of Jacob le Mort, he was appointed to the chair of chemistry. The curators chose Boerhaave because ever since 1702, he had given very successful private lectures on the subject. He assumed his new responsibilities with an oration on chemistry purging itself of its own errors (*De chemia suos errores expurgante*). The tone of the oration is theological, its main issue being the corruption of theology by chemical notions. Boerhaave particularly criticized false (al)chemists who used the Bible as a starting point for their (al)chemical investigations, as if the Bible would hold the secrets of changing metals and making gold. Another problem with chemistry—one that was particularly visible in chemistry for medicine—was that the results of a single experiment were too easily applied to a large group of phenomena. Boerhaave praised the true chemists Roger Bacon and Robert Boyle for bringing chemistry onto the right track again. Their most praiseworthy achievement, according to Boerhaave, was that they had recognized the limits of true chemistry.

Although Boerhaave taught chemistry as a discipline in its own right, the subject was mainly oriented toward medicine. Boerhaave was optimistic about the mechanical method in medicine, but he gradually became more critical of the general (mechanical) laws of nature. He started emphasizing the individual, latent, peculiar powers of bodies. That meant, in regard to medicine, that Boerhaave no longer devoted most attention to the solid parts of the body. Instead, he suggested that 'vital powers' caused the fluids to move through the vessels, thereby invigorating the body with life and motion. With that approach, Boerhaave could maintain that the body was an organic unit, steered by vital forces inherent in the physical substances of the body. He believed that chemical analysis was best suited to investigate the powers of bodies, and chemistry became more important in his teaching program for that reason. Boerhaave's appreciation increased for iatrochemists working in the tradition of Paracelsus and Van Helmont. He particularly admired the natural philosophy of Van Helmont (even though he never warmed to Helmontian remedies).

Among Boerhaave's first activities as a professor of chemistry was refurbishing the chemical laboratory, which was situated in the northwest corner of the Botanical Garden. In 1732, under pressure from the widely circulating—but error-strewn—student publication of his chemistry lectures, Boerhaave published his two-volume *Elementa chemiae*, which was followed by Timothy Dallowe's official English translation in 1735. In order to ensure readers that he had written the book, Boerhaave personally signed all copies of the first edition. For many years, his 'chemistry' remained a standard textbook.

The *Elementa chemiae* consisted of three parts. The first volume was entirely devoted to the history and the theory of chemistry, whereas the shorter second volume concerned chemical procedures. Of particular interest is the fact that Boerhaave presented the classical elements as instruments of chemistry serving the same purpose as utensils, vessels, and *menstrua* (solvents that help to break up a particular substance, so that its latent powers become visible). The passive elements of earth and water form the vessels that the Creator has infused with the active principles of fire and air. The aim of chemistry is to study the changing of bodies by means of motion, which in turn is directed toward finding new appearances and powers. For Boerhaave, that made chemistry the best means of improving natural knowledge. As he put it, 'In physics we can be of good cheer with this guide, in medicine all possible good may be expected from it. It teaches most faithfully how the deepest secrets may be revealed, intricacies be disentangled, how hidden forces of bodies may be discovered, imitated, directed, changed, applied, and perfected' (Boerhaave in Luyendijk-Elshout and Kegel-Brinkgreve, 1983, p. 211).

Boerhaave presented the operations of chemistry in an order and manner most useful to medicine. For instance, following the order of the *Institutiones medicae*, Boerhaave started his account with the vegetative kingdom, because he considered vegetables (after undergoing the process of digestion) to be the building blocks of the body. Moreover, in discussing most of the operations of chemistry, he considered the medicinal virtues and values of the preparation.

'Instructor of All of Europe'

With his appointment to the chair of chemistry, Boerhaave occupied three out of five chairs in the medical faculty. Although the actual number of students declined while Boerhaave was teaching, students from across Europe flocked to Leiden to attend his lectures. Moreover, students took the Boerhaavian method to their home universities (most notably in Edinburgh, Göttingen, and Vienna). Albrecht von Haller praised Boerhaave's pedagogical qualities, calling him 'the instructor of all of Europe'—*communis europae praeceptor*. Boerhaave was particularly praised for his systematization of medicine (theoretical and practical) and chemistry. His most important aim was to teach students the first rudiments and methods of a particular discipline. Hence, he devoted his *Institutiones medicae* mainly to physiology, a rational discipline concerned with the causes of the structure of the body, which studies why human nature is as it is. In clinical medicine, he noted how signs and symptoms are indicative of a particular disease. In chemistry, on the other hand, he did not teach prescribed formulae; he wanted his students to understand what chemistry is and what it does. With respect to remedies, he stressed that it is far more important to understand the nature of diseases and their cures than to learn prescriptions by heart.

So great was Boerhaave's success as a teacher that in 1723, after he had suffered from a long illness, the students and citizens of Leiden celebrated his return to work. Less welcome were the numerous printed editions of student notes of Boerhaave's lectures appearing on the market under his name. The situation greatly annoyed Boerhaave, and when the *Institutiones et experimenta chemiae* was published illegally in 1726 he issued a warning in the Leiden newspaper (the *Leidsche Courant*) stating that he intended to seek out the fraudulent authors, 'in hopes of obtaining legal satisfaction'.

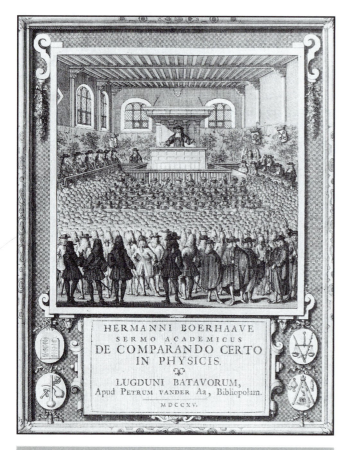

Herman Boerhaave giving a lecture. Engraving with text from *Sermo academicus, de comparando certo in physicis . . .* **Leiden, 1715. Rare Books, Wellcome Library, London.**

In 1727 a second illness left him with a 'chronic complaint', and he decided to resign from his professorships in chemistry and botany. In his farewell oration given on that occasion (*Sermo academicus quem habuit quum honesta missione impetatra botanicam et chemicam professionem publice poneret xxviii Aprilis 1729*), Boerhaave looked back on his life. Nevertheless, he continued teaching medicine (he lectured most notably on nervous diseases), and in 1729 he was named Vice Chancellor of the University for the second time. In his spare time, he untiringly cultivated plants and trees and continued to carry out chemical experiments (for example, he invented a method to purify mercury).

In 1731 the ulcer that Boerhaave suffered from in his youth appeared again. Although he slowly recovered, the first symptoms of his final illness appeared in May 1737. While still pursuing a busy medical practice, Boerhaave felt a tightness in the chest, followed by an abnormal pulsation at the right side of the neck. Gradually, his condition grew worse. He died in September 1738, leaving behind his wife Maria Drolenvaux, whom he had married in 1710, and his daughter Joanna Maria, his only surviving child.

Bibliography

Primary: 1708 [later editions, 1713, 1720, 1727, 1735]. *Institutiones medicae* [English edn. 1714] (Leiden); 1709 [later editions, 1715, 1721, 1728, 1737]. *Aphorismi de cognoscendis et curandis morbis* [English edn., 1724] (Leiden); 1710. *Index plantarum, quae in Horto Academico Lugduno Batavo reperiuntur* (Leiden); 1719. *Libellus de materia medica et remidiorum formulis* [English edn., 1739] (Leiden); 1720. *Index alter plantarum quae in Horto Academico Lugduno-Batavo aluntur* (Leiden); 1732. *Elementa chemiae* [English edn., 1735] (Leiden); 1983. (Luyendijk-Elshout, A. M., and E. Kegel-Brinkgreve, trans. and eds.) *Boerhaave's Orations* (Leiden).

Secondary: Knoeff, Rina, 2002. *Herman Boerhaave (1668–1738). Calvinist, Chemist and Physician* (Amsterdam); Powers, John C., 2001. 'Herman Boerhaave and the Pedagogical Reform of Eighteenth-Century Chemistry.' Unpublished PhD thesis, Indiana University; Cook, Harold J., 2000. 'Boerhaave and the Flight from Reason in Medicine.' *Bulletin for the History of Medicine* 74: 221–240; Cunningham, Andrew, 1990. 'Medicine to Calm the Mind: Boerhaave's Medical System and Why It was Adopted in Edinburgh' in Cunningham, Andrew, and Roger French, eds., *The Medical Enlightenment of the Eighteenth Century* (Cambridge) pp. 40–66; Wright, J. P., 1990. 'Boerhaave on Minds, Human Beings, and Mental Diseases.' *Studies in Eighteenth-Century Culture* 20: 289–302; Lindeboom, Gerrit A., 1968. *Herman Boerhaave. The Man and His Work* (London).

Rina Knoeff

BOISSIER DE LA CROIX DE SAUVAGES, FRANÇOIS
(b. Alais (now Alès), France, 12 May 1706; d. Montpellier, France, 20 February 1767), *medicine.*

Born in Alais, Sauvages was the sixth son of a regimental captain. In his youth, he studied privately with a Dominican priest in Alais. He enrolled at the University of Medicine at Montpellier in 1722. Sauvages studied briefly in Paris in 1730–31, where he associated with Antoine de Jussieu at the Jardin du Roi and conceived a plan for a classification of diseases modeled on work in natural history. Beset with an eye affliction, Sauvages returned to Montpellier in 1731. Although he maintained a private practice and treated patients at the Hôpital-Général, he was principally a medical teacher and theoretician. Sauvages was not awarded a permanent chair at the medical faculty until the 1750s, but he was nonetheless active in the 1730s and 1740s in training students, whose *thèses* incorporated early statements of his views. In 1740 he took over supervision of the Jardin du Roi, heading collecting expeditions in the surrounding countryside. Sauvages contributed regularly to the Société royale des sciences, serving as its interim secretary from 1741–43. His publications earned honors from the learned companies of Paris, Toulouse, and Bordeaux. He continued to teach at the Montpellier faculty until shortly before his death.

Sauvages has often been labeled an 'animist', thanks to his embrace of ideas elaborated by the Halle physician Georg-Ernst Stahl, but his theories also incorporated elements drawn from Isaac Newton and Christian Wolff. Sauvages's unique synthesis was animated by a desire to undercut the influence of Cartesian physicians, whom he labeled 'false mechanicians' for their attempts to explain bodily movements strictly by mechanical and physical principles. Although Sauvages's concept of health and disease was teleological, he was torn in competing directions. Although he argued that many bodily phenomena demonstrated the sway of unvarying 'laws', he also held that the soul made free choices on behalf of health. Drawn to mechanical-geometrical explanation, he found it inadequate to explain clinical phenomena. These tensions were also evident in his efforts at classification.

In his nosology Sauvages argued that to gain firmer ground medicine must rely only on phenomena observable through experience and on reasoning from clear propositions. He urged physicians to adopt the descriptive method of Thomas Sydenham, rather than to search for the causes of disease. Sauvages's nosology revealed both his search for order in medical knowledge and his 'Hippocratic' conviction that illness was characterized not by uniformity, but by singularity. In its final form, his nosology included ten 'classes' of illness subdivided into 'orders' and 'species' that were based on descriptions culled from thousands of historical and contemporary authorities. Acknowledging that treatment could seldom be based solely on knowledge of the 'species' of disease, he nonetheless clung to the belief that medical science would one day discern order in pathological phenomena and develop efficacious treatments.

An important physician in his own right, Sauvages was also the teacher of Théophile de Bordeu and Paul-Joseph Barthez, and therefore central to the emergence of Montpel-lier vitalism. Although his students generally repudiated Sauvages's nosological enterprise, they praised and were strongly influenced by his efforts to undermine mechanistic medicine and to recognize the particularity of the phenomena of life.

Bibliography

Primary: 1752. *Dissertation sur les médicaments qui affectent certaines parties du corps humain plutôt que d'autres; et sur la cause de cet effet* (Bordeaux); 1770. (Gilbert, J.-E., ed.) *Les chefs-d'œuvre de M. Sauvages, ou Recueil de dissertations de cet auteur qui ont remporté le prix dans différentes académies* 2 vols. (Lausanne and Lyon); 1771. *Nosologie méthodique, dans laquelle les maladies sont rangées par classes, suivant le système de Sydenham, et l'ordre des botanistes* 3 vols. (Paris).

Secondary: Williams, Elizabeth A., 2003. *A Cultural History of Medical Vitalism in Enlightenment Montpellier* (Aldershot); Martin, Julian, 1990. 'Sauvages's Nosology: Medical Enlightenment in Montpellier' in Cunningham, Andrew, and Roger French, eds., *The Medical Enlightenment of the Eighteenth Century* (Cambridge) pp. 111–137; Dulieu, Louis, 1969. 'François Boissier de Sauvages (1716–1767).' *Revue d'histoire des sciences* 22: 303–322.

Elizabeth A. Williams

BOND, THOMAS (b. Calvert County, Maryland, USA, 3 May 1713; d. Philadelphia, Pennsylvania, USA, 26 March 1784), *medicine, surgery.*

Bond, son of Quakers Richard Bond, a planter, and Elizabeth Benson Chew, widow of Benjamin Chew, began his medical studies with John Hamilton of Calvert County, and continued his education in Philadelphia, where he became a partner with his half-brother, Samuel Chew, in 1734. He married Susannah Roberts, daughter of the future mayor of Philadelphia, Edward Roberts, in 1735. Susannah died in childbirth in 1737. The following year Bond spent in London, where he met the Quaker physician John Fothergill, and in Paris, where he studied anatomy, medicine, and botany at the Hôtel-Dieu and the Jardin des Plantes. He did not receive an MD degree. He returned to Philadelphia in 1739, and established a medical practice with his younger brother, Phineas Bond. As a physician Bond advocated mild therapies, including hot and cold bathing. He was a renowned surgeon who performed lithotomies, as well as more routine operations including amputations, excision of tumors, and the management of difficult childbirth. In 1742 he married Sarah Weyman, the daughter of Robert Weyman, an Anglican rector in New Jersey. They had seven children; one son, Thomas, Jr., became a physician.

Bond was very involved in public health matters in Philadelphia. In 1741, he was appointed one of the port physicians. He inspected incoming vessels for cases of typhus and yellow fever, and isolated infected individuals. He also oversaw the fumigation of ships and buildings. His interests in public health extended to smallpox inoculation, a new medical practice which he, along with other physicians, publicly recommended in 1737. In 1774, he became a physician to the Society for the Inoculation of the Poor Gratis. In 1779, he lectured on the advantages of inoculation to the American Philosophical Society. This lecture was never published in English, but French and German versions appeared in 1784 and 1787, respectively.

Bond was very active in the civic life of colonial Philadelphia. He was a founding member of the American Philosophical Society in 1743, its vice president from 1769, and, after the American Revolution, he took the lead in its reorganization. Bond was the first to suggest a hospital in Philadelphia, and, with Benjamin Franklin's support, the Pennsylvania Hospital (the first in the United States) was established in 1752. Franklin highlighted Bond's role in his *Autobiography*. Bond placed great emphasis on clinical teaching, and became the first clinical professor at the Pennsylvania Hospital. His apprentices accompanied him on his hospital rounds and to patients' homes. In 1766 he presented a lecture 'on the Utility of Clinical Lectures' to the hospital directors; subsequently, attendance at his lectures became a requirement for the MD degree. Bond died in Philadelphia, and is buried in Christ Church cemetery.

Bibliography

Primary: 1757, 1762. 'Two case histories.' *Medical Observations and Inquiries* 1: 67–80, 2: 265–268; 1784. *Défense de l'inoculation et relation des progress qu'elle a faits à Philadelphie en 1758* (Strasbourg); 1895. 'On the Utility of Clinical Lectures.' reprinted in Morton, Thomas G., and Frank Woodbury, *History of the Pennsylvania Hospital* (Philadelphia) pp. 462–467.

Secondary: Thomson, Elizabeth H., 1958. 'Thomas Bond, 1713–1784: First Professor of Clinical Medicine in the American Colonies.' *Journal of Medical Education* 33: 614–624; Scott, Alison J., 1905–06. 'A Sketch of the Life of Thomas Bond, Clinician and Surgeon.' *University of Pennsylvania Medical Bulletin* 18: 306–318; *ANB*; *DAMB*.

Andrea Rusnock

BONET, THÉOPHILE (b. Republic of Geneva (now Switzerland), 6 March 1620; d. Republic of Geneva, 29 March 1689), *medicine, pathology.*

The Bonets were physicians from father to son for generations. First in the series was Théophile's grandfather, Pierre Bonet, physician to the Duke of Savoy in Turin before moving to Lyon. His father, André Bonet (1554–1639) was also a physician. After the death of his first wife, André moved from Lyon to Geneva and married Marguerite Pinelli-Borzoni in 1612, who was to be Théophile's mother. On 30 December 1617, he became a burgher of Geneva. Théophile and his brother John (Jean) (1614–88) both became physicians. Although little is known of Théophile's life—neither diaries nor letters have been preserved—he grew up in an affluent and cultivated (*lettré*) environment.

After following classes in Geneva's College (*Collège*) and Academy, he left his hometown in search of a medical education. Exactly where he studied is not clear. He may well have traveled to any number of Europe's main universities, which had been the habit of would-be physicians born in Geneva some fifty years earlier. It is more probable that he faithfully studied for three years at the same university, as did other students of his day. What can be ascertained is that he obtained his doctoral degree in medicine from the University of Valence, in France, on 27 November 1643.

Bonet then returned to Geneva, where he set up a practice. In 1652 he married Jeanne Spanheim, daughter of Frédéric Spanheim (1600–49), who was a famous theologian and professor at Geneva's Academy. The same year, he was elected a member of Geneva's parliament. In 1656 Bonet became physician to the town of Neuchâtel, perhaps encouraged by another Geneva physician, Jean Sarasin (1610–76), who had previously occupied the position. Bonet was offered a house, a garden, and quantities of wine and cereals, as well as a modest remuneration for every patient treated. In 1657 he was promoted to the position of ordinary physician to Henri II (Fürsten Henri II).

Also in 1657, having considered that the practice of medicine was badly organized in Neuchâtel, he prepared and wrote a new '*Ordonnance sur l'exercice de la médecine à Neuchâtel*'. That new rule entrusted the town physician with the authority to examine foreign physicians and surgeons, native apothecaries, and midwives. In case of an epidemic, the town physician was made responsible for ensuring that the necessary measures were taken. But Bonet seems to have suffered from the jealousy of certain members of Neuchâtel's ruling classes during his office. Despite his friendship with State Chancellor Georges de Montmollin, in whose house he lived for three years while helping to treat the chancellor's right eye, Bonet decided to leave Neuchâtel after ten years of residence because of the hostile activities of two men—Simon Chevalier, a physician who aspired to become town physician, and an apothecary. He returned to Geneva in 1666, where he established a medical practice. His hearing deteriorated, and in 1670 he resolved to abandon consultations.

Pathological Anatomy and Medical Practice

Abandoning regular practice is deemed to be one of the main causes of Bonet's success as a medical author, because he spent most of his time thereafter collecting and publishing medical data. He excelled in compilation and scholarly endeavors, and between 1670 and 1689 he published no fewer than sixteen volumes that constitute an entire medical encyclopedia. But Bonet is remembered today for one specific volume, the *Sepulchretum sive Anatomia practica*. Its purpose was to propose an overall view of what could be said of the relationship between the observations noted in postmortem dissections and the symptoms of which the patient complained. The book contains 2,934 systematically reported observations that were taken from his own practice and from some 469 medical authors. Beyond the content of the compilation itself, the later success of Bonet's method as it was adopted in nineteenth-century hospital medicine has encouraged many physicians and historians to consider the *Sepulchretum* a cornerstone of medical thought.

A second work, *Mercurius Compitalitius*, was published in Latin in 1683 and translated into English the following year as *A Guide to the Practical Physician*. Therein Bonet proposed a general guide to medical practice for the physician, organized by disease. He also espoused general ethical rules that the physician should observe, both in regard to medical knowledge and in his attitude toward patients. Those recommendations included many professional tactics designed to enhance the image of the physician who must, for example, always offer some remedy in order to answer the patient's expectations, avoid voicing a negative prognosis, and never call on a patient without being invited. Beyond such social rules, Bonet listed numerous precautions to be taken for the patient's own good, among them to observe the patient's bad habits; to instruct, rather than to give orders; and never to disclose the nature of remedies given. Overall, his counseling invited physicians to be critical of ancient therapies and certain superstitious practices that experience had proved to be unsuccessful. Bonet ultimately championed prudence and a critical approach based on learning, experience, and reason.

Bibliography

Primary: 1679. *Sepulchretum sive anatomia practica ex cadaveribus morbo denati* (Geneva); 1684. *A Guide to the Practical Physician; shewing from the most approved Authors, both Ancient and Modern, the truest and safest way of curing all Diseases, Internal and External, whether by Medicine, Surgery or Diet. To which is added An Appendix concerning the Office of a Physician* (London).

Secondary: Buess, H., 1951. 'Théophil Bonet (1620–1689) und die grundsätzliche Bedeutung seines "Sepulchretum in der Geschichte der Pathologischen Anatomie."' *Gesnerus* 8: 32–52; Irons, Ernest E., 1932. 'Théophile Bonet 1620–1689'. *Bulletin of the History of Medicine* 12: 623–664; Gautier, Léon, 1906. *La médecine à Genève jusqu'à la fin du 18e siècle, Mémoires et documents publiés par la société d'histoire et d'archéologie* (Geneva) pp. 251–253.

Philip Rieder

BONTEKOE, CORNELIS (b. Alkmaar, the Netherlands, *c.* 1644; d. Berlin, Germany, 14 January 1685), *medicine.*

Bontekoe, son of Neel Maertens (d. 1649) and Gerrit Jansz. Dekker (d. 1652), who ran a grocery in Alkmaar, started his medical studies at Leiden University on 22 September 1665. Besides studying medicine with Franciscus de le Boë (Sylvius) and Johannes van Horne, Bontekoe studied philosophy with Arnold Geulincx. After graduating with a dissertation entitled *De gangraena et sphacelo* on 6 May 1667, Bontekoe returned to Alkmaar, where he soon got into conflict with local colleagues and apothecaries. He moved to De Rijp and later to the Hague, only to arouse new disputes wherever he went. In the early 1670s, Bontekoe closely studied Descartes' philosophical and physiological works. He enrolled in Leiden University for a second time on 27 April 1674, but on 22 January 1675 he was forbidden to attend any further university disputations, because of his tendency to incite the students against their Aristotelian professors. On 18 December 1675, he was barred from all Leiden classes, whether public or private.

With the publication of his *Tractaat van het excellenste kruyd thee* [Treatise on the Most Excellent Herb of Tea] in 1678, new editions of which appeared in 1679 and 1685, Bontekoe acquired instant fame. After a short period in Amsterdam, he moved to Hamburg and then to Berlin. There he became personal physician and councilor to elector Frederic William of Brandenburg, as well as professor of medicine at Frankfurt an der Oder. In January 1685, Bontekoe fell from the stairs in the house of the painter Jacques Vaillant and suffered a fatal head injury. He was buried in the *Schloßkirche* on 27 January 1685.

In Bontekoe's day, tea offered an alternative to the widespread consumption of wine and beer. He recommended that eight to ten cups of tea should be taken twice daily by those who were not used to the drink. Others could easily take 100 or 200 cups twice. The drink was not considered to be just a simple refreshment. Like other beverages, it was thought to keep the blood warm and the animal spirits flowing, yet without the negative effects of wine and beer. Such dietetic considerations were typical for the Cartesian school, which interpreted the body as a system of tubes, vessels, pores, and valves.

Contrary to some of his iatromechanical contemporaries, however, Bontekoe was no blind follower of Descartes, but insisted on honest experience and methodical reasoning. Puritan views, possibly inspired by his Mennonite background, stood at the center of Bontekoe's ideas on medicine. Convinced that life could be prolonged simply by protecting the body from diseases—as well as from accidents and aging—and holding the uncompromising belief that people are always to blame for their own illnesses, Bontekoe considered medicine as a way to curb the effects of Adam's Fall. Besides dietetic issues, there were moral precepts to consider, because chaste pleasures were considered to be psychosomatic ways of keeping the blood agile.

Moral precepts also included a rather strict pedagogy designed to keep children from surrendering to the lure of the passions. On a broader scale, Bontekoe envisioned a reform of science and of the social institutions connected with it, especially those aspects involving the education of unschooled apothecaries, whom he regarded as the prime agents of death. With his broad readership in the Netherlands and Germany, Bontekoe helped diffuse the idea that the science of medicine was still in its infancy, but that a 'Christian' and 'enlightened' reformation of man might help bring about previously unimagined results.

Bibliography

Primary: 1689. *Alle de philosophische, medicinale en chymische werken* 4 parts in 2 vols. (Amsterdam); 1680–81. *Niew gebouw van de chirurgie of heel-konst* (the Hague); 1688. *Fundamenta medica* (Amsterdam).

Secondary: Ruler, Han van, 2003. 'Bontekoe, Cornelis (*c.* 1644–85)' in Bunge, Wiep van, et al., eds., *The Dictionary of Seventeenth- and Eighteenth-Century Dutch Philosophers*, vol. 1. (Bristol) pp. 128–132; Schweikardt, Christoph, 2003. 'More than Just a Propagandist for Tea. Religious Argument and Advice on a Healthy Life in the Work of the Dutch Physician Cornelis Bontekoe (1647–1685).' *Medical History* 47: 357–368; Baumann, E. D., 1949. *Cornelis Bontekoe (1640–1685). De theedoctor* (Oosterbeek).

Han van Ruler

BORDET, JULES (b. Soignies, Belgium, 13 June 1870; d. Ixelles, Belgium, 6 April 1961), *bacteriology, immunology.*

Bordet was born to Charles Bordet, a schoolteacher, and Célestine Vandenbaele. He lived in Brussels, where he received his medical doctorate in 1892. Twenty-two years old and attracted by the booming studies of bacteriology, he received a scholarship from the Belgian government to work on vaccination, which enabled him to join Elie Mechnikov at the newly founded Pasteur Institute in Paris. There he embarked on a long and successful career in the study of bacteria and immunity.

In 1894 Pfeiffer had described the destruction of cholera vibrios *in vivo* by the peritoneal fluid of immunized guinea pigs. Bordet turned that experiment into a milestone of immunology. He showed that microbial destruction resulted from the action of two substances. One was 'alexine' (a term borrowed from the German biologist Buchner), which was present in the serum of all animals, immunized or not, and was inactivated by heat. The other substance was resistant to heat and was specifically produced in response to germs in the organism (in other words, by vaccination). Nothing was known at the time of the chemical nature of these substances or of their mode of action. Bordet disagreed with Paul Ehrlich's description of their 'fixation' by means of receptors or hypothetical specific sites on the cell surface.

More generally, Bordet established that it was possible to immunize not only with germs, but also with red blood cells. That finding later led Karl Landsteiner (1868–1943) to consider that any chemical substance, properly presented, would trigger an immunologic reaction. Because hemolysis was easy to observe in the test tube, without a microscope, Bordet devised an experimental system to reveal specific antimicrobial immunity. When red blood cells were added to normal serum mixed with a germ suspension, the germs remained unmodified while red cells were hemolyzed. When immune sera were used, germs were destroyed while red cells remained intact. That simple and practical method for diagnosing disease remained in use for a long time, only recently being superseded by more precise methods.

The Nobel Committee awarded its Medicine or Physiology prize to Bordet in 1919 for 'his discoveries in regard to immunity', which illuminated the balance between its specific and nonspecific aspects.

Bordet gave his name to the bacterium (*Bordetella pertussis*) in whooping cough (pertussis), which he described with his brother-in-law Octave Gengou, and initiated the production of a vaccine against the infant scourge. His monumental *Traité de l'immunité dans les maladies infectieuses* (1920), published after further work during the agonizing years of the Great War, provided a fundamental synthesis that he thoroughly updated in 1939.

Reputed to have discussed recent work in immunity until his last breath, Bordet died at the age of eighty. He was a scientist devoted to international cooperation in a time of violent chauvinism among nationalistic teams. In the laboratory of Mechnikov, a supporter of phagocytosis and the role of cells in immunity, Bordet developed research at the intersection of cellular and humoral immunity, which may reflect something of his temperate, conciliating ethos in work and life.

His name is familiar to sociologists of science because the complement-fixation reaction in syphilis (the so-called 'Bordet-Wassermann reaction') inspired the work of the Polish physician Ludwik Fleck (1935), which was revealed to the public by historian Thomas Kuhn. The test was shown to be less sensitive and specific than expected, but the social need for a syphilis test was so strong that it remained in use for three generations. Still more intriguing, the presence of the specific germ was not absolutely required; chemical substances from normal organs could be substituted for the *Treponema*. Those circumstances suggested that so-called 'scientific facts' were 'value-laden' and reflected the collective *Denkstil* [style of thought] of the time.

Bordet became director of the Brussels Pasteur Institute, which opened in 1904. The Brabant Institute, devoted to developing sera and vaccines, is still active today.

Bibliography

Primary: 1901. 'Sur le mode d'action des sérums cytolytiques.' *Annales de l'Institut Pasteur* 15: 303–318; 1909. *Studies in Immunity* (New York); 1920. *Traité de l'immunité dans les maladies infectieuses* (Paris).

Secondary: Mazumdar, Pauline, 1995. *Species and Specificity* (Cambridge); Moulin, Anne Marie, 1991. *Le dernier langage de la médecine* (Paris); Fleck, Ludwik, 1979. *The Genesis and Development of a Scientific Fact* (Chicago); DSB.

Anne Marie Moulin

BORDEU, THÉOPHILE DE (b. Izeste, France, 21 February 1722; d. Paris, France, 24 December 1776), *medicine.*

Bordeu was the son of Antoine, a physician trained in Montpellier. The family was large (Théophile was the eldest of fifteen children) and much concerned about money. Bordeu's brother François was also a physician, and father and sons did everything possible to promote the family's medical reputation. Bordeu studied with the Barnabites at the Collège de Lescar before matriculating at the University of Medicine of Montpellier in 1739. His two *thèses*, *Chilificationis historia* and *De Sensu generice considerato*, drew favorable attention from his teachers; the *De Sensu* presaged his interest in nervous sensibility.

After completing his doctorate (a joint medical and surgical degree) in 1743, Bordeu departed for Pau, where he taught anatomy to the acclaim of students, but to the consternation of locally trained physicians. After a brief return to Montpellier, he moved to Paris, where he studied with the famed surgeon Jean-Louis Petit and saw patients at the Charité hospital. Returning again to Pau, Bordeu assumed a position as superintendent of the waters of Aquitaine, the subject of his first book. With his father he also began a periodical publication that celebrated the virtues of the waters in treating a range of illnesses. Those activities first established Bordeu's reputation and gained for him appointment as a corresponding member of the Academy of Sciences in Paris. While in Pau, Bordeu also worked on the treatise *Recherches anatomiques sur la position des glandes, et sur leur action*, in which he set forth principles of the vitalist physiology for which he was to be principally known.

In 1751 Bordeu settled definitively in Paris. There he began a collaboration with a kinsman, the court physician Louis de Lacaze, that eventually produced three major vitalist texts, including the much-cited *Idée de l'homme physique et moral* of 1755. In Paris, Bordeu frequented the circles of the Encyclopedists, contributing the much-discussed entry 'Crise' to Diderot's venture. Although he made no further contributions to the *Encyclopédie*, he continued his association with Diderot, serving as physician to members of Diderot's household. In the 1750s and 1760s Bordeu became a fashionable physician, developing an extensive clientele of high-born patients, especially women. Although he never held an official position as court physician, he treated many patients at Versailles, including Madame du Barry, who for a time was the 'favorite' of Louis XV. That connection encouraged Bordeu to hope that he would one day gain appointment as First Physician, the remunerative and prestigious post as head of the king's medical entourage, but that ambition was never realized.

The writings of Bordeu's middle and late career were chiefly devoted to topics in practical medicine, including hydrotherapy, lead poisoning, chronic illness, and the diagnostic value of the pulse. He also published several theoretical works, one on the connective ('mucous') tissue and another on the constituents and functions of blood. Between 1761 and 1764 Bordeu was caught up in a scandal set off by the accusation of a rival physician that he had stolen a watch and tobacco case from a patient. Although ultimately exonerated, Bordeu carried the wounds of that affair, and in 1764 he published a polemical history of medicine

aimed in part at those he held responsible. After the affair was resolved he redoubled his efforts to gain renown as both a theoretician and a practitioner of medicine.

In 1774 Bordeu attended Louis XV when the king was fatally stricken with smallpox. After a visit to his native Béarn, Bordeu returned to Paris, where he died at the age of fifty-four. Although in his lifetime Bordeu enjoyed considerable celebrity in medical circles, he has often been better known to history as the fictionalized 'Dr. Bordeu' of Diderot's famous dialogue *Rêve de d'Alembert*, written in 1769. The image it conveyed of Bordeu as a spokesman for Diderot's style of materialism has occasioned considerable misinterpretation of Bordeu's own thinking.

Vitalist Physiology

Bordeu's significance in the history of medicine was ensured principally by his contributions to physiology. He had been a student of the 'animist' theoretician François Boissier de Sauvages at Montpellier, and he absorbed from his teacher a hostility to iatromechanism, especially the Cartesian variety current in the Montpellier of his student days. Bordeu was a devoted student of the medicine of the Ancients, and he sought to recover what he regarded as the spurned legacy of Hippocrates. He was also influenced by the Renaissance physician Joan Baptista van Helmont and by the strong Paracelsian tradition in the Huguenot milieu of Bordeu's native region.

His earliest writings were devoted to an attack on medical mechanism and to promotion of the vitalist principle that there was an absolute distinction between the realm of brute, unorganized matter and that of living beings. Bordeu's first major work sought to undermine the view that glandular action was the result of the mechanical compression of surrounding bone and muscle. Bordeu proposed instead that the glands, like all active components of the body, moved spontaneously in response to peculiar 'forces' or 'tastes' that functioned in harmony with the overall needs of the organism. Orchestrating the ensemble of bodily activities was the general vital force known as 'sensibility'. In defining the nature and influence of sensibility, Bordeu challenged the distinction between sensibility and irritability proposed by the Swiss physiologist Albrecht von Haller. He rejected Haller's finding that sensibility was restricted to nerve fibers and pathways, whereas irritability was a force inherent in muscle fiber. Bordeu argued that sensibility was a diffuse force that pervaded the organism and made use of diverse channels, including the connective tissue (to which he would devote a volume published in 1767).

Bordeu's hostility to Hallerian-style experimentation reflected his conviction that medicine must rest not on experiment, but on clinical observation. Although Bordeu performed experiments of his own design in studying the glands and conducted others in company with his Montpellier colleague, François Bourguignon de Lamure, he questioned the value for medicine of experiments performed on animal subjects, arguing that they were not transferable to human beings. He also held that experiments establishing conditions inimical to the life of the subject yielded results that illuminated pathology and death, but not vitality and life. Bordeu's general physiological framework was adapted from the teleological thinking of the Ancients. It was intended both to discredit mechanistic ideas of bodily function and to undergird a view that medicine's role depended on recognition of the body's 'conserving force'. Bordeu was an important defender of 'expectancy', the view that nature was the ultimate healer and that the physician's role was to aid nature in that task. Bordeu and fellow graduates of Montpellier presented those insights concerning physiology and the character of medicine as the special contribution of a distinctive 'Montpellier school' that constituted a 'modern Cos'.

The Nature of Medicine and the Role of the Physician

Beginning with the works he produced in company with Lacaze, Bordeu elaborated a conception of medical practice that rested on the vitalist principles of the singularity of life and the independence of medicine from 'auxiliary' sciences concerned with strictly physico-chemical phenomena. Urging that the chief task of medicine was the observation of patients in health and sickness, he decried medicine's subjection to mechanics, physics, and chemistry. This view of medicine was in part dependent on Bordeu's insistence on the importance of 'moral' factors in the genesis and cure of illness. He held that only medicine could grasp the complex physical and moral reciprocities that unfolded ceaselessly in the living human organism. Bordeu's therapeutic conceptions made much of the Ancient doctrine of the 'non-naturals', including the 'passions of the soul'. He did not participate in the movement of eighteenth-century materialists to reduce the 'soul' of philosophical and religious tradition to physical structures of brain and nerve. Indeed, he declared his belief in the immaterial, immortal soul and his respect for the truths of revealed religion. Nevertheless, Bordeu argued for the special authority of physicians with respect to 'moral' activities that unfolded in intimate conjunction with physiological processes. Thus, in Bordeu's thinking physiology was not limited to the study of material or physical phenomena—it encompassed feelings and behavior as well. Bordeu referred to physicians as 'legislators' over domains of physical-moral experience that were comprehensible to medicine alone.

At the same time, Bordeu's understanding of medical practice placed great responsibility on the patient for the preservation of his or her own health, which was to be safeguarded through careful attention to the 'non-naturals'. The physician-legislator gave guidance, but patients were called upon to cultivate the habits of diet, exercise, and a general regimen that constituted a 'well-ordered life'. Beyond his tutelary role, the physician's task was largely diagnostic and

prognostic, branches of the medical art to which Bordeu accorded much attention. He attacked the Ancient doctrine of 'crisis', insisting that no illness was reducible to the fatality of numbers and urging that the skilled practitioner must be attuned to variable—often obscure—signs and symptoms. Similarly, his work on the pulse was intended to train physicians in the complex art of distinguishing minute variations in that all-important sign.

With respect to active therapeutics, Bordeu was chiefly devoted to hydrotherapy, arguing for the value of mineral waters in effecting systemic physiological changes. He wrote ardently on behalf of the special value of the waters of his native region, thus mixing therapeutic doctrine with the commercial interests of his medical family. Bordeu participated in the eighteenth-century movement against polypharmacy, and he also decried the overuse of bleeding. That position reflected not only his preference for natural healing, but also his skepticism about the privileged role mechanists accorded the circulation of the blood—especially what he believed to be their tendency to trace all illness to circulatory obstructions. In his history of medicine, the same viewpoint caused him to question the central importance of William Harvey. By contrast, Bordeu was an outspoken defender of inoculation against smallpox. It was a technique he described as having been offered up by nature itself, but one that would succeed only if properly tailored to the circumstances of particular patients.

Bordeu's influence was felt in diverse branches of medicine. His physiological and therapeutic conceptions formed the bedrock of medical vitalism in later eighteenth-century and nineteenth-century France. His work on the connective tissue exerted strong influence on Xavier Bichat and the subsequent development of histology. His emphasis on the variability of distinct physico-moral 'types'—those formed by the influence of occupation, sex, age, and geography—made him a key figure in the development of the medical 'science of man', which spawned anthropology and related social sciences in France. The importance that Bordeu and fellow vitalists accorded the 'passions' in health and sickness also influenced Philippe Pinel, the father of French psychiatry, whose medical training included years of study in Montpellier.

Bibliography

Primary: 1818. (Richerand, A. B., ed.) *Oeuvres complètes de Bordeu* 2 vols. (Paris); 1746. *Lettres contenant des essais sur l'histoire des Eaux minérales du Béarn* (Amsterdam); 1764. *Recherches sur quelques points d'histoire de la médecine* (Liège, Paris); n.d. (Fletcher, Martha W., ed.) *Théophile de Bordeu: Correspondance* 4 vols. (Montpellier).

Secondary: Williams, Elizabeth A., 2003. *A Cultural History of Medical Vitalism in Enlightenment Montpellier* (Burlington, VT); Rey, Roselyne, 2000. *Naissance et développement du vitalisme en France de la deuxième moitié du 18e siècle à la fin du Premier Empire*

(Oxford); Haigh, Elizabeth., 1976. 'Vitalism, the Soul, and Sensibility: The Physiology of Théophile Bordeu.' *Journal of the History of Medicine and Allied Sciences* 31: 30–41; Cornet, Lucien., 1965. 'Un protecteur de Théophile de Bordeu: Le médecin Louis Lacaze (1703–1765).' *Bulletin de la Société des sciences, lettres et arts de Pau* 3d ser., 21: 55–63; DSB.

Elizabeth A. Williams

BORELLI, GIOVANNI ALFONSO   (b. Naples, Italy, 28 January 1608; d. Rome, Italy, 31 December 1679), *physiology, mathematics, physics, astronomy, volcanology.*

Borelli, the son of Miguel Alonso, a Spanish soldier garrisoned at Castel Nuovo, and Laura Borrello (or Porrello), was baptized as Giovanni Francesco Antonio. There is no further documentation until around 1630, when he was studying in Rome as a pupil of the mathematician Benedetto Castelli, probably under the protection of Tommaso Campanella, who had known the young boy when he (Campanella) had been imprisoned at Naples. It was thanks to Castelli—who had been a pupil of Galileo—that Borelli came into contact with Galileo's innovative doctrines. It was probably at this time that Borelli took his mother's maiden name and substituted an Italianized version of his father's name for two of his baptismal names. He probably met Evangelista Torricelli and Famiano Michelini also while in Rome. In 1635, or shortly thereafter, Borelli obtained the public lectureship in mathematics at the University of Messina, on Castelli's recommendation. He soon won renown as a diligent and clever scholar, becoming a member of the Accademia della Fucina. In 1642 he was sent by the Senate of Messina on a yearlong journey to the most important political and cultural centers in Italy to recruit teachers for the University of Messina. He visited Venice—where he stayed for at least two months—Rome, Florence, Naples—where he met Marco Aurelio Severino—Genoa, Bologna, and Padua. While in Bologna he met Bonaventura Cavalieri, who was very impressed by the brilliant mind of the young Neapolitan.

At the beginning of 1643 Borelli returned to Messina, where he remained until 1656. It was in that period that he published his first two works. The first, the *Discorso* against Pietro Emanuele (1646), arose from an argument regarding a geometrical problem suggested by the Genoese mathematician A. Santini. In it Borelli criticized the paralogisms of his adversary and laid down a series of demonstrative rules. His second work was much more important and aroused a great deal of interest. In 1646–48 Sicily was invaded by an epidemic of malignant fevers resulting in very high mortality. When Borelli was asked to express his own opinion regarding the causes of the epidemic and how it could be controlled, he presented his conclusions at the Accademia della Fucina in 1648. Those conclusions were published in 1649 as the *Delle cagioni delle febbri maligne della Sicilia negli anni 1647 e 1648* [On the Causes of the Malignant Fevers of

Sicily in the Years 1647 and 1648], which contained two appendices—one on fevers in general, and the other on digestion. The work is in fact a true iatromechanical manifesto, in which Borelli rejected what were then widely held concepts about malignant fevers.

Instead of the traditional doctrine that good health was the result of a perfect balance between the four elementary qualities of the macrocosm and the four humors of the microcosm, Borelli proposed an atomistic-mechanical interpretation. He totally dismissed the view that malign fevers could derive from a prevalence of heat and dampness in the atmosphere, as well as the idea that they could be caused by astrological influences. Borelli held instead that the pestilence was caused by the violent evaporation of poisonous exhalations—analogous to the 'seeds of pestilence' proposed by the atomist Lucretius—which, when condensed by physical forces, fell to the ground, penetrated the organism, and acted directly on the organs rather than on the humors. Therefore, one could not look for the cure by trying to eliminate an altered humor from the organism. Instead, one must utilize some antidote to poisons, which Borelli identified in sulfur. He considered fever in general to be a healing factor, because it provoked an acceleration of the motion of which life consists—according to his iatromechanical concept. He sustained a physiology based on motion and on the particles and pores, as well as a pathology based on alterations of the normal corpuscular motion. In the appendix on digestion, Borelli stated for the first time that the stomach produced a 'corrosive acid juice', which is capable of dissolving the aliments to their smallest particles.

In February 1656 Borelli was called to the University of Pisa as professor of mathematics. That same year Pisa called Marcello Malpighi to be professor of theoretical medicine, and the Lorraine anatomist Claude Aubry. The three professors soon began to collaborate closely, especially at Borelli's home, which had been transformed into an anatomical laboratory. Lacking manual dexterity in anatomy, Borelli urged the two skilful researchers Malpighi and Aubry to search the bodies of animals for mechanical structures that would have provided an experimental basis for his theories of the corpuscular character of animal matter and the coincidence of life and motion. Lorenzo Bellini, the discoverer of renal tubules, also used to work in Borelli's home laboratory.

It was during that Tuscan period that Borelli produced his mathematical works, the first being the *Euclides restitutus, sive prisca geometriae elementa* (1658), a compendium and clarification of Euclid's *Elementi* in which he reformulated the parallel postulate and the theory of proportions. He then translated an Arab manuscript, conserved in the library of San Lorenzo, that contained the fifth, sixth, and seventh books of Apollonius of Perge's *Conics*. Borelli translated it in Rome in the summer of 1658, with the collaboration of the Maronite scholar Abraham Ecchellensis. Archimedes' *Liber assumptorum* was added to the same codex, but the work was not published until 1661 because of disagreements with Vincenzo Viviani, a former pupil of Galileo and mathematician of the Medici who was also working on the *Conics.*

The hostility between Viviani and Borelli was particularly evident in the activity of the Accademia del Cimento, which had been founded in June 1657 and of which both men were prestigious members. Borelli was the principal animus of the Accademia. There was hardly any experiment to which he had not made an important contribution, including those on the descent of smoke in the Torricellian vacuum, the compressibility of air, the weight of air and its relative density with respect to water, and some phenomena of capillarity. Unfortunately, Borelli's enormous capacity for work and the facility with which he passed from one argument to another created not a little jealousy among his colleagues. Viviani in particular suffered from Borelli's embarrassing presence, which tended to overshadow the contributions of the others.

Borelli was also very interested in astronomy during his stay in Tuscany. In 1664 the appearance of a comet gave him the opportunity to propose one of his most innovative and valid theories—attributing a solid head and an elliptical solar orbit to the comets. His ideas appeared in the *Lettera del movimento della cometa apparsa il mese di dicembre del 1664 in Pisa*, published in 1665 under the pseudonym of Pier Maria Mutoli. In 1666 he dedicated the *Theoricae Mediceorum planetarum ex causis physicis deductae* to Jupiter's satellites, which had been discovered by Galileo in 1610. The *Theoricae Mediceorum* was the result of prolonged and extremely accurate observations carried out with large telescopes. In the process he also anticipated the laws of universal attraction later formulated by Isaac Newton, who did not hesitate to recognize that Borelli had been his own forerunner.

Probably as a consequence of his disagreements with Viviani, Borelli chose to abandon Florence in 1667 and return to Messina, where apparently he had been offered the possibility of a satisfactory salary without any obligation to teach. In 1667 and 1670 he published two works of physics, which represented for him a necessary introduction to a fuller understanding of his doctrine on animal motions. The *De vi percussionis liber* (1667) deals with all of the principal questions of mechanics, as well as impulsive motions; the second book, *De motionibus naturalibus a gravitate pendentibus* (1670), discusses gravity.

In 1669, following a major eruption of Mount Etna, Borelli wrote his famous *Meteorologia Aetnea, seu historia et meteorologia incendii Aetnaei anni 1669* (1670), now considered to be the first work on modern volcanology.

Borelli's peregrinations, however, were not finished. Apparently he let himself get involved (some chroniclers have claimed that he was, in fact, a leader) with an uprising in Messina against the Spanish governor (1670–74). In 1672 a government proclamation banished him and others

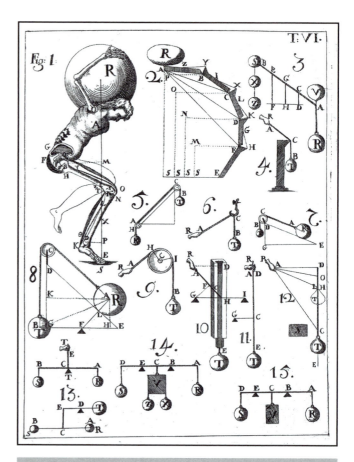

The action of anatomical and mechanical levers and pulleys. Engraving from *De motu animalium* . . . Naples, 1734. Rare Books, Wellcome Library, London.

from the island. Deprived of his pension and his protectors, Borelli returned to Rome with the problem of finding some way of providing for himself. He sought help from friends such as Lucantonio Porzio and Michelangelo Ricci, and he duly became a member of the academy created by Queen Christina of Sweden. There he presented some dissertations, more with the purpose of satisfying the curiosities of Christina than expressing personal scientific interests.

Toward the end of 1667, Borelli accepted the hospitality offered to him by the Piarist Fathers in their Casa di S. Pantaleo, where he taught mathematics at the Scuole Pie, finished a compendium of the *Conics* (1679), and added the finishing touches to his masterpiece, *De motu animalium.* In late 1679 Queen Christina agreed to bear the printing costs, and Borelli dedicated the work to her. He had already corrected the proofs of the first part when he fell ill with pneumonia and died. The Piarists worked with devotion to complete the printing of the *De motu animalium*, which finally came out between 1680 and 1681 and was widely read throughout Europe, establishing Borelli as the father of iatromechanics. *De motu animalium*—like Borelli's other, more important, works—went through many editions.

In the first volume of *De motu animalium,* which appeared in 1680, Borelli dealt with the external motions—the motions produced by the muscles. The second volume dealt with internal motions such as the movements of the muscles themselves, circulation, respiration, the secretion of fluids, and nervous activity. It was published in late 1681. When applying the laws of mechanics to the functions of a living organism, Borelli obtained the most important results in his study of muscular activity in the movement of human limbs, which constitutes the basis of modern muscular mechanics. Borelli also interpreted the flight of birds and the swimming of fish in a physicomechanical sense, i.e., basing his analysis on the laws of the lever and on the shortening of the muscles attached to the skeleton. His analyses of the heart's action and of intestinal movements were less successful, and his attempts to provide a mechanical explanation for those processes that we now know to be of a chemical nature, such as digestion, were an obvious failure. Notwithstanding his application of physical principles, Borelli's observations were above all qualitative, not experimental; the procedure he followed was geometrically constructive, rather than quantitatively analytic. Even though he tried to explain every living phenomenon mechanically, Borelli sometimes made a concession to chemistry, as in his explanation of muscular contraction.

Bibliography

Primary: 1649. *Delle cagioni delle febbri maligne della Sicilia negli anni 1647 e 1648 . . . con una appendice della natura della febbre in comune, et in fine si tratta della digestione de' cibi con nuovo metodo* (Cosenza); 1680–81. *De motu animalium . . . opus posthumum* (Rome).

Secondary: Baldini, Ugo, 1974. 'Giovanni Alfonso Borelli biologo e fisico negli studi recenti.' *Physis* 16: 234–266; Balaguer Perigüell, Emilio, 1971. 'La introducción de la metodologia moderna en biologia: el *De motu animalium* de J. A. Borelli (1608–1679).' *Episteme* 5: 243–262; Belloni, Luigi, 1967. 'Dal Borelli al Malpighi.' *Simposi clinici* 4: xvii–xxiv; Barbensi, Gustavo, 1947. *Borelli* (Trieste); *DSB.*

Giuseppe Ongaro

BOTKIN, SERGEI PETROVICH (b. Moscow, Russia, 5 September 1832; d. Mentona, France, 12 December 1889), *therapeutics.*

Botkin, eleventh child of tea merchant Peter Kononovich Botkin and Anna Ivanovna Postnikova, was brought up by his older brother Vasilii, a writer, who was closely connected to a group of famous intellectuals that included Vissarion Grigorievich Belinsky, Alexander Ivanovich Herzen, and Timofei Nikolaevich Granovskii. Two other Botkin brothers, Mikhail and Dmitrii, were famous artists. Sergei was educated at home first, and then at the private Enessa pension (1847–50) and in Moscow University (1850–55), where he was influenced by the physiologist Ivan Timofeevich Glebov and the surgeon Fedor Ivanovich Inozemtsev. In 1853 he met with Ivan Mikhailovich Sechenov, whose scientific ideas were always close to his own. Botkin went voluntarily to the Crimea in 1855, where he worked under the direction of Nikolay Ivanovich Pirogov in a military hospital for three months.

In February 1856 Botkin traveled to Europe to update his medical knowledge. He visited Berlin, Vienna, Paris, Switzerland, and England; attended lectures by Rudolf Virchow, Ludwig Traube, Johann Oppolzer, and Armand Trousseau; and visited the laboratories of Claude Bernard, Ernst-Felix Hoppe-Seyler, and Carl Ludwig. By virtue of that traveling, Botkin recognized the importance of natural sciences for the development of clinical medicine, and some of his papers were published in *Virchow's Archiv.* In 1858 he married Anastasia Aleksandrovna Krylova (she died in 1875).

Coming to St Petersburg in 1860, Botkin defended his dissertation on the theme 'O vsasyvanii zhira v kishkakh' [On the absorption of fat in the intestines] and was admitted as an adjunct of Professor Pavel Dmitrievich Shipulinskii in the therapeutics clinic of the Medical-Surgical Academy. He assumed that position in 1861and instituted a number of fundamental reforms, among them organizing the first clinical laboratory in Russia. Then he established chemical, physiological (headed by Ivan Petrovich Pavlov from 1878) and bacteriological (1884) laboratories. Botkin believed that it was impossible for a lecturer to acquaint students with all the different manifestations of patients' lives. He felt that it was necessary instead to give to them a general method that would enable the young practitioner to use his knowledge for every sick human.

In 1862 Botkin acquired a reputation as a diagnostician when he recognized thrombosis of the portal vein (near the spleen) before his patient died. He offered a model for research that began with the physical methods (inspection, palpation, auscultation, percussion) and then passed on to the history. Dealing with a case of kidney disease, he analyzed the urine of the patient. The accuracy of diagnosis was to be checked by the dissection of bodies, and it was obligatory in his clinics. Botkin successfully developed the skill required for physical examination of the body. With his hand alone, he could determine the size of the spleen and the immobility of the kidney.

Sharing Sechenov's ideas, during physical examination he emphasized the condition of the nervous system and psyche. He concluded that nervous disorders were a cause of heart illness, and that bronchial asthma and the angina pectoris constituted a variety of neurosis. He underlined the importance of functional interrelations between heart and stomach, and the heart and lungs.

Botkin had a large number of students in his clinics who later became important Russian physicians and chairs of clinical departments in many cities. Among them were Viacheslav Avksentievich Manassein, Nikolai Iakovlevich Chistovich, Vasilii Nikolaevich Sirotinin, Mikhail Vladimirovich Ianovskii, Iuri Timofeevich Chudnovskii, Vasilii Timofeevich Pokrovskii, Iakov Iakovlevich Stol'nikov, and many others. His son, Sergei Sergeevich Botkin, became a physician whose career developed very successfully; he had become head of the therapeutics clinic of the Academy by 1898.

Botkin wanted medicine to be not only an art, but a science that was intended to treat the patient, relieve sufferings, and prevent diseases. He looked at disease as a pathological process in a concrete organism, and he individuated the nature of disease. Beginning in 1867, he began to publish 'Kurs kliniki vnutrennikh bolesny' [Course for an internal disease clinic]. In each volume of that work, Botkin discussed only one clinical case—for example, a case of heart disease, or typhus, or the phenomenon of spleen contraction. The order of reasoning in his book became a model for clinical thinking. According to Botkin, understanding the pathological process makes it possible to foresee the further course of the illness, to establish accurately the treatment necessary, to prevent complications, and to make theoretical conclusions, which also promotes the development of theory about internal pathology.

In the field of cardiology, Botkin called attention to a number of previously unstudied symptoms, offered original methods of research, and identified some remedies. He provided a clinical description of arteriosclerosis and concluded that, if there is a defect of the aortal valves, the diastolic sound could be heard in the area of the third to fourth rib, on the left of the breast (now known as the 'Botkin point', or the fifth auscultation point of the heart). Examining the peripheral blood circulation, he developed a clinical representation of Basedow's (Graves') disease that was characterized by the irregularity of atrium contraction, the contrast between harsh pulsations of the general carotid and faint pulsations of the radial arteries, irritability, and whimpering. Botkin was the author of the theory of neurogenesis of Basedow's disease. In 1875 he and his pupils discovered the spleen's involvement in the process of blood deposition, and in 1884 he offered the idea of the nervous regulation of blood creation. In Botkin's laboratory, Stol'nikov (1879) clamped the kidney artery in experiments with the production of renal hypertensive condition.

Botkin elaborated clinical knowledge of such infectious diseases as typhus, typhoid fever, and recurring typhus, and he distinguished 'catarrhal jaundice' as a particular illness (hepatitis A, known as 'Botkin's disease' in the USSR since 1939). He drew the clinical picture of that disease and noted that it could develop into liver cirrhosis. In Botkin's view, the infectious disease took an atypical course determined by the lifestyle of the individual, especially the use of contaminated food. He believed that there were partial physiological mechanisms in the human organism that gave the individual a chance against illnesses.

He was the first in Russia to draw a clinical picture of myxedema (a complex form of hypothyroidism) and diffused nephritis with a predominance of the interstitial or parenchymatous process.

Botkin and his students often experimented with the medical potential of drugs. They ascertained that sulphoacidic atropine specifically acted on the peripheral nerves, and that substances contained in the leaves of *Digitalis* increased the power of heart contractions rather than decreasing them, as had been thought earlier. In Botkin's clinics the medical properties of *Adonis vernalis* and the diuretic action of *Blattae orientalis* were studied; the beneficial influence of *Grindelia robusta* was elucidated for angina pectoris; and the medical action of potash salts, of tinctures of a May lily of the valley, and other preparations were observed. He considered that when prescribing a medicine, the physician should take the patient's specific features into account and also recommended a rational regime, a diet, and treatment by climate and mineral waters. In 1872 Botkin suggested the Crimea for the treatment of tuberculosis patients.

On 23 October 1865 Botkin organized the Epidemiological Society in St Petersburg and then joined in the editing of *Epidemiologicheskii listok* (1866–68). In 1866 he was appointed a member of the Medical Council of the Ministry of Internal Affairs and the Military-Medical Scientific Committee. Botkin was among those professors of the Medical-Surgical Academy who supported the introduction of medical courses for women in 1872. To benefit those courses, he received money from the estate of the late Kondratiev, a merchant, who donated 20,000 rubles for charitable purposes. In 1872 Botkin was confirmed in the rank of Academician of the Medical-Surgical Academy, and in 1873 he became a physician at the court of Tsar Alexander II.

During the Russo-Turkish War (1877–78) he was headquarters doctor, and thus supervised the organization of therapeutic aid to soldiers. Botkin gave special attention to studying the sick rate during war, to the development of antiepidemic services, to the relocation of hospitals, to the evacuation of sick and wounded soldiers, and to the training of military physicians. Along with Pirogov, he insisted that all administrative authority belonged to physicians in hospitals.

In 1878 Botkin was elected chairman of the Society of Russian Physicians in St Petersburg. Soon the Society took part in the struggle against the consequences of the plague that flashed up in Vetlianka, Astrakhan province. In 1881 Botkin was vice-president of the Commission of Public Health and began to work in the Municipal Duma (parliament) of St Petersburg. In 1886 he was elected trustee of all city hospitals in St Petersburg, and at his initiative free medical aid for the poor was established via a group of Duma physicians. City authorities began to improve the maintenance of hospitals and started to build new ones, including the hospital of the Community of Saint George and the Aleksandrovskaia hospital barracks for contagious patients (now known as the Botkin Hospital). Under his direction, the sanitary inspection of schools was introduced in St Petersburg, and research work on city almshouses began.

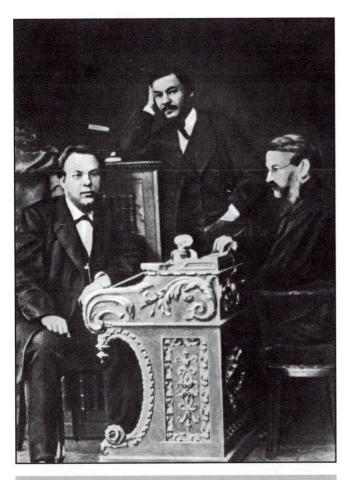

Sergei Petrovich Botkin (seated right, in profile) with Ivan Sechenov (standing center; see biographical entry) and W. Gruber (seated left). Photograph from the Academy Pavlovsky. Wellcome Library, London.

In 1886 Botkin became chairman of the Medical Council commission concerned with the improvement of sanitary conditions and reduction of the death rate in Russia. The activity of Botkin's commission informed the government about the health of the population in the Empire and offered measures for its improvement. In 1887 he suggested separating medicine from the control of the Ministry of Internal Affairs and creating a special administrative system of public health services, but that offer was not accepted. Although the activity of Botkin's commission was important, many hygienists maintained a critical attitude toward it. Feodor Fedorovich Erisman and Evgraf Alekseevich Osipov considered measures suggested for the sanitation of Russia to be insufficient, arguing that beyond sanitary engineering actions, social and economic reforms of the whole of Russian society were important.

On 7 December 1886, Botkin gave a speech at the Medical-Surgical Academy, in which he stated his point of view on the basic problems of medicine and planned the next tasks: 'For the future doctor with a research orientation it is necessary to study nature in the full sense of this word. The knowledge of physics, chemistry, and natural sciences, and the widest education, makes the best preparatory school for studying scientific and applied medicine.'

Botkin was the author of about seventy-five works devoted to problems of therapy, infectious diseases, experimental pathological physiology, and pharmacology. Most of his later lectures were written down and published by his students (Sirotinin, Ianovskii, and others). From 1869 to 1889 Botkin used his own money to publish thirteen volumes of the *Arkhiv kliniki vnutrennykh boleznei*, in which numerous works of his students were published. Beginning in 1881 he issued the *Ezhenedel'naia klinicheskaia gazeta*, which after Botkin's death was edited by Vasily Sirotinin. During the period when Botkin supervised the clinic of the Academy, his students prepared forty doctoral dissertations.

Botkin enjoyed the confidence of the government and pursued an aristocratic lifestyle. He liked to play music, and he appreciated painting. The gatherings for intellectuals and artists at his house on Saturday evenings became well-known, and there were many well-known people among his patients. Twenty-five years of Botkin's professional work were officially recognized in St Petersburg. He was an honorary member of the Moscow and Kazan Universities, and of thirty-five Russian and nine foreign medical societies. He had twelve children from two marriages.

Bibliography

Primary: 1867–75. *Kurs kliniki vnutrennikh boleznei* [Course for Clinics of Internal Illnesses] 3 vols. (St Petersburg); 1887–88. (Sirontinin, Vasiliy Nikolaevich, et al., eds.) *Klinicheskie lektsii* [Clinical Lectures] 3 vols. (St Petersburg); 1950. *Kurs kliniki vnutrennikh boleznei i klinicheskie lektsii* [Course for Clinics of Internal Illnesses and Clinical Lectures] 2 vols. (Moscow).

Secondary: Arinkin, Mikhail Innokentievich, and V. B. Farber, 1948. *S. P. Botkin, 1832–1887* (Moscow); Gukasian, Aram Grigorievich, 1940. 'S. P. Botkin—osnovopolozhnik russkoi kliniki vnutrennikh boleznei' [S. P. Botkin—Founder of the Russian Clinic of Internal Medicine]. *Sovetskaia meditsina* 5–6: 8–12; Lushnikov, Alexander Georgievich, 1969. *S. P. Botkin* (Moscow); Petrov, Boris Dmitrievich, 1982. *S. P. Botkin—zhizn' i deiatel'nost'* [S. P. Botkin—Life and Work] (Moscow).

Dmitry Mikhel

BOUCHARD, CHARLES-JACQUES (b. Montier-en-Der, France, 26 September 1837; d. Lyon, France, 28 October 1915), *clinical medicine, pathology, bacteriology.*

Bouchard attended medical school in Lyon and was an intern there before going to Paris in 1862 to complete his education. In Paris, Bouchard initially worked under Louis Béhier, the chief physician at La Pitié Hospital, and then moved successively to the Charité Hospital (under Alfred Velpeau) and the Salpêtrière Hospital, where he worked under Jean-Martin Charcot. At Charcot's suggestion, Bouchard wrote a doctoral thesis on the origin of cerebral hemorrhages (1867). In his thesis, Bouchard suggested that cerebral hemorrhages were preceded by inflammation of small vessels of the cerebrum, which led to the formation of tiny (miliary) aneurysms—later named 'Charcot-Bouchard aneurysms'.

Between 1868 and 1870, Bouchard completed his clinical training under Béhier, and during that period (in 1869) he became certified as a medical doctor. In 1870 he became head of the Bureau Central de l'Assistance Publique, and in 1876 he moved to the Bicêtre Hospital. Bouchard left the Bicêtre in 1879 for a position at Lariboisière Hospital. He also took up the position of professor of general pathology and therapeutics at the Paris Faculty of Medicine, a position he held until 1910. He became a member of the Academy of Medicine in 1886 and the Academy of Sciences in 1887. Bouchard's increasing clout within the medical Faculty was evidenced in an 1892 confrontation with his former mentor, Charcot. He succeeded in orchestrating the defeat of Charcot's candidate, Joseph Babinski, in the competition for a post of assistant professor (*agrégation*).

Trained in the French clinical tradition that emphasized close observation at the bedside coupled with knowledge of pathological anatomy as revealed through autopsy, Bouchard came of age professionally at a time when the bacteriological theory of infectious disease (associated with discoveries by Louis Pasteur in France and Robert Koch in Germany) was just being developed. Bouchard believed that bacteriology could complement the traditional insights of the clinician and the pathologist, and to that end he established bacteriological laboratories in hospital settings. At Bicêtre, Bouchard began to examine fluid substances collected from patients under his care, and he continued that practice by also setting up a laboratory at Lariboisière Hospital. In those laboratories, he subjected the urine of his patients to chemical and microscope analysis. Whenever a patient bled or developed an abscess, the liquid was drained and subjected to analysis in Bouchard's laboratory.

Bouchard hoped that bacteriology could be used to increase diagnostic accuracy. In 1882, when Koch discovered the tubercle bacillus (the microbe that caused tuberculosis), Bouchard recommended that physicians begin to look for the bacillus in sputum samples from their patients.

Bouchard also supported the introduction of antiseptic agents—that is, chemical substances that either killed the infecting microbe or slowed its rate of multiplication. By performing experiments on patients in hospital wards, Bouchard attempted to determine the therapeutic and toxic levels of various antiseptic agents. He eventually developed antiseptic therapies to treat such diverse conditions as pneumonia, tuberculosis, and typhoid fever.

In 1895, Bouchard published the first edition of his book *Traité de pathologie générale*, which constituted a major attempt to classify infectious diseases. He differentiated infectious diseases into two classes: specific infectious illnesses (with well-defined characteristics and a clearly defined etiology) and nonspecific infectious diseases (caused by various microbes, with the possibility of multiple clinical manifestations). He put forward the notions of 'autointoxication' and 'nutritional slowing' to account for pathogenesis.

Bouchard had a profound impact on French medicine in the late nineteenth and early twentieth centuries, and the many students he trained ensured that his approaches to clinical medicine and pathology had an impact well into the twentieth century.

Bibliography

Primary: 1867. *Recherches sur la pathogénie des hémorrhagies cérébrales.* Doctoral thesis, Paris; 1890. *Actions des produits secrètes par les microbes pathogenèses* (Paris); 1895–1903. *Traité de pathologie générale* (Paris).

Secondary: Contrepois, Alain, 2002. 'The Clinician, Germs and Infectious Diseases: The Example of Charles Bouchard in Paris.' *Medical History* 46: 197–220; Iragui, Vicente J., 1986. 'The Charcot-Bouchard Controversy.' *Archives of Neurology* 43(3): 290–295; Le Gendre, Paul, 1924. *Un médecin philosophe, Charles Bouchard: son œuvre et son temps* (Paris).

J. Rosser Matthews

BOUCHARDAT, APOLLINAIRE (b. L'Isle-sur-Serein, France, 23 July 1806; d. Paris, France, 7 April 1886), *hygiene, pharmacy, diabetes.*

Born into a family of Burgundy winemakers while his father was serving in the French army under Napoleon, Bouchardat worked in his youth in his uncle's pharmacy. In 1827 he received an internship to study pharmacy at the Ecole de Pharmacie de Paris, and two years later he formally embarked on his medical studies. In 1832 he earned his medical degree by writing a doctoral thesis on cholera. In the following year, he passed the competitive examination that permitted him to teach on the Faculty of Medicine in Paris, and he then became chief pharmacist at the Saint Antoine Hospital. In 1834 he became chief pharmacist at the Hôtel Dieu Hospital, a position he would hold for more than two decades. During those years, Bouchardat published in a number of prominent French scientific and medical journals—including *Annales de physique et chimie, Journal de pharmacie,* and the *Comptes rendus de l'Académie des sciences.* In 1850 he was elected to the Academy of Medicine, and in 1852 he was elevated to the chair of hygiene in the Faculty of Medicine. Bouchardat left his position at the Hôtel Dieu in 1855 to concentrate on his scientific research. In 1866 he was elected president of the Academy of Medicine.

Historically, Bouchardat is remembered primarily for his diabetes research and his promotion of hygienic measures. In his diabetic researches, Bouchardat determined that there was a relationship between the consumption of carbohydrates and that glucose-related illness. Consequently, he recommended that diabetics reduce their consumption of sugars and starches and monitor how that change in dietary regimen affected their glucose level—as revealed through daily urinalysis. Because Bouchardat emphasized that the patients learn to monitor these effects themselves, he is also seen as a pioneer in the realm of patient education. Bouchardat did not limit his treatment of diabetes to dietary restrictions, however. He observed that other factors—such as obesity—contributed as well, and consequently he recommended weight reduction and exercise for obese people with diabetes.

By performing experiments with dogs, Bouchardat established the central role of the pancreas in diabetic disease. After binding the pancreatic duct with a ligature, he observed that the dogs lost weight and later were found to have glucose in their urine, indicating the presence of diabetic disease.

In 1881 Bouchardat produced a major work on hygiene—well over 1,000 pages long—in which he attempted to cover all hygienic considerations that might come into play as contributions to disease. The book faithfully reflects the state of the discipline just before wide acceptance of germ theory.

Reflecting his roots in a wine-making family from Burgundy, Bouchardat also produced a number of published monographs on hygienic considerations associated with the consumption of wine, as well as on diseases that could affect vineyards.

For his contributions to the understanding and treatment of diabetes, an award was named in his honor—the Prix Apollinaire Bouchardat. It is awarded annually to a clinician or researcher who makes a significant contribution to the field of diabetology.

Bibliography

Primary: 1881. *Traité d'hygiène publique et privée, basée sur l'étiologie* (Paris); 1883. *De la glycosurie ou Diabète sucré son traitement hygiénique* (Paris).

Secondary: Jörgens, Victor, 2005. 'Apollinaire Bouchardat (1806–1886).' *Diabetologia* 48(1); Chast, F., 2000. 'Apollinaire Bouchardat, Pharmacist, Nutritionist.' *Annales pharmaceutiques françaises* 58 (Supplement 6): 435–442; Baquet, R., 1971. 'Les conseils au diabétiques d'Apollinaire Bouchardat.' *Maroc Medical* 51: 517–520; *Dictionnaire de Biographie Française.*

J. Rosser Matthews

BOURNEVILLE, DÉSIRÉ-MAGLOIRE (b. Garancières (Eure), France, 21 October 1840, d. Paris, France, 29 May 1909), *psychiatry, neurology, nursing, medical journalism, education, politics.*

The eldest of three sons in a Normandy family of small landholders, Bourneville began his medical studies in Paris before he turned nineteen. The psychiatrist Delasiauve, a fellow countryman, gave the young man a chance to do voluntary work at the Bicêtre, along with a job writing for his *Journal de médecine mentale*. During his hospital internship (1865–69), Bourneville served a year under both Delasiauve and Jean-Martin Charcot at the Salpêtrière. He wrote his MD thesis (1870) on clinical thermometry in the diagnosis of cerebral hemorrhage and other neurological conditions. His work during an earlier cholera epidemic had earned commendation, as would his bravery in protecting wounded Communards in 1871.

In 1870 an administrative change at the Salpêtrière resulted in the transfer of epileptic and hysterical patients from Delasiauve's service to a special division under Charcot's direction. Bourneville is usually remembered as Charcot's chief assistant and promoter of the enterprise centered on the clinical characterization of hysteria. He clearly fulfilled that role during the 1870s when he edited Charcot's first lessons on hysteria; founded the weekly journal, *Le progrès médical* (1873); and coauthored the *Iconographie photographique de la Salpêtrière* (1877–80), which was three volumes of text and photographs presenting graphic case histories of hysterical patients. If Charcot was the undisputed leader of the Salpêtrière school, Bourneville was more than just a spokesperson. He likely introduced Charcot to the investigation of hysteria and its broader possibilities for a program of medical positivism. Bourneville had studied the Salpêtrière hysterics during his internship under Delasiauve, at a time when Charcot had little if any experience with functional nervous disease. When those same patients moved to Charcot's service, Bourneville continued to be responsible for charting their clinical course. His own publications put forward the diagnostic criteria for distinguishing hysterical convulsions from epileptic fits.

In 1879 Bourneville won a position as physician and alienist to the Bicêtre, where he would remain for the rest of his career. He was elected to the National Assembly in 1883, after serving for seven years on the Paris municipal council. These offices provided a political base for advancing many health-related proposals, including plans for water purification and improved facilities for the mentally ill. Contemporaries remarked that Bourneville's politics were as radical as the ruddy complexion of the short, rotund figure who represented one of the poorer districts of Paris. At considerable cost to his own political career, he spearheaded a controversial program to replace religious hospital personnel with lay nurses. To that end, he founded nursing schools within the Paris hospitals and even wrote their instructional manuals. He established libraries within hospitals for patients as well as staff.

As physician to Bicêtre, Bourneville established a comprehensive program for severely physically and mentally handicapped children (*aliénés et idiots*). He was a leading expert on their inherited and congenital pathology, and he oversaw the construction of separate housing for such patients at Bicêtre. To the extent possible, children were trained in basic motor and speech skills, bodily hygiene, and manual occupations. Bourneville published a volume on the service each year, the series amounting to nearly thirty volumes in all.

Throughout his career, Bourneville remained an indefatigable author, editor, and publisher. He led the Salpêtrière campaign to debunk claims of religious miracles. In the case of Louise Lateau, the so-called Belgian stigmatic, Bourneville argued that her spontaneous hemorrhages were neither religious marks nor medical frauds, but manifestations of hysteria. As editor of the *Bibliothèque diabolique,* Bourneville published a series of historical monographs that retrospectively diagnosed putative supernatural happenings, such as witchcraft and possession, in medical terms.

Bourneville's aggressive anticlericalism, especially his uncompromising campaign for the laicization of hospital nurses, made him a target for enemies within as well as outside his profession. Voted out of office, vulnerable and increasingly isolated after Charcot's death, and obliged to retire at sixty-five (ironically, he fell victim to his own legislation fixing the retirement age for hospital physicians), Bourneville outlived his era. At age forty-six he had married Maria Breugnon, who died three years before him, leaving an only son. Deposition of their ashes in Père Lachaise cemetery evidenced yet another of Bourneville's secularizing causes—cremation.

Bibliography

Primary: 1875. *Science et miracle. Louise Lateau, ou la stigmatisée belge* (Paris); 1876. *Recherches cliniques et thérapeutiques sur l'épilepsie et l'hystérie* (Paris); 1877–80. (with Regnard, P.) *Iconographie photographique de la Salpêtrière* (Paris); 1895. *Assistance, traitement et éducation des enfants idiots et dégénérés* (Paris).

Secondary: Goetz, Christopher, Michel Bonduelle, and Toby Gelfand, 1995. *Charcot: Constructing Neurology* (New York); Poirier, Jacques, and Jean-Louis Signoret, eds., 1991. *De Bourneville à la sclérose tubéreuse* [15 essays] (Paris).

Toby Gelfand

BOVET, DANIEL (b. Neuchâtel, Switzerland, 23 March 1907; d. Rome, Italy, 8 April 1992), *medicine, chemistry, pharmacology, psychobiology.*

Bovet, son of Pierre Bovet, Professor of Pedagogy at the University of Geneva and his wife, Amy Babut, completed his secondary education in Geneva and graduated from the University of Geneva (1927). He then spent some years as assistant in physiology to F. Batelli, followed by work under Professor Emile Guyenot, while he prepared a thesis on zoology and comparative anatomy for which he was awarded his DSc (1929).

In 1929 he moved to l'Institut Pasteur in Paris (then under the direction of Emile Roux), and worked in Ernest Fourneau's department of therapeutic chemistry, where be remained until 1947. He was charged with reorganizing animal experimentation and, thanks to the daily contact with Fourneau, Bovet acquired a deep knowledge of chemistry and the orientation of his first research. At l'Institut Pasteur he met Filomena Nitti, a doctor in science at the Sorbonne, sister of the bacteriologist F. Nitti, and daughter of the former Italian Prime Minister Francesco Saverio Nitti (obliged to live in exile after the rise of Fascism in Italy). They married and started a very productive program of cooperative research.

In 1944 Bovet discovered pyrilamine (mepyramine), the first antihistamine which, in counteracting the effect of histamine, is effective against allergic reactions. Three years later, a search for a synthetic substitute for curare (a muscle relaxant) led to his discovery of gallamine and other muscle relaxants. Among these are derivatives of succinylcholine, whose curare-like action Bovet was the first to recognize. Curare and its synthetic substitutes had come into surgical use to induce muscle relaxation in conjunction with light anesthesia.

In 1947, the Director of the Italian Superior Institute of Health (ISS) in Rome, Domenico Marotta, asked Bovet to create and direct a Laboratory of Therapeutic Chemistry. He moved to Rome with his wife, and eventually took Italian citizenship. In 1964 he resigned from the ISS and took a chair of pharmacology in the medical school in Sassari, Sardinia. In 1969 he directed a newly founded laboratory of psychobiology and psychopharmacology at the National Research Council in Rome. In 1971 he became a professor of psychobiology at the Faculty of Science of the Rome University 'La Sapienza'.

During these years, Bovet and his coworkers undertook animal studies, investigating the relationships between chemical structure and biological effect. Proceeding by systematic variations and successive simplifications of chemical structure, they succeeded, by degrees, in obtaining simple chemical compounds which proved themselves, from the point of view of specificity and the absence of undesirable side effects, much more useful than naturally occurring substances.

The chemical synthesis of products capable of paralyzing muscle had a large impact in the evolution of modern surgery, as it made possible complicated surgical procedures which often require complete muscular relaxation. Bovet's work in experimental neuropharmacology and psychopharmacology has been particularly important. He showed experimentally that biological amines are the transmitters of nerve impulses in the different tracts of the brain, just as they are the chemical agents linking nerve fibers to peripheral organs. In other words, he produced drugs specifically affecting brain function; the medical world now possesses a number of compounds of this type. Bovet applied the antihistamine drugs in laboratory and clinical studies of the central nervous system. The drugs produced by this research are used for the treatment of Parkinson's, and as tranquillizers.

Important aspects of this research were embodied in Bovet's book written with his wife, *The chemical structure and pharmacodynamic activity of drugs of the vegetative nervous system* (1948). The Bovets and G. B. Marini-Bettòlo published *Curare and Curarelike Agents* (1959).

In 1957, Bovet was awarded the Nobel Prize for Physiology or Medicine 'for his discoveries relating to synthetic compounds that inhibit the action of certain body substances, and especially their action on the vascular system and the skeletal muscles'. In the last part of his scientific career, Bovet developed new methods for the laboratory study of animal behavior, inheritance, and learning. Comparing strains of genetically different mice, he showed differences in the learning and memory pathways. His psychogenetic research concentrated on the synaptic mechanisms of short- and long-term memory and their metabolic structure. He suggested a dualistic or pluralistic mechanism of memory-building. The results of this research were summarized in *Recent advances on learning and retention*, written with F. Bovet-Nitti and A. Oliverio (1969).

In 1946 Bovet was elected a Chevalier of the Legion of Honor of France, and in 1959 a Grand Official of the Order of Merit of the Italian Republic.

Bibliography

Primary: 1937. (with Tréfouël, J., T. Tréfouël, and F. Nitti) 'Chimiothérapie des infections streptococciques par els dérivés du p-aminophénylsulfamide.' *Annales de l'Institut Pasteur* 58: 30–55; 1948. (with Nitti-Bovet, F.) *Structure chimique et activité pharmacodynamique des médicaments du système nerveux végétatif* [The chemical structure and pharmacodynamic activity of drugs of the vegetative nervous system] (Basel); 1959. (with Nitti-Bovet, F., and G. B. Marini-Bettòlo) *Curare and Curare-like Agents* (Amsterdam); 1964. 'The Relationships between Isosterism and Competitive Phenomena in the Field of Drug Therapy of the Autonomic Nervous System and that of the Neuromuscular Transmission.' (Nobel Lecture, December 11, 1957) *Nobel Lectures, Physiology or Medicine 1942–1962* (Amsterdam) pp. 552–558.

Secondary: Oliverio, A., 1994. 'Daniel Bovet.' *Biographical Memoirs of Fellows of the Royal Society* 39: 60–70; Bignami, G., ed., 1993. 'Special issue in honour of the late Daniel Bovet (Ricordo di Daniel Bovet).' *Annali dell'Istituto di Sanità* vol. 29, supplement 1 (Rome); Bovet, D., 1989. *Une chimie qui guérit. Histoire de la découverte des sulfamides* (Paris): Bovet, D., 1974. 'Daniel Bovet (Autobiografia)' in Macorini, Edgardo, ed., *Scienziati e tecnologi contemporanei* (Milan) pp. 161–162.

Bernardino Fantini

BOWDITCH, HENRY INGERSOLL (b. Salem, Massachusetts, USA, 9 August 1808; d. Boston, Massachusetts, USA, 14 January 1892), *medicine, public health.*

The son of Nathaniel Bowditch and Mary Ingersoll, Bowditch received his education in Boston at Harvard College and Harvard Medical School. Following his graduation in 1832, Bowditch joined a growing stream of American physicians traveling to Paris to study with the eminent physician, Pierre Louis. Bowditch spent nearly two years shadowing Louis in the hospital wards. While in Paris he kept company with his peer, Oliver Wendell Holmes, who returned from Paris to an influential career that paralleled Bowditch's in Boston. Also in Paris in 1833, Bowditch met his future wife, Olivia Yardley, a visiting student from England. They continued a transatlantic romance and, overcoming parental objections, wed in New York City in 1838.

Bowditch's early medical career was partly eclipsed by his outspoken and active opposition to slavery, a stance that he attributed to witnessing the attack on abolitionist William Lloyd Garrison in the streets of Boston in 1835. Bowditch fought fiercely in the cause. A member of the Warren Street Chapel, Bowditch first lobbied the chapel to house antislavery meetings, and later resigned in protest of the members' attempts to exclude colored children, as well as their censure of his abolitionist speeches. Appointed as a physician at Massachusetts General Hospital in 1838, Bowditch offered his resignation in 1841 to protest his being prohibited from admitting colored patients to the hospital. He apparently won his point, since the hospital's trustees formally declined his resignation and soon advanced him to the position of visiting physician. He remained in the hospital service until 1863. Bowditch proudly recounted a story of how, on the heels of the Fugitive Slave Act of 1850, he drove through the streets of Boston bringing William Craft, an escaped slave, to rejoin Craft's wife, Ellen. He and Craft sat together, making a show of being heavily armed with pistols and a revolver to discourage interference.

Bowditch gradually established a reputation as an expert in lung disease. One of his earliest publications, *The Young Stethoscopist* (1846), became a standard text for generations of students learning the new art of diagnosing lung disease through auscultation. Perhaps Bowditch's most enduring contribution to medicine was his championing of an improved procedure, called thoracentesis, for draining pathological fluid from the space around the lungs. Starting in the early 1850s, Bowditch's careful observational studies and persuasive advocacy helped to advance this simple and safe technique ahead of a riskier but widely favored alternative, both among American and European colleagues. In 1859, Bowditch succeeded George C. Shattuck as the Jackson Professor of Clinical Medicine at Harvard Medical School.

Bowditch's expertise with pulmonary disease also provided his entry into more extensive, later work advocating for reform of public health. In the 1850s he began an extensive survey of the incidence of consumption, or pulmonary tuberculosis, in New England, and made his report to the Massachusetts Medical Society in 1862, emphasizing the need for sanitary reform to combat the disease. In 1869, when the legislature created the Massachusetts State Board of Health, Bowditch became its first chairman and served on the Board for ten years. He and George Derby represented the Board's active wing, and met with recurring disappointment in their efforts to spur intervention in the problems that the Board documented. Bowditch's advocacy for the public health continued unabated. In the wake of the 1878 epidemic of yellow fever, the federal government briefly roused to attention to create the first national quarantine act and the short-lived National Health Board, where Bowditch served briefly. Bowditch also joined the American Medical Association at its founding in 1847, and served in 1876 as its President.

Bibliography

Primary: 1852. 'On pleuritic effusions and the necessity of paracentesis for their removal.' *American Journal of the Medical Sciences* 23: 320–350; 1862. *Consumption in New England* (Boston).

Secondary: Bowditch, Vincent Y., 1902. *Life and correspondence of Henry Ingersoll Bowditch* 2 vols. (Boston); *DAMB*.

Christopher Crenner

BOWLBY, (EDWARD) JOHN MOSTYN (b. London, England, 26 February 1907; d. Isle of Skye, Scotland, 2 September 1990), *child psychiatry.*

Bowlby, the son of a military surgeon, was one of six children and received his education at the Royal Naval College in Dartmouth, Devon. He studied medicine at the University of Cambridge, where he became acquainted with developmental psychology, and at University College Hospital, London. He received his MD from Cambridge in 1939, and commenced his training in psychiatry at the Maudsley Hospital, London. From 1936 to 1940 he was on the staff of the London Child Guidance Clinic, and volunteered at a progressive school for maladjusted children, where he made extensive observations on isolated and anxious children. At the same time, he underwent psychoanalysis with Joan Rivière (1883–1962), a close associate of Melanie Klein (1882–1960), which sensitized him to the importance of the early emotional experiences of children. From 1940 to 1945, Bowlby served in the RAMC. In 1946 he was appointed director of the Department of Children and Parents at the Tavistock Clinic and Institute, where he remained until his retirement in 1972. At the Tavistock he undertook his most original work—on attachment theory, or the development of emotional bonds between mothers and children.

From the beginning of his career, Bowlby felt that psychoanalysts placed too much emphasis on the inner emotional and fantasy world of children, and neglected the significance of actual events on emotional development. He was particularly interested in the emotional consequences of periods of separation from mothers or mother-substitutes. In one of his first studies, he investigated young children who were hospitalized, institutionalized, or undergoing a prolonged separation from their parents for other reasons. The results of this research were presented in a film, *A Two-Year-Old Goes to Hospital*, released in 1952, which had a significant influence in changing hospital practices by allowing more extended visiting hours for parents. In 1950, the World Health Organization invited Bowlby to investigate the mental health of homeless children in postwar Europe, which allowed him to further investigate the effects of maternal separation and deprivation on growing children.

In the 1950s Bowlby and his associates formulated the tenets of attachment theory, which assumed that a sustained, warm, and intimate relationship between mothers and children was essential for healthy emotional development. To develop an alternative theoretical perspective not dependent on psychoanalysis, Bowlby became interested in ethology, which depends on extensive observations made in naturalistic settings. On the basis of his observations of interactions between mothers and children, Bowlby concluded that there were three phases in the response of children to separation. The first response was protest, motivated by separation anxiety; the second despair, motivated by grief and mourning; and the third a phase of detachment and denial, which was essentially a defense mechanism. According to Bowlby, excessive separation anxiety in children was generally motivated by adverse family experiences.

Bowlby's views on the nature of the emotional development of children, and the consequences of separation from parental figures, only became influential during the later part of his career. He is currently recognized as one of the most influential child psychiatrists of the twentieth century.

Bibliography

Primary: 1951. *Maternal Care and Mental Health* (Geneva) [1953, abridged as *Child Care and the Growth of Love* (London)]; 1969–1980. *Attachment and Loss* 3 vols. 1969. *Attachment* (vol. 1); 1973. *Separation: Anxiety and Anger* (vol. 2); 1980. *Loss: Sadness and Depression* (vol. 3) (London); 1988. *A Secure Base: Parent-Child Attachment and Healthy Human Development* (New York).

Secondary: Holmes, Jeremy, 1993. *John Bowlby and Attachment Theory* (London and New York); Dijken, Suzan van, 1988. *John Bowlby, His Early Life: A Biographical Journey into the Roots of Attachment Theory* (London and New York); *Oxford DNB*.

Hans Pols

BOYLE, EDWARD MAYFIELD (b. Freetown, Sierra Leone, 1878; d. Baltimore, Maryland, USA, 21 November 1936), *medicine, radiology.*

Boyle was born into the Krio cultural matrix of the British colony of Freetown, Sierra Leone. He grew up in Freetown and attended public schools at a time when there was already an established, elite cultural and medical tradition. It is likely that Boyle's chosen route toward medicine was guided by the strong influence of the Church Missionary Society in Sierra Leone; the medical achievements of fellow countryman John Easmon (his cousin); and the growing national awareness of medical opportunities abroad, especially those in North America.

Given those influences, it is perhaps not surprising that Boyle did not follow the traditional medical training route for Africans. He traveled instead to the United States in the 1890s and studied at the Agricultural and Mechanical (A&M) College in Alabama from 1896 to 1898. Boyle matriculated at Howard University (Washington, D.C.) in 1898 to study theology, but he switched to the College of Medicine in 1900. When he received his MD in 1902, Boyle became the first African to graduate from Howard University's College of Medicine.

Throughout his professional career, Boyle was licensed as a practitioner in several states: Maryland (1903), Pennsylvania (1906), and the District of Columbia (1909). He studied clinical medicine under William Osler at Johns Hopkins Medical School in 1904. Boyle studied diseases of the heart at Harvard University with Max Kahn and clinical diagnostic radiology with Joseph C. Bloodgood at Johns Hopkins. He completed further courses in radiology at Bellevue, Beth Israel, and Lincoln Hospitals in New York City and at the College of the City of New York. In spite of his numerous achievements, however, British colonial medical policy prevented Boyle from returning to Sierra Leone to practice medicine in anything but the most limited fashion.

Married to Bertha Stokes Boyle of Washington, D.C., Boyle left three children in the United States when he died at the comparatively early age of fifty-eight. He was buried in Baltimore, Maryland.

Bibliography

Primary: 1912. 'A Comparative Physical Study of the Negro.' *Journal of the National Medical Association* 4: 124–130; 1925. 'Anaphylaxis in its Relation to Hay-Fevered Asthma.' *Journal of the National Medical Association* 17: 1.

Secondary: Oestreich, Alan E., ed., 1996. *A Centennial History of African Americans in Radiology* (Takoma Park, MD); Patton, Adell Jr., 1996. *Physicians, Colonial Racism, and Diaspora in West Africa* (Gainesville, FL); Patton, Adell Jr., 1982. 'Howard University and Meharry Medical Schools in the Training of African Physicians, 1868–1978' in Harris, Joseph E., ed., *Global Dimensions of the African Diaspora* (Washington, DC) pp.142–162; Patton, Adell Jr., 1982. 'Document: E. Mayfield Boyle: 1902 Howard University Medical School Graduate Challenge to British Medical Policy in West Africa.' *Journal of Negro History* 67(1): 41–51; Miller, Kelly, 1916. 'The Historic Background of the Negro Physician.' *Journal of Negro History* 1/2: 99–109.

Adell Patton Jr.

BOYLSTON, ZABDIEL (b. Muddy River [now Brookline], Massachusetts, USA, 9 March 1680; d. Brookline, Massachusetts, USA, 1 March 1766), *surgery, smallpox inoculation.*

Boylston, son of physician and farmer Thomas Boylston and Mary Gardner, studied medicine with his father (who died when Zabdiel was fifteen), and with the Boston surgeon and physician John Cutler. He did not receive an MD degree.

Bolyston established a successful medical and surgical practice, which he ran from an apothecary shop he opened in Boston in the early 1700s. An entrepreneur, Boylston developed and sold medicines and medical equipment, as well as sugar and spices in his shop. His business and medical practice made him an affluent man. In 1706 he married Jerusha Minot, daughter of John Minot and Elizabeth Brick of Dorchester. Zabdiel and Jerusha had eight children.

In April 1721 a ship from the West Indies carrying a passenger sick with smallpox arrived in Boston. Initially authorities tried to contain the disease through isolation and sanitation, but these measures failed to halt its spread. On 6 June 1721 the Reverend Cotton Mather, one of the leading divines in Boston, circulated 'An Address to the Physicians of Boston', urging physicians to try the practice of inoculation. The procedure consisted of inserting pus taken from a pustule on a smallpox patient into a small incision made in the arm or leg of a healthy individual, thereby inducing a usually mild case of smallpox and protecting that individual from natural smallpox. Mather had learned about inoculation from an African slave named Onesimus, and later read published reports in the *Philosophical Transactions* by Italian physicians who had observed the practice in Constantinople. The Boston physicians did not respond to Mather's request, so Mather wrote Boylston directly, and sent excerpts from the *Philosophical Transactions*. On June 26 Boylston tried the procedure on his son (age six), his thirty-six-year-old black slave Jack, and Jack's son (age thirty months). All three recovered without difficulties.

There was strong opposition to inoculation, and Boylston and Mather were ostracized. One of the leading critics was the Edinburgh MD William Douglass, who argued that inoculation spread smallpox. Other objections focused on religious concerns (that the practice intervened in Divine Providence) and on ethical issues (that it was wrong to deliberately infect a healthy individual). Boylston and Mather continued to defend the practice, despite threats to themselves and their families. The epidemic ended one year later in the spring of 1722, by which time 5,889 people had suffered from smallpox, and 844 had died. Boylston had inoculated 246 individuals, of whom six had died.

News of Boylston's inoculations spread to England, where the practice was advocated by Lady Mary Wortley Montagu and physicians associated with the Royal Society. The large number of successful inoculations performed by Boylston helped persuade London physicians and patients to try the practice. Boylston was invited to London to share his experiences. He arrived in 1725 and stayed two years, giving lectures to the Royal Society and the Royal College of Physicians. He was the first Americanborn physician elected a Fellow of the Royal Society. While in London, Boylston wrote a pamphlet summarizing his experiences with inoculation.

Boylston returned to Boston and resumed his lucrative medical practice. In the 1730 smallpox epidemic in Boston, he once again led inoculation efforts. In 1740, he retired to his farm in Brookline, and spent his remaining years breeding horses.

Bibliography

Primary: 1726. *Historical Account of the Small-Pox Inoculated in New England, Upon All Sorts of Persons, Whites, Blacks, and of All Ages and Constitutions* (London and Boston).

Secondary: Mager, Gerald Marvin, 1975. 'Zabdiel Boylston: Medical Pioneer of Colonial Boston.' PhD thesis, University of Illinois; Blake, John B., 1952. 'The Inoculation Controversy in Boston, 1722.' *New England Quarterly* 25: 489–506; *DAMB*.

Andrea Rusnock

BRAHMACHARI, UPENDRANATH   (b. Jamalpur, Bihar, India, 7 June 1875; d. Calcutta, India, 6 February 1946), *medicine, pharmacology.*

Upendranath, son of Nilmani Brahmachari, a medical officer of the East Indian Railway, graduated with honors in mathematics from Hooghly College (1893) and received an MSc in chemistry from Presidency College, Calcutta (1894). He attended Calcutta Medical College (1894–98) and received an MB, followed by the MD (1902) and a PhD in physiology (1904). With Professor McCay as his advisor, Brahmachari worked on hemolysis for his PhD thesis.

Brahmachari joined the Provincial Medical Service (1899–1900) and served Dacca Medical School as teacher of pathology and materia medica (1901–04). While there, he built up a good practice and collaborated with the superintendent, Sir Neil Campbell. He lectured in medicine at the Campbell Medical School, Calcutta (1905–23), and worked as an additional physician at the Calcutta Medical College Hospital (1923–27). Brahmachari retired in 1927, but continued as honorary professor of tropical medicine at the Carmichael Medical College. He was married and had two sons and two daughters.

Brahmachari is best known for his lifelong studies of *kala-azar* (black fever, or visceral leishmaniasis) and his discovery of urea stibamine (1921) for its treatment. Soon after the introduction of tarter emetic, he started using the better-tolerated drug, sodium antimonyl tartrate. Brahmachari pointed out that when the drug was injected intravenously, the same cells in the spleen that harbored the kala-azar parasite picked up the particles of antimony. The two contending agents thus came in closest contact with each other in those tissue cells, which destroyed the parasites in the speediest way.

Nevertheless, Brahmachari was not content with those drugs and the mode of treatment because there were certain toxic effects, and the treatment was tedious and lengthy. At Campbell Medical School from 1915 to 1921, he carried out many experiments in a small room lacking such basic facilities as a water tap and gas connection. There he first synthesized several new inorganic antimonials and achieved some clinical success with colloidal metallic antimony. Dissatisfied with those results, he turned his attention to organic aromatic antimonials. He experimented with various salts, and in 1920 prepared for the first time in India several organic compounds of antimony. In 1921, he synthesized stibalinic acid with urea and produced a potential remedy for the treatment of kala-azar. It is possible that he might have been trying to get painless antimonial compounds suitable for intramuscular administration. Ultimately led by the knowledge that urea in combination with certain drugs reduces pain when injected, he prepared that compound and named it urea stibamine. It shortened the course of treatment and could cure intractable cases. For seven years he generously supplied urea stibamine to the Kala-azar Commission in Assam for treatment of the disease.

Brahmachari also discovered post–kala-azar dermal leishmanoid (PKDL), a skin lesion that developed in certain cases of kala-azar after completion of antimonial treatment and apparent cure. He also contributed to the knowledge of a range of other diseases, including malaria, filariasis, diabetes, leprosy, and meningitis, as well as hematological disorders. Brahmachari made an outstanding contribution to the treatment of 'quarantine fever' in India. Simultaneously a doctor and a chemist, he also contributed to medicine through his studies of the quinoline and acidine compounds.

As a successful physician, Brahmachari commanded public confidence. He was knighted in 1934.

Bibliography

Primary: 1932. *Reports of the Kala-azar Commission, India, Report No. II (1926–30)* (Calcutta).

Secondary: Chattopadhyay, Anjana, 2002. *Biographical Dictionary of Indian Scientists* (New Delhi); Chakraborty, Arun Kumar, 1989. *Chikitsa Bijnane Aviskar O Kolkata* [Bengali] (Calcutta).

Achintya Kumar Dutta

BRAID, JAMES   (b. Ryelaw, Kinross, Scotland, 19 June 1795; d. Chorlton upon Medlock, Manchester, England, 25 March 1860), *surgery, hypnotism.*

The son of a humble landowner in Fife, Braid was apprenticed to a surgeon in Leith and attended classes at Edinburgh University in 1812–14 before obtaining his LRCSEd in 1815. He married young, in 1813, and had a son (who would also become a surgeon) and a daughter by his wife Margaret. In 1825, after nine years as surgeon to Lord Hopetoun's lead mines in Lanarkshire, Braid set up in private practice at Dumfries. Shortly thereafter, on the advice of a patient, he moved to Manchester where he remained for the rest of his life. By 1828 he was established in a town-center practice, and had gained a reputation for competence both in surgery in general, and in the treatment of clubfoot in particular. On the latter he published in *Lancet* and other medical journals.

Braid's interest in 'hypnosis'—the word he coined—began in November 1841 after he attended a demonstration by the French mesmerist, Charles Lafontaine (1803–92). By the end of that month he had mastered the technique (using eye fixation to induce hypnotic states), formulated his own views on the phenomenon, and begun publicly lecturing on the subject. The lectures formed the basis of his only full-length book, *Neurypnology, or, The Rationale of Nervous Sleep* (London, 1843), in which he maintained that 'mesmeric sleep' was not attributable to the transfer of 'mesmeric fluid' or 'animal magnetism' from operator to patient, but rather was a peculiar nervous state, different from sleep and probably involving changes in cerebral circulation.

At first, Braid explained hypnotic phenomena in the physiological terms of phrenology; indeed, he referred to the mesmeric stimulation of the cerebral 'organs' as 'phrenomesmerism'. Because mesmerized subjects appeared to him to behave exactly in accord with the characteristics attributed to specific phrenological faculties when those faculties were 'touched' by the hypnotist, Braid inadvertently gave a new lease of life to phrenological theory. At the same time, he advanced an understanding of mesmerism that required no reference to occult forces.

However, Braid gradually revised his views. In *The Power of the Mind over the Body* (1846), *Magic, Witchcraft, Animal Magnetism, Hypnotism, and Electro-Biology* (1852), *Hypnotic Therapeutics, Illustrated by Cases* (1853), and other less significant articles and pamphlets, he abandoned all mention of phrenomesmerism, and moved away from physiological explanation. Although he continued to regard 'hypnotic sleep' as divided into two stages, he now redefined these states as 'sub-hypnotic' and 'double consciousness'—the latter being an extension of the former's suspension of critical faculties, and the place where imagination, under the sway of suggestion, took control. Braid continued to believe that hypnosis was beneficial in the treatment of physical ailments by the changes it wrought in blood circulation. But he now also postulated the direct influence of the mind, as stimulated by appropriate suggestions, on particular mental and physiological functions.

Braid's work on hypnosis gained some recognition from the British medical profession during his lifetime, but it was largely forgotten thereafter. It was only toward the end of the nineteenth century, and primarily in France, that it was taken up because of Braid's emphasis on 'suggestion' as the clue to hypnotic and related phenomena. He came to be hailed as a forerunner to the Nancy School of hypnotism, although his actual influence on it was slight. Ironically, his influence was greater and more direct on the rival school of the Salpêtrière in Paris, where the great neurologist Jean-Martin Charcot (1825–93) was to make hypnotism scientifically acceptable. Charcot took up Braid's ideas and methods via the writings in the 1860s of a number of French medical men (nicknamed the 'Braidists')

who borrowed directly from Braid's *Neurypnology*. Like Braid in the 1840s, therefore, the Salpêtrière school tended to regard hypnotism as having physiologically definable stages (catalepsy, lethargy, and somnambulism) which could be initiated and terminated by particular stimuli. Braid's place in the history of hypnosis thus remains, in equal measure, important and ambiguous.

Bibliography

Secondary: Gault, A., 1992. *A History of Hypnotism* (Cambridge); Kravis, N. M., 1988. 'James Braid's Psychophysiology: A Turning Point in the History of Psychiatry.' *American Journal of Psychiatry* 145: 1191–1206; *Oxford DNB*.

Roger Cooter

BRAVO DE SOBREMONTE, GASPAR (b. San Cristóbal del Monte, Cantabria, Spain, 1603; d. Madrid, Spain, March 1683), *medicine*.

The son of a gentleman, Bravo de Sobremonte used to boast about his lineage, an old family from the northern mountains of Spain, and he never relinquished the hereditary and honorary titles of Alderman of San Cristóbal de Sobremonte and Mayor of the Valderrebible Valley, where his birthplace was.

He did his primary studies in Aguilar de Campoo, a modest village, although the most important of those near San Cristóbal. Then he moved to Valladolid, in order to study in one of the three most important Castilian universities, together with Alcalá and Salamanca; there he studied logic and philosophy (1623–26) and medicine and surgery (1626–30). Afterward, he did the compulsory medical practice with an eminent doctor (1630–32) and sat the examination of King's physician (1632), thus obtaining his license to practice medicine throughout the Castilian territory.

While studying, he was a collegian of the College of Physicians of San Raphael in Valladolid (1626), where he reached the position of Vice-Rector (1630), Rector (1630), and Elector for his lifetime.

In Valladolid he gained the degrees of Bachelor of Arts (1626), Bachelor of Medicine (1630), Graduate in Medicine (January 1637), and Doctor in Medicine (February 1637). His extraordinary lectures were *De elementis* (1631), *De facultatibus* (1632), and *De influxu partium principum* (1633). He was Professor of Arts (1632, 1636), then of Surgery (1637), Method (1640), Vespers (1646), and he was both chairs of Prime, Hippocrates (1650) and Avicenna (1655), the most important in Medicine. In 1657 he was appointed Royal Physician, and he left Valladolid and moved to Madrid, where he died after several years service for Philip IV and Charles II. He was married twice, to Luisa Pérez (d. 1647) and Ana María Argos de Aramburu.

He owned a large book collection, with more than 1,000 volumes in 1649, thirty-four years before dying. He always tried to have updated information about the latest medical advances, following the neo-Hippocratic tendency that dominated from the second half of the sixteenth century in the University of Valladolid, whose motto was 'to respect the ancient doctrines, interpreting them according to the modern theoretical outlooks'. The result was Bravo de Sobremonte's dense work, which includes open support for Harvey's theory of blood circulation, lymphatic circulation, *perspiratio insensibilis*, the concepts of acrimony and *fermentatio*, and the use of chemical remedies such as the antimony, among others. His argument in favor of Peruvian bark clearly shows his frame of mind: 'The principle *contraria-contrariis* does not only refer to contrary qualities, but it also means contrary to disease' (1684, vol. V, p. 13).

His work includes a medical topography of Madrid: *De Mantue Carpetanotum salubritate & situ*; the autopsy of King Philip IV's corpse, with a detailed description of his renal calculi and the kidney injuries found; several medical histories; and a discussion of new diseases such as the *Plica*. However, he made no significant contribution to legal medicine in his study of the signs of torture; instead he hoped to refute the superstition saying that a corpse, under certain circumstances, could accuse the murderer.

Thanks to his considered criticism of novelties, he was highly influential in Spanish medicine and was acknowledged as a great doctor in Europe.

Bibliography

Primary: 1654–84. *Opera Medicinalia* 5 vols. (Lyon); 1649. *Resolutionem et consultationem medicorum circa universam totius philosophiae doctrina* (Valladolid); 1662. *Resolutionem et consultationem medicorum, tertia editio* (Lyon).

Secondary: Rojo Vega, Anastasio, 2003. 'Miguel Polanco y la Restauración de la Medicina. Siglo XVII.' *Medicina & historia*, n. 4. Cuarta época 2: 2–15; López Piñero, José M., 1973. 'Harvey's Doctrine of the Circulation of the Blood in Seventeenth-Century Spain.' *Journal of the History of Medicine* 28: 230–242; Granjel, Luis S., 1960. *La obra de Gaspar Bravo de Sobremonte* (Salamanca).

Anastasio Rojo
(trans. Ana Sáez Hidalgo)

BRAZIL, VITAL

BRAZIL, VITAL (b. Mineiro da Campanha, São Paulo State, Brazil, 28 April 1865; d. Rio de Janeiro, Brazil, 8 May 1950), *medicine, bacteriology.*

Brazil's patriotic parents, José and Mariana dos Santos Pereira, gave him his unusual name in honor of his country. Young Vital rose from modest origins to become, as his obituary in *Estado do São Paulo* (9 May 1950) put it, 'one of the greatest Brazilians of our time', distinguished by his presence on the 10,000 Cruzeiro currency note. After Oswaldo Cruz, he is arguably Brazil's most famous international medical personality.

Graduating from Rio de Janeiro's medical school in 1891 through his and his family's great sacrifices, Vital Brazil began his medical career as a private practitioner in up-country São Paulo State, where he encountered numerous cases of poisonous snakebite among his patients. In his spare time he worked in his makeshift laboratory to study venom typologies, inspired by an article on the same subject by the great Pasteurian Albert Calmette. Convinced that the serotherapy of the Pasteur Institute was the key to effective treatment of snakebite and infections, Brazil joined the São Paulo Bacteriological Institute as student and assistant to state bacteriologist Adolfo Lutz (1897). At the coffee port of Santos in 1899, Brazil diagnosed the first appearance of the third pandemic of bubonic plague on Brazilian soil. He contracted the disease himself, but recovered after receiving treatment with antiplague serum manufactured by the Pasteur Institute of Paris. When supplies ran short, the State of São Paulo requisitioned a farm called Butantán, six miles from the city of São Paulo, to begin the production of antiplague serum locally. Vital Brazil was appointed to head the project (1899).

At Butantán, Brazil supervised the production of protective sera against diphtheria, tetanus, and bubonic plague, while continuing his research on snake venom. The first antiplague sera were ready in 1901, and in that same year he published his initial articles on snake venom. Appreciative of Vital Brazil's work at the Serotherapy Institute, the Brazilian Congress of Medicine and Surgery sent him to Europe (1903) to meet Calmette and others working in his field.

In the 1920s, leading up to his retirement in 1927, Brazil extended his studies to the physiological actions of spider and toad venoms, and he lectured widely to inform the general public of the availability of serotherapy. Within a decade of his visit to Europe, the dynamic but modest Brazilian had become the world's foremost authority on antivenomous serotherapy, and his laboratory had become recognized as one of the world's leading centers for the study and production of poisonous snake antidotes—products that would save thousands of Brazilian lives.

Bibliography

Primary: 1899. 'A peste bubônica em Santos. Trabalho do Instituto Bacteriológico de São Paulo.' *Revista Médica de São Paulo* 2: 343–355; 1941. *Memória histórica do Instituto de Butantán* (São Paulo).

Secondary: Hawgood, Barbara, 1992. 'Pioneers of Anti-venomous Serotherapy: Dr. Vital Brazil (1865–1950).' *Toxicon* 30: 573–579; Vital Brazil, Oswaldo, 1987. 'History of the primordia of snake-bite accident serotherapy.' *Memórias do Instituto de Butantán* 49: 7–20.

Myron Echenberg

BRÈS, MADELEINE

BRÈS, MADELEINE (b. Bouillargues [near Nîmes], France, 1839; d. Montrouge, Paris, France, 1925), *medical education, maternal health, infant welfare.*

Brès was the daughter of a wheelwright named Gébelin who worked in the provincial hospitals. That early exposure to medicine sparked her interest in health care. She married at fifteen and was widowed soon after, which compelled her to earn her living as a midwife. In 1866 she wrote to the dean of the Paris medical school, Adolphe Wurtz, asking for admission to the Paris School of Medicine. She had picked an opportune time for her request. Both Wurtz and the Minister of Education, Victor Duruy, were considering a plan to admit women to the school in order to counteract Empress Eugénie's request to open a school for women missionary physicians. Brès was told that to be considered she must first obtain the equivalent of a baccalaureate degree, although there was still the issue of overcoming the reluctance of the medical faculty to admit women. Mary Putnam, a young American physician then attending the Paris clinics in a number of French hospitals, did much to overcome that reluctance.

After Brès obtained the necessary preliminary degree, she was admitted to the school in January 1868, along with Mary Putnam (later Jacobi), an Englishwoman named Elizabeth Garrett (later Anderson), and a Russian woman, Mme Goncharev—all three of whom had first qualified as physicians in their own countries. She began her medical studies, which were somewhat delayed by the Prussian army's siege of Paris and by the Paris Commune that followed. During the Franco-Prussian War and the Commune, Brès served as a provisional *interne* at the La Pitié under Paul Broca, who raised her to that position because of the scarcity of trained physicians. In spite of Broca's support for her application, the faculty of the Paris medical school refused to recognize her qualifications as hospital resident or to let her take the examinations to properly qualify herself for hospital work. Women did not have the opportunity to take the prestigious examinations for the *internat* until 1886, when Paul Bert, then Minister of Public Instruction, went over the head of the medical faculty to permit Augusta Klumpke and Blanche Edwards-Pilliet to compete for positions.

Although the medical degrees awarded to Elizabeth Garrett and Mary Putnam preceded hers, on 3 June 1875 Brès became the first French woman to earn a Paris degree. Her thesis on the breast and breast feeding analyzed the changes in milk composition in nursing women during the development of the infant. A portrait of Brès by Jean Béraud shows her defending her thesis before a committee of the Faculté.

In 1885 Brès founded a free crèche for infants of working-class families up to the age of three (renamed Crèche Madeleine Brès eight years later), into which she poured most of her earnings. She conducted 'causeries maternelles' in order to teach women who were working in crèches or as baby nurses, and she edited a journal from 1883 to 1885 on the hygiene of women and children (*L'Hygiène de la Femme et l'Enfant*). Brès wrote a book about bottle feeding (*L'allaitment artificiel et le biberon*) and another about childcare and hygiene (*Mamans et bébés*) in 1899. At the turn of the century, she was celebrated as the 'dean' of women physicians in France, but as she grew older her earnings dried up. Poor and almost blind at the end of her life, she died at Montrouge, a Paris suburb.

Bibliography

Primary: 1875. *De la mammelle et de l'allaitement.* Thesis, Paris; 1889. *L'allaitement artificiel et le biberon* (Paris); 1899. *Mamans et bébés* (Paris); 1883–1895. (editor) *L'Hygiène de la Femme et l'Enfant.*

Secondary: Lipinska, Mélanie, 1900. *Les femmes médecins depuis l'antiquité jusqu'à nos jours* (Paris); Schultze, Caroline, 1888. *La femme médecin au XIXe siècle.* Thesis, Paris.

Joy Harvey

BREUER, JOSEF

BREUER, JOSEF (b. Vienna, Austria, 15 January 1842; d. Vienna, 20 June 1925), *medicine, physiology, psychoanalysis.*

Breuer was the son of Leopold Breuer, a teacher of religion at the Vienna Israelite Congregation who belonged to the first generation of Jews to break out of the ghetto's intellectual isolation and acquire a Western education. Following private schooling with his father, Breuer attended the Academic Gymnasium and then began his study of medicine at the University of Vienna in 1859. Breuer graduated in 1867 and soon became the assistant of the internist Johann von Oppolzer. He established himself as a general practitioner in 1871 and received the university title of docent in internal medicine in 1875, an office that he resigned in 1885.

With time, Breuer developed into one of Vienna's most esteemed and popular physicians. The admiration he received also became apparent in the large number of university colleagues who consulted him and in his appointment to the Academy of Sciences in 1894.

In addition to his activity as a general practitioner, Breuer continued the physiological researches for which he is to this day numbered among the great physiologists of the nineteenth century. As an assistant, he and Ewald Hering had already discovered the reflex self-regulation of breathing (the Hering-Breuer reflex) in 1868. Breuer also conducted investigations of the structure and functioning of the ear labyrinth's semicircular canals. He built his work on the research of the physiologist Goltz, who in 1870 found that the semicircular canals constitute an organ that perceives the head's movement in space. Breuer discovered that the rotational movement of the endolymph, a thick fluid in the semicircular canal, is activated by the rotational movement of the head and affects the nerve receptors in the semicircular canals' ampullae. The perpendicular positioning of the three semicircular canals makes it possible to perceive movement along all three spatial axes. Working independently, the physicist Ernst Mach and the Scottish chemist A. Crum Brown simultaneously found the same explanation for the semicircular canals' functioning (the Mach-Breuer endolymph flow theory).

In 1880, Breuer's attention was drawn to the unusual condition of a young woman named Bertha Pappenheim. She became known as 'Anna O.' in a study Breuer and Sigmund Freud published in 1895 under the title *Studies on*

Hysteria. The young woman had displayed severe symptoms of hysteria, including hemiplegia, aphasia, nervous coughing, and a refusal to eat. Breuer began treating Anna O. with hypnosis. He discovered that her hysterical symptoms disappeared in a waking state after he had succeeded in inducing her to repeat their first appearance verbally while under hypnosis, thus dissipating the energy of the accompanying effects that had been transformed into symptoms. In a phase during which she could speak only English, Anna O. herself later referred to the process as the 'talking cure' and 'chimney sweeping'. In *Studies on Hysteria,* that form of treatment was termed the 'cathartic method'. It laid the cornerstone for psychoanalysis, which would later be developed by Sigmund Freud.

The friendship between Breuer and Freud broke up soon after publication of *Studies on Hysteria* because of personal and professional differences, among them Breuer's refusal to recognize Freud's postulations regarding the role of childhood seduction in the etiology of hysteria.

Although personal contact between Freud and Breuer ceased completely, Freud throughout his life remained aware of the significant achievements that his former friend Breuer had made in the development of psychoanalysis.

Bibliography

Primary: 1868. 'Die Selbststeuerung der Athmung durch den Nervus vagus.' *Sitzungsberichte der Akademie der Wissenschaften, Wien, Mathematisch-naturwissenschaftliche Klasse* 58(2): 909–937; 1874. 'Über die Function der Bogengänge des Ohrlabyrinths'. *Medizinische Jahrbücher* 4: 72–124; 1895. (with Freud, Sigmund) *Studien über Hysterie* (Leipzig and Vienna) [translations: 2004. *Studies in Hysteria,* trans. Nicola Luckhurst (London); 1955. *The Standard Edition of the Complete Psychological Works of Sigmund Freud, vol. ii, Studies on Hysteria,* trans. James and Alix Strachey (London)].

Secondary: Hirschmüller, Albrecht, 1989. *The Life and Work of Josef Breuer: Physiology and Psychoanalysis* (New York and London); *DSB*.

Christian Huber
(trans. Christopher Barber)

BRIGHAM, AMARIAH (b. New Marlboro, Massachusetts, USA, 26 December 1798; d. Utica, New York, USA, 8 September 1849), *psychiatry.*

Brigham, son of Massachusetts farmer John Brigham and Phoebe Clark, had a difficult childhood. After the death of both his parents when he was eleven, he moved to upstate New York to live with an uncle who was a doctor. Ten months later, the uncle also died. Brigham took a series of occasional jobs—in a bookstore, as a teacher in an Albany, New York, school—and then prepared for a medical career, largely through apprenticeships in New Marlboro and in Canaan, Connecticut, supplemented by attending one term of lectures in New York City.

When Brigham attempted to earn his living from the practice of medicine, he joined a seriously overcrowded profession, and his early efforts in Massachusetts, in Enfield and Greenfield, met with little success. This prompted him to leave for a year in Europe, where he first encountered medical men specializing in the treatment of mental disorders. In 1831 he returned to the United States, and resumed his efforts to build a practice, this time in Hartford, Connecticut.

Hartford was then home to one of the first asylums in America. The Hartford Retreat, as its name implies, was modeled on the York Retreat in England. Unlike its inspiration, however, the Connecticut institution had been founded largely upon medical initiative, and had employed a physician as superintendent from its opening in 1824. Not surprisingly, it had also made a substantial place for medical therapies alongside and in combination with psychosocial interventions. Its second superintendent, however, Silas Fuller, was largely an absentee, and the lay steward and matron sought to create an expanded role for themselves. Faced with administrative turmoil, the Retreat's managers forced the resignation of all three officers in 1840, and appointed Brigham as the new head of the asylum.

Brigham had published three books in this period, all of them touching on mental and nervous disease: *Remarks on the Influence of Mental Cultivation and Mental Excitement upon Health* (1832); *Observations on the Influence of Religion on the Health and Physical Welfare of Mankind* (1835); and *An Inquiry Concerning the Diseases and Functions of the Brain, the Spinal Cord, and the Nerves* (1840). His skepticism about religious enthusiasm, and his view that such extremism fostered mental instability, echoed long-standing beliefs among alienists, although such claims were inevitably controversial in a period where revivalist religion was enjoying great successes in the new American republic. Yet his claims were, it seems, part of his appeal to the asylum's managers.

Brigham left the Hartford Retreat in 1842 for the far bigger challenge of opening and running the state asylum at Utica, New York. At both establishments, he continued his emphasis on a combination of medical and moral treatment. He was also active in forming a new professional organization of asylum doctors, the Association of Medical Superintendents of American Institutions for the Insane, which first met in Philadelphia in 1844. That same year, he began publishing America's first specialist journal devoted to asylum medicine, the *American Journal of Insanity,* subsidizing its operations from his own pocket, and having it printed at the asylum by the patients. The journal is the direct ancestor of the modern *American Journal of Psychiatry,* a name change that took place in 1921.

Brigham's health began to fail in 1848. He took a journey to the South the following year, but his decline continued, and by early September he was dead.

Bibliography

Primary: 1832. *Remarks on the Influence of Mental Cultivation and Mental Excitement upon Health* (Hartford, CT) (reprint, 1973); 1835. *Observations on the Influence of Religion on the Health and Physical Welfare of Mankind* (Boston) (reprint, 1973); 1840. *An Inquiry Concerning the Diseases and Functions of the Brain, the Spinal Cord, and the Nerves* (New York) (reprint, 1973).

Secondary: Carlson, Eric T., 1956. 'Amariah Brigham: I. Life and Works.' *American Journal of Psychiatry* 112: 831–836; Carlson, Eric T., 1957. 'Amariah Brigham: II. Psychiatric Thought and Practice.' *American Journal of Psychiatry* 113: 911–916; *DAMB*.

Andrew Scull

BRIGHT, RICHARD (b. Bristol, England, 28 September 1789; d. London, England, 16 December 1858), *medicine, pathology, nephrology.*

The extensive—and undoubtedly justified—attention given to Paris as the center of pathological anatomy in the early nineteenth century, particularly through the works of historian Erwin Ackerknecht, philosopher Michel Foucault, and others, has perhaps tended to withhold attention from clinical-pathological explorations in Great Britain. Certainly a remarkable contributor in this domain was Richard Bright, one of the 'Great Men of Guy's', whose observations laid the foundation for the modern understanding of renal disease, and who added chemical correlation to the findings at bedside and at the *sectio cadaveris.*

Bright was the son of Richard Bright of Bristol and Sarah Heywood. The Brights were a prominent family of merchant-venturers and bankers, and the family affluence allowed the young Bright to enjoy an extended period of medical study, and to defer the building of a private practice in favor of what would later be termed 'research'. Bright's initial schooling (1795–1808) took place first at a school conducted by John Prior Estlin at Bristol, then with the Reverend Lant Carpenter in Exeter, in which setting Bright eventually served as a sort of senior pupil and teacher. Yet in these years he did not shine as a scholar, and seemed to suffer periods of 'lassitude' and melancholy, of the sort not unknown in adolescence. He did, however, acquire a fondness for natural history—particularly geology, the passion of his father—and no doubt the strict tutelage of that time had its effect; for Bright emerged as a broadly knowledgeable young man, a capable linguist, and a skilled draftsman.

Having chosen medicine as his career (to his father's initial displeasure), Bright fashioned his professional training through study at Edinburgh and lectures and clinical work at Guy's Hospital (which at the time for instructional purposes was allied with St Thomas's Hospital as the 'United Borough Hospitals'). Guy's physician William Babington (1756–1833), for whom Bright served as 'clerk', and surgeon Astley Cooper (1768–1841) most influenced Bright. He returned for a time to the University of Edinburgh, and

received his MD in 1813, having submitted a thesis on 'contagious erysipelas'. An adventurous interruption to Bright's medical studies was an expedition to Iceland with his friend Henry Holland and Sir George Mackenzie (1780–1848). Bright contributed several charming sketches and chapters on the natural history of the island to MacKenzie's book, *Travels to the Island of Iceland During the Summer of the Year 1810* (1811). All who have written about Bright cite his interest in geology and other descriptive sciences, and his keen eye and pen, as foundational for his work in clinical-pathological correlation.

He next worked at the Carey Street Dispensary (1814) under Thomas Bateman (1778–1821), then at the Lock Hospital (1815), and from 1816 until 1819 at the Fever Hospital, all in London. During a good part of 1814 and 1815, Bright indulged his fondness for travel with an extensive wandering through Austria and Hungary. He was always the active traveler and sharp observer, combining some medical learning with his interests in geology, linguistics, and the vagaries of human social behavior. Calling at baronial castles while also inspecting mines, prisons, and tribes of gypsies, Bright filled up notebooks and, in 1818, published *Travels from Vienna through Lower Hungary; with Some Remarks on the State of Vienna During the Congress in the Year 1814*, which included some pleasing illustrations by his own hand. The 762-page volume won favorable reviews and substantial readership. He delayed his return home to join other Guy's doctors at Brussels caring for wounded soldiers following Waterloo. Back in England, he commenced practice and became assistant physician to Guy's Hospital in 1820, then physician in 1824.

Although practice and teaching occupied much of his time, Bright used the opportunities afforded by the 'museum of disease' that was Guy's to carry out the clinical-pathological work that led to the magisterial *Reports of Medical Cases*, published in two sections (three actual volumes) 1827–31. He carried out many autopsies himself, and others were done by Thomas Hodgkin (1798–1866), perhaps the leading early British student of 'morbid anatomy', and then lecturer on this subject and museum curator at Guy's.

Richard Bright's most notable contribution led to one of the first eponymous diseases, the *morbus Brightii*, or Bright's disease. Through correlation of observations made at the bedside of patients showing 'dropsical effusion' (edema), examination of their urine for coagulability (albuminuria), and the findings at autopsy, Bright demonstrated that those dropsical patients with albuminous urine had kidney disease. Something like this had been hinted at by the work of John Blackall (1771–1860) and William Charles Wells (1757–1817), but Bright made the linkage conclusive through use of pathological anatomy and the accumulation of many cases. He delineated three forms of the morbid appearance of the diseased kidneys, but withheld judgment as to whether these were distinct diseases or several stages of one disorder. The case histories and handsome colored engravings of the *Reports of Medical Cases*, those documenting albuminous renal disease and much else, made it a landmark of the golden period of premicroscopic clinical-anatomical correlation. The rich observations and plates illustrating neurological disease which made up much of the second volume reveal sophistication in this realm: Bright was among the first to clearly describe the locus of brain lesions in convulsive disorders and strokes.

During the years when he was adducing his clinical and pathological observations, a British 'school' of clinical chemistry arose, and Bright apparently perceived that a fuller elaboration of kidney disease might benefit from this new facet of medical science. He turned first to William Prout (1785–1850) and John Bostock (1773–1846, lecturer in chemistry at Guy's), whose findings appeared as notes or letters in the *Reports*. Later, Guy's physician George Owen Rees (1813–89) provided much of the chemical data. Quite possibly for the first time, a sort of 'research agenda' occupied a teaching hospital, as albuminous nephritis became the house disease at Guy's. Bright published additional clinical and pathological observations and therapeutic ideas, Rees and others did further chemical work, and pupils were sent into the wards to see how many patients showed coagulable urine.

In 1842 Bright gained permission to assign, during the summer, the beds of the 'clinical wards' (i.e., what might be called the 'teaching beds') entirely for the investigation of kidney disease. There was set up 'a room between the two wards for the meeting of the physicians and pupils . . . and a small laboratory . . . fitted up and decorated entirely for our purposes'. The information compiled from this summer project appeared in a lengthy report in the *Guy's Hospital Reports* of 1843. This remarkable and precocious study brings to mind the 'metabolic ward', or set of research beds, within teaching hospitals of a hundred years later, although no claim can be made that Guy's in 1842 actually raised that idea.

Guy's has continued as a center of nephrology (the later name for the specialty centered on medical renal disease) until the present day. Bright himself, however, found it increasingly difficult to sustain both investigative work and a growing, high-caste (although not entirely so) private practice, and withdrew from his major role at Guy's in 1844. By then, he had also experienced several bouts of illness himself, and the deaths of several of his children. His work on renal disease had, of course, established his reputation internationally long before he ceased visits to the deadhouse.

In 1822 Bright had married Martha Babington, daughter of Guy's senior physician, William Babington. Whereas this union could be imagined as careerist in motivation, in fact, ample evidence shows that the affection was real and deep, and Martha's death in 1823 following the birth of their child devastated the new husband and father. He dealt with his grief in good part through work. In 1826 he married Elizabeth (Eliza) Follett; they had seven children, six of whom

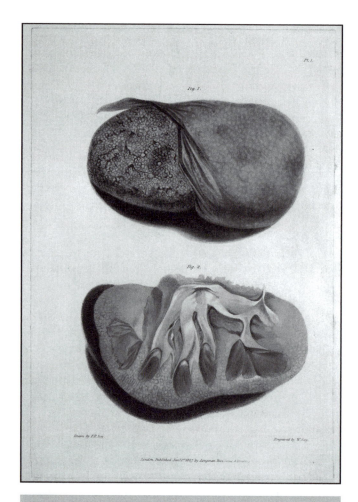

'Bright's' disease of the kidney. Colored stipple engraving from *Reports of medical cases . . .* London, 1827–31. Rare Books, Wellcome Library, London.

survived childhood. Bright was devoted to his large family, although family letters reveal considerable marital tension created largely by Bright's absences and delays in joining the family on summer holidays; this occurred when he acceded to demands of his London practice, and to his quiet but intense determination to further clinical-pathological knowledge.

As a young man, Bright could seem diffident and lacking in confidence, and occasionally such tendencies reappeared even in his mature years of accomplishment. An American pupil at Guy's in a memoir described him as 'kindness itself' to his ward patients, and he seems to have been generally well-liked. His reputation as physician and gentleman knew no blemish. Bright's work and contributions illustrate something of the 'practical' British style of clinical-anatomical correlation (for him, morbid anatomy yielded clear insights to guide therapy).

We also see in his career how affluence, private practice, and active investigation interrelated in a period before medicine—at least British medicine—offered any sort of structure to nourish research, or to sustain a physician mainly interested in this pursuit. Alternatively, one might interpret the career described above as illustrative of how research and publication can serve to establish reputation and build practice. No doubt something of the latter occurred; but there seems little doubt that Richard Bright was suffused with a passion to build knowledge, move a new sort of medicine forward, and enhance the standing of his hospital and medical school.

Bibliography

Primary: 1818. *Travels from Vienna through Lower Hungary with Some Remarks on the State of Vienna During the Congress of the Year 1814* (Edinburgh); 1827–1831. *Reports of Medical Cases Selected with a View of Illustrating the Symptoms and Cure of Diseases by a Reference to Morbid Anatomy* (London); 1836. 'Cases and observations illustrative of renal disease accompanied with the secretion of albuminous urine.' *Guy's Hospital Reports* 1: 338–379; 1839. (with Addison, Thomas) *Elements of the Practice of Medicine* (London).

Secondary: Berry, Diana, and Campbell Mackenzie, 1992. *Richard Bright, 1789–1858: Physician in an Age of Revolution and Reform* (London); Bright, Pamela, 1983. *Dr. Richard Bright (1789–1858)* (London); Peitzman, Steven J., 1981. 'Bright's Disease and Bright's Generation: Toward Exact Medicine at Guy's Hospital.' *Bulletin of the History of Medicine* 55: 307–321; *DSB*; *Oxford DNB*.

Steven J. Peitzman

BRISTOWE, JOHN SYER (b. Camberwell, Surrey, England, 19 January 1827; d. Dixton, Monmouth, Wales, 20 August 1895), *medicine.*

Bristowe was the eldest son of John Syer Bristowe, a medical practitioner, and Mary Chesshyre. He was educated at King's College, London, and entered St Thomas's Hospital in 1846. He qualified MRCS and LSA in 1849, MB in 1850, and MD in 1852. His first appointment was as house surgeon at St Thomas's in 1849, but he moved to medicine in 1854 when he was elected physician and lecturer on materia medica. He spent his whole career at the hospital holding, in turn, lectureships in general anatomy and physiology, then pathology in succession to John Simon. In 1876 he became lecturer in medicine, a post he held until his death. He was elected FRCP in 1858, giving the Croonian Lectures in 1872 and the Lumleian Lectures in 1879, and he became a FRS in 1881. He was active in numerous metropolitan medical societies, worked for many institutions as a consulting physician, and served on charitable bodies. Bristowe married Miriam Isabella Stearns in 1856 and they had five sons and five daughters.

Bristowe is principally remembered for his work in public health, both as an investigator for the Medical Department of the Privy Council, and as Medical Officer of Health (MOH) for Camberwell, London. Early in his career he investigated local epidemics and undertook special studies for the Department, including those on phosphorous poisoning in the manufacture of matches (1862); on the carriage of infection by rags (1865); and on the cattle plague with John Burdon Sanderson (1865).

His most famous study was made with Timothy Holmes in 1863 into the sanitary condition of English hospitals. The enquiry was prompted by the debate over the resiting of St Thomas's Hospital: Florence Nightingale and other sanitarians wanted to move it to the healthier countryside, but metropolitan consultants wanted it to remain in the capital. The Bristowe-Holmes report confounded the sanitarians by suggesting that case selection, not environment, was the dominant factor in hospital mortality. Thus, a hospital in a heavily populated, urban-industrial area would inevitably admit more serious cases and have higher mortality than a country hospital, where there was less pressure on admissions. Bristowe maintained his increasingly demanding role in Camberwell for thirty-nine years, from 1856 until his death. In the 1880s, with John Tripe, he was responsible for demonstrating the local dangers of smallpox hospitals, and this work led to the reorganization and relocation of isolation hospitals in London.

Bristowe was best known to contemporaries as the author of *A Treatise on the Theory and Practice of Medicine*, a much used textbook that was first published in 1876 and went through seven editions to 1890. As a practicing physician, he was best known for his work on diseases of the nervous system, especially brain tumors, cerebral syphilis, general paralysis of the insane, and hysteria. However, typically for the time, he was not a specialist, but practiced and published across medicine. He was famed for his diagnostic acumen, known both for being slow and meticulous over most cases, yet able to diagnose others instantly and at a distance. He was reputed to be a therapeutic nihilist, a view that seems to have arisen from his insistence on using only drugs of proven value, although he was famed for prescribing infusion of gentian when no particular drug was indicated. Bristowe was a renowned teacher, celebrated for his memory, his attention to detail, and his ability to relate individual cases to each other.

Bristowe was a central figure in metropolitan medicine for nearly half a century. He was serious and rigid, with his renowned skepticism seen to define his character. However, he was held in some affection by his colleagues, and as someone, to quote an obituarist, 'whose whole life was a protest against authorized quackery, the ignorant, the pretentious, and the insincere'.

Bibliography

Primary: 1876. *A Treatise on the Theory and Practice of Medicine* (London); 1880. *The Physiological and Pathological Relations of the Voice and Speech* (London); 1888. *Clinical Lectures and Essays on Diseases of the Nervous System* (London).

Secondary: Hardy, Anne, 1993. *The Epidemic Streets: Infectious Disease and the Rise of Preventive Medicine, 1856–1900* (Oxford); 1896. 'In memoriam—John Syer Bristowe.' *St Thomas's Hospital Reports* 23: xvii–xxv; *Oxford DNB*.

Michael Worboys

BRIUKHONENKO, SERGEI SERGEEVICH (b. Kozlov, Russia, 30 April [12 May] 1890; d. Moscow, Russia, 20 April 1960), *physiology.*

Briukhonenko was born into the family of a railway engineer in the Russian province of Tambov. The atmosphere of his family was filled with intellectual and artistic interests, and Sergei himself was a gifted musician and artist. From 1905 the family lived in Moscow, where Briukhonenko studied in a classical gymnasium and entered the Department of Natural Sciences at the Moscow University in 1908. The next year he passed into the Medical Faculty, where he focused on bacteriology under the guidance of Professor G. Gabrichevskii.

Briukhonenko graduated from the university in 1914, just before the beginning of World War I, and he soon joined the Russian Army. The severe war experience (he served as a military physician for three years and was awarded medals) and the death of his wife and son during the typhus epidemic strongly influenced his medical practices. In 1919 Briukhonenko started working as an assistant in Moscow University's Clinic of Therapy and Pathology. It was headed by Professor F. Andreev, who was known for his works on revival. That collaboration played an important role in extending and improving the practice of resuscitation in Russia; Andreev supported Briukhonenko's desire to develop a system of artificial blood circulation.

For decades physicians had tried to find a way to keep a patient alive while working on the heart. Today, the heart-lung machine takes over the functions of the heart and lungs during open-heart surgery and allows a surgeon to carefully stop the heart, while the rest of the patient's body continues to receive oxygen-rich blood. The surgeon can then perform delicate work on the heart without interference from bleeding or the heart's pumping motion. When the procedure is over, the surgeon restarts the heart and disconnects the heart-lung machine. The invention of the heart-lung machine has been one of the truly revolutionary changes in medical equipment.

In September 1925 at the Second Congress of Russian Pathologists in Moscow, Briukhonenko demonstrated the world's first working model of a heart-lung machine—twelve years before the invention of it by John H. Gibbon (1937). Briukhonenko's experimental machine was called an 'avtozektor'. It used two roller pumps and was designed to replace the heart and lung action of a dog. Bayer-205 (germanin) was suggested for blood stabilization. Its valuable property in triggering artificial hemophilia was discovered during Briukhonenko's research in cooperation with A. Steppun and H. Zeiss at the Moscow Research Institute for Chemistry and Pharmacology.

During the next years Briukhonenko performed many public demonstrations with the help of an avtozektor, 'reviving' a severed dog's head ten minutes after death. He became a very popular person in the USSR, heading the Laboratory of Experimental Therapy at the Institute of Blood Transfusion (1930). It was later transformed (1935) into the Research Institute of Experimental Physiology and Therapy, with a staff of 150. The scientific program of the laboratory covered a wide range of problems dealing with human and animal resuscitation and the relevant medical equipment. Using a new model of Briukhonenko's avtozektor, Professor N. Terebinsky performed the first open-heart operation in the world in 1931, on a dog. Beginning in 1940, Briukhonenko and his collaborators started to perform their revival techniques on corpses at the Sklifossovskii Institute for Medical Emergency in Moscow, but World War II interfered with the transfer of the experimental results into clinical practice.

Briukhonenko spent the last years of his life as a vice-president in a new institute—Experimental Surgery Facilities and Instruments. He obtained fame through his inventions—for example, when Professor A. Vishnevskii performed the first human open-heart operation in the USSR (27 November 1957) with the support of Briukhonenko's avtozektor. But Briukhonenko never achieved worldwide recognition.

Bibliography

Primary: 1964. *Iskusstvennoe krovoobrashchenie* [Artificial Blood Transfusion] (Moscow).

Secondary: Sirotkina, M.G., and V. S. Gutkin, 1972. *S. S. Briukhonenko* (Moscow); Probert, W., and D. Melrose, 1960. 'An Early Russian Heart-Lung Machine.' *British Medical Journal* ii: 1047–1048.

Marina Sorokina

BROCA, (PIERRE) PAUL (b. Sainte-Foy-la-Grande, France, 28 June 1824; d. Paris, France, 8 July 1880), *medicine, surgery, aphasiology, anthropology.*

Usually known as Paul, Broca was born into a family of French Calvinists (Huguenots) in the same year when the reactionary King Charles X took the throne and began to restore the old royal order of French society. That probably did not go down well with Paul's father, Jean-Pierre Broca (called Benjamin), a physician whose nonconformist family had been in the area east of Bordeaux for centuries. He was kind, pleasant, volatile, and restless, with a reputation for devotion to the poor. Paul's mother, Annette Thomas Broca, was the daughter of a Calvinist minister. Her family background and personal outlook were also strongly republican. She was rather more strict and serious than her husband, well-educated, and a perfectionist.

At the age of eight, after three years of elementary school, Broca entered the Calvinist collège in Sainte-Foy-la-Grande. He was remembered as a brilliant student. At age sixteen, he took his bachelor of letters in preparation for medical education, since that was his parents' wish for his career. In truth, he actually preferred engineering. He took a mathematics degree by examination at Toulouse, but then his

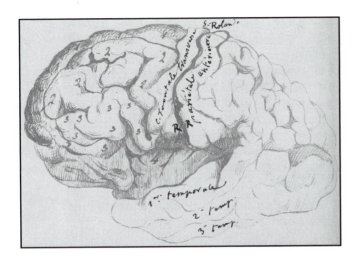

Brain of a thirteen-year-old boy who fell from a height. Cerebral matter issued from the left frontal fracture, resulting in partial aphasia. Drawing by Broca, May 1863, from Ange Duval, *Observations d'aphémie pour server a la determination du siege de la faculté de langage . . .* **Paris, 1864. Wellcome Library, London.**

younger sister died. On the theory that he could return to practice medicine in Sainte-Foy, he gave up his engineering ambitions. At the age of seventeen, he went to Paris to study medicine.

Broca thrived in the intensely competitive environment of Parisian medicine. After two years, he won appointment as *externe* [student] to the surgeon Philippe-Frédéric Blandin at the Hôtel Dieu. In December 1844 he finished at the top of the *concours* [examination] for appointment as an *interne* in the Paris hospitals. His first post was at the Bicêtre with the psychiatrist François Leuret, who was interested in comparative neuroanatomy. Another assignment was with the surgeon-anatomist Pierre-Nicholas Gerdy at the Charité. In the course of various intrigues, he was appointed *interne* to Blandin in 1847 and allowed a fourth year of the internship through 1848. February through June of 1848 saw the Parisian populist revolution that resulted in the short-lived 'second republic' of France. Broca considered himself to be a 'moderate' republican. He saw some action as a soldier, and especially as an interne at the Hôtel Dieu, but mainly he forged ahead with his work and his career. His appointment as prosector of anatomy in 1848 brought him students and improved finances.

Metastatic Cancer and the Microscope

Broca's doctoral thesis of 1849 was the next major step in his ascension through the ranks. Before the introduction of the achromatic microscope in 1830, microscopes were of limited general use. Using the new instruments, Schleiden and Schwann had announced the cell theory in 1838–39, but the theory's centrality to pathology was not established until Virchow's publication of his *Cellular Pathologie* in 1858. At considerable expense, Broca bought a microscope in 1847. He used it to prove the phenomenon of the venous spread of cancer cells, an idea that he inherited from Hermann Lebert. Late in 1849, months after submission of his thesis, Broca learned about a prize for a memoir on cancer that was being offered by the Académie de Médecine. The entry was due on 29 February 1850. Literally with much help from his friends, and with little sleep, he met the deadline and won the Prix Portal.

The next critical step in Broca's academic progression was his success in the very public *agrégation* [examination] of 1853, which gave him the title of *professeur agrégé* [roughly, assistant professor] and an appointment as hospital surgeon to the central bureau of Paris. Those positions, and his reputation as a rising young star, brought him enough clinical activity and income so that he began to look for a wife. Much to his mother's relief and satisfaction, Paul Broca married Adèle-Augustine Lugol (1835–1914), a fellow Huguenot, in 1857. She was the orphaned daughter of Jean-Guillaume Lugol, the inventor of Lugol's (iodine) solution. Their daughter Pauline was born in 1858, son Auguste in 1859, and youngest son André in 1863. Auguste became a prominent Parisian pediatric surgeon, and André a professor of medical physics in Paris.

Anthropology Leads to Aphasia

As a youth in Sainte-Foy, Broca had taken an interest in paleontology. His first encounter with practical anthropology occurred in 1847, when he was appointed to a commission to excavate an old cemetery. Studying the comparative anatomy of apparently extinct animals led easily to questions about transmutation of species. Broca and others wanted to discuss those controversial matters at meetings of the Société de Biologie, but he found that the group did not want to go there. He thus began to organize another scientific society that would be more willing to go where true science seemed to lead. The Société d'Anthropologie held its first official meeting in 1859, the same year as the publication of Darwin's *Origin of Species*. Broca served as Secretary (later General Secretary) of the Société for the rest of his life. From its beginning, one of the main subjects of interest to the group was craniology and brain anatomy.

During the spring of 1861, there was much debate about brain size and intelligence at the Société de Anthropologie, which led to a related discussion about the relative importance of the size of the frontal lobes. In such debates at that time, the old bogeyman of phrenology was always in the background. Phrenology seemed to have been discredited in the 1840s, and with it all theories of cerebral localization—but not quite. The prominent and colorful physician Jean-Baptiste Bouillaud still accepted Gall's localization of the 'faculty of language' in the frontal lobes bilaterally. Bouillaud's son-in-law and disciple, Ernst Aubertin, was an active member of the Société, and he brought up the issue of language localization. Aubertin acknowledged that finding an autopsied case of complete destruction of both frontal lobes in a person who had still been speaking after the lesion would invalidate the phrenological localization of language. Broca participated in these debates, but not as a strong partisan.

On 12 April 1861, a fifty-one-year-old epileptic man named Leborgne was transferred to Broca's surgical service at the Bicêtre; he was dying of gangrene of the leg. Leborgne was known to the hospital staff as 'Tan', because that was the only word he could say. Broca examined Tan and established that he understood some visual language by hand signals. He then invited Aubertin to see the patient, and Aubertin agreed that Tan was an acceptable test case. Tan obligingly died on 17 April 1861. Only hours later, Broca showed the brain at a meeting of the Société d'Anthropologie. After it was hardened in alcohol for two months, the brain was then shown to the more prestigious Société Anatomique.

In essence, there was a large area of softening in the left anterior sylvian region, mainly involving the frontal lobe. Since Tan's documented clinical course had evolved slowly over the years, Broca reasoned that the pathological process had started in the center of the demonstrated lesion. Six months later, another patient (Lelong) with a similar story came to autopsy; his lesion was more restricted to the second and, especially, the third left frontal gyri. Hence, the lateral portion of the third (lateral) frontal gyrus is known as 'Broca's area'. Broca's original term for the expressive language deficit associated with lesions of that area was 'aphémie' [aphemia], but the term 'aphasia', proposed by Armand Trousseau in 1864, quickly supplanted it.

Aphasia Leads to Cerebral Localization and Dominance

Broca continued to collect cases of aphasia. In 1863 he had eight cases, and he noted that it was 'remarkable how in all these patients the lesion was on the left side'. By 1865 he had dozens of cases, and he was prepared to state that 'We speak with the left hemisphere.' ['Nous parlon avec l'hémisphere gauche.'] Thus, Broca made two fundamental contributions: (1) he established the validity of cerebral/cortical localization in a scientific form that transcended phrenology, and (2) he demonstrated the phenomenon of cerebral dominance for language. It should be noted that the idea of a 'faculty' of language, as Broca used it, did not include any motor element. A 'faculty' was strictly an 'intellectual' entity.

Needless to say, there have been arguments about both contributions. The controversy that arose in the 1860s was about priority for discovering cerebral dominance. Gustave Dax, a physician in Montpellier, claimed that his long-dead father, Marc Dax, had presented a paper on left cerebral dominance for language in 1836 in Montpellier. Current scholarship concludes that Marc Dax probably recognized the phenomenon, whether or not the paper was actually presented, but Broca gets the lion's share of the credit for discovering and promulgating knowledge of left cerebral dominance for language. With regard to localization, the most famous disagreement came from the Parisian neurologist Pierre Marie, who in 1906 published a drawing of Leborge's unsliced brain and concluded that the area of brain damage was far more extensive than Broca had said. However, another French group subsequently 'sliced' the brain by computed tomography in 1980, and they concluded that 'Broca was right.' (Signoret et al., 1984)

Back to Anthropology and Comparative Neuroanatomy

After 1865 Broca's interest in language disorders and localization continued, but his primary scientific focus was on anthropology. Because anthropological research so often raised issues about evolution and related questions, its growth was generally opposed by the conservative element in the French establishment. Broca's appointments as member of the Academy of Medicine and as Professor in the Faculty of Medicine, both in 1867, strengthened the position of the entire field. Eventually, in the 1870s, Broca was able to teach research methods to large numbers of investigators in formal classes. He invented more than two dozen instruments for measuring skeletal remains, especially the skull. In addition to his acknowledged role as founder of French anthropology, he actively encouraged the development of the field in other countries.

In France, the decade of the 1870s began with the disastrous Franco-Prussian War of 1870–71. During the second siege of Paris, Broca took part in a daring and successful plot to remove 75,000,000 francs from Paris to the Administration of Public Assistance outside the city, by moving the cash concealed in a potato cart. For most of the remainder of the 1870s, comparative neuroanatomy was at the center of his attention. In 1878 Broca published his conception of the 'limbic lobe', a circuit of deep cerebral structures that he associated with the sense of smell. In 1937 James Papez elaborated on that concept and proposed that the limbic lobe was a major part of the cerebral mechanism for elaboration of emotions.

In February 1880 Broca was elected to the French Senate as a representative of science, despite strong conservative opposition. He enjoyed the honor for only five months. His sudden death was thought to be due to an acute myocardial infarction.

Bibliography

Primary: 1861. 'Remarques sur le siège de la faculté du langage articulé, suivies d'une observation d'aphémie.' *Bulletin de la Société Anatomique de Paris* 36 (2e série): 6, 330–357; 1865. 'Du siège de la faculté du langage articulé dans l'hémisphère gauche du cerveau.' *Bulletin de la Société d'Anthropologie* 6: 377–393; 1878. 'Le grand lobe limbique et la scissure limbique dans le série des mammifère.' *Revue d'Anthropologie* 1 (2e série): 385–498.

Secondary: Finger, Stanley, and Daniel Roe, 1996. 'Gustave Dax and the Early History of Cerebral Dominance.' *Archives of Neurology* 53: 806–812; Greenblatt, Samuel H., 1984. 'The Multiple Roles of Broca's Discovery in the Development of the Modern Neurosciences.' *Brain and Cognition* 3: 249–258; Signoret, Jean-Louis, Paul Castaigne, François Lhermitte, René Abelanet, and Pierre Lavorel, 1984. 'Rediscovery of Leborgne's Brain: Anatomical Description with CT Scan.' *Brain and Language* 22: 303–319; Schiller, Francis, 1979. *Paul Broca. Founder of French Anthropology, Explorer of the Brain* (Berkeley); 1881. 'Paul Broca, Honorary Member.' *Journal of the Anthropological Institute* 10: 242–260; *DSB.*

Samuel H. Greenblatt

BRODIE, BENJAMIN COLLINS   (b. Winterslow, Wiltshire, England, 8 June 1783; d. Surrey, England, 21 October 1862), *surgery.*

Brodie was the fourth child, and third son, of Rev Peter Bellinger Brodie, parish rector, who had previously been educated at Worcester College, Oxford. Brodie's mother was Sarah, daughter of Benjamin Collins, banker of Salisbury. Brodie received his early general and classical education from his father. When he was eighteen he went to London, principally to study anatomy. He initially attended the lectures of John Abernethy (1764–1831) at St Bartholomew's Hospital; then, in 1801 and 1802, those of James Wilson (1780–1821) at the Great Windmill Street School. In 1803 he became a pupil of Sir Everard Home (1756–1832) at St George's Hospital, and was appointed his House Surgeon in 1805. He also gained the MRCS that year. He was later appointed demonstrator to the Anatomical School at St George's.

When his demonstratorship terminated, Brodie assisted Home in his private operations and comparative anatomical research, and this is said to have stimulated his subsequent work on scientific subjects. He continued his anatomical studies under Wilson, and lectured and demonstrated at the Great Windmill Street School until 1812. He was elected assistant surgeon at St George's and served from 1808 until 1822, when he was elevated to surgeon. In 1819 he had been appointed professor of comparative anatomy and physiology to the RCS. He was elected FRS in 1810, and awarded the Society's Copley Medal in 1811 because of the quality of his Croonian Lecture: 'On the influence of the brain on the action of the heart and the generation of animal heat'. At this time he also published 'On the effects produced by certain vegetable poisons (Alcohol, Tobacco, Woorara, &c)'. He was elected the Society's president from 1858 until he resigned in 1861 because of his failing eyesight.

Brodie saw a case of spontaneous dislocation of the hip as a house surgeon, and studied other diseases of joints, later writing a book on this topic. He was a distinguished surgeon, said to have been cool and very knowledgeable, and his surgical practice prospered. During this period, he published numerous papers and several books, including some on the urinary organs and others on nervous diseases. He was also recognized as an outstanding diagnostician. He attended George IV and assisted in the removal of a sebaceous cyst from his scalp. He later attended George IV at Windsor during his fatal illness. When William IV succeeded George IV, Brodie was made sergeant-surgeon to the King in 1832, and a baronet in 1834. On Victoria's accession to the throne, he was made sergeant-surgeon to the Queen.

Brodie served as president of the RCS in 1844 and, in 1858, as first President of the General Medical Council. He was elected a member of numerous foreign medical societies, and took an active part in various learned societies in London. Upon his death in 1862, his eldest son succeeded to the baronetcy, and was appointed professor of chemistry at Oxford in 1865.

Bibliography

Primary: 1818. *Pathological and Surgical Observations on Diseases of the Joints* (London); 1854. *Psychological Inquiries* (London) [published anonymously].

Secondary: Holmes, T., 1897. *Sir Benjamin Collins Brodie* (London); Hawkins, C., 1865. *The Works of Sir Benjamin Brodie . . . with an Autobiography.* 3 vols. (London); Acland, H. W., 1864. *Biographical Sketch of Sir Benjamin Brodie* (London); Anon. 1862. 'Sir Benjamin Brodie, Bart., F.R.S.' *Lancet* ii: 452–457; [Anon.] 1862. 'Death of Sir Benjamin Brodie, Bart., F.R.S.' *British Medical Journal* ii: 446–448; *DSB; Oxford DNB; Plarr's Lives.*

Matthew Howard Kaufman

BROUARDEL, PAUL   (b. St Quentin, France, 13 February 1837; d. Paris, France, 23 July 1906), *forensic medicine, public health, hygiene, medical jurisprudence.*

Brouardel's father, Auguste, was a professor of secondary education in St Quentin. Paul Brouardel studied at the Faculty of Medicine of Paris under the physiologist Étienne-Jules Marey, interned at the Cochin hospital, and received his doctorate in 1865. He then served on the staff of the St Antoine and Pitié hospitals. He succeeded Tardieu to the chair of legal medicine at the Paris faculty in 1879 and later served as Dean of the Faculty (1887-1901). He edited or sat on the editorial board of numerous important medical journals and serial publications. Most notably, he was principal editor of the *Annales d'hygiène et de médecine légale* (from 1879) and co-edited, with Augustin Gilbert, the ten-volume *Traité de médecine et de thérapeutique* (1895–1902). He was involved in nearly every hygiene and professional organization of note in the late nineteenth century, including the national public health council (CCHP), which he chaired (1884–1903), and the first national antituberculosis committee, which he founded (1899). He was head of the Association Générale des Médecins de France (1902–06), honorary president of the Union des Syndicats Médicaux (from 1889), and a member of the Academy of Medicine (1881) and the Academy of Science (1892).

Brouardel played an important, often pivotal role in three areas: forensics and jurisprudence, germ theory and public health, and medical legislation. In the 1880s he reorganized and expanded the morgue services in Paris; set foundations for forensic criminology by creating a taxonomy of the postmortem signs of accidental death and criminal acts; and further delineated parameters for the criminalization of abortion. Brouardel is credited with first drawing attention to child abuse, rape, and molestation by his exposition of forensic evidence—work that was brought to the attention of a young Sigmund Freud through their joint association with Charcot. He produced professional and judicial guidelines for malpractice, as well as standards for expert medical witnessing.

Brouardel made a substantial contribution to the medical profession's acceptance of the Pastorian revolution. His conversion to germ theory evidently occurred during his early hospital years in the 1860s. At the famous debates in the Academy of Medicine in 1887, Brouardel was an important spokesperson for Pasteur, even to the extent of covering up the postmortem diagnosis of a child who had died of rabies. Through the *Traité* and other works, Brouardel established germ theory in diagnosis and therapeutics. Within the CCHP he began a nascent program of modern epidemiology, sending out young researchers such as André Chantemesse and Léon Thoinot to investigate the role of drinking water in the transmission of typhoid and cholera. As dean, Brouardel promoted the teaching of bacteriology at the Paris Faculty and worked to reform medical education to include more experimental science. He used his array of political connections to launch a campaign for a Pasteurian public health law (ultimately passed in eviscerated form in 1902). Brouardel played a central, if controversial, role in other aspects of medical politics, including the Medical Practice Act of 1892 and the Medical Assistance Act of 1893.

Bibliography

Primary: 1895 (with Thoinot, L.) *La fièvre typhoïde* (Paris); 1895–1902. *Traité de médecine et de thérapeutique* 10 vols. (Paris); 1897. *L'infanticide* (Paris); 1903. *La profession médicale au commencement du XXe siècle* (Paris); 1906. *Cours de médecine légale* 13 vols. (Paris).

Secondary: Aisenberg, Andrew, 1999. *Contagion: Disease, Government and the Social Question in Nineteenth Century France* (Stanford); Hildreth, Martha L., 1987. *Doctors, Bureaucrats and Public Health in France, 1888–1902* (New York); Léonard, Jacques, 1986. 'Comment peut-on être Pasteurien?' in Salomon-Bayet, Claire, ed., *Pasteur et la Révolution Pastorienne* (Paris) pp. 145–179; Masson, Jeffrey Moussaiff, 1984. *The Assault on Truth. Freud's Suppression of the Seduction Theory* (New York and Toronto).

Martha Hildreth

BROUSSAIS, FRANÇOIS-JOSEPH-VICTOR (b. St Malo, France, 17 December 1772; d. Paris, France, 18 November 1838), *medical theory, therapeutics.*

Broussais was born in St Malo, on the Brittany coast, and spent his early years in the nearby village of Pleurtuit. His family had practiced the healing arts for several generations—his father as a surgeon, one of his grandfathers as a pharmacist, and one of his great-grandfathers as a physician. Broussais seems to have enjoyed a close relationship with his father, sharing not only the latter's interest in medicine but also his Voltairean and anticlerical attitudes, and his strong support for the ideals of the French Revolution.

Broussais was sent for his secondary education to the College of the Cordeliers in the inland town of Dinan, not far from St Malo. One of his fellow students was the future Romantic writer, statesman, and Christian apologist, François-René de Chateaubriand (1768–1848). Many years later, Broussais was mentioned without rancor in Chateaubriand's memoirs of his school days, notwithstanding the fact that by then Broussais was known as a champion of materialism.

In 1792 Broussais broke off his studies to enlist in the Republican army and fight against the *chouans*—Breton counterrevolutionary insurgents encouraged by the local clergy. He served in the army until 1794 and then, after training at the Hôtel Dieu hospital of St Malo and the School of Naval Surgery at Brest, he was appointed surgeon second class and assigned to a frigate at the end of 1795. As he was embarking on his commission he received news that his parents had been murdered by *chouans,* and the emotional impact of that devastating event further intensified his lifelong antiroyalist and anticlerical stance.

Broussais left the navy in 1798, after saving enough money to support himself while studying medicine at the 'school of health' in Paris, founded during the Revolution. There his principal teachers were François Chaussier (1746–1828), professor of anatomy and physiology, and Philippe Pinel (1745–1826), professor of medicine. In addition, he followed the private courses of his near-contemporary Marie-François-Xavier Bichat (1771–1802), and apparently became Bichat's friend before the latter's premature death.

Broussais completed his medical studies in 1802 with a thesis on fevers, which he dedicated to Pinel. He remained in Paris and entered private practice, but had only modest success in attracting a clientele. On the advice of a senior military medical officer, René Nicolas Dufriche Desgenettes (1762–1837), he joined the army medical service in 1803. During the next eleven years he served with the armies of Napoleon in the Low Countries; in Germany, Austria and Italy; and in Spain, where he was posted for six years.

While on military service, Broussais continued to pursue the research agenda that Bichat and others had established for the medical school and hospital system of Paris.

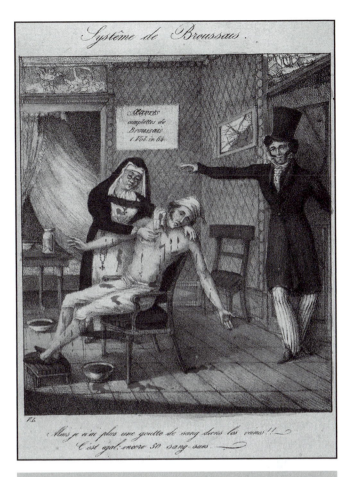

Systême de Broussais.

Broussais instructs a nurse to continue bleeding a pallid, blood-smeared patient. Lithograph with watercolor, Iconographic Collection, Wellcome Library, London.

That approach, which depended on ready access to large numbers of patients, involved establishing correlations between the clinical symptoms of diseases and the pathological alterations of internal tissues revealed in subsequent autopsies. But whereas the investigations of Parisian doctors were largely confined to impoverished urban hospital patients, Broussais claimed that his studies gave a much broader and more representative picture of symptoms and their associated tissue lesions. After all, he had examined military as well as civilian patients, the relatively prosperous as well as the poor and malnourished, those in cities as well as the countryside, and patients in both hot and cold climates.

The first results of Broussais' studies were published in 1808 in his *History of the Phlegmasies or Chronic Inflammations*. In that work he argued that inflammations of the lungs and gastrointestinal tract were the most common causes of death, and in accordance with the methodology of Bichat he identified within those two organ systems the specific inflamed tissues that were associated with each set of symptoms. Although it was not widely acclaimed, the book was praised by Desgenettes, and it helped to secure the latter's

patronage for Broussais after the fall of Napoleon and the disbanding of the imperial armies in 1814.

The former monastery of Val-de-Grace in Paris had become a military hospital in 1796, and clinical teaching was conducted there until 1800. In 1815 it was reorganized to become a school of military medicine as well as a hospital, with the teaching program to commence in 1816. Desgenettes was named professor in chief, and through his influence Broussais was appointed as the second professor. Val-de-Grace provided Broussais with a secure institutional base that was independent of the Paris medical school, now renamed the Faculty of Medicine. Furthermore, his clinical course was open to the public, so he was able to attract civilian students and thus compete with the Faculty.

Concurrent with his first year of teaching at Val-de-Grace, Broussais published his *Examination of the Generally Accepted Medical Doctrine and the Modern Systems of Nosology* as a direct attack on the orthodoxy of the Faculty of Medicine. Written in a highly polemical style, the book denounced the approach of Pinel, and others, that made nosological systems—classifications of diseases based on the resemblances of symptoms—the central focus of medical theory. For Broussais, diseases arose from disturbances of normal physiological functioning caused by 'irritations', or excessive external stimuli. Those irritations, if prolonged, would lead to inflammation, and when inflammation became chronic it produced permanent lesions in the inflamed tissues. To regard symptom complexes as diseases was to engage in 'ontology', or the reification of phenomena that were only superficial effects of underlying pathological conditions. The prime example of ontology in Broussais' sense was the concept of 'essential fevers', or fevers presumed to arise in the whole organism without having a localized cause in the tissues of some particular organ.

Broussais' *Examination* and its theory of 'physiological medicine' quickly polarized the French medical community, with many students and younger physicians being attracted to Broussais' approach. For several years he lectured to overflow audiences, and his courses repeatedly had to be moved into larger halls to accommodate the crowds. His fundamental doctrine—that most diseases are forms of gastroenteritis caused by inflammation, and that copious bloodletting by means of leeches provides the most effective therapy in such cases—was also widely adopted, although it was never without its critics.

The sources of Broussais' popularity lay partly in medical theory and partly in political symbolism. On the medical side, the theoretical focus of Parisian medicine after Bichat was on the localization of diseases in specific tissues. The concept of 'essential fevers' was therefore a glaring anomaly, and Broussais' explanation of such fevers as the results of inflammation of the gastrointestinal tract provided an appropriate resolution of the problem. In addition, his claim to have derived that explanation from extensive clinical and autopsy experience fit with the most highly regarded methodology of medical research. Finally, on the political side, Broussais' attack on 'ontology' was couched in the language of materialism, and that made adherence to his medical theory an expression of opposition to the restored Bourbon regime and its alliance with the Catholic Church.

The political connotations of Broussais' position were reinforced in successive editions of the *Examination*—the second edition being published in 1821, the year after Broussais succeeded Desgenettes as chief at Val-de-Grace, and the third edition in 1829–34. The title of the work was simplified, and the invective became more extreme as Broussais cast his critical eye over the whole of medicine since Hippocrates, expanding each new edition to approximately twice the length of its predecessor.

Broussais also applied the principles of his 'physiological medicine' to psychology and psychiatry in 1828, with a book entitled *On Irritation and Madness* that attacked the philosophical psychology of Victor Cousin (1792–1867) and others on the grounds of their 'spiritualism', another form of 'ontology'. Broussais defended the materialist view that consciousness and thought are the results of brain activity, and that disturbances of physiological processes in the brain are the causes of mental illness.

Although the Bourbon government had purged the Faculty of Medicine of 'liberal' members in 1822, it exercised less political control over the Academy of Medicine, and Broussais was elected to membership in 1823. The Revolution of 1830 and the fall of the Bourbons brought the Orléanist king Louis-Philippe to power. The new government included many officials favorable to Broussais, and in 1831 he was appointed to a specially created chair of general pathology and therapeutics at the Faculty of Medicine. In the following year the government reestablished the Academy of Moral and Political Sciences, which had been abolished by Napoleon in 1801, and Broussais became a member of the section for philosophy. He also was named Inspector General of the military medical service, and Commander of the Legion of Honor.

Just as Broussais' career reached those heights, the cholera epidemic of 1832 severely undermined the credibility of his medical theory. His doctrine of gastrointestinal inflammation did nothing to explain the specific features of the epidemic, and his preferred therapy of extensive bloodletting was not only ineffectual against cholera but manifestly harmful. By that time Broussais had attracted a large number of influential patients, the most important of whom was Casimir-Pierre Périer (1777–1832), Louis-Philippe's chief minister. Périer's rapid decline and death from cholera in May 1832, while under Broussais' care, dealt a heavy blow to the latter's prestige.

When interest in physiological medicine waned, Broussais achieved new popularity through his lectures on phrenology. He had been active in the founding of the Society of Phrenology in 1831, becoming its first secretary-general. His phrenological lectures again drew large audiences, first

at Val-de-Grace and then at the Faculty of Medicine. Materialism was still an attractive component of his teaching for many, but since the Revolution of 1830 it had lost its political connotation of opposition to the Bourbons. Broussais' lectures at the Faculty of Medicine were published in 1836, and at the time of his death he was revising his treatise *On Irritation and Madness* to incorporate phrenological theory.

He was well enough to read a memoir to the Academy of Moral and Political Sciences at the beginning of October 1838, but afterward he succumbed quickly to rectal cancer and died in the middle of the following month. His funeral attracted a large turnout, especially of medical students, and the cortege paused at the monument to Napoleon in the Place Vendome. Broussais's entire medical career had depended upon the army, which was still associated with the glory of Napoleon despite changes in the political climate.

Both the 'physiological medicine' of Broussais and the theory of phrenology that he embraced toward the end of his life are doctrines that no longer have any currency, and his therapeutic reliance on leeches seems archaic. Nevertheless, his critique of 'ontology' had a lasting effect on medical thinking. By arguing that all pathological phenomena arise from the alteration of normal physiological processes, Broussais took the final step in discrediting the concept of diseases as independent entities and prepared the way for the 'experimental pathology' of Claude Bernard (1813–78) and the 'cellular pathology' of Rudolf Virchow (1821–1902).

Bibliography

Primary: 1808. *Histoire des phlegmasies ou inflammations chroniques, fondée sur de nouvelles observations de clinique et d'anatomo-pathologie* (Paris); 1816. *Examen de la doctrine médicale généralement adoptée et des systèmes modernes de nosologie* (Paris); 1821. *Examen des doctrines médicales et des systèmes de nosologie* (2nd edn.) 2 vols. (Paris); 1828. *De l'irritation et de la folie* (Paris); 1829–34. *Examen des doctrines médicales et des systèmes de nosologie* (3rd edn.) 4 vols. (Paris); 1836. *Cours de phrénologie* (Paris).

Secondary: Albury, W. R., 1998. 'Corvisart and Broussais: Human Individuality and Medical Dominance' in Hannaway, Caroline, and Ann Le Berge, eds., *Constructing Paris Medicine* (Amsterdam) pp. 221–250; Braunstein, Jean-François, 1986. *Broussais et le matérialisme: médecine et philosophie au XIXe siècle* (Paris); Foucault, Michel, 1972. *Naissance de la clinique* (2nd edn.) (Paris) pp. 177–198; Ackerknecht, Erwin H., 1967. *Medicine at the Paris Hospital, 1794–1848* (Baltimore) pp. 61–80; DSB.

W. R. Albury

BROWN, JOHN (baptized Buncle, Berwickshire, Scotland, 17 May 1735; d. London, England, 17 October 1788), *medicine.*

Brown, son of Archibald Brown, a weaver, was educated at the parish school of Duns. He was apprenticed to a weaver at the age of ten, but he was such an outstanding student that he was allowed to return to school. By the age of thirteen he became a teaching assistant, and by the age of eighteen, a tutor in a local laird's household.

Around 1758 Brown began attending lectures in philosophy and divinity at the University of Edinburgh, and by 1760 he had turned his attention to medicine, joining the Royal Medical Society, the main student society. Brown supported himself during his extensive medical studies through his knowledge of Latin, tutoring students, coaching them through their required oral examinations, and translating theses required for graduation. In 1765 he opened a boarding house, which contributed to his popularity among students. He also married, and the couple eventually had eight children.

Brown acquired a patron in the popular and influential professor, William Cullen (1710–90). Cullen hired Brown as tutor to his children, and it may have been Cullen's intercession that led other members of the medical faculty to give Brown free admission to their lectures. But patronage relationships were a series of delicate balances, which might go awry when the patron and client disagreed over the efforts of the former or the merits of the latter. In 1776 the professorship of Institutes of Medicine was vacant, and Brown claimed that Cullen had promised to support him for it. Cullen seems not so much to have denied the claim as to have refused to take it seriously. The resulting quarrel split the Royal Medical Society into Cullen and Brown supporters, and spilled over into Edinburgh newspapers.

Brown obtained his MD from the University of St Andrews in order to give private lectures in medicine, in which he developed what became known as the Brunonian system, which stated that there was a fundamental life force, which he called the 'exciting power'. This exciting power was located in the nervous system, and was acted upon by the environment in what we would now call a feedback loop. Brown divided all diseases into two categories: 'asthenic', which were caused by insufficient exciting power and had to be treated by strong stimulants, notably opium and alcohol; and 'sthenic', which were caused by an excess of the exciting power, and required mild bloodletting and purging to reduce the stimulation. As one commentator explained it, the exciting power, which sustained life, was like fire in a chimney, requiring both fuel and air to burn. Too little of either and the fire would die down, corresponding to asthenic diseases; but too much of either would lead the fire to burn too brightly and consume all its fuel, corresponding to sthenic diseases. Brown's exciting power can be thought of as an intermediary between eighteenth-century concepts of 'irritability' and nineteenth-century vitalism, which held that living processes could not be reduced to mathematical or physical formulae.

The quarrel with Cullen and the rest of the medical faculty hindered Brown's success in Edinburgh and, in 1786, he and his family moved to London, where he died two years later. After his death, the controversy surrounding Brunonianism died down. His *Elementa Medicina*, first published in

Latin in 1780, was translated into English, French, Italian, and German in the 1790s, and was part of the medical literature informing both *naturphilosophie* and homeopathy in the early nineteenth century.

Bibliography

Primary: 1804. (Brown, William Cullen, ed.) *The Works of Dr. John Brown* (London); 1795. (Beddoes, Thomas, ed.) *The Elements of Medicine: a new edition, revised and corrected with a biographical preface* (London).

Secondary: Bynum, W. F., and Roy Porter, eds., 1988. *Brunonianism in Britain and Europe* (London); Thomson, John, 1859. *An account of the life, lectures, and writings of William Cullen* (Edinburgh); *Oxford DNB*.

Lisa Rosner

BROWN-SÉQUARD, CHARLES-ÉDOUARD   (b. Port Louis, Mauritius, 8 April 1817; d. Paris, France, 1 April 1894), *medicine, physiology, neurology, endrocrinology.*

Brown-Séquard's father, Edward Brown, was a merchant sea captain from Philadelphia who died at sea before his son was born. His mother, Charlotte Séquard, was of French descent. Mauritius had been French property until 1814, when it became British. That fact would have an influence on Brown-Séquard's life: he was raised in a French cultural environment and language, but became a British citizen. In 1838 he and his mother moved to Paris, where he studied medicine and worked in the private laboratory of the physiologist Martin-Magron. In 1846 he wrote his MD thesis (Brown-Séquard, 1846), still using the name Brown—he added his mother's name a few years later. In 1848 he worked at the *Charité* hospital and became secretary of the *Société de Biologie*. When Louis Napoleon became emperor in 1852, Brown-Séquard chose to leave France, probably because of his republican sympathies. Between 1852 and 1878 he lectured, practiced, or experimented in London, Paris, and several cities in the United States, crossing the ocean many times. Considered an expert in epilepsy, he was invited to work at the newly founded National Hospital for the Paralysed and Epileptic in London (1860–63). He was a teacher to John Hughlings Jackson (1835–1911) there, but because he preferred to do more experimental work, he left after a few years. With interruptions, he lectured at Harvard University during the period 1864 to 1866. Brown-Séquard finally settled in Paris in 1878, succeeding Claude Bernard (1813–78) at the Collège de France. He married three times and became a widower as many times, but he had a daughter and a son.

Brown-Séquard is best known for his experimental work with hemisections of the spinal cord. His discovery that pathways for pain sensation cross to the contralateral side after entering the spinal cord opposed the dominant ideas of Charles Bell and François-Achille Longet. Brown-Séquard's name is still attached to the clinical syndrome resulting from such injuries in human beings. These patients suffer from ipsilateral paresis and hypesthesia and contralateral hypalgesia below the level of the injury. He also investigated the function of the vasomotor nerves, an area in which he competed with Claude Bernard (1852). Other fields in which he worked include the function of the adrenal glands, artificially induced hereditary epilepsy, and the effects of testicular extracts. The latter work, although controversial and sensational, initiated research in endocrinology.

From his experimental and clinical work on the spinal cord and subsequent observations of cerebral lesions, Brown-Séquard challenged prevailing theories of circumscribed localizations in the brain (e.g., Broca, Fritsch, Hitzig, and Ferrier). His theory was based on distant action [*action à distance*] and networks [*réseau de cellules anastomosées*], a dynamic concept of nervous system function based on inhibition and excitation [*dynamogénie*]. He ascribed the effect of stimulation or damage to the nervous system to the working of these principles, and he explained changes in the nervous system on the basis of various combinations of these phenomena. For example, inhibition of one part of the nervous system is often accompanied by excitation in another part. He defended his theories on several occasions, e.g., during meetings of the *Société de Biologie*, where he debated with Jean-Martin Charcot. In 1893 Charles Scott Sherrington referred to part of Brown-Séquard's work, stating that he had been able to confirm the principle of inhibition and excitation. In his last years, he caused a sensation by his claims for the rejuvenating effects of testicular extracts.

Bibliography

Primary: 1846. *Recherches et expériences sur la physiologie de la moelle épinière.* MD thesis (Paris); 1860. *Physiology and Pathology of the Central Nervous System* (London).

Secondary: Bonduelle, Michel, 2001. 'Charles-Édouard Brown-Séquard.' *Revue neurologique* 157: 234–238; Koehler, Peter J., 1994. 'Brown-Séquard's Spinal Epilepsy.' *Medical History* 38: 189–203; Aminoff, Michael J., 1993. *Brown-Séquard. A Visionary of Science* (New York); Olmsted, J. M. D., 1953. *Charles-Édouard Brown-Séquard: A Nineteenth-century Neurologist and Endocrinologist* (Baltimore).

Peter Koehler

BROWNE, THOMAS   (b. London, England, 19 November 1605; d. Norwich, England, 19 October 1682), *medicine, literature.*

Browne was the third child and eldest son of Thomas and Anne Browne. His father was a silk merchant in the City of London. Browne was eight years old when his father died. In the following year, his mother married Sir Thomas Dutton, a soldier. The family fortune was not well managed by the executors of his father's will, but there remained sufficient funds to send Browne to Winchester for seven years, and

then on to Oxford where he took his BA (1626) and MA (1629). While at Oxford he studied not only the traditional classic texts required of those reading medicine, but also the newly introduced subjects of anatomy and botany.

In 1630 Browne set out to travel and to complete his medical education. He went first to Montpellier, and in 1632, to Padua. Finally, in 1633, he traveled to Leiden, where he took his MD.

Thomas Browne had an insatiable appetite for facts, and a remarkable ability to recall them. He was also a gifted linguist, speaking, as he said, 'no less than six languages'. He returned to England in 1634. It was at this time that he decided to take stock of his life, his experiences, and his beliefs by writing a personal journal. He wrote, he claimed, for himself alone, with no thought of publication. The book he produced, *Religio Medici*, turned out to be a gem of seventeenth-century prose. A pirated edition of the book was published in 1642, and this stimulated Browne to publish an authentic version in 1643.

By this time Browne was established as a physician in Norwich, having moved there in 1637. In 1641 he married Dorothy, the daughter of Edward Mileham, a local worthy. They had twelve children, seven of whom survived into adult life. They were a devoted family. Edward, the eldest child, became a physician in London and a member of the Royal Society, to whose proceedings Browne also contributed through his correspondence with Edward.

Browne's *Pseudodoxia Epidemica* [Vulgar Errors] was published in 1646. It was a formidable work covering the causes of errors in varying fields of knowledge. It was widely read and admired, and was reprinted in his lifetime. Today it gives us insight into Browne's erudition and imagination, and pleasure from his writing; but it is otherwise not an easy read.

After the publication of *Vulgar Errors*, Browne did not publish again for ten years. Then in 1658, following the discovery of Saxon burial urns near Walsingham in Norfolk, he was moved to do so. *Hydriotaphia—Urn-Burial* is a meditation on death and the Christian belief in immortality. It is a suitable subject for the rich music of Browne's prose, and he makes good use of it. The book was published together with another shorter piece, *The Garden of Cyrus*. This is a strange collection of speculations on the subject of patterns to be found in nature. It is inventive, almost playful at times, but most modern readers are likely to remain bemused.

There were no further major publications during Browne's lifetime. *Christian Morals* was published posthumously, as was *A Letter to a Friend*, although the latter was written some ten years before his death. *Letter* gives us a rare glimpse of Browne as a concerned physician caring for a young man dying from tuberculosis.

Browne became a celebrated national figure, and was knighted by Charles II on his visit to Norwich in 1671. He continued in active medical practice until he died in 1682 at age seventy-seven. The continuing affection in which

Browne is held depends in part on a sense of companionship with an erudite, warm-hearted country doctor who transcends time and place.

Bibliography

Primary: 1964. (Keynes, Geoffrey, ed.) *The Works of Sir Thomas Browne* (London).

Secondary: Bennett, Joan, 1962. *Sir Thomas Browne* (Cambridge); *Oxford DNB*.

Ian Tait

BRUCE, DAVID   (b. Melbourne, Australia, 29 May 1855; d. London, England, 27 November 1931), *tropical medicine, bacteriology, parasitology.*

Bruce was the only son of David Bruce, an engineer from Edinburgh, Scotland, and Jane Hamilton. His family moved back to his mother's hometown of Sterling, Scotland, when Bruce was five. He attended Sterling High School and, after a few years in business, entered the University of Edinburgh (1876) with the intention of studying zoology. He eventually chose medicine. Bruce graduated MB CM (1881) and went to work for Herbert Stanley Stone at Reigate, Surrey, where he met Mary Elizabeth Sisson Steel (1849–1931), the daughter of Stone's predecessor in the practice. They married in 1883. Mary traveled with Bruce, and participated in his research. In their long and fruitful partnership in science, Mary coauthored thirty of the more than 172 articles contributed by Bruce.

Bruce joined the Army Medical Service, graduating top of his class from the Army Medical School at Netley (1883). He was posted to Malta in 1884, and plunged into research on the mysterious fever prevalent among the British troops there. After conducting postmortem examinations, Bruce successfully isolated and cultivated the suspect microorganism from the spleens of the victims. He went on to prove, by experimenting on monkeys, that this microorganism, now known as *Brucella melitensis*, was the cause of Malta fever. While on leave (1888), Bruce and his wife worked in Robert Koch's laboratory in Berlin. Bruce returned to England and accepted an assistant professorship of pathology at Netley (1889).

In 1894 Bruce was posted to Pietermaritzburg, South Africa, to investigate a disease called 'nagana', which was decimating the cattle in Zululand. The disease had been associated with the tsetse fly, but its exact cause and nature were unknown. In the blood of the affected animals, Bruce discovered a parasite which he initially thought to be a filaria, but later decided was a trypanosome—*Trypanosoma brucei*. Bruce described the life history of the tsetse fly and established, by conducting experiments on dogs and horses, that the parasite was transmitted to domestic animals through the bite of the fly. He also suspected that some wild game were infected with the parasite, although he could not verify his conjecture.

Back in England, Bruce was appointed medical advisor to the Army Medical Services Department (1901). He supervised the sleeping sickness commission of the Royal Society, and went to Uganda to investigate the disease (1903). Joseph E. Dutton (1874–1905) had discovered a microorganism in the blood of a fever patient which he named *Trypanosoma gambiense* (1902). Aldo Castellani, moreover, had observed trypanosomes in the cerebrospinal fluid of some sleeping sickness patients, although he initially dismissed its relevance to the disease. After a fraught period of research, the commission concluded that sleeping sickness was caused by *T. gambiense* transmitted by tsetse flies. Over the next decade, Bruce continued to work on the natural history of trypanosomes, especially his hypothesis that some domestic and wild animals were their reservoir.

When World War I broke out, Bruce was appointed Commandant of the Royal Army Medical College at Millbank. He presided over the pathological committee of the War Office, and headed a commission investigating tetanus and trench fever. The commission supported anti-typhoid inoculation of the troops. Bruce also recommended the immediate injection of tetanus antiserum for wounded soldiers. Bruce was elected FRS (1899), knighted (1908), and created KCB (1918). He served as president of the Royal Society of Tropical Medicine and Hygiene (1917–1919), and as president of the British Association for the Advancement of Science (1924). Bruce died a few days after the death of his wife, during Lady Bruce's funeral.

Bibliography

Primary: 1887. 'Note on the discovery of the microorganism in Malta Fever.' *Practitioner* 39: 161–170; 1888. 'The Micrococcus of Malta Fever.' *Practitioner* 40: 241–249; 1895. *Preliminary Report on the Tsetse Fly Disease or Nagana in Zululand* (Durban).

Secondary: Grogono, Basil J. S., 1995. 'Sir David and Lady Bruce.' *Journal of Medical Biography* 3: 79–83, 125–132; *DSB*; *Oxford DNB*.

Shang-Jen Li

BRÜCKE, ERNST WILHELM VON   (b. Berlin, Germany, 6 September 1819; d. Vienna, Austria, 7 January 1892), *physiology.*

Brücke, son of the portrait painter Johann Gottfried Brücke, studied medicine in Heidelberg and Berlin, where he completed his dissertation (1842) under the direction of the anatomist and physiologist Johannes Müller. In 1843 Brücke became Müller's assistant, a position held previously by Theodor Schwann and Jacob Henle. Brücke's Habilitation was accepted in 1844, and he began teaching as a Privatdozent at the Berlin medical faculty. The subject of his lectures was physiology.

Along with his close friends Hermann Helmholtz, Emil Du Bois-Reymond, and Carl Ludwig, Brücke belonged to a group of young scientists for whom physics and chemistry

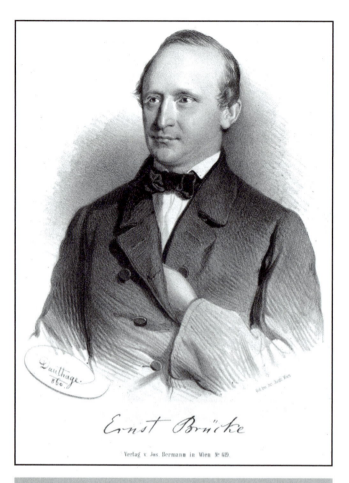

Ernst Wilhelm von Brücke. Lithograph by A. Dauthage, 1860. Iconographic Collection, Wellcome Library, London.

were the unshakeable models for the investigation of life. 'Brücke and I, we have sworn to each other to demonstrate the basic truth that no other forces operate in living organisms except physicochemical ones,' wrote Du Bois-Reymond in an 1842 letter to Eduard Hallmann. The two 'organic physicists' saw themselves as the avant-garde of a new experimental physiology that they felt obligated to defend against the conservatives—the faculty of the Berlin medical school, whom they perceived as vitalistic and hostile to experimentation.

Brücke's early research work in particular shows how productive the physicalistic program was. Between 1841 and 1848 he published nearly twenty journal articles. Most of them appeared in two leading journals of that time—Müller's *Archiv für Anatomie, Physiologie und wissenschaftliche Medicin* and Poggendorff's *Annalen der Physik und Chemie*. Brücke also shared his friends' enthusiasm for esthetics and worked as a teacher of anatomy at the Berlin Academy of Fine Arts (1846–48), a position that Helmholtz and Du Bois-Reymond filled after him.

During the years under Müller, the optical apparatus of the eye was at the center of Brücke's investigations. He pub-

lished on vitreous bodies (1843–45), studied the role of the retina's rods and cones (1844), and described the fibers of the ciliary muscle (1846). In order to investigate the absorption of light waves through the eye's optical media (1845–46), Brücke inventively used the new photographic method that had been introduced by the Paris painter and physicist Louis Jacques Mandé Daguerre a few years earlier. Continuing Müller's research on *Augenleuchten* [luminosity of the eye], Brücke demonstrated (1845–47) that the phenomenon is caused by reflections of light in the background of the eye—the so-called *tapetum lucidum*, a thin layer behind the retina. In 1847 he finished his *Anatomische Beschreibung des menschlichen Augapfels*. That small monograph, dedicated to Müller and published by the famous Berlin publisher of science and literature, Georg Reimer, became a standard work for contemporary ophthalmologists. Altogether, Brücke's optical works laid the foundation for the invention of the eye mirror ophthalmoscope, constructed by Helmholtz in 1851. Brücke himself summarized that fascinating story of discovery four decades later, in a book entitled *Das Augenleuchten und die Erfindung des Augenspiegels* (1893).

In 1848, on the recommendation of Johannes Müller and Alexander von Humboldt, Brücke became a professor of physiology and pathology at Königsberg University. In a primitive laboratory he studied *Mimosa pudica* and described the hydrostatic power driving the plant's movements. A year later Brücke received a call to Vienna, where he assumed the chair of physiology and microscopical anatomy at the Josephinum, an academy where military physicians received their training. Since no space for research and teaching existed there, Brücke was allowed to convert the Josephinum's library into a physiological laboratory and to use an old kitchen as a chemical laboratory. With support from the Austrian Ministry of Education, scientific instruments were bought and technical devices were developed to run a mechanical workshop.

In 1854, Brücke's physiological institute moved into the building of an abandoned gun factory. The Josephinum's laboratory was taken over by Carl Ludwig, who moved from Zurich to Vienna in 1855. During the next ten years the two friends and colleagues worked in a fruitful scientific collaboration, primarily in the fields of cardiovascular physiology and physiological chemistry. In 1865 Ludwig moved to Leipzig, where he established a new institute building for experimental physiology—the biggest research institute of its kind at that time. Brücke's like-minded ambitions failed, however. In contrast to Leipzig or Berlin, where Du Bois-Reymond opened a new physiological institute in 1877, the laboratory working conditions in Vienna remained provisional for a long time. Only in 1885 was Brücke's institute connected to the city's gas, water, and electricity supply. For nearly half a century, the physiological institute of the Vienna medical faculty remained housed in a converted gun factory.

Brücke's more than 150 publications contributed to nearly every basic field in physiology. He worked on the electrophysiology of nerves and muscles; the lymphatic system; the coagulation of blood; the resorption of fat, carbohydrates and proteins in the digestive tract; and many other themes. Most of his studies combined anatomical, microscopical, physical, and chemical methods. His studies on pepsin and peptic digestion (1859–61) became classics in the history of biochemistry and enzyme research. In his two-volume *Vorlesungen über Physiologie,* published in 1873–74, Brücke demonstrated to his students the great diversity of research in physiology.

Brücke also pioneered in vocal physiology and linguistics. He studied the mechanism of speech and the structure of language by analyzing the multiple parts of the mouth, the larynx, and the pharynx, and he demonstrated how each structure played its role in phonation. In his *Grundzüge der Physiologie und Systematik der Sprachlaute* (1856–76), Brücke developed an artificial sign language for linguists and teachers of deaf-mutes. His monograph *Die physiologischen Grundlagen der neuhochdeutschen Verskunst* (1871) is a speech analysis of poetry writing. Brücke's investigations on language structure and vocal articulation are prime examples of a very basic idea in nineteenth-century physiology, namely, that all various forms of esthetic or artistic expression can be analyzed by scientific methods. Together with Helmholtz, who became famous with his fundamental investigations of musical acoustics, Brücke was the major representative of that scientific reductionism.

Physiology and art, and the interrelationships between the two, formed an integral part of Brücke's work and drove his research interests throughout his life. As with his linguistic studies on poetry, he analyzed works of visual art in terms of optics and color sensation. Following in his father's footsteps, Brücke himself practiced painting during yearly journeys to Italy. In his book *Über Ergänzungsfarben und Kontrastfarben* (1865), he developed a color theory for painters, colorists, and artisans.

In the 1860s Brücke became a member of the directory board of the newly established Vienna *Kunstgewerbemuseum.* In his role as the museum's adviser, he published *Die Physiologie der Farben für die Zwecke der Kunstgewerbe.* It deals with questions of taste, style, and aesthetic values and their translation into decorative artifacts. The book went through two editions (1866, 1887) and was translated into French and English. Just as successful on the international market was his book on the esthetics of the human body, *Schönheit und Fehler der menschlichen Gestalt* (1891, 1893, 1905), which was written for artists and artistically inclined amateurs. Brücke and most of his generation, including his friends Helmholtz and Du Bois-Reymond, enthusiastically praised ideal art and did not recognize the new artist movements of his time and their anti-idealistic sense of beauty, for which Vienna became a center at the turn of the twentieth century.

Bibliography

Primary: 1847. *Anatomische Beschreibung des menschlichen Augapfels* (Berlin); 1873–74. *Vorlesungen über Physiologie* 2 vols. (Vienna); 1891. *Schönheit und Fehler der menschlichen Gestalt* (Vienna); 1978. (Brücke, Hans, ed.) *Ernst Wilhelm von Brücke— Briefe an Emil Du Bois-Reymond* (Graz).

Secondary: Schickore, Jutta, 2000. 'Locating Rods and Cones: Microscopic Investigations of the Retina in Mid-Nineteenth-Century Berlin and Würzburg.' *Science in Context* 13(1): 137–152; Lenoir, Timothy, 1997. 'The Politics of Vision: Optics, Painting, and Ideology in Germany, 1845–95' in Lenoir, Timothy, ed., *Instituting Science. The Cultural Production of Scientific Disciplines* (Stanford) pp.131–178; Lesky, Erna, 1965. *Die Wiener Medizinische Schule im 19. Jahrhundert* (Graz); *DSB.*

Sven Dierig

BRUNFELS, OTTO

BRUNFELS, OTTO (b. Mainz, Germany, *c.* 1489; d. Berne, Switzerland, 23/25 November 1534), *botany, medicine.*

Brunfels was the son of the cooper Johann Brunfels, but nothing is known about his mother. Otto grew up in Mainz, where he earned an MA at the university in 1508 or 1509, and then entered the Carthusian order. Between 1519 and 1521, he was a member of the Carthusian monastery in Strasbourg, where he came into contact with humanists and later leaders in the Reformation, such as Caspar Hedio and Martin Bucer.

After he fled from the monastery in the summer of 1521, Brunfels was initially active as a priest in the service of Ulrich von Hutten in Steinau, near Steinheim. He was forced to leave that position in April 1522, at the instigation of the Carthusian monastery in Strasbourg. On his way to Switzerland, he remained for a time as an ordained preacher in Neuenburg (Breisgau), where he spoke out clearly in support of the new teachings of the Reformation. In March 1524, Brunfels was granted the right of burgher in the now Protestant city of Strasbourg, where he married Dorothea Heiligenhensin in July 1524. She would later play an important role in the posthumous publication of his manuscripts. In 1528 he was appointed to teach at the former Carmelite School in Strasbourg, and around 1532–33 he received a doctorate in medicine from the University of Basel. At the end of 1533, Brunfels moved to the city of Berne to become municipal physician. He died there in 1534.

Brunfels left a large number of theological, pedagogical, botanical, medical, and pharmaceutical writings. However, it was as a botanist that he achieved fame. With his *Herbarum vivae eicones ad naturae imitationem,* edited in three volumes, and his two-volume *Contrafayt Kreüterbuoch,* all published after 1530 and in part posthumously, Brunfels became—along with Hieronymus Bock and Leonhart Fuchs—one of the three 'German fathers of botany'. In his *Herbarum vivae eicones,* Brunfels described more than 230 plants, most of which could be found in the vicinity of the city of Strasbourg. His descriptions emphasized the therapeutic applications of the various plants, following the classical authorities Dioscorides, Pliny, and Galen, as well as Arab and several contemporary Italian authors.

Brunfels' *Kreüterbuoch* is a German version of the *Herbarum vivae eicones*. Almost all its illustrations were taken from the *Herbarum*, and another fifty were added. The German text was made tighter and more concisely structured than the original Latin *Herbarum* text. It contained brief information on nomenclature, the appearance of the plant, its typical locations, the season when the plant could be found, and its medical utility. But the *Herbarum vivae eicones* and the *Kreüterbuoch* did not become famous because of their text; rather, their fame was due to their accurate, true-to-nature illustrations. The woodcuts by the artist Hans Weiditz represented the plants in a degree of exact reproduction unparalleled at the time and became a standard of excellence for subsequent works in botany.

Brunfels' other numerous writings were less influential. He wrote more than twenty-five treatises on theology and pedagogy, translated ancient medical authors, and edited contemporary works on practical medicine (such as Lorenz Fries's *Spiegel der Artzney*) and anatomy (Alessandro Benedetti's *De historia corporis humani*). In his posthumously published *Reformation der Apotecken*, Brunfels developed a set of regulations for pharmacists for the city of Bern that were based on the Strasbourg model, and he presented one of the first dispensatories in Switzerland.

Bibliography

Primary: 1530–36. *Herbarum vivae eicones ad naturae imitationem, summa cum diligentia & artificio effigiatae, una cum effectibus earundem, in gratiam veteris illius, & iamiam renascentis herbariae medicinae* . . . 3 vols. (Strasbourg); 1532–37. *Contrafayt Kreuterbuch: Nach rechter vollkommener art u. Beschreibungen der alten . . . ärtzt, vormals in teutscher sprachnye gesehen* . . . 2 vols. (Strasbourg); 1536. *Reformation der Apotecken* (Strasbourg).

Secondary: Mittelheiser, Marguerite, 1985. *Les Kreuterbücher [Kräuterbücher] d' Otto Brunfels* (Strasbourg); Dilg, Peter, 1979. 'Die "Reformation der Apotecken" (1536) des Berner Stadtarztes Otto Brunfels.' *Gesnerus* 36: 181–205; Baader, Gerhard, 1978. 'Mittelalter und Neuzeit im Werk von Otto Brunfels.' *Medizinhistorisches Journal* 13: 186–203; DSB.

Jürgen Helm and Karin Stukenbrock

BRUNTON, THOMAS LAUDER (b. Hiltonshill, Roxburghshire, Scotland, 14 March 1844; d. London, England, 16 September 1916), *medicine, pharmacology*.

Brunton, the third son of James Brunton and his second wife, Agnes, was educated privately before entering the University of Edinburgh, where he was influenced by James Carmichael and graduated MB CM. After graduation he served as a house physician at Edinburgh Infirmary (1866–67), and received his BSc and MD (1868) and DSc (1870).

Brunton went to study pharmacology in Vienna with Ernst Brücke (1819–1892), and in Berlin with Meyer. He then studied physiological chemistry with Willy Kuhne (1837–1900) in Amsterdam, before working in the physiology laboratory of Carl Ludwig in Leipzig.

After returning to London in 1870, Brunton was appointed lecturer in materia medica and pharmacology at the Middlesex Hospital (1870–71), and in 1871 took up the same post at St Bartholomew's Hospital, London. At St Bartholomew's he became a respected lecturer, and gradually moved up the professional hierarchy, serving as casualty physician (1871–75), assistant physician (1875–97), and physician (1897–1904), receiving a baronetcy in 1900.

It was his work in physiology and pharmacology that established his reputation. Brunton was actively involved in vivisection and physiological research, with his early interest in the problems of digestion, secretion, and cardiac action shaping his work. His diagnostic approach owed much to an interpretation of symptoms based on disordered physiology, and was often viewed with skepticism. He contributed to the *Handbook for the Physiological Laboratory* (1873) with John Scott Burdon Sanderson (1828–1905), and was a founder of the Physiological Society. Brunton publicly defended vivisection, arguing that many of the benefits produced by medicine had been derived by animal experimentation.

Despite his early contribution to physiology, it was his pharmacological research that increasingly absorbed Brunton's professional energies. His MD had concentrated on the beneficial effects of digitalis on the stressed heart, and his work on the physiology and therapy of cardiovascular disease, the diuretic effects of mercury, and the action of enzymes contributed to the development of experimental pharmacology. For Brunton, pharmacology had to be closely linked to physiology, and in his *Textbook of Pharmacology, Therapeutics and Materia Medica* (1885), he emphasized the physiological actions of pure drugs. The work established his reputation, and his *Textbook* was the first to consider pharmacology a science.

Brunton believed in the need for rational therapeutics based on pharmacological research, and wanted to establish therapeutics as a science, a view he propounded in his lectures to the RCP. It was an approach reflected in his pioneering work on angina, and the action of amyl nitrite in relieving the symptoms. Brunton had discovered that bloodletting relieved his patient's angina, and reasoned that dilation of the blood vessels would do the same. After experiments on himself, he tried amyl nitrite on angina patients with success, introducing a new class of remedies—the vasodilators—into medicine.

However, Brunton also advocated nonmedical methods. He wrote widely on the importance of environment, exercise, rest, and massage, and advocated schemes in favor of national health, school hygiene, and military training, helping to found the National League for Physical Education and Improvement (1906).

Brunton's other published work covered a wide range of areas, from the treatment and bacteriology of cholera, through death in chloroform anesthesia, to the benefits of artificial respiration and the possibility of blood transfusion. Throughout, he advocated extensive research and experimentation, placing greater emphasis on this than practical hospital work, often leading him to miss clinical signs in patients.

Brunton was a scientific practitioner who wanted to use the laboratory to enhance treatment and diagnosis. At St Bartholomew's, he carried out numerous experiments in a makeshift laboratory he had established in the hospital's scullery. He felt that too much research was done imperfectly in the wards, and argued that research laboratories were essential to the proper functioning of a medical school. His published work was influential in linking the practice of medicine with the sciences upon which it was based, but it was his contribution to establishing pharmacology as a science that had the most impact.

Bibliography

Primary: 1885. *Textbook of Pharmacology, Therapeutics and Materia Medica* (London); 1907–1911. *Collected Papers on Circulation and Respiration* (London); 1910. *On the Physiological Basis of Physical Education* (London); 1914. *Therapeutics of the Circulation* (London).

Secondary: Sharpey-Schafer, E., 1927. *History of the Physiological Society* (London); *DSB*; *Oxford DNB*.

Keir Waddington

BRYCE, LUCY MEREDITH

BRYCE, LUCY MEREDITH (b. Lindfield, New South Wales, Australia, 12 June 1897; d. Melbourne, Australia, 30 July 1968), *hematology.*

Bryce was the eldest child of Robert Bryce, merchant and importer, and his wife Margaret Annie Lucy, née Doak, of Sydney. She was educated at Melbourne Church of England Girls' Grammar School and the University of Melbourne, where she took out a science degree in 1918. She went on to graduate MB BS in the stellar class of 1922 that included (Sir) Macfarlane Burnet, (Sir) Rupert Willis, (Dame) Kate Campbell, and (Dame) Jean Macnamara

Bryce was always interested in medical research, and after graduation she became one of the first staff members at the Walter and Eliza Hall Institute of Medical Research. There she began to work with a remarkable South Australian nurse, Mrs Fanny Eleanor Williams, who had worked in the army pathology laboratory on the Greek island of Lemnos during World War I—first under William Upjohn and later under Charles Martin, head of the Lister Institute in London. There Williams saw first-hand what blood transfusions could do. She traveled to London with Martin, where he trained her in methods of bacteriological investigation, and then returned to France with him and won the Royal Red Cross for her work in his pathology department. After the war, Williams became one of the inaugural staff at the Hall Institute, where she remained until she retired in 1957.

Fanny Williams was described as 'the channel through which serological techniques developed in Melbourne', and she instructed Lucy Bryce in the techniques of antigen typing and bacteriological analysis. In 1925–26 Bryce extended her training with a research post at the Lister Institute in London, and in 1928 she was appointed as the first bacteriologist and clinical pathologist at the (Royal) Melbourne Hospital. In 1934 she entered private practice as a clinical pathologist, but she continued part-time research at the Hall Institute (1934–46) and at the Commonwealth Serum Laboratories (1939–44), and was honorary director of pathology at the Queen Victoria Hospital. During World War II she was visiting specialist with the rank of major at the 115th Australian General Hospital in Heidelberg.

Lucy Bryce's first year as pathologist at the Melbourne Hospital saw her chasing compatible blood donors among patients' relatives and workmates in 'panic parties' for emergency transfusions. Early in 1929 the medical superintendent, Eric Cooper, suggested she set up a blood transfusion service similar to the one recently established by the Red Cross in London. That was to be her defining life's work. The Victorian Division of the Australian Red Cross agreed to organize a panel of blood donors who were prepared to attend hospitals when required, with Bryce as honorary director carrying out the serology and laboratory testing, as well as the medical care of the donors. Later she introduced blood storage techniques developed during the Spanish Civil War. Her leadership of the Red Cross Blood Transfusion Service, as it became known, was meticulous and inspirational.

Lucy Bryce was author or coauthor of forty-three scientific articles in bacteriology and hematology, but she will be remembered most for her pioneering work with Rachel Jakobowicz on blood typing and the Rhesus (Rh) factor, and for their joint work with Dame Kate Campbell on hemolytic disease in the newborn. Bryce also published a history of the transfusion service up to 1959, entitled *An Abiding Gladness* (1965). At the time of her death, she was working on a book about her travels in southeast Europe in the 1920s.

She retired as honorary director of the blood transfusion service in 1954 but, despite failing health following a stroke, continued as chairman of the transfusion committee until 1966. She had been appointed CBE in 1951. Bryce died on 30 July 1968 and was cremated.

Bibliography

Primary: 1965. *An Abiding Gladness: The Background of Contemporary Blood Transfusion During the Years 1929–1959 in the Victorian Division of the Australian Red Cross Society* (Melbourne).

Secondary: Klugman, Matthew, 2004. *Blood Matters: A Social History of the Victorian Red Cross Blood Transfusion Service* (Melbourne); *AuDB*.

Janet McCalman

BUCHAN, WILLIAM (b. Ancrum, Roxburghshire, Scotland, c. 1728; d. London, England, 25 February 1805), *medicine, popular medicine.*

Buchan, son of a small estate owner and farmer, was educated at Jedburgh grammar school and Edinburgh University, transferring his studies from theology to medicine. In this progressive environment where he also studied botany, mathematics, and astronomy, he was taught by John Rutherford (1695–1779), Robert Whytt (1714–66), the two Alexander Monros (*primus*, 1697–1767, and *secundus*, 1733–1817), and William Cullen (1710–90). Leaving Edinburgh about 1758, Buchan settled in Yorkshire where he became medical officer to a new branch of the Foundling Hospital at Ackworth (1759), and published his MD thesis, *De infantum vita conservanda* (1761). He married Elizabeth Peter (1760), and moved to practice medicine in Sheffield (1762) before returning to Edinburgh (1766). William and Elizabeth had a daughter and two sons, one of whom, Alexander Peter Buchan, became a physician.

Elizabeth was a distant relative of Sir John Pringle to whom Buchan dedicated the second and subsequent editions of his *Domestic Medicine; or, The Family Physician* (1769), an early work in this genre in English, and the most enduringly popular. Embracing a democratic, Enlightenment medical populism that saw accessible knowledge and skill as essential for human progress, *Domestic Medicine* expounded to the lay reader a philosophy of health pursued through reason, temperance, hygiene, and obedience to Nature's laws. Although the first edition was said to have been heavily edited (or rewritten) by the intellectual Edinburgh printer, William Smellie (1740–95), whose imprint it bears, there were at least 142 revised or reprinted English language editions between 1769 (Edinburgh) and 1871 (Philadelphia). There were also European and Scandinavian editions, and from Catherine the Great of Russia, Buchan received a gold medal. *Domestic Medicine* was particularly popular in the United States, where it was 'Americanized' to the diseases and climate of that continent. The third English edition (1774) included chapters on venereal disease, sensory disorders, hygiene, infectious and occupational diseases, childcare, and an index of medicines. Although in later years, Buchan bitterly complained of plagiarism, he was reputed to have long since sold the copyright for £700. *Domestic Medicine* simply moved with the times, the author's name acting as a marketing brand.

Domestic Medicine appealed to the self-consciously improving middle classes (the price being six shillings) with its emphasis on rational treatment and cleanliness, and the dismissal of superstition, *Dreckapotheke*, quackery, and faith healing. It was an extraordinarily secular work. In the second edition, for example, all references to Jesuit's bark were changed to Peruvian bark. The inclusion of a section on children's ailments, almost certainly inspired by Buchan's experience at Ackworth, exemplified the growing awareness of childhood as a distinct developmental period, as well as a consciousness that excessive infant mortality was remediable. Despite the book's title and the author's recognition that medical knowledge was widely diffused, he attempted to set reasonable boundaries between orthodox medicine and lay treatment, or selfhealing. In doing this, he was accepted in both camps.

Buchan was elected FRCPEd (1772). On the death of his friend, John Gregory (1773), professor of the Institutes of Medicine, he applied unsuccessfully for the position, which went to Gregory's son, James (1778). Buchan moved to London the same year, where he practiced medicine for the rest of his life, most notably at the Chapter Coffee House near St Paul's Cathedral, the meeting place for the city's *literati*. In his commitment to render 'Medicine more open to mankind' (Buchan, 1774, p. xxi), he published *Observations Concerning the Prevention and Cure of the Venereal Disease* (1796), in which he lamented the fact that some people still believed the pox could be cured by transmitting it to someone else. Other books in the genre included *On the Offices and Duties of a Mother* (1800), and *Advice to Mothers* (1803). None achieved the popularity of *Domestic Medicine*.

Although little is known of Buchan's own domestic life, colleagues described him as a man of athletic build, convivial and compassionate. He died at his son's house, and was buried in Westminster Abbey.

Bibliography

Primary: 1769. *Domestic Medicine; or, The Family Physician* (Edinburgh) [2nd edn., 1772, 3rd edn., 1774]; 1796. *Observations Concerning the Prevention and Cure of the Venereal Diseases* (London); 1803. *Advice to Mothers on the Subject of Their Own Health; and on the Means of Promoting the Health, Strength, and Beauty of their Offspring* (London).

Secondary: Rosenberg, Charles E., 1983. 'Medical text and social context: explaining William Buchan's Domestic Medicine.' *Bulletin of the History of Medicine* 57: 22–42; Blake, John B., 1977. 'From Buchan to Fishbein: The Literature of Domestic Medicine' in Risse, Guenter B., Ronald L. Numbers, and Judith Walzer Leavitt, eds., *Medicine Without Doctors: Home Health Care in American History* (New York); Lawrence, C. J., 1975. 'William Buchan: Medicine Laid Open.' *Medical History* 19: 20–35; *Oxford DNB*.

Carole Reeves

BUCK, PETER HENRY (aka TE RANGI HIROA) (b. Urenui, New Zealand, 1877?; d. Honolulu, Hawaii, 1 December 1951), *Maori medicine, public health administration, anthropology.*

Buck was the son of a Maori mother and William Henry Buck, an Irish-born settler. That mixed ancestry allowed Buck to move comfortably among both European and indigenous New Zealanders. In 1904 he was the first Maori to graduate in medicine from the Otago Medical School, five years after Maui Pomare completed his studies at the American Missionary Medical College in Chicago. (In 1949 Buck commented that Pomare had been his role model: 'Resplendent in the top hat, frock coat, and striped trousers that characterized the profession in those days, he visited Wirepa and me in Dunedin and cheered us on the way to acquire similar symbols of success.')

From 1905 to 1909 Buck worked alongside Pomare as medical officer to the Maori in the recently established Department of Public Health, where they fought to improve basic sanitary and infant welfare practices, and began to collect Maori health statistics. Buck was also responsible for designing a model pah (settlement) and hygiene exhibit for the 1907 New Zealand International Exhibition of Arts and Industries. The two men were instrumental in convincing government to pass the Tohunga Suppression Act of 1907, which outlawed traditional native healers. In 1909, however, Buck was persuaded to resign his post and enter parliament as one of four statutory Maori MPs.

Despite that change of career, he remained committed to health. His 1910 MD thesis—'Medicine Amongst the Maoris, in Ancient and Modern Times'—sought to educate his fellow doctors in Maori concepts of disease. The text contained three distinct parts: ancient Maori medicine, the impact of civilization, and the contemporary condition of the race. Three years later he was active in treating an outbreak of smallpox among North Island Maori. During World War I Buck served as medical officer with the Maori contingent at Gallipoli and in Europe. There he began the study of physical anthropology, measuring Maori troops and modeling his subsequent report on that of the British Association on Anthropomorphic Investigation (1919).

In 1919 Buck returned to the restructured Department of Public Health as Director of the Division of Maori Hygiene. His efforts to revive the prewar Maori councils that had been charged with enforcing sanitary rules and observances were largely frustrated by lack of staffing and funds. With the blessing of the Director General of Health, he devoted ever more of his time to anthropology and hygiene, which he saw as essential for 'the proper understanding and betterment of Native Races'. One example of that approach was his article on pre-European Maori diet in the *New Zealand Dental Journal* (1925), linking the adoption of European foods to the deterioration in Maori dental health.

In 1927, tired of working late to pursue his anthropological interests and convinced that others could undertake his health work 'equally well or better', Buck resigned to become an ethnologist at the Bishop Museum in Hawaii. Within a decade he had risen to become the Museum's director, a role he retained until his retirement. Buck was knighted in 1946 for services to science and literature, a designation that perhaps undervalued his contribution to Maori health.

In *The Coming of the Maori* (1949), Buck argued that by 1930 the Maori no longer needed 'a special ambassador of their own blood' in order to understand health matters.

Subsequent events proved him wrong, though Buck's part in helping to reverse the Maori population decline after 1900 ensured that he would continue to be acknowledged as a role model for Maori health professionals.

Bibliography

Primary: Hiroa, Te Rangi, 1922–23. 'Maori Somatology: Racial Averages.' *Journal of the Polynesian Society* 31: 37–44, 145–153, 159–170, 32: 21–28, 189–199; 1925. 'The Pre-European Diet of the Maori.' *New Zealand Dental Journal* 20: 203–217.

Secondary: Dow, D. A., 1999. *Maori Health & Government Policy 1840–1930* (Wellington); Condliffe, J. B., 1971. *Te Rangi Hiroa: The Life of Sir Peter Buck* (Christchurch).

Derek A. Dow

BUDD, WILLIAM (b. North Tawton, Devonshire, England, 14 September 1811; d. Walton-in-Gordano, Somerset, England, 9 January 1880), *medicine, epidemiology.*

Budd was the fifth in a family of ten children born to Samuel Budd, a surgeon, and Catherine Wreford. Of the six sons who studied medicine, the best known are William and George Budd (1808–82). William's medical education (1828–38) included London, Paris, and Edinburgh, from where he graduated with a gold medal, although he was unimpressed with the teaching compared with Paris. During three visits to Paris (1829, 1833–34, 1836), he studied under Pierre Bretonneau (1778–1826) and Pierre Louis (1787–1872), who both worked on continued fever which Louis named typhoid fever (1829). In Paris that year, Budd suffered a severe attack of the fever.

Practicing in North Tawton (population 1,300), he observed a typhoid epidemic (1839) and concluded that the disease was contagious, being transmitted via intestinal discharges. Budd later argued for specificity, as in the smallpox model. In contrast, the anticontagionist view, disseminated by Charles Murchison (1830–79), held that it emanated from putrefying organic material or water-borne organic impurities. In Budd's view, sewage contamination of water might propagate typhoid, but only when the sewage contained the specific typhoid poison. He suffered a further bout of the infection (1840) just as he began service with the Seaman's Hospital Society aboard HMS Dreadnought at Greenwich, London.

After convalescence, he settled into practice in Bristol (1841), and was appointed physician to St Peter's Hospital, an English Poor Law institution (1842). By 1847 he was physician to the Bristol Royal Infirmary, and in April of that year married Caroline Mary Hilton. They had six daughters and three sons; the youngest, George Turnavine Budd, becoming a doctor in Plymouth, Devon. Budd taught medicine at Bristol Medical School (1845–55) and was president (1855–56) of Bristol's branch of the Provincial Medical and Surgical Association (later the British Medical Association).

Budd's commitment to the prevention of epidemic disease was manifest in his friendship with David Davies, Bristol's first medical officer of health; in his seat on the board of the Bristol Waterworks Company; and in his evidence presented to the Health of Towns Commission (1845), which showed that Bristol had England's third highest mortality rate after Liverpool and Manchester. He became an advocate of disinfection (using chloride of lime and perchloride of iron), used in the Bristol cholera epidemics of 1849 (1,979 deaths), 1854 (430 deaths), and 1866 (twenty-nine deaths). His pamphlet on the particulate nature of cholera (1849) was published almost simultaneously with John Snow's theory of an infectious cholera agent passing from the intestines into the public water supply, although Snow was more interested in transmission patterns than the role of contagious agents (Snow, 1849).

Budd's credibility was undermined when he and other Bristol doctors claimed the cholera poison to be a fungus, a notion soon disproved, making him forever cautious about the nature of infectious agents. During the third cholera epidemic, Budd spoke of the 'enormous multiplication which these poisons undergo in the living body'. It was, he suggested, 'this multiplication and the disturbances attaching to it that . . . constitutes the disease and destroys life' (Budd, 1866). Unlike William Farr, and to some extent Snow, Budd was not a statistical epidemiologist, although his contribution was recognized in his election as FRS (1871). He also differed from many in that he was interested in animal epidemic diseases, considering them models for the study of contagious epidemics in humans. His belief that animal epidemics could be halted by slaughter of infected herds was dubbed by the *Times* newspaper as 'the Pole-axe Theory of Dr Budd'.

Many of Budd's articles were drafted long before publication, and his major work on typhoid (1873) was largely based on previously published papers. In it can be seen evidence of his skills as a draftsman and photographer. Described by contemporaries as vivacious, eloquent, imaginative, and genial, of a good height with a strong-looking robust body, Budd was rendered hemiplegic by a stroke in 1873. He died in the same year that Carl Joseph Eberth (1835–1926) described a bacillus he had found in the intestinal lesions of typhoid fever patients.

Bibliography

Primary: 1839. *On the Causes of Fevers* [1984. Smith, Dale C., ed. (Baltimore)]; 1849. *Malignant Cholera: Its Mode of Propagation, and Its Prevention* (London); 1856. 'On intestinal fever: its mode of propagation.' *Lancet* ii: 694–695; 1863. 'Variola ovina, sheep's small-pox: or the laws of contagious epidemics illustrated by an experimental type.' *British Medical Journal* ii: 141–150; 1866. *Memoranda on Asiatic Cholera: Its Mode of Spreading, and its Prevention*, 2nd edn. (Bristol); 1873. *Typhoid Fever: Its Nature, Mode of Spreading, and Prevention* (London).

Secondary: Pelling, Margaret, 1978. *Cholera, Fever and English Medicine, 1825–1865* (Oxford and New York); McFarlan, A. M., 1959. *William Budd and Cholera in Bristol* (Bristol); Goodall, E. W., 1936. *William Budd, MD Edin, FRS: The Bristol Physician and Epidemiologist* (London); [Anon.], 1880. 'Obituary, William Budd, MD.' *Lancet* i: 148–149; Snow, John, 1849. *On the Mode of Communication of Cholera* (London); *DSB*; *Oxford DNB*.

Carole Reeves

BÜCHNER, FRIEDRICH KARL CHRISTIAN LUDWIG
(b. Darmstadt, Germany, 29 March 1824; d. Darmstadt, 1 May 1899), *medicine, medical philosophy*.

Büchner was the younger brother of Georg Büchner, the poet. As his father wished, Ludwig (as he was known) studied medicine at Giessen, Strassburg, Würzburg, and Vienna without giving up his former studies of philosophy. He received his MD in 1848 with a thesis on the nervous system. He worked as a practitioner at Darmstadt, and actively participated in the attempt of a bourgeois revolution in 1848–49. From 1852 he was an intern at Tübingen, where he qualified as a university lecturer in 1854 and taught at the university as Privatdozent. His work *Kraft und Stoff* (1855) was the first book based on his studies on natural science and philosophy to be published. It was a bestseller; within fifty years the book was printed twenty-one times and translated into more than ten languages. Although its theoretical standard did not go beyond earlier literature of a materialistic and atheistic orientation, it was a good survey on the actual development of natural science for the ordinary reader. Büchner's book made such a splash that we cannot picture international philosophical discussion without it. It inserted the direct participation of special sciences into the actual philosophical and political debate of its time. Büchner's philosophy can be summarized in one sentence: Ludwig Büchner was a representative of mechanistic materialism.

According to Büchner, natural science is the base for any philosophy. Reality is a reflection of natural science. There is only one 'Seiendes' (ontological principle), which is both 'Kraft' (force or energy) and 'Stoff' (matter). *Kraft* and *Stoff* are only two forms of manifestation of one and the same existence. The *Kraft* is movement of the *Stoff* or cause of such. Matter and movement are eternal. *Stoff*, *Kraft* and mind are merely different expressions for one 'Seiendes'. Any dualism of mind and matter, soul and body, has to be fought against. Nature follows strict laws; i.e., there is only causality but no teleology. Immaterial phenomena do not exist. Metaphysics are antiquated. Man is a product of nature, a product of evolution. In his volition and his activities he is determined by nature. As it is the case with life, thinking is solely a special form of the general movement of nature, too. Soul is a collective term for the brain functions. The human soul is the brain itself and hence mortal. God is nothing more than nature itself.

Due to massive criticism of his book *Kraft und Stoff,* Büchner had to give up his academic career. Subsequently he worked as a physician and writer at Darmstadt. During the years 1872–73, his scientific lecture tours took him all over Germany and even to North America. Moreover, Ludwig Büchner was widely known as the founder of the German alliance of freethinkers (1881), and as the cofounder of the *Freier Deutscher Hochstift* (1859) in Frankfurt am Main. Last of all, he was the first person to publish a survey on the complete works of his brother Georg.

Bibliography

Primary: 1855. *Kraft und Stoff* (Frankfurt am Main) [Eng. edn., 1864. 15th enlarged edn., 1883 (Leipzig)]; 1857. *Natur und Geist* (Frankfurt am Main); 1869. *Der Mensch und seine Stellung in der Natur* (Leipzig); 1874. *Der Gottesbegriff und seine Bedeutung in der Gegenwart* (Leipzig); 1889. *Das künstige Leben und die moderne Wissenschaft* (Leipzig); 1894. *Am Sterbelager des Jahrhunderts* (Berlin); 1894. *Darwinismus und Sozialismus* (Leipzig); 1900. *Im Dienste der Wahrheit* (Giessen).

Secondary: Faber, Heiko, 2002. *Ludwig Büchner (1824–1899) und der naturwissenschaftliche Materialismus in der zweiten Hälfte des 19. Jahrhunderts* (Heidelberg); Gregory, Frederick, 1977. *Scientific Materialism in Nineteenth-Century Germany* (Dordrecht), DSB.

Wolfgang U. Eckart

BUFALINI, MAURIZIO (b. Cesena, Italy, 4 June 1787; d. Florence, Italy, 31 March 1875), *medicine.*

Bufalini attended grammar school in Cesena and Rimini, and the Faculty of Medicine in Bologna. Then he studied in Pavia, with Antonio Scarpa, and in Milan, where vitalistic doctrine and the theories of John Brown on excitability prevailed.

He returned to Cesena to practice medicine, and then was appointed lecturer in clinical medicine at the prestigious University of Bologna (1813). In the same year he published an essay in which he criticized vitalistic theory and Brownism. That piece provoked so much outrage that he abandoned teaching, returning to private practice. In Cesena, he continued to elaborate his conception of medical science in *Fondamenti della patologia analitica* (1819) and *Sulla nuova dottrina medica italiana* (1825), and he provoked further polemics with his new essay (1832).

In 1835 he was appointed to the chair of medicine at the medical school of Santa Maria Nuova in Florence. However, even there Bufalini's ideas bruised collegial elbows. It was in regard to epidemics, above all, that he argued with Pietro Betti, who was responsible for all of the *lazzaretti* [hospitals] of Tuscany during the epidemic of cholera in 1854–55.

He occupied the chair of medicine in the post-doctoral *Istituto di Studi Superiori* of Florence, founded in 1859. Together with Francesco Puccinotti, another great reformer of Italian medicine, Bufalini was the main supporter of that prestigious Institute and served as its superintendent (1863–67) when Florence was the capital of Italy.

For Bufalini, life represented a complex phenomenon that could be defined only through understanding all of its details. Medical science must be based on the examination of facts, and one cannot pretend to infer the 'science of illnesses' from the science of health, nor the 'science of disorder from the science of order'. He elaborated a system of medicine that was articulated in four phases: the classification of diseases (nosology), the analysis of symptoms and signs (semiotics), the investigation of causes (etiology), and the observation of the effect of drugs (therapeutics). Bufalini called this method 'experimental', connecting it to the Galilean tradition. It was analytical and synthetic at same time: whatever was distilled at the ends of the observation must then be integrated into an orderly system. Accordingly, he titled the medical journal he founded in 1847 *Sperimentale.*

He also endured accusations of materialism and atheism from Abbot Fabriani (1826), but in fact Bufalini believed religion to be the base of the moral life. Moral development, according to Bufalini, derived from education. Emulation must stimulate individual activity without extinguishing the impulses to solidarity. With all that in mind, he endorsed the rise of kindergartens, in which emulation and competition should be combined with solidarity.

Bufalini dedicated himself to politics as well. Stressing the relationship between freedom and science, he defended the absolute freedom of the press and of association. In 1831 and then again in 1848 he was elected to two important appointments in the Papal State, but he preferred the title of senator in Tuscany. With the annexation of Tuscany to the Kingdom of Sardinia—in effect, with the unification of Italy—he became a senator in the new kingdom, but his old age did not allow him to participate actively in Parliament.

Bufalini's school left a great heritage in research and academic teaching, as well as in the practice of medicine. Nevertheless, he remained a controversial figure. Some of his supporters reproached Bufalini's easy enthusiasm for theoretical experimentalism when faced with a lack of effective experiments. However, according to the clinician Augusto Murri, Bufalini 'opened the era of medicine that scrutinized the patient with observation, with the knife and the laboratory retort, the microscope and the machines'.

Bibliography

Primary: 1819. *Fondamenti della patologia analitica* (Pavia); 1863. *Istituzioni di patologia medica* (Florence).

Secondary: 1990. (Pancaldi, Giuliano, ed.) *Maurizio Bufalini: medicina, scienza e filosofia* (Bologna); 1951. 'Onoranze a Maurizio Bufalini.' *Rivista di storia delle scienze mediche e naturali* 42: 131–215.

Patrizia Guarnieri

BUIAL'SKII, IL'IA VASIL'EVICH (b. Vorob'evka, Chernigov gubernia [province], Russia, 26 June 1789; d. St Petersburg, Russia, 8 December 1866), *anatomy, surgery.*

Buial'skii finished Chernigov seminary (1809) and the Medical-Surgical Academy in St Petersburg (1814), where he remained after graduation as a dissector in the department of anatomy and as an adjunct of surgery in the clinic (1817–21). He was a professor of the St Petersburg Medical-Surgical Academy (1825), the head of the department of normal anatomy, and a member of a series of foreign medical societies.

Buial'skii was the greatest practitioner of 'pre-Pirogovist' surgery in Russia. His fundamental works were devoted to normal, topographic, and pathological anatomy; vascular surgery; and the surgical treatment of urinary calculus. His best compositions, beginning with a dissertation on aneurisms, were about the surgery of blood vessels.

Buial'skii advocated the study of anatomy by the method of ice sculpture (frozen corpses) and laid the foundation for topographic anatomy in Russia. He developed methods of injection and embalming and created a unique museum of preparations that were transferred to the Medical-Surgical Academy.

His most prominent published work was the atlas *Anatomiko-khirurgichsekie tablitsy, ob"iasniaiushchie proizvodstvo operatsii pereviazyvaniia bol'shikh arterii* [Anatomical-surgical tables, explaining the production of the operation for the dressing of main arteries] (1828). The artistically executed drawings in fourteen tables were reproduced to natural size from his personal preparations. This was the first Russian atlas and manual of operative surgery. The edition was acquired by almost all European universities and earned high praise from contemporaries.

The second part of the atlas—*Anatomiko-patologicheskie i khirurgicheskie tablitsy gryzh* [Anatomical-pathological and surgical tables of ruptures]—came out in 1835. The third part, devoted to lithotripsy and lithotomy, was published in 1852. All three parts were in folio format and were distinguished by the high quality of artistic execution; the best artist-engravers took part in their creation. Because the printing of these editions was expensive, the author did not publish tables for all of operative surgery.

Buial'skii also wrote the first manual in Russia on forensic medicine (1824), a textbook on human anatomy (1844), and a study aid on plastic anatomy for artists (1860). As an anatomist he paid the greatest attention to details, emphasizing their applied significance. Above all, Buial'skii's anatomical studies emphasized the importance of the surgical relationship of body parts (blood vessels and others). Part of his scientific work was devoted to describing anomalies of development.

In 1846 Buial'skii published the pioneering work in Russia 'O perelivanii krovi' ('About blood transfusion') with a detailed investigation of attempts in a given area, predicting a great future for the method. However, because of the inade-quate science of the time and the risk for the health of the patient, he did not perform a single blood transfusion himself.

The surgical talent of Buial'skii shone especially after he became first consultant to the Mariinskii hospital (1831–64). The majority of his various operations—from plastic and bone surgery to ruptures and lithotomy—were carried out within the walls of that hospital, where the outpatient clinic treated from 30,000 to 40,000 people annually. In addition, he was the surgeon for the Tsarkoe lycée (1833) and the chief doctor for all the cadet buildings (1835).

Buial'skii also had a large obstetrical and gynecological practice, and he published 'Anatomiko-patologicheskie rassmotrenie vnematochnoi beremennosti' ['The anatomical-pathological examination of extra-uterine pregnancy'] in 1843. He was the first in Russia to perform the operation for vaginal fistulas, and he suggested a series of surgical instruments (the 'Buial'skii spatula' and others) for that procedure.

He was one of the first Russian surgeons to apply chloroform (August 1848) and ether (May 1847) as anesthetics, and to use plaster casts for fractures. He was the virtuoso of a broad range of operative techniques, including the development of a series of surgical operations (resection of the upper jaw, the operation for vascular aneurisms, and others).

From 1831 to 1866, Buial'skii taught anatomy at the Academy of Art, where his lectures were heard by many famous artists. He personally prepared muscles in a frozen corpse, from which a plaster copy was taken by the sculptor Peter Klodt to make the celebrated statue 'The Lying Body' (1836).

In his capacity as manager of the St Petersburg surgical instrument factory (1829–41), Buial'skii made a significant contribution to improving the production of surgical instrumentation. He developed and produced more than twenty-five specialized sets.

The opinions of Buial'skii on the general principles of therapy for pathological processes differed little from others at the time. A fundamental role during treatment was assigned to 'diversionary means' such as anti-inflammatory methods, leeches, blood-letting, Spanish fly, and purgatives.

Bibliography

Primary: 1833. Rossiskii gosudarstvennyi istorichekii arkhiv [Russian State Historic Archive]. 'Delo o lechenii profesorom Buial'skim vospitanika Voeikova' ['File about the treatment by Professor Buial'skii of pupil Voeikov']. F. II, op. 134, d. 784a (St Petersburg).

Secondary: 1998. *Professors of the Military Medical (Medico-surgical) Academy (1798–1998)* (St Petersburg); Popov, V., and E. Dyskin, 1990. *I. V. Buial'skii i ego rol' v razvitii otechestvennoi anatomii i sudebnoi meditsiny.* [I. V. Buial'skii and his role in the development of homeland anatomy and forensic medicine] (Leningrad); Margorin, E., 1948. *Il'ia Buial'skii* (Leningrad).

Mikhail Poddubnyi

BURDENKO, NIKOLAI NILOVICH

BURDENKO, NIKOLAI NILOVICH (b. Kamenka, Penza *gubernia* [province], Russia, 22 May [3 June] 1876; d. Moscow, USSR, 11 November 1946), *neurosurgery, military field surgery, military medicine.*

Burdenko, the founder of neurosurgery in the Soviet Union, was even better known as head surgeon of the Red Army throughout World War II. Born into a Russian-Ukrainian family, he entered Tomsk University in 1898. After expulsion in 1901 for political involvement, he was redirected to the more liberal Iur'ev (Tartu) University, from which he graduated in 1906. While he was a medical student, his service on the front-line staff of the Red Cross during the Russo-Japanese War (1904–05) was an important formative experience.

After graduation, Burdenko worked first as a practicing doctor in the Riga city hospital. In1908 he returned to Iur'ev University, defending his dissertation a year later on 'Materialy k voprosu o posledstviiakh pereviazki venae portae' [Materials on the problem about the consequences of dressing portal veins].

From 1910 he worked as a sessional lecturer in the department of surgery at Iur'ev University, refining his clinical practice and his technique in surgical operations on the central nervous system. Burdenko was an established medical scientist by the beginning of World War I, but he also became a remarkable field surgeon, developing methods for operating on wounds of the central nervous system under field conditions.

He spent the early Soviet years in Voronezh, then moved to Moscow in 1923, after which his career rose meteorically. He was already director of the faculty surgical clinic at the First Moscow State University in 1924, but by 1938 he chaired the Academic Medical Council of the Commissariat of Health, and the following year he was elected a full member of the Academy of Medical Sciences. Most importantly, he was appointed chief surgeon of the Red Army at the beginning of World War II.

Burdenko's first major contribution to Soviet medicine was during the interwar years, with the creation of neurosurgery as a distinct field based on his sophisticated, nuanced, and deeply considered research and practice. His many innovations included the 'Burdenko method', which stratified the hard brain membrane (dura mater) to remedy defects; the 'Burdenko-Pussel operation', which corrected defects of the brain stem; and an operative method on tumors of the III and IV ventricles of the brain. Most important of all, he assembled a brilliant team of neurosurgeons in Moscow, an achievement that was institutionally formalized in 1934 by the creation of the Central Institute of Neurosurgery (now the N. N. Burdenko Institute of Neurosurgery).

Burdenko's second major contribution was in military medicine, especially field surgery. Although in poor health himself throughout World War II, he immersed himself in the problems of specialized care and shock. Through his detailed and commanding wartime directives and manuals, Burdenko apprised Soviet medicine of the latest advances in the 'pharmaceutical revolution' (especially the sulfonamides and penicillin), thus positioning Soviet doctors to use the new drugs effectively.

Along with Efim Ivanovich Smirnov, Burdenko extended the tradition of Pirogov in improving the organization of military surgical care and treatment. They shifted the focus of military medical care from mass evacuation of the wounded far to the rear, as practiced in World War I, to treatment in front-line organizations. Their great success was gauged by the high proportion of wounded soldiers who were returned to the front. That gauge itself is disquieting, because it reveals the instrumental need to find front-line troops from wherever possible—a perspective that Burdenko shared and to which he contributed. Nevertheless, the fact that 75 percent of wounded Soviet troops were sent back to the front lines attests to the effectiveness of Burdenko's leadership and the military medical system that he helped develop.

Bibliography

Primary: 1951. *N.N. Burdenko. Sobranie sochinenii.* [Collected Works] (Moscow); 1950. *Materialy k biografii N. N. Burdenko* [Materials for a Biography of N. N. Burdenko] (Moscow).

Secondary: Mirskii, Mark Borisovich, 1983. *Istseliaiiushchi skal'pelem. Akademik N.N. Burdenko* [The Healing Scalpel. Academician N. N. Burdenko] (Moscow); Bagdasar'ian, S. M., 1948. *Nikolai Nilovich Burdenko. Zhizn' i deiatel'nost'* [Nikolai Nilovich Burdenko. Life and Work] (Moscow).

Chris Burton

BURKITT, DENIS PARSONS

BURKITT, DENIS PARSONS (b. near Enniskillen, Northern Ireland, 28 February 1911; d. Gloucester, England, 23 March 1993), *surgery, cancer research, tropical medicine, nutrition.*

Early Life

Burkitt's family was firmly protestant, his grandfather having been a Presbyterian pastor. He was educated at Dean Close School, Cheltenham, but returned to Ireland and Trinity College Dublin to study engineering, the profession of his successful father, James Parsons Burkitt. He claimed that he was an unpromising student without direction, the loss of one eye in a childhood accident being all that distinguished him. But his father knew his son. Years later, Burkitt found a letter sent by his tutor to his father, in which the tutor doubted the young man's ability to gain a degree. James Burkitt had marked the letter to be kept, feeling that his son had been underestimated. It did not take long for the young Burkitt to find his own direction, but exactly half a century later, a new letter offering him Honorary Fellowship of the College, the highest award that could be bestowed, confirmed his father's prediction.

Change in Direction

After being invited to a Christian bible group and enjoying the possessing company of the members, Burkitt realized that he had no real faith, and so he committed his life to Jesus Christ. His faith firm and his motivation strengthened, he soon felt the call to become a doctor, left engineering behind, and embarked upon his new vocation with enthusiasm and conviction.

After qualification as a doctor in 1935, Burkitt immediately trained in surgery and became FRCSEd in 1938. Feeling a strong commitment to overseas work and a desire to help the most underprivileged, he applied to the Colonial Medical Service. He was rejected more than once because of his age, doubts about the capabilities of a one-eyed surgeon, and (he believed) his robust faith. He was gravely disappointed, but World War II soon afterward gave him the opportunity to work overseas. Burkitt served in the Royal Army Medical Corps from 1942 to 1945, stationed in East Africa, Ceylon, and Singapore. He married his wife, the nurse Olive Rogers, during a brief period of leave at that time, although they were not to see each other again for two and a half years.

Burkitt's Lymphoma

With his wartime experience, Burkitt was accepted into the Colonial Medical Service in 1947. His first posting was as a district medical officer to Lira Hospital in Northwest Uganda, where he did everything, including supervising the rural dispensaries. After only a year at Lira, he was transferred to Mulago Hospital, which was linked with Makerere College, Kampala, as one of its three surgeons.

It was in 1957 that Hugh Trowell, senior government physician in Uganda, asked him to examine the head and neck tumors of a five-year-old boy. When a girl with identical signs was admitted a few weeks later, and he saw a similar case at Jinja, east of Kampala, he realized that the tumor was possibly a previously undescribed cancer. But Burkitt was puzzled, because in all the cases examined at autopsy, there was also tumor in ovary, thyroid, or other tissues. A. G. Oettle was visiting Kampala then, and he said that the jaw tumor was not seen in South Africa. Burkitt felt sure that there must be a geographical limit and so, with the help of Olive, he dispatched 1,200 questionnaire letters about the occurrence of facial tumors in children to doctors all over Africa. Preliminary investigation suggested a tumor belt stretching across Africa, ten degrees north and ten degrees south of the equator.

With his two colleagues—E. H. Williams, a missionary doctor from Arua in West Nile, and the Canadian Clifford Nelson—Burkitt made a 10,000-mile safari in East, Central, and South Africa to find out where the tumor was seen. The MRC gave him a grant of £250 for that expedition, and his own experience as a district medical officer stood him in good stead. He was able to relate to and understand the problems of the hospital staff that the team visited. He reported the first results of his research to a 1958 meeting of the Association of Surgeons of East Africa in Kampala and,

with Professor J. N. P. (Jack) Davies, again in the *British Journal of Surgery* and *The Medical Press* (Dublin). Burkitt realized that the jaw tumor was found only where there was enough rainfall and temperature, in the same way as malaria. He suggested that an insect carried an infectious agent responsible for the disease. Despite little interest in his initial reports, the third and classic paper, published in *Cancer* with G. T. O'Conor (1961), awakened significant interest. It signaled a new stage in Burkitt's career and created awareness of the childhood cancer that is now known as Burkitt's lymphoma.

The early 1960s were seminal. Michael Epstein attended one of Burkitt's lectures in 1961; suspecting a viral cause for the lymphoma, he asked Burkitt for a sample to work on. Three years later he isolated what is now known as the Epstein-Barr virus. The proposed connection with an insect vector was found to be indirect, and eventually the correct chain of events was established. Burkitt's lymphoma occurs only in the hot, wet, tropical areas where malaria is hyperendemic and childhood immunity is depressed by malarial infection. These conditions allow expression of the oncogenic potential of the Epstein-Barr virus which, combined with other factors, transforms lymphocytes into malignant cells and causes the lymphoma. Burkitt also found that the tumor melted away when the patient was treated with methotrexate (cyclophosphamide is used now), and that it could be cured. It was a triumph of detective work and logical thinking, and it represented the first time a virus had been found to cause a human cancer. The work gave a great stimulus to cancer research and changed the direction of future investigation. Burkitt's lymphoma survey is still regarded as one of the pioneering studies of geographical pathology.

All of that work was carried out part-time while Burkitt fulfilled his role as a government surgeon. It was only in 1962 that he laid down his scalpel and joined the MRC, before returning to London in 1966 and pursuing further studies of the geographical distribution of cancer and other diseases in Africa and beyond.

Fiber and Western Diseases

In London, Burkitt met Peter Cleave, an eccentric retired naval surgeon who got him interested in the link between diet and disease. Cleave published a grandiose but lucidly argued hypothesis that it was the high proportion of refined food in the diet that was responsible for many of the common diseases of the developed world. Burkitt saw that this could explain his observations as to the rarity of diseases such as gallstones, hemorrhoids, diabetes, and bowel cancers in Africa, and he added his distinguished authority to those already advocating the importance of dietary fiber. Working with Hugh Trowell and Alec Walker, he developed and extended existing hypotheses, arguing that in the nineteenth century infectious and deficiency

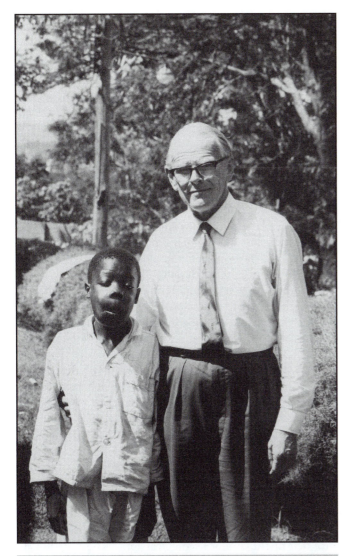

Denis Parsons Burkitt with a young patient suffering from Burkitt's lymphoma, Kampala, Uganda, early 1960s. Photograph from Archives and Manuscripts, Wellcome Library, London. Reproduced with permission of Olive Burkitt.

diseases were due to factors in the environment that could be controlled, and that the chronic noninfectious diseases of the twentieth century could similarly be eradicated. The specific focus was the idea that there must be some common causative element in colonic disease, particularly colon cancer.

Walker first drew attention to the role of fiber in deficiency diseases and observed, along with Burkitt, that Africans produce several times more fecal material than westerners, and with less discomfort. Support seemed to be provided by N. S. Painter's observations; he found that symptoms of colonic diverticulitis included an increase in intralumenal pressure, which was inversely related to dietary fiber intake. When patients ate bran, it was found

that pressure returned to normal and symptoms subsided. Burkitt, Trowell, and Walker emphasized the positive health benefit of the fiber that was removed in the process of refining food. Further research on stools and transit times in the intestinal tract demonstrated man's maladaptation to the type of diet now common in the West, which has replaced a more natural diet, high in fiber.

Burkitt published his second citation classic in 1971 (*Cancer* 28: 3–13), linking bowel cancer to a low-fiber diet. Several books with Trowell followed. No true laboratory or biochemical link between dietary fiber and the diseases mentioned underpinned their study, and the work relied on anecdotal evidence rather than the detailed epidemiological studies that characterized Burkitt's mapping of lymphoma. Nevertheless, the enthusiasm of Burkitt and Trowell held the hypothesis together until others took a more detailed interest in the passage of fiber through the gut. Some of the original hypothesis has now been dropped or modified, but thanks to Burkitt, the science of nutrition was galvanized. He crusaded for the rest of his life to encourage increased consumption of vegetable fiber, acquiring the nickname 'Bran Man' while reshaping the contents of breakfast tables around the developed world. He talked endlessly about our maladaptation to the diet of the developed world. Despite the fact that no clinically proven relationship with disease had been demonstrated, he expressed his beliefs without doubting their correctness, and much of what he suggested did have a strong element of truth.

Honors and Christian Humility

Burkitt was honored in many places and by many national and scientific institutions, the most significant probably being his election as FRS in 1972. He was appointed CMG in the same year and received the Gold Medal of the BMA in 1978. The Royal College of Physicians and Surgeons in Canada summarized his achievements wonderfully when they awarded him an Honorary Fellowship in 1992: 'It is impossible to grasp the number of lives that have been improved or saved and will continue to be improved as a result of Dr Burkitt's epidemiological acumen and his missionary zeal when promoting our health'.

His deep and vibrant faith was fundamental in all he did; he showed great humility in every area of his life. He proved over and over again, when events were difficult, what he had been told by his mother as a boy: 'Disappointment, His appointment—you only need change one letter'. On his office wall he displayed the Apostle Paul's words, 'What do you possess that was not given to you? If then you really received it all as a gift, why take the credit to yourself?' Burkitt lived by his simple faith, grateful for everything he had achieved but refusing to take credit for it. His students were said to always comment on his down-to-earth attitude and modest character, reflected very clearly in the following passage that he chose to inscribe in his books:

Attitudes are more important than abilities

Motives are more important than methods

Character is more important than cleverness

Perseverance is more important than power

And the heart takes precedence over the head.

Burkitt's remarkable ability to construct hypotheses relating to the etiology of the diseases he observed led him to publish citation classics in two unrelated medical fields. He continued editing, writing, and lecturing right up to the last days of his life.

Bibliography

Primary: 1958–59. 'A Sarcoma Involving the Jaws in African Children.' *British Journal of Surgery* 46: 218–223; Epstein, M. Anthony, and M. Barry, 1964. 'Cultivation In Vitro of Human Lymphoblasts from Burkitt's Malignant Lymphoma.' *Lancet* i: 252–253; 1971. 'Epidemiology of Cancer of the Colon and Rectum.' *Cancer* 28: 3–13; 1993. 'Direction Determines Destination.' *Nucleus* (April): 6–11 (www.cmf.org.uk).

Secondary: Epstein, Anthony, and M. A. Eastwood, 1995. 'Denis Parsons Burkitt.' *Biographical Memoirs of Fellows of the Royal Society* 41: 88–102; Fergusson, Andrew, 1993. 'D. P. Burkitt CMG, MD, FRCSED, FRS.' *British Medical Journal* 306(6883): 996; Heaton, Kenneth, 1993. 'Denis Burkitt.' *Lancet* 341(8850): 951–952; Blythe, Max, 1990. Denis Burkitt in interview with Max Blythe. Oxford Brookes University School of Biological and Molecular Sciences and the Royal College of Physicians (recorded 10 December 1990); Kellock, Brian, 1985. *The Fibre Man: The Life Story of Dr. Denis Burkitt* (Tring); Gelmser, Bernard, 1970. *Mr. Burkitt and Africa* (New York).

Amy Gardiner and Eldryd Parry

BURNET, (FRANK) MACFARLANE (b. Traralgon, Victoria, Australia, 3 September 1899; d. Port Fairy, Australia, 31 August 1985), *virology, immunology, disease ecology.*

The son of Frank Burnet, a bank manager, and Hadassah Mackay, Burnet grew up in rural Victoria, acquiring a Scottish yearning for education, a sense of Presbyterian rectitude, and a love of beetles. He remained a bug hunter for most of his life. While a medical student at the University of Melbourne, Burnet developed his biological interests under zoology professor Wilfred Agar, an admirer of Alfred North Whitehead's arguments against reductionism. After graduation (MB BS 1922; MD 1924), Burnet trained in pathology at the Melbourne Hospital and the Walter and Eliza Hall Institute, where he studied animal and bacterial viruses (phage). After completing a PhD at the University of London, he returned to Melbourne in 1928 as assistant director of the Hall Institute. In 1944, resisting a call from Harvard, he became director of the Institute and professor of experi-

mental medicine at the University of Melbourne. By the time he retired in 1965, the Hall Institute was the premier research institute in Australia.

Burnet demonstrated imagination and skill in the laboratory. Working with Jean Macnamara, he differentiated strains of the poliomyelitis virus, and he excelled in growing influenza virus in the chorioallantoic membrane of the chick. His work on biological aspects of virus growth and the prevention of virus infections was celebrated; in 1935 Burnet identified the agent of Q fever (*Coxiella burnetti*). The demand for field studies of disease outbreaks, such as psittacosis, meant that his research was never limited to esoteric bench work. Living and working in a settler society, with its population problems and a fragile environment, led him toward a broader ecological perspective on disease.

Burnet was introduced to the latest evolutionary theories by H. G. Wells and Julian Huxley's *The Science of Life* (1930), which provided 'that ecological slant to the study of human disease' that came to characterize his work. Burnet's *Biological Aspects of Infectious Disease* (1940) examined infectious disease 'along ecological lines as a struggle for existence between man and microorganisms'. Evolutionary biology allowed him to integrate masses of laboratory and epidemiological observations, which distinguished his science from the mere reductionism of most laboratory researchers and the routinism of microbe hunters, whom he frequently disparaged. Burnet saw himself as a naturalist fallen among medical scientists. Later editions, retitled *The Natural History of Infectious Disease*, gave more attention to urbanization, overpopulation, human mobility, and biological warfare. This book inspired many other scientists to view microbes ecologically.

Burnet regarded immunology as a branch of medical science that might embrace ecological approaches. In 1949 he proposed a theory of acquired immunological tolerance, a hypothesis confirmed by Peter Medawar, with whom he shared the 1960 Nobel Prize in Physiology or Medicine. In the late 1950s, Burnet also developed a clonal selection theory of antibody formation; he wanted his 'biological' explanation of the immune response to replace older 'chemical' theories. In 1957, driven by intellectual enthusiasm, he told his subordinate investigators at the Hall Institute to swing from virology into immunology.

Increasingly stern and authoritarian, Burnet became the arbiter of support for scientific investigation in Australia. In the 1960s and 1970s he controlled medical research in the territory of Papua New Guinea, attempting to transform it into a laboratory for ecological studies. Realizing that his ecological vision lacked a means of explaining human social life and culture, Burnet flirted with ethnology and sociobiology, especially in *Dominant Mammal* (1970). The eugenic enthusiasms of his youth led to an abiding concern with the quality and quantity of population, topics on which he frequently broadcast and wrote after the Nobel Prize gave him a platform. Knighted in 1951, he was awarded the Order of

Merit and the Royal Society's Royal and Copley Medals, among many other honors. The Macfarlane Burnet Institute at Monash University is named for him. His autobiographical reflections can be found in *Changing Patterns* (1968) and *Credo and Comment* (1979).

Bibliography

Primary: 1953. *The Natural History of Infectious Diseases* (Cambridge).

Secondary: 1968. *Changing Patterns: An Atypical Autobiography* (Melbourne).

Warwick Anderson

BURTON-BRADLEY, BURTON GYRTH (b. Sydney, Australia, 18 November 1914; d. Port Moresby, Papua New Guinea, 31 January 1994), *psychiatry.*

Burton-Bradley, the son of Alan Burton-Bradley and grandson of Henry Burton Bradley, one of the first solicitors to practice in Sydney, graduated MB BS at the University of Sydney in 1944 and worked for four years as a country general practitioner in New South Wales. From 1949 to 1950 he was connected to the Australian military mission to Germany. He worked at the Brisbane Mental Hospital from 1950 to 1957, gaining a Diploma in Psychological Medicine from the University of Melbourne in 1956. From 1957 to 1959 he worked as a Colombo Plan psychiatrist in Singapore, as Lecturer in Psychological Medicine at the University of Malaya, and as medical superintendent of the Woodbridge Mental Hospital, where he encountered patients from a wide variety of cultural backgrounds.

In 1959 Burton-Bradley moved to Papua New Guinea, then under Australian control, where he remained for the rest of his life. Until 1975 he was director of Papua New Guinea's mental health division, and the only psychiatrist for a population of more than 2.5 million people. When he arrived there were no psychiatric facilities, but by 1975 he had established a mental health service with a staff of more than 150 physicians, psychologists, social workers, occupational therapists, and psychiatric nurses, mostly trained by Burton-Bradley. His work was seen by the World Health Organization as a model for the organization of psychiatric facilities in a developing country.

Unlike most physicians, he stayed in Papua New Guinea when it gained independence in 1975, and in 1978 he was appointed professor of psychiatry at the University of Papua New Guinea. During his stay in Papua New Guinea, Burton-Bradley acquainted himself with anthropological writings and conducted research in transcultural psychiatry, investigating mental illness in more than forty distinct language groups in rural areas and detailing how mental illness was characterized by the indigenous population. He also investigated the obstacles to psychiatric treatment that were posed by cultural difference, and by differences in language and social organization. His writings on transcultural psychiatry and the local cargo cult have been widely recognized.

Burton-Bradley published more than 200 papers on topics as diverse as cargo cults, betel and kava addiction, traditional mental health practices among ethnic groups in Papua New Guinea, the effects of sociocultural transition on mental health, suicide, amok (indiscriminate homicidal frenzy), the marginality of mixed-race individuals in urban Papua New Guinea, traditional mental health systems in Papua New Guinea, and art therapy in a transcultural context. In 1966 he received a Diploma in Tropical Medicine and Hygiene from the University of Sydney for his work on mixed-race ethnopsychiatry, and in 1969 he received an MD from the University of New South Wales for his work on transcultural psychiatry.

Burton-Bradley was a consultant and advisor to the South Pacific Commission from 1966 and to the World Health Organization from 1977. He frequently gave advice on the development of psychiatric services in the region and came to be known as the 'father of Melanesian psychiatry'. He contributed to forensic psychiatry and advised the local government and courts in cases of serious crimes. Burton-Bradley was knighted in 1990 for his pioneering work in psychiatry in Papua New Guinea.

Bibliography

Primary: 1973. (with Lidz, Ruth W., and Theodor Lidz) 'Cargo Cultism: A Psychosocial Study of Melanesian Millenarianism.' *Journal of Nervous and Mental Diseases* 157: 370–388; 1974. (with Torrey, E. Fuller, and Barbara B. Torrey) 'The Epidemiology of Schizophrenia in Papua New Guinea.' *American Journal of Psychiatry* 131: 567–573; 1975. *Stone Age Crisis: A Psychiatric Appraisal* (The Abraham Flexner Lectures in Medicine) (Nashville, TN); 1978. (with Billig, Otto) *The Painted Message* (Cambridge, MA).

Secondary: Goddard, Michael, 1992. 'Bedlam in Paradise: A Critical History of Psychiatry in Papua New Guinea.' *Journal of Pacific History* 27: 55–72; [Anon.], 1991. 'Sir Burton G. Burton-Bradley.' *Australian and New Zealand Journal of Psychiatry* 25: 191–196.

Hans Pols

BUSTAMANTE VASCONCELOS, MIGUEL ENRIQUE (b. Oaxaca, Oaxaca, Mexico, 2 May 1898; d. Mexico City, Mexico, 4 January 1986), *public health, history of medicine.*

Bustamante, the eldest of fourteen siblings, was born into a cultured, liberal family in the city of Oaxaca, one of the most historical areas of Mexico. His mother decided that he should study medicine, so he moved to the capital. He was the first Mexican to earn a Doctorate in Public Health (1928). In addition, it was from one of the foremost medical centers of the time—Johns Hopkins University—thanks to a scholarship from the Rockefeller Foundation. Later, that organization helped him establish sanitary units and study different forms of parasitosis. In addition to his concern for public health, Bustamante was a historian of medicine, an interest he attributed to the influence of William Henry Welch.

Bustamante's main contribution was to improve rural hygienic conditions through an integrated national policy that included a program of hygiene education involving federal, state, and municipal sanitary services. It brought together doctors, nurses, engineers, and inspectors and covered geographical, economic, historical, and cultural questions. When published in 1934, those ideas had an enormous impact, and they are still reprinted today. The application of Bustamante's program was facilitated by the establishment of the Coordinated Sanitary Services for Health and Assistance.

Bustamante was active in an era of Mexico's history when the country created institutions concerned with health and hygiene. With President Lázaro Cárdenas, he organized the Six-Year Plan (1933), which was designed to provide the nation with infrastructure for education and medicine. Bustamante drafted the Sanitary Codes and the Law of Coordination and Cooperation of Health Services, and he participated in creating the Institute for Health and Tropical Diseases (ISET, 1939), where he served as director. That was the first site in Mexico where infectious and parasitic diseases were studied scientifically. Bustamante also recognized that medical necessities differed in various zones of the country, a finding that led him to promote the elaboration of a national medical geography.

Bustamante identified onchocerciasis in southwestern Mexico. He also studied yellow fever, spotted fever and its vector in Mexico (*Rhipicephalus sanguineus*, 1942–43), typhus, and several serums, vaccines, and antihelminthics. He was an important promoter of campaigns to combat smallpox, typhus, whooping cough, uncinariasis, leptospirosis, poliomyelitis, salmonella, treponematosis, and malaria, and he was instrumental in eradicating *Aëdes aegypti*.

From the late 1950s to the early 1960s, he served as Subsecretary of Health and Assistance, Secretary of the Council of General Health, and President of the National Academy of Medicine. Internationally, Bustamante participated in the International Sanitary Conference that drafted the World Health Constitution, and he served as General Secretary of the Pan-American Sanitary Office and editor of its *Bulletin* for many years. He presided over the Commission of Administration, Finances, and Legal Issues of the XII Assembly of the WHO and the Executive Council of the United Nations Children's Fund.

Bustamante felt that it was fundamental for young medical students to have contact with sick people in their own social milieu. To accomplish that objective, he founded the Departments of Public Health, Medical Sociology, and Epidemiology at the National University of Mexico. He was also an important advocate for the need to learn about the lessons of the past, and coauthored a four-volume history of public health in Mexico.

He insisted that simply providing medical attention was not enough; it was necessary also to improve people's living conditions, and he was convinced that communication among physicians and social scientists was very important. Bustamante had a modern view of public health and was a humanist, keenly aware of his social duty. Those who knew him remember him as a simple, cordial man.

Bibliography

Primary: 1925. *Probable existencia de la oncocercosis en Chiapas* (Mexico City); 1934. *La Coordinación de los Servicios Sanitarios Federales y Locales como Factor de Progreso Higiénico en México* (México City); 1960 (with Amézquita, José Alvarez, Antonio López Picazos, and Francisco Fernández del Castillo). *Historia de la Salubridad y la Asistencia en México* (México City) [English trans. 1968].

Secondary: Carrillo, Ana María, 2003. 'Miguel Bustamante' in *Ciencia y tecnología en México en el siglo XX* (Mexico) pp. 143–158; Birn, Anne E., 1997. 'Miguel Enrique Bustamante (1898–1986)' in Magner, Lois N., ed., *Doctors, Nurses and Medical Practitioners: A Bio-Bibliographical Sourcebook* (Westport, CT) pp. 30–36.

Ana Cecilia Rodríguez de Romo

IBN BUṬLĀN, AL-MUKHTAR B. AL-ḤASAN B. ʿABDŪN B. SAʿDŪN
(b. Baghdad, Iraq, ?; d. Antioch [now Antakya, Turkey], 2 September 1066), *medicine, philosophy, theology.*

Ibn Buṭlān was a Christian physician, a cleric, and probably a priest as well. After his training under Christian masters such as the renowned Nestorian priest, physician, and philosopher Ibn al-Ṭayyib, he taught medicine and philosophy in Baghdad. Ibn Buṭlān left his native city in January 1049 for a journey to Cairo, although he also visited other cities such as Antioch, Laodicea, Jaffa, and Aleppo, in which he advised the governor on the healthiest location of a hospital to be built there. Once in Cairo, he became engaged in a vitriolic debate with Ibn Riḍwān (988–1068), at the time chief physician of Egypt, which resulted in a remarkable medico-philosophical controversy comprising ten essays in which the two adversaries tried to exhibit their entire erudition in Greek medicine and philosophy. The rhetorical nature of the discussion—namely, whether the mature chicken is of a warmer nature than the young chicken—and the attacks against one another were moved, first, by Ibn Buṭlān's need to become publicly known in the new city in which he wanted to settle down, and second, to prevent Ibn Riḍwān's reputation and position from being threatened, or shared, by a foreign newcomer. Nevertheless, it appears from the controversy that Ibn Buṭān refused to follow slavishly the doctrines of the Ancients, which he had mastered. After three or four years in Cairo, he moved in 1054 to Constantinople, where he witnessed a terrible pestilential epidemic. About one year later, he returned to Syria, alternating between Aleppo and Antioch, where he is said to have supervised the building of a hospital in 1063. Eventually he became a monk and retired to a monastery in Antioch, where he died on 2 September 1066.

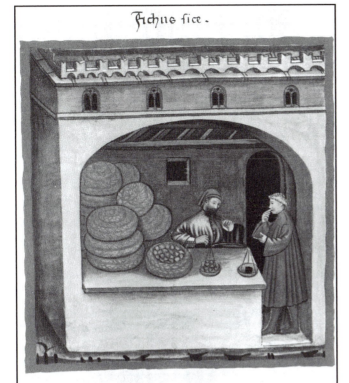

 Fichus fice.

Nature .c.η.f.m j. melior ex eis. tautainse rotitor unnamieni. petrou η presuatura tosicho noumetiη. opulatioi wscenbη. remotio noume mea. cur nueibη η amigdalis Dulcibη.

Apothecary dispensing siropus acetosus (medicated syrup) or dried figs, *Tacuinum sanitatis*, fourteenth century. From *Chemist and Druggist*, 28 June 1930: 798. Wellcome Library, London.

The originality of his literary production on medicine includes a popular and influential *Almanac of Health* in a tabular format entitled *Taqwīm al-siḥḥa*. Known in the Western tradition as *Tacuini Sanitatis*, it was translated into Latin by Farāj ibn Sālim from Sicily in the thirteenth century and was first printed in 1531. In 1533 it was also translated into German by Michael Herr. Ibn Buṭlān is also the author of the satirical work *Da'wat al-aṭibbā'* [The Physicians' Dinner Party]. Written in Constantinople in 1058 and dedicated to a Marwanid ruler, this work is described by J. Schacht as 'a witty skit on quacks, their ignorance and arrogance, with remarks on the ethics of the medical profession'. Ibn Buṭlān also wrote on other unusual topics, such as an essay on how to buy slaves and how to detect bodily defects (*Risālat fī shira' al-raqīq wa-taqlīb al-'abīd*), and a *Compendium for Monasteries and Monks* (*Kunnash al-adyirah wa-r-ruhbān*), a medical guide for Christian monks also known as *On the*

Management of Diseases for the Most Part Through Common Foodstuffs and Available Medicaments, Specifically for the Use of Monks of the Monasteries and Whoever is Far from the City. Toward 1063 he also worked on a Discourse 'on the reason why the skilled physicians have changed the treatment of most diseases which were formerly treated with hot remedies, advising in their place a cooling treatment . . . and how this new system has gradually gained ground in 'Iraq and the neighbouring countries' because of changes in climate and vegetation. Regarding the controversy with Ibn Riḍwān, as a means to draw the attention of Egyptian physicians, and against his own views, in the first essay Ibn Buṭlān supported the opinion of his fellow pupil al-Yabrūdī, who had refuted the most widely accepted hypothesis some time before in Cairo. Ibn Riḍwān's rhetorical answer was followed by a long discourse intended to undermine his adversary's authority. Divided in seven parts, the last one consisted in a description of Ibn Riḍwān's medical mistakes. In turn, the Egyptian physician not only replied in writing, but also successfully exhorted his colleagues to ignore Ibn Buṭlān and to treat him as an irresponsible fool, after which he is said to have left Cairo in wrath.

Bibliography

Primary: Schacht, Joseph, and Meyerhof, Max, 1937. *The Medico-Philosophical Controversy between Ibn Butlan and Ibn Ridwan. A Contribution to the History of Greek Learning among the Arabs* (Cairo); 1985. *Da'wat al-aṭibbā'* [The Physicians' Dinner Party]. (Edited from Arabic manuscripts and with an introduction by Klein-Franke, F.) (Wiesbaden); Jadon, S. Y., 1968. 'The Arab Physician Ibn Buṭlān's (d. 1066) Medical Manual for the Use of Monks and Country People [Arabic].' Unpublished PhD dissertation, University of California, Los Angeles, 2 vols.; Elkhadem, Hosam, 1990. *Le "Taqwim al-sihha" (Tacuini sanitatis) d'Ibn Buṭlān: Un traité médical du XIe siècle. Histoire du texte, édition critique, traduction, commentaire* (Leuven, Belgium) (Académie royale de Belgique, Classe des lettres, Fonds René Draguet, vol. 7).

Secondary: Schacht, Joseph, 2003. *The Encyclopaedia of Islam* (new edn., 11 vols. Leiden, 1960–2002) III, pp. 740–742; Conrad, Lawrence I., 1995. 'Scholarship and social context: a medical case from the eleventh-century Near-East' in Bates, Don, ed., *Knowledge and the Scholarly Medical Traditions* (Cambridge) pp. 84–100; Levey, Martin, 1965. 'Some Eleventh-Century Medical Questions Posed by Ibn Buṭlān and Later Answered by Ibn Ithirdī.' *Bulletin of the History of Medicine* 39: 495–507; Meyerhof, M., and Schacht, J., 1936–1937. 'Une controverse médico-philosophique au Caire en 441 de l'Hégire (1050 ap. J.C.); avec un aperçu sur les études grecques dans l'Islam.' *Bulletin de l'Institute d'Egypte* 19: 29–43.

Cristina Álvarez Millán